The GALE
ENCYCLOPEDIA of
SURGERY

A GUIDE FOR PATIENTS AND CAREGIVERS

The GALE ENCYCLOPEDIA of SURGERY

A GUIDE FOR PATIENTS AND CAREGIVERS

VOLUME

1

A - F

ANTHONY J. SENAGORE, M.D., EXECUTIVE ADVISOR
CLEVELAND CLINIC FOUNDATION

GALE®

THOMSON
★
™
GALE

Detroit • New York • San Diego • San Francisco • Cleveland • New Haven, Conn. • Waterville, Maine • London • Munich

Gale Encyclopedia of Surgery: A Guide for Patients and Caregivers

Anthony J. Senagore MD, Executive Adviser

Project Editor
Kristine Krapp

Editorial
Stacey L. Blachford, Deirdre Blanchfield, Madeline Harris, Chris Jeryan, Jacqueline Longe, Brigham Narins, Mark Springer, Ryan Thomason

Editorial Support Services
Andrea Lopeman, Sue Petrus

Indexing
Synapse

Illustrations
GGS Inc.

Permissions
Lori Hines

Imaging and Multimedia
Leitha Etheridge-Sims, Lezlie Light, Dave Oblender, Christine O'Brien, Robyn V. Young

Product Design
Michelle DiMercurio, Jennifer Wahi

Manufacturing
Wendy Blurton, Evi Seoud

LIBRARY OF CONGRESS CATALOGING-IN-PUBLICATION DATA

Gale encyclopedia of surgery : a guide for patients and caregivers /
  Anthony J. Senagore, [editor].
     p. cm.
       Includes bibliographical references and index.
       ISBN 0-7876-7721-3 (set : hc) — ISBN 0-7876-7722-1 (v. 1) — ISBN
       0-7876-7723-X (v. 2) — ISBN 0-7876-9123-2 (v. 3)
       Surgery—Encyclopedias. 2. Surgery—Popular works. I. Senagore,
         Anthony J., 1958-

RD17.G34 2003
617'.91'003—dc22   2003015742

This title is also available as an e-book.
ISBN: 0-7876-7770-1 (set)
Contact your Gale sales representative for ordering information.

Printed in Canada
10 9 8 7 6 5 4 3 2 1

CONTENTS

LIST OF ENTRIES

PLEASE READ—
IMPORTANT INFORMATION

The *Gale Encyclopedia of Surgery* is a medical reference product designed to inform and educate readers about a wide variety of surgeries, tests, drugs, and other medical topics. The Gale Group believes the product to be comprehensive, but not necessarily definitive. While the Gale Group has made substantial efforts to provide information that is accurate, comprehensive, and up-to-date, the Gale Group makes no representations or warranties of any kind, including without limitation, warranties of merchantability or fitness for a particular purpose, nor does it guarantee the accuracy, comprehensiveness, or timeliness of the information contained in this product. Readers should be aware that the universe of medical knowledge is constantly growing and changing, and that differences of medical opinion exist among authorities.

INTRODUCTION

The *Gale Encyclopedia of Surgery: A Guide for Patients and Caregivers* is a unique and invaluable source of information for anyone who is considering undergoing a surgical procedure, or has a loved one in that situation. This collection of 465 entries provides in-depth coverage of specific surgeries, diagnostic tests, drugs, and other related entries. The book gives detailed information on 265 surgeries; most include step-by-step illustrations to enhance the reader's understanding of the procedure itself. Entries on related topics, including anesthesia, second opinions, talking to the doctor, admission to the hospital, and preparing for surgery, give lay readers knowledge of surgery practices in general. Sidebars provide information on who performs the surgery and where, and on questions to ask the doctor.

This encyclopedia minimizes medical jargon and uses language that laypersons can understand, while still providing detailed coverage that will benefit health science students.

Entries on surgeries follow a standardized format that provides information at a glance. Rubrics include:

Definition
Purpose
Demographics
Description
Diagnosis/Preparation
Aftercare
Risks
Normal results
Morbidity and mortality rates
Alternatives
Resources

Inclusion criteria

A preliminary list of surgeries and related topics was compiled from a wide variety of sources, including professional medical guides and textbooks, as well as consumer guides and encyclopedias. Final selection of topics to include was made by the executive adviser in conjunction with the Gale editor.

About the Executive Adviser

The Executive Adviser for the *Gale Encyclopedia of Surgery* was Anthony J. Senagore, MD, MS, FACS, FASCRS. He has published a number of professional articles and is the Krause/Lieberman Chair in Laparoscopic Colorectal Surgery, and Staff Surgeon, Department of Colorectal Surgery at the Cleveland Clinic Foundation in Cleveland, Ohio.

About the contributors

The essays were compiled by experienced medical writers, including physicians, pharmacists, nurses, and other health care professionals. The adviser reviewed the completed essays to ensure that they are appropriate, up-to-date, and medically accurate. Illustrations were also reviewed by a medical doctor.

How to use this book

The **Gale Encyclopedia of Surgery** has been designed with ready reference in mind.

- Straight **alphabetical arrangement** of topics allows users to locate information quickly.
- **Bold-faced terms** within entries and **See also terms** at the end of entries direct the reader to related articles.
- **Cross-references** placed throughout the encyclopedia direct readers from alternate names and related topics to entries.
- A list of **Key terms** is provided where appropriate to define unfamiliar terms or concepts.
- A sidebar describing **Who performs the procedure and where it is performed** is listed with every surgery entry.
- A list of **Questions to ask the doctor** is provided wherever appropriate to help facilitate discussion with the patient's physician.

- The **Resources** section directs readers to additional sources of medical information on a topic. Books, periodicals, organizations, and internet sources are listed.
- A **Glossary** of terms used throughout the text is collected in one easy-to-use section at the back of book.
- A valuable **Organizations appendix** compiles useful contact information for various medical and surgical organizations.
- A comprehensive **General index** guides readers to all topics mentioned in the text.

Graphics

The *Gale Encyclopedia of Surgery* contains over 230 full-color illustrations, photos, and tables. This includes over 160 step-by-step illustrations of surgeries. These illustrations were specially created for this product to enhance a layperson's understanding of surgical procedures.

Licensing

The Gale Encyclopedia of Surgery is available for licensing. The complete database is provided in a fielded format and is deliverable on such media as disk or CD-ROM. For more information, contact Gale's Business Development Group at 1-800-877-GALE, or visit our website at www.gale.com/bizdev.

CONTRIBUTORS

Laurie Barclay, M.D.
Neurological Consulting Services
Tampa, FL

Jeanine Barone
Nutritionist, Exercise Physiologist
New York, NY

Julia R. Barrett
Science Writer
Madison, WI

Donald G. Barstow, R.N.
Clinical Nurse Specialist
Oklahoma City, OK

Mary Bekker
Medical Writer
Willow Grove, PA

Mark A. Best, MD, MPH, MBA
Associate Professor of Pathology
St. Matthew's University
Grand Cayman, BWI

Maggie Boleyn, R.N., B.S.N.
Medical Writer
Oak Park, MIn

Susan Joanne Cadwallader
Medical Writer
Cedarburg, WI

Diane Calbrese
*Medical Sciences and Technology
  Writer*
Silver Spring, MD

Richard H. Camer
Editor
International Medical News Group
Silver Spring, MD

Rosalyn Carson-DeWitt, M.D.
Medical Writer
Durham, NC

Lisa Christenson, PhD
Science Writer
Hamden, CT

Rhonda Cloos, RN
Medical Writer
Austin, TX

Angela Costello
Medical writer
Cleveland, OH

**Esther Csapo Rastegari, RN,
  BSN, EdM**
Medical Writer
Holbrook, MA

**L. Lee Culvert, BS,
  Biochemistry**
Health Writer
Alna, ME

Tish Davidson, AM
Medical Writer
Fremont, CA

Lori De Milto
Medical Writer
Sicklerville, NJ

Victoria E. DeMoranville
Medical Writer
Lakeville, MA

Altha Roberts Edgren
Medical Writer
Medical Ink
St. Paul, MN

Lorraine K. Ehresman
Medical Writer
Northfield, Quebec, Canada

**L. Fleming Fallon, Jr., MD,
  DrPH**
Professor of Public Health
Bowling Green State University
Bowling Green, OH

Paula Ford-Martin
Freelance Medical Writer
Warwick, RI

Janie Franz
Freelance Journalist
Grand Forks, ND

Rebecca J. Frey, PhD
Freelance Medical Writer
New Haven, CT

Debra Gordon
Medical Writer
Nazareth, PA

Jill Granger, M.S.
Sr. Research Associate
Dept. of Pathology
University of Michigan Medical
  Center
Ann Arbor, MI

Laith F. Gulli, M.D.
M.Sc., M.Sc.(MedSci), M.S.A.,
  Msc.Psych, MRSNZ
FRSH, FRIPHH, FAIC, FZS
DAPA, DABFC, DABCI
*Consultant Psychotherapist in
  Private Practice*
Lathrup Village, MI

Stephen John Hage, AAAS, RT(R), FAHRA
Medical Writer
Chatsworth, CA

Maureen Haggerty
Medical Writer
Ambler, PA

Robert Harr, MS, MT (ASCP)
Associate Professor and Chair
Department of Public and Allied
  Health
Bowling Green State University
Bowling Green, OH

Dan Harvey
Medical Writer
Wilmington, DE

Katherine Hauswirth, APRN
Medical Writer
Deep River, CT

Caroline Helwick
Medical Writer
New Orleans, LA

Lisette Hilton
Medical Writer
Boca Raton, FL

René A. Jackson, RN
Medical Writer
Port Charlotte, FL

Nadine M. Jacobson, RN
Medical Writer
Takoma Park, MD

Randi B. Jenkins, BA
Copy Chief
Fission Communications
New York, NY

Michelle L. Johnson, M.S., J.D.
*Patent Attorney and Medical
  Writer*
ZymoGenetics, Inc.
Seattle, WA

Paul A. Johnson, Ed.M.
Medical Writer
San Diego, CA

Cindy L. A. Jones, Ph.D.
Biomedical Writer
Sagescript Communications
Lakewood, CO

**Linda D. Jones, BA, PBT
  (ASCP)**
Medical Writer
Asheboro, NY

Crystal H. Kaczkowski, MSc.
Health Writer
Chicago, IL

Beth A. Kapes
Medical Writer
Bay Village, OH

Jeanne Krob, M.D., F.A.C.S.
Physician, Writer
Pittsburgh, PA

Monique Laberge, PhD
Sr. Res. Investigator
Dept. of Biochemistry &
  Biophysics, School of Medicine
University of Pennsylvania
Philadelphia, PA

Richard H. Lampert
Senior Medical Editor
W.B. Saunders Co.
Philadelphia, PA

Victor Leipzig, Ph.D.
Biological Consultant
Huntington Beach, CA

Lorraine Lica, PhD
Medical Writer
San Diego, CA

John T. Lohr, Ph.D.
*Assistant Director, Biotechnology
  Center*
Utah State University
Logan, UT

Jennifer Lee Losey, RN
Medical Writer
Madison Heights, MI

Jacqueline N. Martin, MS
Medical Writer
Albrightsville, PA

Nancy F. McKenzie, PhD
Public Health Consultant
Brooklyn, NY

Mercedes McLaughlin
Medical Writer
Phoenixville, CA

**Christine Miner Minderovic,
  BS, RT, RDMS**
Medical Writer
Ann Arbor, MI

Mark A. Mitchell, M.D.
Freelance Medical Writer
Bothell, WA

Erika J. Norris, MD, MS
Medical Writer
Oak Harbor, WA

Teresa Norris, R.N.
Medical Writer
Ute Park, NM

Debra Novograd, BS, RT(R)(M)
Medical Writer
Royal Oak, MI

Jane E. Phillips, PhD
Medical Writer
Chapel Hill, NC

J. Ricker Polsdorfer, M.D.
Medical Writer
Phoenix, AZ

**Elaine R. Proseus, M.B.A./T.M.,
  B.S.R.T., R.T.(R)**
Medical Writer
Farmington Hills, MI

Robert Ramirez, B.S.
Medical Student
University of Medicine &
  Dentistry of New Jersey
Stratford, NJ

Martha S. Reilly, OD
*Clinical Optometrist/ Medical
  Freelance Writer*
Madison, WI

Toni Rizzo
Medical Writer
Salt Lake City, UT

Richard Robinson
Freelance Medical Writer
Sherborn, MA

Nancy Ross-Flanigan
Science Writer
Belleville, MI

Belinda Rowland, Ph.D.
Medical Writer
Voorheesville, NY

Laura Ruth, Ph.D.
*Medical, Science, & Technology
  Writer*
Los Angeles, CA

Kausalya Santhanam, Ph.D.
Technical Writer
Branford, CT

Joan Schonbeck
Medical Writer
Nursing Department
Massachusetts Department of
  Mental Health
Marlborough, MA

Stephanie Dionne Sherk
Freelance Medical Writer
University of Michigan
Ann Arbor, MI

Lee A. Shratter, MD
Consulting Radiologist
Kentfield, CA

Jennifer Sisk
Medical Writer
Havertown, PA

Allison J. Spiwak, MSBME
Circulation Technologist
The Ohio State University
Columbus, OH

Kurt Sternlof
Science Writer
New Rochelle, NY

Margaret A Stockley, RGN
Medical Writer
Boxborough, MA

Dorothy Stonely
Medical Writer
Los Gatos, CA

Bethany Thivierge
Biotechnical Writer/Editor
Technicality Resources
Rockland, ME

Carol Turkington
Medical Writer
Lancaster, PA

Samuel D. Uretsky, Pharm.D.
Medical Writer
Wantagh, NY

Ellen S. Weber, M.S.N.
Medical Writer
Fort Wayne, IN

Barbara Wexler
Medical Writer
Chatsworth, CA

Abby Wojahn, RN, BSN, CCRN
Medical Writer
Milwaukee, WI

Kathleen D. Wright, R.N.
Medical Writer
Delmar, DE

Mary Zoll, Ph.D.
Science Writer
Newton Center, MA

Michael V. Zuck, Ph.D.
Medical Writer
Boulder, CO

Abdominal ultrasound

Definition

Abdominal ultrasound uses high frequency sound waves to produce two-dimensional images of the body's soft tissues, which are used for a variety of clinical applications, including diagnosis and guidance of treatment procedures. Ultrasound does not use ionizing radiation to produce images, and, in comparison to other diagnostic imaging modalities, it is inexpensive, safe, fast, and versatile.

Purpose

Abdominal ultrasound is used in the hospital radiology department and emergency department, as well as in physician offices, for a number of clinical applications. Ultrasound has a great advantage over x-ray imaging technologies in that it does not damage tissues with ionizing radiation. Ultrasound is also generally far better than plain x rays at distinguishing the subtle variations of soft tissue structures, and can be used in any of several modes, depending on the area of interest.

As an imaging tool, abdominal ultrasound generally is indicated for patients afflicted with chronic or acute abdominal pain; abdominal trauma; an obvious or suspected abdominal mass; symptoms of liver or biliary tract disease, pancreatic disease, gallstones, spleen disease, kidney disease, and urinary blockage; evaluation of ascites; or symptoms of an abdominal aortic aneurysm.

Specifically:

• Abdominal pain. Whether acute or chronic, pain can signal a serious problem—from organ malfunction or injury to the presence of malignant growths. Ultrasound scanning can help doctors quickly sort through potential causes when presented with general or ambiguous symptoms. All of the major abdominal organs can be studied for signs of disease that appear as changes in size, shape, or internal structure.

• Abdominal trauma. After a serious accident such as a car crash or a fall, internal bleeding from injured abdominal organs is often the most serious threat to survival. Neither the injuries nor the bleeding may be immediately apparent. Ultrasound is very useful as an initial scan when abdominal trauma is suspected, and it can be used to pinpoint the location, cause, and severity of hemorrhaging. In the case of puncture wounds, from a bullet for example, ultrasound can locate the foreign object and provide a preliminary survey of the damage. (**CT scans** are sometimes used in trauma settings.)

• Abdominal mass. Abnormal growths—tumors, cysts, abscesses, scar tissue, and accessory organs—can be located and tentatively identified with ultrasound. In particular, potentially malignant solid tumors can be distinguished from benign fluid-filled cysts. Masses and malformations in any organ or part of the abdomen can be found.

• Liver disease. The types and underlying causes of liver disease are numerous, though jaundice tends to be a general symptom. Sometimes, liver disease manifests as abnormal laboratory results, such as abnormal **liver function tests**. Ultrasound can differentiate between many of the types and causes of liver malfunction, and it is particularly good at identifying obstruction of the bile ducts and cirrhosis, which is characterized by abnormal fibrous growths and altered blood flow.

• Pancreatic disease. Inflammation of the pancreas—caused by, for example, abnormal fluid collections surrounding the organ (pseudocysts)—can be identified by ultrasound. Pancreatic stones (calculi), which can disrupt proper functioning, can also be detected.

• Gallstones. Gallstones are an extremely common cause of hospital admissions. In the non-emergency or non-acute setting, gallstones can present as abdominal pain, or fatty-food intolerance. These calculi can cause painful inflammation of the gallbladder and obstruct the bile ducts that carry digestive enzymes from the gallbladder and liver to the intestines. Gallstones are readily identifiable with ultrasound.

LOGIQ 700
GE MEDICAL SYSTEMS
19CFG

DEC-13-93 09:22:31
14cm   326s
ABD-GEN
CINE 0097
54DR
8G

15.4

15.4
CM/s

TIC=1.2 MI=0.9

An ultrasound screen shows a patient's kidney. *(Photograph by Brownie Harris. The Stock Market. Reproduced by permission.)*

• Spleen disease. The spleen is particularly prone to injury during abdominal trauma. It may also become painfully inflamed when infected or cancerous. The spleen can become enlarged with some forms of liver disease.

• Kidney disease. The kidneys are also prone to traumatic injury and are the organs most likely to form calculi, which can block the flow of urine and cause further systemic problems. A variety of diseases causing distinct changes in kidney morphology can also lead to complete kidney failure. Ultrasound imaging has proved extremely useful in diagnosing kidney disorders, including blockage and obstruction.

• Abdominal aortic aneurysm. This is a bulging weak spot in the abdominal aorta, which supplies blood directly from the heart to the entire lower body. A ruptured aortic aneurysm is imminently life-threatening. However, it can be readily identified and monitored with ultrasound before acute complications result.

• Appendicitis. Ultrasound is useful in diagnosing appendicitis, which causes abdominal pain.

Ultrasound technology can also be used for treatment purposes, most frequently as a visual aid during surgical procedures—such as guiding needle placement to drain fluid from a cyst, or to guide biopsies.

Description

Ultrasound includes all sound waves above the frequency of human hearing—about 20 thousand hertz, or cycles per second. Medical ultrasound generally uses frequencies between one and 10 megahertz (1–10 MHz). Higher frequency ultrasound waves produce more detailed images, but they are also more readily absorbed and so cannot penetrate as deeply into the body. Abdominal ultrasound imaging is generally performed at frequencies between 2–5 MHz.

An ultrasound scanner consists of two parts: the transducer and the data processing unit. The transducer both produces the sound waves that penetrate the body and receives the reflected echoes. Transducers are built around piezoelectric ceramic chips. (Piezoelectric refers to electricity that is produced when you put pressure on certain crystals such as quartz.) These ceramic chips react to electric pulses by producing sound waves (transmitting) and react to sound waves by producing electric pulses (receiving). Bursts of high-frequency electric pulses supplied to the transducer cause it to produce the scanning sound waves. The transducer then receives the returning echoes, translates them back into electric pulses, and sends them to the data processing unit—a computer that organizes the data into an image on a television screen.

Because sound waves travel through all the body's tissues at nearly the same speed—about 3,400 miles per hour—the microseconds it takes for each echo to be received can be plotted on the screen as a distance into the body. (The longer it takes to receive the echo, the farther away the reflective surface must be.) The relative strength of each echo, a function of the specific tissue or organ boundary that produced it, can be plotted as a point of varying brightness. In this way, the echoes are translated into an image.

Four different modes of ultrasound are used in medical imaging:

• A-mode. This is the simplest type of ultrasound in which a single transducer scans a line through the body with the echoes plotted on screen as a function of depth. This method is used to measure distances within the body and the size of internal organs.

• B-mode. In B-mode ultrasound, which is the most common use, a linear array of transducers simultaneously scans a plane through the body that can be viewed as a two-dimensional image on screen.

• M-Mode. The M stands for motion. A rapid sequence of B-mode scans whose images follow each other in sequence on screen enables doctors to see and measure range of motion, as the organ boundaries that produce reflections move relative to the probe. M-mode ultrasound has been put to particular use in studying heart motion.

• Doppler mode. Doppler ultrasonography includes the capability of accurately measuring velocities of moving material, such as blood in arteries and veins. The principle is the same as that used in radar guns that measure the speed of a car on the highway. Doppler capability is most often combined with B-mode scanning to produce images of blood vessels from which blood flow can be directly measured. This technique is used extensively to investigate valve defects, arteriosclerosis, and hypertension, particularly in the heart, but also in the abdominal aorta and the portal vein of the liver.

The actual procedure for a patient undergoing an abdominal ultrasound is relatively simple, regardless of the type of scan or its purpose. Fasting for at least eight hours prior to the procedure ensures that the stomach is empty and as small as possible, and that the intestines and bowels are relatively inactive. This also helps the gallbladder become more visible. Prior to scanning, an acoustic gel is applied to the skin of the patient's abdomen to allow the ultrasound probe to glide easily across the skin and to better transmit and receive ultrasonic pulses. The probe is moved around the abdomen's surface to obtain different views of the target areas. The patient will likely be asked to change positions from side to side and to hold the breath as necessary to obtain the desired views. Usually, a scan will take from 20 to 45 minutes, depending on the patient's condition and anatomical area being scanned.

Ultrasound scanners are available in different configurations, with different scanning features. Portable units, which weigh only a few pounds and can be carried by hand, are available for bedside use, office use, or use outside the hospital, such as at sporting events and in ambulances. Portable scanners range in cost from $10,000 to $50,000. Mobile ultrasound scanners, which can be pushed to the patient's bedside and between hospital departments, are the most common configuration and range in cost from $100,000 to over $250,000, depending on the scanning features purchased.

Preparation

A patient undergoing abdominal ultrasound will be advised by his or her physician about what to expect and how to prepare. As mentioned above, preparations generally include fasting.

Aftercare

In general, no aftercare related to the abdominal ultrasound procedure itself is required. Discomfort during the procedure is minimal.

Risks

Properly performed, ultrasound imaging is virtually without risk or side effects.

Results

As a diagnostic imaging technique, a normal abdominal ultrasound is one that indicates the absence of the suspected condition that prompted the scan. For example, symptoms such as abdominal pain radiating to the back suggest the possibility of, among other things, an abdominal aortic aneurysm. An ultrasound scan that indicates the absence of an aneurysm would rule out this life-threatening condition and point to other, less serious causes.

Because abdominal ultrasound imaging is generally undertaken to confirm a suspected condition, the results of a scan often will confirm the diagnosis, be it kidney stones, cirrhosis of the liver, or an aortic aneurysm. At that point, appropriate medical treatment as prescribed by a patient's physician is in order.

Ultrasound scanning should be performed by a registered and trained ultrasonographer, either a technolo-

KEY TERMS

Accessory organ—A lump of tissue adjacent to an organ that is similar to it, but which serves no important purpose (if it functions at all). While not necessarily harmful, such organs can cause problems if they are confused with a mass, or in rare cases, if they grow too large or become cancerous.

Ascites—Free fluid in the abdominal cavity.

Benign—In medical usage, benign is the opposite of malignant. It describes an abnormal growth that is stable, treatable, and generally not life-threatening.

Biopsy—The surgical removal and analysis of a tissue sample for diagnostic purposes. Usually the term refers to the collection and analysis of tissue from a suspected tumor to establish malignancy.

Calculus—Any type of hard concretion (stone) in the body, but usually found in the gallbladder, pancreas, and kidneys. Calculi (the plural form) are formed by the accumulation of excess mineral salts and other organic material such as blood or mucous. They can cause problems by lodging in and obstructing the proper flow of fluids, such as bile to the intestines or urine to the bladder.

Cirrhosis—A chronic liver disease characterized by the degeneration of proper functioning—jaundice is often an accompanying symptom. Causes of cirrhosis include hepatitis, alcoholism, and metabolic diseases.

Common bile duct—The branching passage through which bile—a necessary digestive enzyme—travels from the liver and gallbladder into the small intestine. Digestive enzymes from the pancreas also enter the intestines through the common bile duct.

Computed tomography scan (CT scan)—A specialized type of x-ray imaging that uses highly focused and relatively low-energy radiation to produce detailed two-dimensional images of soft-tissue structures, such as the brain or abdomen. CT scans are the chief competitor to ultrasound and can yield higher quality images not disrupted by bone or gas. They are, however, more cumbersome, time consuming, and expensive to perform, and they use ionizing radiation.

Doppler—The Doppler effect refers to the apparent change in frequency of sound-wave echoes returning to a stationary source from a moving target. If the object is moving toward the source, the frequency increases; if the object is moving away, the frequency decreases. The size of this frequency shift can be used to compute the object's speed—be it a car on the road or blood in an artery.

Frequency—Sound, whether traveling through air or the human body, produces vibrations—molecules bouncing into each other—as the shock wave travels along. The frequency of a sound is the number of vibrations per second. Within the audible range, frequency means pitch—the higher the frequency, the higher a sound's pitch.

Ionizing radiation—Radiation that can damage living tissue by disrupting and destroying individual cells at the molecular level. All types of nuclear radiation—x rays, gamma rays, and beta rays—are potentially ionizing. Sound waves physically vibrate the material through which they pass, but do not ionize it.

Jaundice—A condition that results in a yellow tint to the skin, eyes, and body fluids. Bile retention in the liver, gallbladder, and pancreas is the immediate cause, but the underlying cause could be as simple as obstruction of the common bile duct by a gallstone or as serious as pancreatic cancer. Ultrasound can distinguish between these conditions.

Malignant—The term literally means growing worse and resisting treatment. It is used as a synonym for cancerous and connotes a harmful condition that generally is life-threatening.

Morphology—Literally, the study of form. In medicine, morphology refers to the size, shape, and structure rather than the function of a given organ. As a diagnostic imaging technique, ultrasound facilitates the recognition of abnormal morphologies as symptoms of underlying conditions.

gist or a physician (radiologist, obstetrician/gynecologist). Ultrasound scanning in the emergency department may be performed by an emergency medicine physician, who should have appropriate training and experience in ultrasonography.

Resources

BOOKS

Dendy, P. P., and B. Heaton. *Physics for Diagnostic Radiology.* 2nd ed. Philadelphia: Institute of Physics Publishing, 1999.

Kevles, Bettyann Holtzmann. *Naked to the Bone: Medical Imaging in the Twentieth Century.* New Brunswick, New Jersey: Rutgers University Press, 1997.

Zaret, Barry L., ed. *The Patient's Guide to Medical Tests.* Boston: Houghton Mifflin Company, 1997.

PERIODICALS

Kuhn, M., R. L. L. Bonnin, M. J. Davey, J. L. Rowland, and S. Langlois. "Emergency Department Ultrasound Scanning for Abdominal Aortic Aneurysm: Accessible, Accurate, Advantageous." *Annals of Emergency Medicine* 36, No. 3 (September 2000): 219-23.

Sisk, Jennifer. "Ultrasound in the Emergency Department: Toward a Standard of Care." *Radiology Today* 2, No. 1 (June 4, 2001): 8-10.

ORGANIZATIONS

American College of Radiology. 1891 Preston White Drive, Reston, VA 20191-4397. (800) 227-5463. <http://www.acr.org>.

American Institute of Ultrasound in Medicine. 14750 Sweitzer Lane, Suite 100, Laurel, MD 20707-5906. (301) 498-4100. <http://www.aium.org>.

American Registry of Diagnostic Medical Sonographers. 600 Jefferson Plaza, Suite 360, Rockville, MD 20852-1150. (800) 541-9754. <http://www.ardms.org>.

American Society of Radiologic Technologists (ASRT). 15000 Central Avenue SE, Albuquerque, NM 87123-2778. (800) 444-2778. <http://www.asrt.org>.

Radiological Society of North America. 820 Jorie Boulevard, Oak Brook, IL 60523-2251. (630) 571-2670. <http://www.rsna.org>.

Society of Diagnostic Medical Sonography. 12770 Coit Road, Suite 708, Dallas, TX 75251-1319. (972) 239-7367. <http://www.sdms.org>.

Jennifer E. Sisk, M.A.
Lee A. Shratter, M.D.

Abdominal wall defect repair

Definition

Abdominal wall defect repair is a surgery performed to correct one of two birth defects of the abdominal wall: gastroschisis or omphalocele. Depending on the defect treated, the procedure is also known as omphalocele repair/closure or gastroschisis repair/closure.

Purpose

For some unknown reason, while in utero, the abdominal wall muscles do not form correctly. And, when the abdominal wall is incompletely formed at birth, the internal organs of the infant can either protrude into the

---

WHO PERFORMS THE PROCEDURE AND WHERE IS IT PERFORMED?

Abdominal wall defect surgery is performed by a pediatric surgeon. A pediatric surgeon is specialized in the surgical care of children. He or she must have graduated from medical school, and completed five years of postgraduate **general surgery** training in an accredited training program. A pediatric surgeon must complete an additional accredited two-year fellowship program in **pediatric surgery** and be board-eligible or board-certified in general surgery. (Board certification is granted when a fully trained surgeon has taken and passed first a written, then an oral examination.) Once the general surgery boards are passed, a fellowship-trained pediatric surgeon becomes eligible to take the Pediatric Surgery examination. Other credentials may include membership in the American College of Surgeons, the American Pediatric Surgical Association, and/or the American Academy of Pediatrics. Each of these organizations require that fellows meet well-established standards of training, clinical knowledge, and professional conduct.

If prenatal screening indicates that abdominal wall defects are present in the fetus, delivery should occur at a hospital with an intensive care nursery (NICU) and a pediatric surgeon on staff.

---

umbilical cord (omphalocele) or to the side of the navel (gastroschisis). The size of an omphalocele varies—some are very small, about the size of a ping pong ball, while others may be as big as a grapefruit. **Omphalocele repair** is performed to repair the omphalocele defect in which all or part of the bowel and other internal organs lie on the outside of the abdomen in a hernia (sac). Gastroschisis repair is performed to repair the other abdominal wall defect through which the bowel thrusts out with no protective sac present. Gastroschisis is a life-threatening condition that requires immediate medical intervention. Surgery for abdominal wall defects aims to return the abdominal organs back to the abdominal cavity, and to repair the defect if possible. It can also be performed to create a pouch to protect the intestines until they are inserted back into the abdomen.

Demographics

Abdominal wall defects occurs in the United States at a rate of one case per 2,000 births, which means that some 2,360 cases are diagnosed per year. Mothers below the age of 20 are four times as likely as mothers in their late twenties to give birth to affected babies.

Description

Abdominal wall defect surgery is performed soon after birth. The protruding organs are covered with dressings, and a tube is inserted into the stomach to prevent the baby from choking or breathing in the contents of the stomach into the lungs. The surgery is performed under general anesthesia so that the baby will not feel pain. First, the pediatric surgeon enlarges the hole in the abdominal wall in order to examine the bowel for damage or other birth defects. Damaged portions of the bowel are removed and the healthy bowel is reconnected with stitches. The exposed organs are replaced within the abdominal cavity, and the opening is closed. Sometimes closure of the opening is not possible, for example when the abdominal cavity is too small or when the organs are too large or swollen to close the skin. In such cases, the surgeon will place a plastic covering pouch, commonly called a silo because of its shape, over the abdominal organs on the outside of the infant to protect the organs. Gradually, the organs are squeezed through the pouch into the opening and returned to the body. This procedure can take up to a week, and final closure may be performed a few weeks later. More surgery may be required to repair the abdominal muscles at a later time.

Diagnosis/Preparation

Prenatal screening can detect approximately 85% of abdominal wall defects. Gastroschisis and omphalocele are usually diagnosed by ultrasound examinations before birth. These tests can determine the size of the abdominal wall defect and identify the affected organs. The

surgery is performed immediately after delivery, as soon as the newborn is stable.

Aftercare

After surgery, the infant is transferred to an **intensive care unit** (ICU) and placed in an incubator to keep warm and prevent infection. Oxygen is provided. When organs are placed back into the abdominal cavity, this may increase pressure on the abdomen and make breathing difficult. In such cases, the infant is provided with a breathing tube and ventilator until the swelling of the abdominal organs has decreased. Intravenous fluids, **antibiotics**, and pain medication are also administered. A tube is also placed in the stomach to empty gastric secretions. Feedings are started very slowly, using a nasal tube as soon as bowel function starts. Babies born with omphaloceles can stay in the hospital from one week to one month after surgery, depending on the size of the defect. Babies are discharged from the hospital when they are taking all their feedings by mouth and gaining weight.

Risks

The risks of abdominal wall repair surgery include peritonitis and temporary paralysis of the small bowel. If a large segment of the small intestine is damaged, the baby may develop short bowel syndrome and have digestive problems.

Normal results

In most cases, the defect can be corrected with surgery. The outcome depends on the amount of damage to the bowel.

Morbidity and mortality rates

The size of the abdominal wall defect, the extent to which organs protrude out of the abdomen, and the presence of other birth defects influence the outcome of the surgery. The occurrence of other birth defects is uncommon in infants with gastroschisis, and 85% survive. Approximately half of the babies diagnosed with omphalocele have heart defects or other birth defects, and approximately 60% survive to age one.

Alternatives

Gastroschisis is a life-threatening condition requiring immediate surgical intervention. There is no alternative to surgery for both gastroschisis and omphalocele.

Resources

BOOKS

Iannucci, Lisa. *Birth Defects*. Berkeley Heights: Enslow Publishers Inc., 2000.

KEY TERMS

Abdomen—The portion of the body that lies between the thorax and the pelvis. It contains a cavity with many organs.

Amniotic membrane—A thin membrane that contains the fetus and the protective amniotic fluid surrounding the fetus.

Anesthesia—A combination of drugs administered by a variety of techniques by trained professionals that provide sedation, amnesia, analgesia, and immobility adequate for the accomplishment of the surgical procedure with minimal discomfort, and without injury, to the patient.

Gastroschisis—A defect of the abdominal wall caused by rupture of the amniotic membrane or by the delayed closure of the umbilical ring. It is usually accompanied by protrusion of abdomen organs.

Hernia—The protrusion or thrusting forward of an organ or tissue through an abnormal opening into the abdominal sac.

Omphalocele—A hernia that occurs at the navel.

Peritonitis—Inflammation of the membrane lining the abdominal cavity. It causes abdominal pain and tenderness, constipation, vomiting, and fever.

Short bowel syndrome—A condition in which digestion and absorption in the small intestine are impaired.

Ultrasound—An imaging technology that that allow various organs in the body to be examined.

Umbilical ring—An opening through which the umbilical vessels pass in the fetus; it is closed after birth and its site is indicated by the navel.

PERIODICALS

Kurchubasche, Arlet G. "The fetus with an abdominal wall defect." *Medicine & Health/Rhode Island* 84 (2001): 159–161.

Lenke, R. "Benefits of term delivery in infants with antenatally diagnosed gastroschisis." *Obstetrics and Gynecology* 101 (February 2003): 418–419.

Sydorak, R. M., A. Nijagal, L. Sbragia, et al. "Gastroschisis: small hole, big cost." *Journal of Pediatric Surgery* 37 (December 2002): 1669–1672.

White, J. J. "Morbidity in infants with antenatally-diagnosed anterior abdominal wall defects." *Pediatric Surgery International* 17 (September 2001): 587–591.

ORGANIZATIONS

American Academy of Pediatrics. 141 Northwest Point Boulevard, Elk Grove Village, IL 60007-1098. (847) 434-4000. <http://www.aap.org>.

OTHER

"Abdominal Defects." Medical and Scientific Information Online, Inc. [cited April 8, 2003]. <http://www.cpdx.com/cpdx/abdwall.htm>.

National Birth Defects Prevention Network. January 27, 2003 [cited April 8, 2003]. <http://www.nbdpn.org>.

Monique Laberge, Ph.D.

Abdominoplasty

Definition

Also known as a tummy tuck, abdominoplasty is a surgical procedure in which excess skin and fat in the abdominal area is removed and the abdominal muscles are tightened.

Purpose

Abdominoplasty is a cosmetic procedure that treats loose or sagging abdominal skin, leading to a protruding abdomen that typically occurs after significant weight loss. Good candidates for abdominoplasty are individuals in good health who have one or more of the above conditions and who have tried to address these issues with diet and **exercise** with little or no results.

Women who have had multiple pregnancies often seek abdominoplasty as a means of ridding themselves of loose abdominal skin. While in many cases diet and exercise are sufficient in reducing abdominal fat and loose skin after pregnancy, in some women these conditions may persist. Abdominoplasty is not recommended for women who wish to have further pregnancies, as the beneficial effects of the surgery may be undone.

Another common reason for abdominoplasty is to remove excess skin from a person who has lost a large amount of weight or is obese. A large area of overhanging skin is called a pannus. Older patients are at an increased risk of developing a pannus because skin loses elasticity as one ages. Problems with hygiene or wound formation can result in a patient who has multiple hanging folds of abdominal skin and fat. If a large area of excess tissue is removed, the procedure is called a panniculectomy.

In some instances, abdominoplasty is performed simultaneously or directly following gynecologic surgery such as **hysterectomy** (removal of the uterus). One study found that the removal of a large amount of excess abdominal skin and fat from morbidly obese patients dur-

Abdominoplasty (tummy tuck) surgery. Portions of the lower abdominal tissues have been removed and the navel repositioned. The remaining skin flaps will be sutured. *(Photography by MM Michele Del Guercio. Reproduced by permission.)*

ing gynecologic surgery results in better exposure to the operating field and improved wound healing.

Contraindications

Certain patients should not undergo abdominoplasty. Poor candidates for the surgery include:

- Women who wish to have subsequent pregnancies.
- Individuals who wish to lose a large amount of weight following surgery.
- Patients with unrealistic expectations (those who think the surgery will give them a "perfect" figure).
- Those who are unable to deal with the post-surgical scars.
- Patients who have had previous abdominal surgery.
- Heavy smokers.

Demographics

According to the American Academy of Plastic Surgeons, in 2001 there were approximately 58,567 abdominoplasties performed in the United States, relating to 4% of all plastic surgery patients and less than 0.5%

of all plastic surgery procedures. Female patients accounted for 97% of all abdominoplasties. Most patients were between the ages of 35 and 50 (58%), with patients under 35 accounting for 20% and patients over 50 accounting for 22%. Eighty-two percent of all plastic surgery patients during 2001 were white, 7% were Hispanic, 5% were African American, and 5% were Asian American.

Description

The patient is usually placed under general anesthesia for the duration of surgery. The advantages to general anesthesia are that the patient remains unconscious during the procedure, which may take from two to five hours to complete; no pain will be experienced nor will the patient have any memory of the procedure; and the patient's muscles remain completely relaxed, lending to safer surgery.

Once an adequate level of anesthesia has been reached, an incision is made across the lower abdomen. For a complete abdominoplasty, the incision will stretch from hipbone to hipbone. The skin will be lifted off the abdominal muscles from the incision up to the ribs, with a separate incision being made to free the umbilicus (belly button). The vertical abdominal muscles may be tightened by stitching them closer together. The skin is then stretched back over the abdomen and excess skin and fat are cut away. Another incision will be made across the stretched skin through which the umbilicus will be located and stitched into position. A temporary drain may be placed to remove excess fluid from beneath the incision. All incisions are then stitched closed and covered with dressings.

Individuals who have excess skin and fat limited to the lower abdomen (i.e., below the navel) may be candidates for partial abdominoplasty. During this procedure, the muscle wall is not tightened. Rather, the skin is stretched over a smaller incision made just above the pubic hairline and excess skin is cut away. The incision is then closed with stitches. The umbilicus is not repositioned during a partial abdominoplasty; its shape, therefore, may change as the skin is stretched downward.

Additional procedures

In some cases, additional procedures may be performed during or directly following abdominoplasty. **Liposuction**, also called suction lipectomy or lipoplasty, is a technique that removes fat that cannot be removed by diet or exercise. During the procedure, which is generally performed in an outpatient surgical facility, the patient is anesthetized and a hollow tube called a cannula is inserted under the skin into a fat deposit. By physical manipulation, the fat deposit is loosened and sucked out of the body. Liposuction may be used during abdominoplasty to remove fat deposits from the torso, hips, or other areas. This may create a more desired body contour.

Some patients may choose to undergo breast augmentation, reduction, or lift during abdominoplasty. Breast augmentation involves the insertion of a silicone- or saline-filled implant into the breast, most often behind the breast tissue or chest muscle wall. A **breast reduction** may be performed on patients who have large breasts that cause an array of symptoms such as back and neck pain. Breast reduction removes excess breast skin and fat and moves the nipple and area around the nipple (called the areola) to a higher position. A breast lift, also called a mastopexy, is performed on women who have low, sagging breasts, often due to pregnancy, nursing, or aging. The surgical procedure is similar to a breast reduction, but only excess skin is removed; **breast implants** may also be inserted.

Breast reconstruction

A modified version of abdominoplasty may be used to reconstruct a breast in a patient who has undergone mastectomy (surgical removal of the breast, usually as a

WHO PERFORMS THE PROCEDURE AND WHERE IS IT PERFORMED?

Abdominoplasty is usually performed by a plastic surgeon, a medical doctor who has completed specialized training in the repair or reconstruction of physical defects or the cosmetic enhancement of the human body. In order for a plastic surgeon to be considered board certified by the American Board of Plastic Surgery, he or she must meet a set of strict criteria (including a minimum of five years of training in **general surgery** and plastic surgery) and pass a series of examinations. The procedure may be performed in a hospital **operating room** or a specialized outpatient surgical facility.

treatment for cancer). Transverse rectus abdominis myocutaneous (TRAM) flap reconstruction may be performed at the time of mastectomy or as a later, separate procedure. Good candidates for the surgery include women who have had or will have a large portion of breast tissue removed and also have excess skin and fat in the lower abdominal region. Women who are not in good health, are obese, have had a previous abdominoplasty, or wish to have additional children are not considered good candidates for TRAM flap reconstruction.

The procedure is usually performed in three separate steps. The first step is the TRAM flap surgery. In a procedure similar to traditional abdominoplasty, excess skin and fat is removed from the lower abdomen, then stitched into place to create a breast. The construction of a nipple takes place several months later to enable to the tissue to heal adequately. Finally, once the new breast has healed and softened, tattooing may be performed to add color to the constructed nipple.

Costs

Because abdominoplasty is considered to be an elective cosmetic procedure, most insurance policies will not cover the procedure, unless it is being performed for medical reasons (for example, if an abdominal hernia is the cause of the protruding abdomen).

A number of fees must be taken into consideration when calculating the total cost of the procedure. Typically, fees include those paid to the surgeon, the anesthesiologist, and the facility where the surgery is performed. If liposuction or breast surgery is to be performed, additional costs may be incurred. The average cost of abdominoplas-

QUESTIONS TO ASK THE DOCTOR

- How long have you been practicing plastic surgery?
- Are you certified by the American Board of Plastic Surgeons?
- How many abdominoplasties have you performed, and how often?
- What is your rate of complications?
- How extensive will the post-surgical scars be?
- What method of anesthesia will be used?
- What are the costs associated with this procedure?
- Will my insurance pay for part or all of the surgery?
- Do you provide revision surgery (i.e., if I experience suboptimal results)?

ty is $6,500, but may range from $5,000–9,000, depending on the surgeon and the complexity of the procedure.

Diagnosis/Preparation

There are a number of steps that the patient and plastic surgeon must take before an abdominoplasty may be performed. The surgeon will generally schedule an initial consultation, during which a **physical examination** will be performed. The surgeon will assess a number of factors that may impact the success of the surgery. These include:

- the patient's general health
- the size and shape of the abdomen and torso
- the location of abdominal fat deposits
- the patient's skin elasticity
- what medications the patient may be taking

It is important that the patient come prepared to ask questions of the surgeon during the initial consultation. The surgeon will describe the procedure, where it will be performed, associated risks, the method of anesthesia and pain relief, any additional procedures that may be performed, and post-surgical care. The patient may also meet with a staff member to discuss how much the procedure will cost and what options for payment are available.

The patient will also receive instructions on how to prepare for abdominoplasty. Certain medications should be avoided for several weeks before and after the surgery; for example, medications containing **aspirin** may interfere with the blood's ability to clot. Because tobacco can interfere with blood circulation and wound healing, smokers are recommended to quit for several weeks before and after the procedure. A medicated antibacterial soap may be prescribed prior to surgery to decrease levels of bacteria on the skin around the incision site.

Aftercare

The patient may remain in the hospital or surgical facility overnight, or return home the day of surgery after spending several hours recovering from the procedure and anesthesia. Before leaving the facility, the patient will receive the following instructions on post-surgical care:

- For the first several days after surgery, it is recommended that the patient remain flexed at the hips (i.e., avoid straightening the torso) to prevent unnecessary tension on the surgical site.
- Walking as soon as possible after the procedure is recommended to improve recovery time and prevent blood clots in the legs.
- Mild exercise that does not cause pain to the surgical site is recommended to improve muscle tone and decrease swelling.
- The patient should not shower until any drains are removed from the surgical site; sponge baths are permitted.
- Work may be resumed in two to four weeks, depending on the level of physical activity required.

Surgical drains will be removed within one week after abdominoplasty, and stitches from one to two weeks after surgery. Swelling, bruising, and pain in the abdominal area are to be expected and may last from two to six weeks. Recovery will be faster, however, in the patient who is in good health with relatively strong abdominal muscles. The incisions will remain a noticeable red or pink for several months, but will begin to fade by nine months to a year after the procedure. Because of their location, scars should be easily hidden under clothing, including bathing suits.

Risks

There are a number of complications that may arise during or after abdominoplasty. Complications are more often seen among patients who smoke, are overweight, are unfit, have diabetes or other health problems, or have scarring from previous abdominal surgery. Risks inherent to the use of general anesthesia include nausea, vomiting, sore throat, fatigue, headache, and muscle sore-

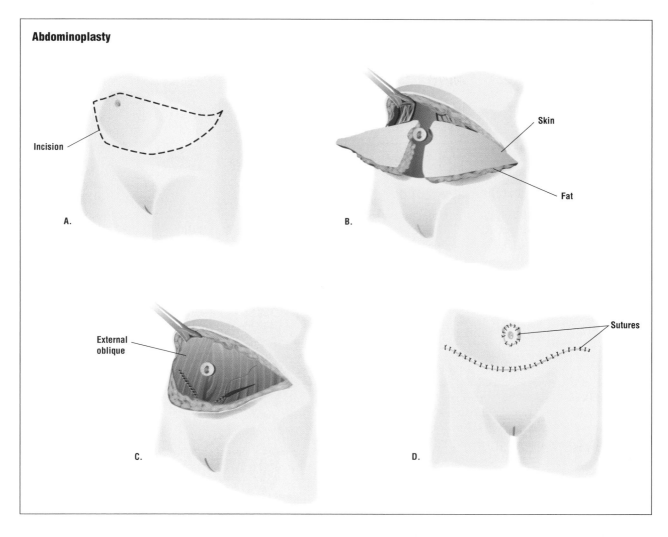

Abdominoplasty

Incision

Skin

Fat

A.

B.

External oblique

Sutures

C.

D.

In an abdominoplasty, or tummy tuck, an incision is made in the abdomen (usually from hip bone to hip bone). Excess skin and fat is removed (B). The muscles may be tightened (C). The navel will be placed into the proper position (D), and the major incision closed beneath it. *(Illustration by GGS Inc.)*

ness; more rarely, blood pressure problems, allergic reaction, heart attack, or stroke may occur.

Risks associated with the procedure include:

- bleeding
- wound infection
- delayed wound healing
- skin or fat necrosis (death)
- hematoma (collection of blood in a tissue)
- seroma (collection of serum in a tissue)
- blood clots
- pulmonary embolism (a blood clot that travels to the lungs)

- numbness to the abdominal region or thighs (due to damage to nerves during surgery)

Normal results

In most cases, abdominoplasty is successful in providing a trimmer abdominal contour in patients with excess skin and fat and weak abdominal muscles. A number of factors will influence how long the optimal results of abdominoplasty will last, including age, skin elasticity, and physical fitness. Generally, however, good results will be long-lasting if the patient remains in good health, maintains a stable weight, and exercises regularly. One study surveying patient satisfaction following abdominoplasty indicated that 95% felt their symptoms (excess skin and fat) were improved, 86% were satisfied with the results of the surgery, and 86% would recommend the procedure to a friend.

Morbidity and mortality rates

The overall rate of complications associated with abdominoplasty is approximately 32%. This percentage, however, is higher among patients who are overweight; one study placed the complication rate among obese patients at 80%. Rates are also higher among patients who smoke or are diabetic. The rate of major complications requiring hospitalization has been reported at 1.4%.

Alternatives

Before seeking abdominoplasty, an individual will want to be sure that loose and excess abdominal skin and fat cannot be decreased through a regimen of diet and exercise. Abdominoplasty should not be viewed as an alternative to weight loss. In fact, some doctors would suggest that a patient be no more than 15% over his or her ideal body weight in order to undergo the procedure.

Liposuction is a surgical alternative to abdominoplasty. There are several advantages to liposuction. It is less expensive (an average of $2,000 per body area treated compared to $6,500 for abdominoplasty). It also is associated with a faster recovery, a need for less anesthesia, a smaller rate of complications, and significantly smaller incisions. What liposuction cannot do is remove excess skin. Liposuction is a good choice for patients with localized deposits of fat, while abdominoplasty is a better choice for patients with excess abdominal skin and fat.

Resources

PERIODICALS

Hensel, J. M., J. A. Lehman, M. P. Tantri, M. G. Parker, D. S. Wagner, and N. S. Topham. "An Outcomes Analysis and Satisfaction Surgery of 199 Consecutive Abdominoplasties." *Annals of Plastic Surgery,* 46, no. 4 (April 1, 2001): 357–63.

Vastine, V. L., et al. "Wound Complications of Abdominoplasty in Obese Patients." *Annals of Plastic Surgery,* 41, no. 1 (January 1, 1999): 34–9.

ORGANIZATIONS

American Academy of Cosmetic Surgery. 737 N. Michigan Ave., Suite 820, Chicago, IL 60611. (312) 981-6760. <http://www.cosmeticsurgery.org>.

American Board of Plastic Surgery, Inc. 7 Penn Center, Suite 400, 1635 Market St., Philadelphia, PA 19103-2204. (215) 587-9322. <http://www.abplsurg.org>.

American Society of Plastic Surgeons. 444 E. Algonquin Rd., Arlington Heights, IL 60005. (888) 4-PLASTIC. <http://www.plasticsurgery.org>.

OTHER

"2001 Statistics." *American Society of Plastic Surgeons,* 2003 [cited April 8, 2003]. <http://www.plasticsurgery.org/public_education/2001statistics.cfm>.

"Abdominoplasty." *American Society of Plastic Surgeons,* 2003 [cited April 8, 2003]. <http://www.plasticsurgery.org/public_education/procedures/Abdominoplasty.cfm>.

Gallagher, Susan. "Panniculectomy: Implications for Care." *Perspectives in Nursing,* 2003 [cited April 8, 2003]. <http://www.perspectivesinnursing.org/v3n3/panniculectomy.html>.

"Training Requirements." *American Board of Plastic Surgery,* July 2002 [cited April 8, 2003]. <http://www.abplsurg.org/training_requirements.html>.

"Tummy Tuck." *The American Society for Aesthetic Plastic Surgery,* 2000 [cited April 8, 2003]. <http://www.surgery.org/q1>.

Zenn, Michael R. "Breast Reconstruction: TRAM, Unipedicled." *eMedicine,* December 13, 2001 [cited April 8, 2003]. <http://www.emedicine.com/plastic/topic141.htm>.

Stephanie Dionne Sherk

ABO blood typing *see* **Type and screen**

Abortion, induced

Definition

Induced abortion is the intentional termination of a pregnancy before the fetus can live independently. An abortion may be elective (based on a woman's personal choice) or therapeutic (to preserve the health or save the life of a pregnant woman).

Purpose

An abortion may be performed whenever there is some compelling reason to end a pregnancy. An abortion is termed "induced" to differentiate it from a spontaneous abortion in which the products of conception are lost naturally (also called a miscarriage).

An abortion is considered to be elective if a woman chooses to end her pregnancy, and it is not for maternal or fetal health reasons. Some reasons a woman might choose to have an elective abortion are:

- Continuation of the pregnancy may cause emotional or financial hardship.
- The woman is not ready to become a parent.
- The pregnancy was unintended.
- The woman is pressured into having one by her partner, parents, or others.
- The pregnancy was the result of rape or incest.

A therapeutic abortion is performed in order to preserve the health or save the life of a pregnant woman. A health care provider might recommend a therapeutic abortion if the fetus is diagnosed with significant abnormalities or not expected to live, or if it has died *in utero*. Therapeutic abortion may also be used to reduce the number of fetuses if a woman is pregnant with multiples; this procedure is called multifetal pregnancy reduction (MFPR).

A therapeutic abortion may be indicated if a woman has a pregnancy-related health condition that endangers her life. Some examples of such conditions include:

- severe hypertension (high blood pressure)
- cardiac disease
- severe depression or other psychiatric conditions
- serious kidney or liver disease
- certain types of infection
- malignancy (cancer)
- multifetal pregnancy

Demographics

Abortion has been a legal procedure in the United States since 1973. Since then, more than 39 million abortions have taken place. It is estimated that approximately 1.3–1.4 million abortions occur in the United States annually. Induced abortions terminate approximately half of the estimated three million unplanned pregnancies each year and approximately one-fifth of all pregnancies.

In 2000 an estimated 21 out of 1,000 women aged 15–44 had an abortion. Out of every 100 pregnancies that year that ended in live birth or abortion, approximately 24 were elective terminations. The highest abortion rates in 2000 occurred in New Jersey, New York, California, Delaware, Florida, and Nevada (greater than 30 per 1,000 women of reproductive age). Kentucky, South Dakota, Wyoming, Idaho, Mississippi, Utah, and West Virginia had the lowest rates (less than seven per 1,000 women).

In 2000 and 2001, the highest percentage of abortions were performed on women between the ages of 20 and 30, with women ages 20–24 having the highest rate (47 per 1,000 women). Adolescents ages 15–19 accounted for 19% of elective abortions, while 25% were performed on women older than 30. Approximately 73% of women having an abortion had previously been pregnant; 48% of those had a previous abortion.

Non-hispanic, white women reported the highest percentage of abortions in 2000 and 2001 (41%). African American women accounted for 32%, Hispanic women for 20%, Asian and Pacific Islander women for 6%, and Native American women for 1%. The highest abortion rates occurred among African American women (49 per 1,000 women), with Hispanic and Asian women also reporting higher-than-average rates (33 and 31 per 1,000 women, respectively). The rate was the lowest among white women (13 per 1,000 women).

Description

Abortions are safest when performed within the first six to 10 weeks after the last menstrual period (LMP). This calculation is used by health care providers to determine the stage of pregnancy. About 90% of women who have abortions do so in the first trimester of pregnancy (before 13 weeks) and experience few complications. Abortions performed between 13 and 24 weeks (during the second trimester) have a higher rate of complications. Abortions after 24 weeks are extremely rare and are usually limited to situations where the life of the mother is in danger.

Although it is safer to have an abortion during the first trimester, some second trimester abortions may be inevitable. The results of genetic testing are often not available until 16 weeks gestation. In addition, women, especially teens, may not have recognized the pregnancy or come to terms with it emotionally soon enough to have a first trimester abortion. Teens make up the largest group having second trimester abortions.

Very early abortions cost between $200 and $400. Later abortions cost more. The cost increases about $100 per week between the thirteenth and sixteenth week. Second trimester abortions are much more costly because they often involve more risk, more services, anesthesia, and sometimes a hospital stay. Private insurance carriers may or may not cover the procedure. Federal law prohibits federal funds (including **Medicaid**) from being used to pay for an elective abortion.

Medical abortions

Medical abortions are brought about by taking medications that end the pregnancy. The advantages of a first trimester medical abortion are:

- The procedure is non-invasive; no **surgical instruments** are used.
- Anesthesia is not required.

Abortion, induced

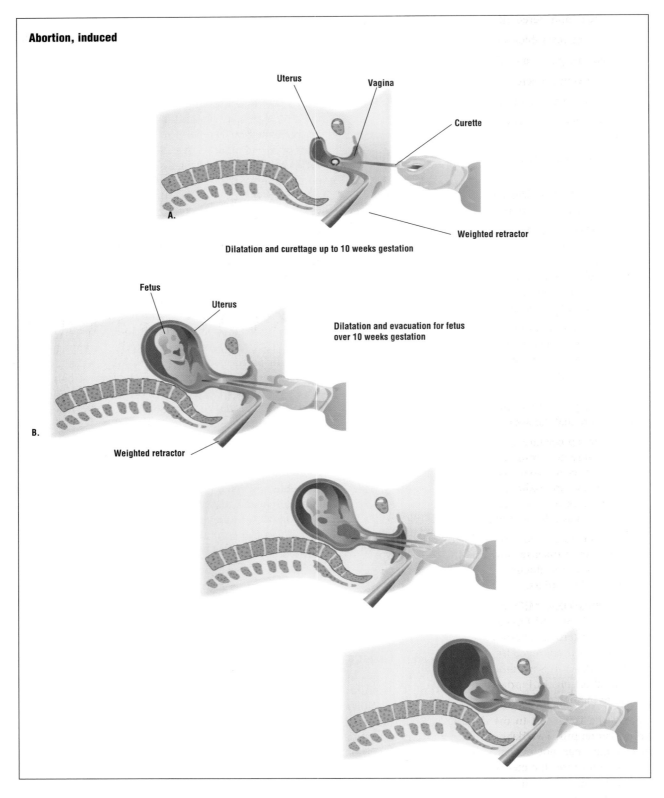

Uterus

Vagina

Curette

Weighted retractor

A.

Dilatation and curettage up to 10 weeks gestation

Fetus

Uterus

Dilatation and evacuation for fetus
over 10 weeks gestation

B.

Weighted retractor

A dilatation and curettage is used to perform an abortion up to 10 weeks gestation (A). Over 10 weeks, the physician may use dilatation and evacuation to achieve the abortion (B). *(Illustration by GGS Inc.)*

- Drugs are administered either orally or by injection.
- The outcome resembles a natural miscarriage.

   Disadvantages of a medical abortion are:

- The effectiveness decreases after the seventh week.
- The procedure may require multiple visits to the doctor.
- Bleeding after the abortion lasts longer than after a surgical abortion.
- The woman may see the contents of her womb as it is expelled.

As of 2003, two drugs were available in the United States to induce abortion: methotrexate and mifepristone.

METHOTREXATE. Methotrexate (Rheumatrex) targets rapidly dividing fetal cells, thus preventing the fetus from further developing. It is used in conjunction with misoprostol (Cytotec), a prostaglandin that stimulates contractions of the uterus. Methotrexate may be taken up to 49 days after the first day of the last menstrual period.

On the first visit to the doctor, the woman receives an injection of methotrexate. On the second visit, about a week later, she is given misoprostol tablets vaginally to stimulate contractions of the uterus. Within two weeks, the woman will expel the contents of her uterus, ending the pregnancy. A follow-up visit to the doctor is necessary to assure that the abortion is complete.

With this procedure, a woman will feel cramping and may feel nauseated from the misoprostol. This combination of drugs is approximately 92–96% effective in ending pregnancy. Approximately 50% of women will experience the abortion soon after taking the misoprostol; 35–40% will have the abortion up to seven days later.

Methotrexate is not recommended for women with liver or kidney disease, inflammatory bowel disease, clotting disorders, documented immunodeficiency, or certain blood disorders.

MIFEPRISTONE. Mifepristone (RU-486), which goes by the brand name Mifeprex, works by blocking the action of progesterone, a hormone needed for pregnancy to continue. It was approved by the Food and Drug Administration (FDA) in September 2000 as an alternative to surgical abortion. Mifepristone can be taken up to 49 days after the first day of a woman's last period.

On the first visit to the doctor, a woman takes a mifepristone pill. Two days later she returns and, if the miscarriage has not occurred, takes two misoprostol pills, which causes the uterus to contract. Approximately 10% will experience the abortion before receiving the dose of misoprostol.

Within four days, 90% of women have expelled the contents of their uterus and completed the abortion. With-

in 14 days, 95–97% of women have completed the abortion. A third follow-up visit to the doctor is necessary to confirm through observation or ultrasound that the procedure is complete. In the event that it is not, a surgical abortion is performed. Studies show that 4.5–8% of women need surgery or a blood **transfusion** after taking mifepristone, and the pregnancy persists in about 1%. Surgical abortion is then recommended because the fetus may be damaged. Side effects include nausea, vaginal bleeding, and heavy cramping. The bleeding is typically heavier than a normal period and may last up to 16 days.

Mifepristone is not recommended for women with ectopic pregnancy or an intrauterine device (IUD), or those who have been taking long-term steroidal therapy, have bleeding abnormalities, or on blood-thinners such as Coumadin.

Surgical abortions

MANUAL VACUUM ASPIRATION. Up to 10 weeks gestation, a pregnancy can be ended by a procedure called manual vacuum aspiration (MVA). This procedure is also called menstrual extraction, mini-suction, or early abortion. The contents of the uterus are suctioned out through a thin plastic tube that is inserted through the cervix; suction is applied by a syringe. The procedure generally lasts about 15 minutes.

A 1998 study of women undergoing MVA indicated that the procedure was 99.5% effective in terminating pregnancy and was associated with a very low risk of complications (less than 1%). Menstrual extractions are safe, but because the amount of fetal material is so small at this stage of development, it is easy to miss. This results in an incomplete abortion that means the pregnancy continues.

DILATATION AND SUCTION CURETTAGE. Dilation and suction curettage may also be called D & C, suction dilation, vacuum curettage, or suction curettage. The procedure involves gentle stretching of the cervix with a series of dilators or specific medications. The contents of the uterus are then removed with a tube attached to a suction machine, and walls of the uterus are cleaned using a narrow loop called a curette.

Advantages of an abortion of this type are:

• It is usually done as a one-day outpatient procedure.

• The procedure takes only 10–15 minutes.

• Bleeding after the abortion lasts five days or less.

• The woman does not see the products of her womb being removed.

Disadvantages include:

• The procedure is invasive; surgical instruments are used.

• Infection may occur.

The procedure is 97–99% effective. The amount of discomfort a woman feels varies considerably. Local anesthesia is often given to numb the cervix, but it does not mask uterine cramping. After a few hours of rest, the woman may return home.

DILATATION AND EVACUATION. Some second trimester abortions are performed as a dilatation and evacuation (D & E). The procedures are similar to those used in a D & C, but a larger suction tube must be used because more material must be removed. This increases the amount of cervical dilation necessary and increases the risk and discomfort of the procedure. A combination of suction and manual extraction using medical instruments is used to remove the contents of the uterus.

OTHER SURGICAL OPTIONS. Other surgical procedures are available for performing second trimester abortions, although are rarely used. These include:

• Dilatation and extraction (D & X). The cervix is prepared by means similar to those used in a dilatation and evacuation. The fetus, however, is removed mostly intact although the head must be collapsed to fit through the cervix. This procedure is sometimes called a partial-birth abortion. The D & X accounted for only 0.17% of all abortions in 2000.

• Induction. In this procedure, an abortion occurs by means of inducing labor. Prior to induction, the patient may have rods inserted into her cervix to help dilate it or receive medications to soften the cervix and speed up labor. On the day of the abortion, drugs (usually prostaglandin or a salt solution) are injected into the uterus to induce contractions. The fetus is delivered within eight to 72 hours. Side effects of this procedure include nausea, vomiting, and diarrhea from the prostaglandin, and pain from uterine contractions. Anesthesia of the sort used in childbirth can be given to reduce pain. Many women are able to go home a few hours after the procedure.

• Hysterotomy. A surgical incision is made into the uterus and the contents of the uterus removed through the incision. This procedure is generally used if induction methods fail to deliver the fetus.

Diagnosis/Preparation

The doctor must know accurately the stage of a woman's pregnancy before an abortion is performed. The doctor will ask the woman questions about her menstrual cycle and also do a **physical examination** to confirm the stage of pregnancy. This may be done at an office visit before the abortion or on the day of the abortion.

Pre-abortion counseling is important in helping a woman resolve any questions she may have about having the procedure. Some states require a waiting period (most often of 24 hours) following counseling before the abortion may be obtained. Most states require parental consent or notification if the patient is under the age of 18.

Aftercare

Regardless of the method used to perform the abortion, a woman will be observed for a period of time to make sure her blood pressure is stable and that bleeding is controlled. The doctor may prescribe **antibiotics** to reduce the chance of infection. Women who are Rh negative (lacking genetically determined antigens in their red blood cells that produce immune responses) should be given an injection of human Rh immune globulin (RhoGAM) after the procedure unless the father of the fetus is also Rh negative. This prevents blood incompatibility complications in future pregnancies.

Bleeding will continue for about five days in a surgical abortion and longer in a medical abortion. To decrease the risk of infection, a woman should avoid intercourse, tampons, and douches for two weeks after the abortion.

A follow-up visit is a necessary part of the woman's aftercare. Contraception will be offered to women who wish to avoid future pregnancies, because menstrual periods normally resume within a few weeks.

Risks

Complications from abortions can include:

- uncontrolled bleeding
- infection
- blood clots accumulating in the uterus
- a tear in the cervix or uterus
- missed abortion (the pregnancy is not terminated)
- incomplete abortion where some material from the pregnancy remains in the uterus

Women who experience any of the following symptoms of post-abortion complications should call the clinic or doctor who performed the abortion immediately:

- severe pain
- fever over 100.4°F (38.2°C)
- heavy bleeding that soaks through more than one sanitary pad per hour

---

KEY TERMS

Curette—A spoon-shaped instrument used to remove tissue from the inner lining of the uterus.

Endocarditis—An infection of the inner membrane lining of the heart.

Fibroid tumors—Non-cancerous (benign) growths in the uterus; they occur in 30–40% of women over age 40 and do not need to be removed unless they are causing symptoms that interfere with a woman's normal activities.

Lupus erythematosus—A chronic inflammatory disease in which inappropriate immune system reactions cause abnormalities in the blood vessels and connective tissue.

Prostaglandin—Responsible for various hormonal reactions such as muscle contraction.

Rh negative—Lacking the Rh factor, genetically determined antigens in red blood cells that produce immune responses. If an Rh negative woman is pregnant with an Rh positive fetus, her body will produce antibodies against the fetus's blood, causing a disease known as Rh disease. Sensitization to the disease occurs when the women's blood is exposed to the fetus's blood. Rh immune globulin (RhoGAM) is a vaccine that must be given to a woman after an abortion, miscarriage, or prenatal tests in order to prevent sensitization to Rh disease.

- foul-smelling discharge from the vagina
- continuing symptoms of pregnancy

Normal results

Usually the pregnancy is ended without complication and without altering future fertility.

Morbidity and mortality rates

Serious complications resulting from abortions performed before 13 weeks are rare. Of the 90% of women who have abortions in this time period, 2.5% have minor complications that can be handled without hospitalization. Less than 0.5% have complications that require a hospital stay. The rate of complications increases as the pregnancy progresses.

Only one maternal death occurs per 530,000 abortions performed at eight weeks gestation or less; this increases to one death per 17,000 abortions performed from 16 to 20 weeks, and one death per 6,000 abortions performed over 20 weeks.

Alternatives

Adoption is an option for pregnant women who do not want to raise a child but are unwilling or unable to have an abortion. Adoption agencies, crisis pregnancy centers, family service agencies, family planning clinics, or state social service agencies are available for women to contact for more information about the adoption process.

Resources

PERIODICALS

Centers for Disease Control and Prevention. "Abortion Surveillance—United States, 1999." *Morbidity and Mortality Weekly Report* 51 (2002): SS09.

Finer, L. B. and S. K. Henshaw. "Abortion Incidence and Services in the United States in 2000." *Perspectives on Sexual and Reproductive Health* 35 (2003): 6–15.

Jones, R. K., J. E. Darroch, and S. K. Henshaw. "Patterns in the Socioeconomic Characteristics of Women Obtaining Abortions in 2000–2001." *Perspectives on Sexual and Reproductive Health* 34 (2002): 226–35.

ORGANIZATION

Alan Guttmacher Institute. 1120 Connecticut Ave., NW, Suite 460, Washington, DC 20036. (202) 296-4012. <http://www.agi-usa.org>.

Centers for Disease Control and Prevention, Division of Reproductive Health. 4770 Buford Highway, NE, Mail Stop K-20, Atlanta, GA 30341-3717. (770) 488-5200. <http://www.prochoice.org>.

National Abortion Federation. 1755 Massachusetts Ave., NW, Suite 600, Washington, DC 20036. (202) 667-5881. <http://www.prochoice.org>.

Planned Parenthood Federation of America. 810 Seventh Ave., New York, NY 10019. (212) 541-7800. <http://www.plannedparenthood.org>.

OTHER

"Abortion After the First Trimester." *Planned Parenthood Federation of America*. July 2001 [cited February 26, 2003]. <http://www.plannedparenthood.org/library/facts/abotaft 1st_010600.html>.

"Choosing Abortion: Questions and Answers." *Planned Parenthood Federation of America*. February 2003 [cited February 26, 2003]. <http://www.plannedparenthood.org/ABORTION/chooseabort1.html>.

"Manual Vacuum Aspiration." *Reproductive Health Technologies Project*. 2002 [cited February 26, 2003]. <http://www.rhtp.org/early/early_manvac.htm>.

"Medical Abortion: Questions and Answers." *Planned Parenthood Federation of America*. June 2002 [cited February 26, 2003]. <http://www.plannedparenthood.org/abortion/medicalabortion.html>.

Roche, Natalie E. "Therapeutic Abortion." *eMedicine*. May 22, 2002 [cited February 26, 2003]. <http://www.emedicine.com/med/topic3311.htm>.

"Surgical Abortion: Questions and Answers." *Planned Parenthood Federation of America*. April 23, 2003 [cited February 26, 2003]. <http://www.plannedparenthood.org/ABORTION/surgabort1.html>.

Trupin, Suzanne R. "Abortion." *eMedicine*. December 2, 2002 [cited February 26, 2003]. <http://www.emedicine.com/med/topic5.htm>.

Debra Gordon
Stephanie Dionne Sherk

Abscess incision and drainage

Definition

An abscess is an infected skin nodule containing pus. It may need to be drained via an incision (cut) if the pus does not resolve with treatment by **antibiotics**. This allows the pus to escape, the infection to be treated, and the abscess to heal.

Purpose

An abscess is a pus-filled sore, usually caused by a bacterial infection. The pus is comprised of both living and dead organisms. It also contains destroyed tissue due to the action of white blood cells that were carried to the area to fight the infection. Abscesses are often found in the soft tissue under the skin such as the armpit or the groin. However, they may develop in any organ, and are commonly found in the breast and gums. Abscesses are far more serious and call for more specific treatment if they are located in deep organs such as the lung, liver, or brain.

Because the lining of an abscess cavity tends to interfere with the amount of drug that can penetrate the source of infection from the blood, the cavity itself may require draining. Once an abscess has fully formed, it often does not respond to antibiotics. Even if the antibiotic does penetrate into the abscess, it does not function as well in that environment.

Demographics

Abcess drainage is a minor and common surgical procedure that is often performed in a professional medical office. Accurate records concerning the number of procedures are kept in private medical office rather than hospital records. For these reasons, it is impossible to accurately tally the number of abscess incision and drainage procedures performed in a year. The procedure increases in frequency with increasing age.

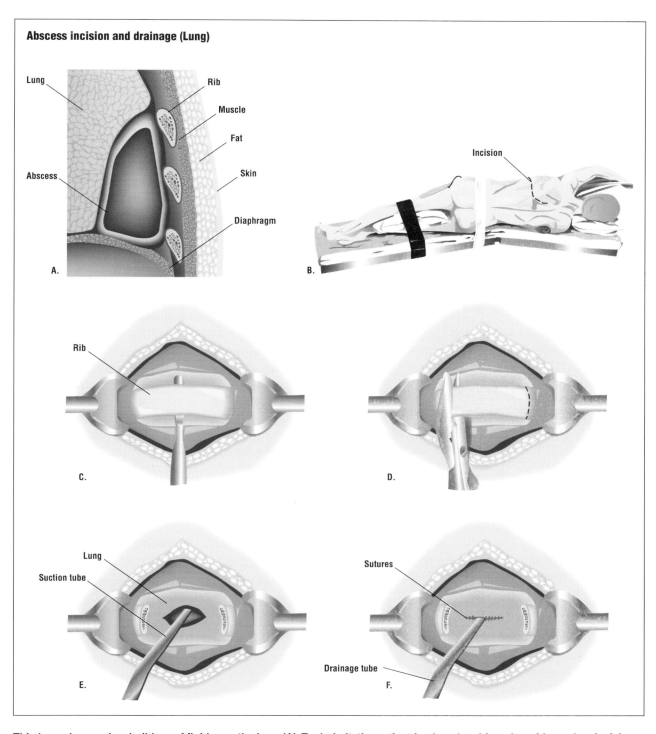

Abscess incision and drainage (Lung)

A.

Lung
Rib
Muscle
Fat
Skin
Abscess
Diaphragm

B.

Incision

C.

Rib

D.

E.

Lung
Suction tube

F.

Sutures
Drainage tube

This lung abscess is a build-up of fluid near the lung (A). To drain it, the patient is placed on his or her side, and an incision is made (B). A rib is exposed (C) and cut (D). The fluid in the abscess is suctioned (E), and the incision is closed around a temporary drainage tube (F). *(Illustration by GGS Inc.)*

Description

A doctor will cut into the lining of an abscess, allowing the pus to escape either through a drainage tube or by leaving the cavity open to the skin. The size of the incision depends on the volume of the abscess and how quickly the pus is encountered.

WHO PERFORMS THE PROCEDURE AND WHERE IS IT PERFORMED?

Abscesses are most commonly incised and drained by general surgeons. Occasionally, a family physician or dermatologist may drain a superficial abscess. These procedures may be performed in a professional office or in an outpatient facility. The skin and surrounding area may be numbed by a topical anesthetic.

Brain abscesses are usually drained by neurosurgeons. Thoracic surgeons drain abscesses in the lung. Otolaryngologists drain abscesses in the neck. These procedures are performed in a hospital **operating room.** General anesthesia is used.

QUESTIONS TO ASK THE DOCTOR

- How many abscess incision and drainage procedures has the physician performed?
- What is the physician's complication rate?

Cells normally formed for the surface of the skin often migrate into an abscess. They line the abscess cavity. This process is called epithelialization. This lining prevents drugs from reaching an abscess. It also promotes recurrence of the abscess. The lining must be removed when an abscess is drained to prevent recurrence.

Once an abscess is opened, the pus drained, and the epithelial lining removed, the doctor will clean and irrigate the wound thoroughly with saline. If it is not too large or deep, the doctor may simply pack the abscess wound with gauze for 24–48 hours to absorb the pus and discharge.

If it is a deeper abscess, the doctor or surgeon may insert a drainage tube after cleaning out the wound. Once the tube is in place, the surgeon closes the incision with simple stitches and applies a sterile dressing. Drainage is maintained for several days to help prevent the abscess from reforming. The tube is removed, and the abscess allowed to finish closing and healing.

Diagnosis/Preparation

An abscess can usually be diagnosed visually, although an imaging technique such as a computed tomography (CT) scan or ultrasound may be used to confirm the extent of the abscess before drainage. Such procedures may also be needed to localize internal abscesses such as those in the abdominal cavity or brain.

Prior to incision, the skin over an abscess will be cleansed by swabbing gently with an antiseptic solution.

Aftercare

Much of the pain around an abscess will be gone after the surgery. Healing is usually very rapid. After the

drainage tube is removed, antibiotics may be continued for several days. Applying heat and keeping the affected area elevated may help relieve inflammation.

Risks

Any scarring is likely to become much less noticeable as time goes on, and eventually become almost invisible. Occasionally, an abscess within a vital organ (such as the brain) damages enough surrounding tissue that there is some permanent loss of normal function.

Other risks include incomplete drainage and prolonged infection. Occasionally, an abscess may require a second incision and drainage procedure. This is frequently due to retained epithelial cells that line the abscess cavity.

Normal results

Most abscesses heal after drainage alone. Others may require more prolonged drainage and antibiotic drug treatment.

Morbidity and mortality rates

Morbidity associated with an abscess incision and drainage is very uncommon. Post-surgical problems are usually associated with infection or an adverse reaction to antibiotic drugs prescribed. Mortality is virtually unknown.

Alternatives

There is no reliable alternative to surgical incision and drainage of an abscess. Heat alone may cause small superficial abscesses to resolve. The degree of epithelialization usually determines if the abscess reappears.

See also Incision care; Wound care.

Resources

BOOKS

Bland, K. I., W. G. Cioffi, and M. G. Sarr. *Practice of General Surgery.* Philadelphia: Saunders, 2001.

KEY TERMS

White blood cells—Cells that protect the body against infection.

Braunwald, E., Longo, D. L., and J. L. Jameson. *Harrison's Principles of Internal Medicine, 15th Edition.* New York: McGraw-Hill, 2001.

Goldman, L., and J. C. Bennett. *Cecil Textbook of Medicine, 21st Edition.* Philadelphia: Saunders, 1999.

Schwartz, S. I., J. E. Fischer, F. C. Spencer, G. T. Shires, and J. M. Daly. *Principles of Surgery, 7th Edition.* New York: McGraw Hill, 1998.

Townsend, C., K. L. Mattox, R. D. Beauchamp, B. M. Evers, and D. C. Sabiston. *Sabiston's Review of Surgery, 3rd Edition.* Philadelphia: Saunders, 2001.

PERIODICALS

Cmejrek, R. C., J. M. Coticchia, and J. E. Arnold. "Presentation, Diagnosis, and Management of Deep-neck Abscesses in Infants." *Archives of Otolaryngology Head and Neck Surgery,* 128(12) 2002: 1361–1364.

Douglass, A. B., and J. M. Douglass. "Common Dental Emergencies." *American Family Physician,* 67(3) 2003: 511–516.

Usdan, L. S., and C. Massinople. "Multiple Pyogenic Liver Abscesses Associated with Occult Appendicitis and Possible Crohn's Disease." *Tennessee Medicine,* 95(11) 2002: 463–464.

Wang, L. F., W. R. Kuo, C. S. Lin, K. W. Lee, and K. J. Huang. "Space Infection of the Head and Neck." *Kaohsiung Journal of Medical Sciences,* 18(8) 2002: 386–392.

ORGANIZATIONS

American Academy of Otolaryngology-Head and Neck Surgery. One Prince St., Alexandria, VA 22314-3357. (703) 836-4444. <http://www.entnet.org/index2.cfm>.

American College of Surgeons. 633 North St. Clair Street, Chicago, IL 60611-32311. (312) 202-5000; Fax: (312) 202-5001. Web site: <http://www.facs.org>. E-mail: <postmaster@facs.org>.

American Medical Association. 515 N. State Street, Chicago, IL 60610. (312) 464-5000. <http://www.ama-assn.org>.

American Osteopathic College of Otolaryngology-Head and Neck Surgery. 405 W. Grand Avenue, Dayton, OH 45405. (937) 222-8820 or (800) 455-9404; Fax (937) 222-8840. Email: info@aocoohns.org.

American Society of Colon and Rectal Surgeons. 85 W. Algonquin Rd., Suite 550, Arlington Heights, IL 60005. (847) 290-9184; Fax: (847) 290-9203. <http://www. fascrs.org>. Email: ascrs@fascrs.org.

OTHER

American Society of Colon and Rectal Surgeons, (April 4, 2003). <http://www.fascrs.org/brochures/anal-abscess. html>.

Merck Manual, (April 5, 2003). <http://www.merck.com/pubs/ mmanual/section6/chapter74/74a.htm>.

National Library of Medicine, (April 4, 2003). <http://www. nlm.nih.gov/medlineplus/ency/article/001353.htm>.

Oregon Health and Science University, (April 4, 2003). <http:// www.ohsu.edu/cliniweb/C1/C1.539.830.25.html>.

Vanderbilt University Medical Center, (April 4, 2003). <http:// www.mc.vanderbilt.edu/peds/pidl/neuro/brainabs.htm>.

L. Fleming Fallon, Jr, MD, DrPH

Acetaminophen

Definition

Acetaminophen is a medicine used to relieve pain and reduce fever.

Purpose

Acetaminophen is used to relieve many kinds of minor aches and pains, including headaches, muscle aches, backaches, toothaches, menstrual cramps, arthritis, and the aches and pains that often accompany colds. It is suitable for control of pain following minor surgery, or for **post-surgical pain** after the need for stronger pain relievers has been reduced. Acetaminophen is also used in combination with narcotic **analgesics** both to increase pain relief and reduce the risk that the narcotics will be abused.

Description

This drug is available without a prescription. Acetaminophen (APAP) is sold under various brand names, including Tylenol, Panadol, Aspirin-Free Anacin, and Bayer Select Maximum Strength Headache Pain Relief Formula. Many multi-symptom cold, flu, and sinus medicines also contain acetaminophen. Persons are advised to check the ingredients listed on the container to see if acetaminophen is included in the product.

Acetaminophen is also included in some prescription-only combinations. These usually contain a narcotic in addition to acetaminophen; it is combined with oxycodone in Percocet, and is included in Tylenol with Codeine.

Studies have shown that acetaminophen relieves pain and reduces fever about as well as **aspirin**. But differences between these two common drugs exist. Acetaminophen is less likely than aspirin to irritate the stomach. However, unlike aspirin, acetaminophen does not reduce the redness, stiffness, or swelling that accompany arthritis.

Recommended dosage

The usual dosage for adults and children age 12 and over is 325–650 mg every four to six hours as needed. No more than 4 g (4,000 mg) should be taken in 24 hours. Because the drug can potentially harm the liver, people who drink alcohol in large quantities should take considerably less acetaminophen and possibly should avoid the drug completely.

For children ages six to 11 years, the usual dose is 150–300 mg, three to four times a day. People are advised to check with a physician for dosages for children under six years of age.

Precautions

A person should never take more than the recommended dosage of acetaminophen unless told to do so by a physician or dentist.

Because acetaminophen is included in both prescription and non-prescription combinations, it is important to check the total amount of acetaminophen taken each day from all sources in order to avoid taking more than the recommended maximum dose.

Patients should not use acetaminophen for more than 10 days to relieve pain (five days for children) or for more than three days to reduce fever, unless directed to do so by a physician. If symptoms do not go away, or if they get worse, the patient should contact a physician. Anyone who drinks three or more alcoholic beverages a day should check with a physician before using this drug and should never take more than the recommended dosage. People who already have kidney or liver disease or liver infections should also consult with a physician before using the drug. Women who are pregnant or breastfeeding should also consult with a physician before using acetaminophen.

Smoking cigarettes may interfere with the effectiveness of acetaminophen. Smokers may need to take higher doses of the medicine, but should not take more than the recommended daily dosage unless told to do so by a physician.

Many drugs can interact with one another. People should consult a physician or pharmacist before combining acetaminophen with any other medicine, and they should not use two different acetaminophen-containing products at the same time, unless instructed by a physician or dentist.

Some products, such as Nyquil, contain acetaminophen in combination with alcohol. While these products are safe for people who do not drink alcoholic beverages, people who consume alcoholic drinks regu-larly, even in moderation, should use extra care before using acetaminophen-alcohol combinations.

Acetaminophen interferes with the results of some medical tests. Before having medical tests done, a person should check to see whether taking acetaminophen would affect the results. Avoiding the drug for a few days before the tests may be necessary.

Side effects

Acetaminophen causes few side effects. The most common one is lightheadedness. Some people may experience trembling and pain in the side or the lower back. Allergic reactions do occur in some people, but they are rare. Anyone who develops symptoms such as rash, swelling, or difficulty breathing after taking acetaminophen should stop taking the drug and get immediate medical attention. Other rare side effects include yellow skin or eyes, unusual bleeding or bruising, weakness, fatigue, bloody or black stools, bloody or cloudy urine, and a sudden decrease in the amount of urine.

Overdoses of acetaminophen may cause nausea, vomiting, sweating, and exhaustion. Very large overdoses can cause liver damage. In case of an overdose, a person is advised to get immediate medical attention.

Interactions

Acetaminophen may interact with a variety of other medicines. When this happens, the effects of one or both of the drugs may change or the risk of side effects may be greater. Among the drugs that may interact with acetaminophen are alcohol, non-steroidal anti-inflammatory drugs (NSAIDs) such as Motrin, oral contraceptives, the anti-seizure drug phenytoin (Dilantin), the blood-thinning drug warfarin (Coumadin), the cholesterol-lowering drug cholestyramine (Questran), the antibiotic Isoniazid, and zidovudine (Retrovir, AZT). People should check with a physician or pharmacist before combining acetaminophen with any other prescription or nonprescription (over-the-counter) medicine.

Resources

BOOKS

Brody, T.M., J. Larner, K.P. Minneman, and H.C. Neu. *Human Pharmacology: Molecular to Clinical, 2nd ed.* St. Louis: Mosby Year-Book, 1998.

Griffith, H.W., and S. Moore. *2001 Complete Guide to Prescription and Nonprescription Drugs.* New York: Berkely Publishing Group, 2001.

OTHER

"Acetaminophen." Federal Drug Administration. Center for Drug Evaluation and Research. [cited May 2003] <http://

KEY TERMS

Arthritis—Inflammation of the joints; the condition causes pain and swelling.

Fatigue—Physical or mental weariness.

Inflammation—A response to irritation, infection, or injury, resulting in pain, redness, and swelling.

www.fda.gov/cder/foi/nda/2000/75077_Acetaminophen. pdf>.

"Acetaminophen." Medline Plus Drug Information. [cited May 2003] <http://www.nlm.nih.gov/medlineplus/druginfo/ medmaster/a681004.html>.

"Acetaminophen, Systemic." Medline Plus Drug Information. [cited May 2003] <http://www.nlm.nih.gov/medlineplus/ druginfo/uspdi/202001.html>.

Nancy Ross-Flanigan
Sam Uretsky

Acid reducers *see* **Gastric acid inhibitors**

Adenoidectomy

Definition

An adenoidectomy is the surgical removal of the adenoids—small lumps of tissue that lie in the back of the throat behind the nose.

Purpose

The adenoids are removed if they block breathing through the nose and if they cause chronic earaches or deafness. The adenoids consist of lymphoid tissue—white blood cells from the immune system. They are located near the tonsils, two other lumps of similar lymphoid tissue. In childhood, adenoids and tonsils are believed to play a role in fighting infections by producing antibodies that attack bacteria entering the body through the mouth and nose. In adulthood however, it is unlikely that the adenoids are involved in maintaining health, and they normally shrink and disappear. Between the ages of two and six, the adenoids can become chronically infected, swelling up and becoming inflamed. This can cause breathing difficulties, especially during sleep. The swelling can also block the eustachian tubes that connect the back of the throat to the ears, leading to hearing problems until the blockage is relieved. The purpose of an adenoidectomy is thus to remove infected adenoids. Since they are often associated with infected tonsils, they are often removed as part of a combined operation that also removes the tonsils, called a T&A (**tonsillectomy and adenoidectomy**).

Demographics

Demographics information is difficult to provide because adenoidectomy is routinely performed in an outpatient setting, for which demographic data are not well recorded. Good information is available from the 1970s and 1980s when the surgery was performed in an inpatient setting. In the United States in 1971, more than one million combined T&As, tonsillectomies alone, or adenoidectomies alone were performed, with 50,000 of these procedures consisting of adenoidectomy alone. In 1987, 250,000 combined or single procedures were performed, with 15,000 consisting of adenoidectomy alone. Now, almost all adenoidectomies are performed on an outpatient basis unless other medical problems require hospital admission or an overnight stay. T&A is considered the most common major surgical procedure in the United States.

Description

An adenoidectomy is performed under general anesthesia. The surgeon removes the adenoids from behind the palate. Stitches are usually not required.

Excision through the mouth

The adenoids are most commonly removed through the mouth after placing an instrument to open the mouth and retract the palate. A mirror is used to see the adenoids behind the nasal cavity. Several instruments can then be used to remove the adenoids.

• Curette removal. The most common method of removal is using the adenoid curette, an instrument that has a sharp edge in a perpendicular position to its long handle. Various sizes of curettes are available.

• Adenoid punch instrument. An adenoid punch is a curved instrument with a chamber that is placed over the adenoids. The chamber has a knife blade sliding-door to section off the adenoids that are then housed in the chamber and removed with the instrument.

• Magill forceps. A Magill forceps is a curved instrument used to remove residual adenoid, usually located deeper in the posterior nasal cavity, after attempted removal with curettes or adenoid punches.

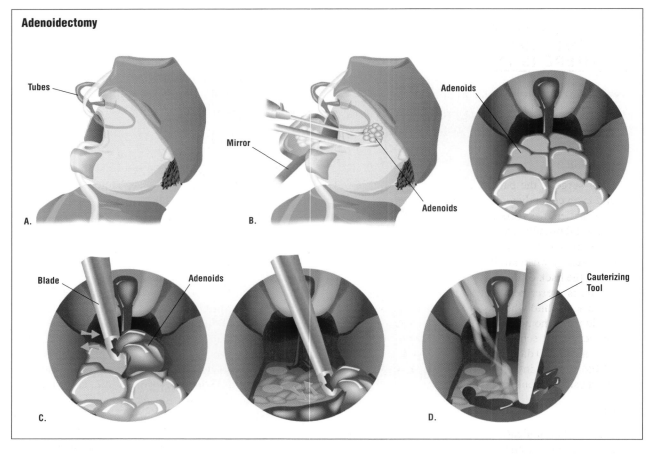

Adenoidectomy

A.

B.

Tubes

Mirror

Adenoids

Adenoids

Blade

Adenoids

Cauterizing Tool

C.

D.

Patient's mouth is held open with tubes (A). A mirror is used to visualize the adenoids during the procedure (B). The adenoids are removed with a side-to-side or front-to-back motion (C). Bleeding is controlled with a cauterizing tool (D). *(Illustration by GGS Inc.)*

• Electrocautery with a suction Bovie. The adenoids can also be removed by electrocautery with a suction Bovie, an instrument with a hollow center to suction blood and a rim of metal to achieve coagulation.

• Laser. The Nd:YAG laser has also been used to remove the adenoids. However, this technique has caused scarring of tissue and is usually avoided.

Excision through the nose

Adenoids may also be removed through the nasal cavity with a surgical suction instrument called a microdebrider. With this procedure, bleeding is controlled either with packing or suction cautery.

Diagnosis/Preparation

The primary methods used to determine whether adenoids need removal are:

• medical history

• physical examination

• throat bacterial cultures

• x rays

• blood tests

When the patient arrives at the hospital or the day-surgery unit, a nurse or a doctor will ask questions concerning the patient's general health to make sure he or she is fit to undergo surgery. They will also check that the patient has not had anything to eat or drink and will record pulse and blood pressure. The doctor or nurse must be informed if the patient has had any allergic or unusual reactions to drugs in the past. The patient will be asked to put on a hospital gown and to remove any loose orthodontic braces, false teeth, and jewelry. In the past, an adenoidectomy usually called for an overnight stay in hospital. However, it is increasingly more common to have this operation on an outpatient basis, meaning that the patient goes home on the same day. The surgery is usually performed early in the morning to allow a sufficient observation period after the operation.

Aftercare

After surgery, the patient wakes up in the recovery area and is given medication to reduce swelling and pain. When the patient has recovered from surgery, he or she is sent home and usually given a week's course of **antibiotics** to be taken by mouth. The patient may also develop a sore throat, especially when swallowing or speaking, or moderate pain at the back of the nose and throat, for which pain medication is prescribed. Normally, the pain goes away after a week. A child who has undergone an adenoidectomy should rest at home for at least one week to avoid possible infections at school. Swimming should not be allowed for at least 10 days after the operation. If there is any sign of bleeding or infection (fever, increased pain), the treating physician should be immediately contacted.

Risks

Risks and complications include those generally associated with surgery and anesthesia. Very few complications are known to occur after this operation, except, very rarely, bleeding (which occurs in 0.4% of cases). Bleeding is more a concern with a very young child because he or she often will not notice. For this reason, a child is always kept in observation at the hospital or clinic for a few hours after the operation. If bleeding does occur, the surgeon may insert a pack of gauze into the nose to stop the blood flow for subsequent removal after a day or two. The other possible complications are those associated with any operation, including infection of the operated area, which may result in light bleeding, increased pain, and fever. Infection is usually treated with antibiotics and bed rest.

Normal results

Adenoidectomy is an operation that has very good outcomes, and patients are expected to make a full and quick recovery once the initial pain has subsided. Adenoid tissue rarely regrows, but some instances have been reported. The exact mechanism is unknown but may be related to incomplete removal.

Alternatives

There is no good evidence supporting any curative non-surgical therapy for chronic infection of the adenoid.

Antibiotics have been used for as long as six weeks in lymphoid tissue infection, but with failure to eradicate the bacteria. With reported incidences of drug-resistant bacteria, use of long-term antibiotics is not a recommended alternative to surgical removal of infected adenoids.

Some studies indicate some benefit from using topical nasal steroids. Studies show that while using the medication, the adenoids may shrink up to 10% and help relieve nasal blockage. However, once the steroid medication is stopped, the adenoids can again enlarge and continue to cause symptoms. In a child with nasal obstructive symptoms, a trial of topical nasal steroid spray and saline spray may be attempted for controlling symptoms.

Resources

BOOKS

Bluestone, C. D. *Pediatric otolaryngology* Philadelphia: Saunders, 2003.

Lee, K. J. *Essential otolaryngology: head and neck surgery.* New York: McGraw-Hill Medical Pub. Division, 2003.

Markel, H. and F. A. Oski. *The Practical Pediatrician: The A to Z Guide to Your Child's Health, Behavior, and Safety.* New York: W. H. Freeman and Co., 1995.

PERIODICALS

Felder-Puig, R., A. Maksys, C. Noestlinger, et al. "Using a children's book to prepare children and parents for elective ENT surgery: results of a randomized clinical trial." *International Journal of Pediatrics and Otorhinolaryngology* 67 (January 2003): 35–41.

Homer, J. J., J. Swallow, and P. Semple. " Audit of pain management at home following tonsillectomy in children." *Journal of Laryngology and Otology* 115 (March 2001): 205–208.

Kokki, H. and R. Ahonen. "Pain and activity disturbance after paediatric day case adenoidectomy." *Paediatric Anaesthesiology* 7 (1997): 227–231.

KEY TERMS

Adenoids—Small lumps of lymphoid tissue near the tonsils on the walls of the upper throat behind the nose.

Anesthesia—A combination of drugs administered by a variety of techniques by trained professionals that provide sedation, amnesia, analgesia, and immobility adequate for the accomplishment of the surgical procedure with minimal discomfort, and without injury, to the patient.

Antibodies—Proteins that are produced normally by specialized white blood cells after stimulation by a foreign substance (antigen) and that act specifically against the antigen in an immune response.

Electrocautery—The cauterization of tissue using electric current to generate heat.

Immune system—Mechanism that protects the body from foreign substances, cells and pathogens by producing the immune response, a concerted defense involving the thymus, spleen, lymph nodes, white blood cells including the B cells and T cells, and antibodies.

Lymphoid tissue—Tissue that contains white blood cells of the immune system.

Tonsillectomy—Surgical removal of the tonsils.

Tonsils—Two lumps of lymphoid tissue located on either side of the back of the throat.

Kvaerner, K. J., P. Nafstad, and J. J. Jaakkola. "Otolaryngological surgery and upper respiratory tract infections in children: an epidemiological study." *Annals of Otology, Rhinology and Laryngology* 111 (November 2002): 1034–1039.

McClay, J. E. "Resistant bacteria in the adenoids: a preliminary report." *Archives of Otolaryngology: Head and Neck Surgery* 123 (May 2000): 625–629.

ORGANIZATIONS

American Academy of Otolaryngology - Head and Neck Surgery. One Prince Street, Alexandria, VA 22314. (703) 806-4444. <http://www.entnet.org>.

American College of Surgeons. 633 N. Saint Claire St., Chicago, IL 60611. (312) 202-5000. <http://www.faacs.org>.

OTHER

American College of Surgeons. "Tonsillectomy and Adenoidectomy." February 21, 2003 [cited April 23, 2003]. <http://www.facs.org/public_info/operation/aboutbroch. html>.

BUPA. "Adenoidectomy." [cited April 23, 2003]. <http://www. bupa.com>.

Texas Pediatric Surgical Associates. "Adenoids and Adenoidectomy." [cited April 23, 2003]. < http://www.pedisurg.com/ PtEducENT/adenoids.htm>.

Monique Laberge, Ph.D.

Admission to the hospital

Definition

Hospital admission involves staying at a hospital for at least one night or more.

Purpose

Staying in the hospital overnight is done because the individual is too sick to stay at home, requires 24-hour nursing care, and/or is receiving medications and undergoing tests and/or surgery that can only be performed in the hospital setting.

Description

An individual may be admitted to the hospital for a positive experience, such as having a baby, or because they are undergoing an **elective surgery** or procedure, or because they are being admitted through the emergency department. Being admitted through the emergency department is the most stressful of these circumstances because the event is unexpected and may be a major life crisis.

Before the person is taken to their room, admitting procedures are performed. The person's personal data is recorded and entered into the hospital's computer system. This data may include:

- name
- address
- home and work telephone number
- date of birth
- place of employment
- occupation
- emergency contact information, or the names and telephone numbers of those individuals the hospital should contact if the person being admitted needs emergency care or their condition worsens significantly
- insurance coverage
- reason for hospitalization
- allergies to medications or foods
- religious preference, including whether or not one wishes a clergy member to visit

There may be several forms to fill out. One form may be a detailed medical and medication history. This history will include past hospitalizations and surgeries. Having this information readily available will make the process move faster, and can allow a family member or friend who is accompanying the person to help fill out the forms more easily. The hospital may ask if there are any advance directives. This refers to forms that have been filled out indicating what medical decisions one wants others to make on their behalf. One form is called a **living will** and clearly tells which specific resuscitation efforts the person does or does not want to have performed on them in order to save or extend their life. Another form may be a durable power to attorney. This is a form stating whom the patient wishes to make medical decisions for them if they themselves are unable to do so, such as if they are in a coma. Some hospitals have blank forms that the individual can use to make these designations, others may just ask if the forms have been filled out, and if so to add a copy of them into the person's medical record. They are considered legally binding, and an attorney can assist in filling them out. During the time spent in admitting, a plastic bracelet will be placed on the person's wrist with their name, age, date of birth, room number, and medical record number on it. A separate bracelet is added that lists allergies. Forms are completed and signed, so that the patient is giving full consent to have the hospital personnel take care of them while they are in the hospital during that particular hospital stay. Subsequent hospital stays require new consent forms.

Once all the admitting information has been completed, the next step is usually being taken to one's room. Most people stay in a semi-private room, which means that there are two people to a room. In some circumstances, a person's medical condition may require staying in a private room. If there are private rooms available, and the individual is willing to pay the extra cost (insurance companies generally only cover the cost of a semi-private room), it may be possible to have a private room. Most hospital rooms are set up so that one bed is closer to the door, and the other is next to a window. There are curtains that can be drawn completely around the bed so that some degree of privacy is possible. Once taken to a room, the nurse taking care of the patient will go over the medical and medication history, and orient the person to the room. This means that they will explain how to adjust bed height, how to use the nurse call button, show where the bathroom is located, and explain how to use the bedside telephone and television. The cost for the telephone and television are not usually covered by insurance. There is usually a calendar in the room, to help the patient keep track of the date, as it can be disorienting to be in an unfamiliar place, especially

over several days or weeks. There may be limitations on using the bathroom, if the person's doctor feels that the patient's condition is such that they should not get out of bed. These kinds of decisions are made with the person's safety and medical condition in mind. If the person is not thinking clearly, perhaps because of some medication they are receiving, the side rails of the bed may be put up, to prevent falling out of bed. The nurse will review the doctor's orders, such as what tests have been scheduled, whether or not they can get out of bed for the bathroom or to walk around the unit, what medications they will be getting, and whether or not there are restrictions on what they can eat. The hospital will supply towels, sheets, and blankets, but some people like to bring something personal with them from home. Because of the risk of infections being transferred from one patient to another, one may prefer to leave things at home. If one does choose to bring in something personal, it should be washed with warm or hot water and soap to make sure that germs are not brought home from the hospital.

Sometimes when people are admitted to the hospital they need extremely close observation that can only be given in specialized care called an **intensive care unit**. Because of the severity of their condition, visiting hours are more restricted than in the regular rooms. It may be that only one or two people can visit at a time, and only for a few minutes at a time. Once the person's condition improves, they may then be transferred to a room with a less rigid visitation policy. If an individual has a surgical procedure performed, they will spend a few hours in a recovery area. This is to make sure that the person's condition is stable before returning to the regular room. Visiting is limited in the recovery area, and the person may spend most of the time sleeping, as the effects of the surgical anesthesia wear off.

If the person entering the hospital is a child, the parents or guardian will fill out the hospital forms. Most hospitals allow parents and guardians to stay overnight in the hospital with the child, and to be with them 24 hours a day. Many hospitals have special areas for children to play in, and even areas in which they do not have anything done to them which is painful, so they can completely relax.

Preparation

If the hospitalization is prearranged, there are preparations that will make the process go more smoothly. It is helpful to have a list of all medications currently being taken, the dosages, how often they are taken, and the reason for taking them. The list should also include any allergies to food and medications, including a description of the reaction, and when the food or medication was last

KEY TERMS

C-PAP machine—A continuous positive airway pressure machine used at night to alleviate sleep apnea. A mask is placed over the nose and room air is blown into the patient's airway, keeping the airway from collapsing, and alleviating snoring and periods of stopping breathing during the night.

Elective surgery—Elective surgery is surgery that is planned and anticipated. For example, a person may have a medical condition that requires surgery to fix an ongoing problem. Their condition may have developed over weeks or months, and through discussion with their doctor they come to agree that the time is now best for taking care of this condition. The surgery is scheduled, and the person has advanced notice that they will be spending some time in the hospital.

taken. The list should include over-the-counter (OTC) and prescription medications, vitamins, supplements, and herbal and home remedies.

If the hospital stay involves surgery in which there is the potential for significant blood loss, it may be possible to arrange to have blood drawn and stored so that in the event of a **transfusion**, the individual receives his or her own blood.

If the hospital stay is an extended one, a list of family and friends, with their telephone numbers, can make it easier to stay in touch with people who can come and visit, or offer support by telephone. It is not a good idea to bring anything of value to the hospital as there are many times when one could be out of the room. However, it may be helpful to have some pocket change available if one needs to make some small purchases at the hospital gift shop, such as a newspaper. If one is going to visit someone in the hospital, change or one dollar bills to use at vending machines may come in handy.

A small bag can be brought into the hospital that contains:

- night clothes (The hospital supplies their own, but some people like to wear familiar clothing; some people use the hospital outfits to decrease the chance of staining their own clothing or bringing germs home from the hospital.)
- a robe
- slippers
- clothes for the return trip home

- reading material for the hospital stay
- hobby materials such as knitting or a book of crossword puzzles
- reading glasses
- personal care items such as comb, brush, and toothbrush (most hospitals supply these items, but many individuals prefer to have their own from home)

It is best not to bring in any medication from home unless it has been prearranged with the physician and hospital staff prior to hospitalization. This is to prevent an error from occurring by having the person taking one dose from their own medicine and then being given another dose from the hospital pharmacy.

Resources

BOOKS

Perry, Anne Griffin. *Clinical Nursing Skills and Techniques.* Mosby, 1998.

ORGANIZATIONS

American Hospital Association. One North Franklin, Chicago, IL 60606. (312) 422-3000. <http://www.aha.org>.
Nemours Center for Children's Health Media. <http://kids health.org>.

Esther Csapo Rastegari, R.N., B.S.N., Ed.M.

Adrenal gland removal *see* **Adrenalectomy**

Adrenalectomy

Definition

Adrenalectomy is the surgical removal of one or both adrenal glands. The adrenal glands are paired endocrine glands—one located above each kidney—that produce hormones such as epinephrine, norepinephrine, androgens, estrogens, aldosterone, and cortisol. Adrenalectomy is usually performed by conventional (open) surgery; however, in selected patients, surgeons may use **laparoscopy**. With laparoscopy, adrenalectomy can be accomplished through four very small incisions.

Purpose

Adrenalectomy is usually advised for patients with tumors of the adrenal glands. Adrenal gland tumors may be malignant or benign, but all typically excrete excessive amounts of one or more hormones. When malignant, they

Adrenalectomy

A.

B.
Right adrenal gland
Left adrenal gland
Right kidney
Left kidney
Inferior vena cava
Aorta
Incision

C.
Duodenum
Vena cava
Tumor
Adrenal gland
Renal vein

D.
Adrenal vein
Vena cava
Adrenal gland
Renal vein

E.
Liver
Adrenal gland
Kidney

To remove the adrenal glands, an incision is made below the patient's ribcage (A). The adrenal gland, which sits on top of the kidney (B), is visualized (C). The vein emerging from the gland is tied off and cut (D), and the adrenal gland is removed (E). *(Illustration by GGS Inc.)*

are usually neuroblastoma cancers. A successful procedure will aid in correcting hormone imbalances, and may also remove cancerous tumors before they invade other parts of the body. Occasionally, adrenalectomy may be recommended when hormones produced by the adrenal glands aggravate another condition such as breast cancer.

Demographics

Neuroblastoma is one of the few cancer types known to secrete hormones. It occurs most often in children, and it is the third most common cancer that occurs in children. In the united States, approximately 7.5% of the childhood cancers diagnosed in 2001 were neuroblastomas, affecting one in 80,000 to 100,000 children. Close to 50% of cases of neuroblastoma occur in children younger than two years old. The disease is sometimes present at birth, but is usually not noticed until later. Approximately one-third of neuroblastomas start in the adrenal glands. According to some reports, African-American children develop the disease at a slightly higher rate than Caucasian children (8.7 per million compared to 8.0 per million cases diagnosed).

Description

Open adrenalectomy

The surgeon may operate from any of four directions, depending on the exact problem and the patient's body type.

In the anterior approach, the surgeon cuts into the abdominal wall. Usually the incision will be horizontal, just under the rib cage. If the surgeon intends to operate on only one of the adrenal glands, the incision will run under just the right or the left side of the rib cage. Sometimes a vertical incision in the middle of the abdomen provides a better approach, especially if both adrenal glands are involved.

In the posterior approach, the surgeon cuts into the back, just beneath the rib cage. If both glands are to be removed, an incision is made on each side of the body. This approach is the most direct route to the adrenal glands, but it does not provide quite as clear a view of the surrounding structures as the anterior approach.

In the flank approach, the surgeon cuts into the patient's side. This is particularly useful in massively obese patients. If both glands need to be removed, the surgeon must remove one gland, repair the surgical wound, turn the patient onto the other side, and repeat the entire process.

The last approach involves an incision into the chest cavity, either with or without part of the incision into the abdominal cavity. It is used when the surgeon anticipates a very large tumor, or if the surgeon needs to examine or remove nearby structures as well.

Laparoscopic adrenalectomy

This technique does not require the surgeon to open the body cavity. Instead, four small incisions (about 0.5 in [1.27 cm] diameter each) are made into a patient's flank, just under the rib cage. A laparoscope enabling the surgeon to visualize the inside of the abdominal cavity on a television monitor is placed through one of the incisions. The other incisions are for tubes that carry miniaturized versions of surgical tools. These tools are designed to be operated by manipulations that the surgeon makes outside the body.

Diagnosis/Preparation

Most aspects of preparation are the same as in other major operations. In addition, hormone imbalances are often a major challenge. Whenever possible, physicians will try to correct hormone imbalances through medication in the days or weeks before surgery. Adrenal tumors may cause other problems such as hypertension or inadequate potassium in the blood, and these problems also should be resolved if possible before surgery is performed. Therefore, a patient may take specific medicines for days or weeks before surgery.

Most adrenal tumors can be imaged very well with a CT scan or MRI, and benign tumors tend to look different on these tests than do cancerous tumors. Surgeons may order a CT scan, MRI, or scintigraphy (viewing of the location of a tiny amount of radioactive agent) to help locate exactly where the tumor is located.

The day before surgery, patients will probably have an enema to clear the bowels. In patients with lung problems or clotting problems, physicians may advise special preparations.

Aftercare

Patients stay in the hospital for various lengths of time after adrenalectomy. The longest hospital stays are required for open surgery using an anterior approach; hospital stays of about three days are indicated for open surgery using the posterior approach or for laparoscopic adrenalectomy.

The special concern after adrenalectomy is the patient's hormone balance. There may be several sets of required lab tests to define hormone problems and monitor the results of drug treatment. In addition, blood pressure problems and infections are more common after removal of certain types of adrenal tumors.

As with most open surgery, surgeons are also concerned about blood clots forming in the legs and traveling to the lungs (venous thromboembolism), bowel problems, and postoperative pain. With laparoscopic adrenalectomy, these problems are somewhat less prevalent, but they are still present.

Risks

The risks of adrenalectomy include major hormone imbalances, caused by the underlying disease, the surgery, or both. These can include problems with healing, blood pressure fluctuations, and other metabolic problems.

Other risks are typical of many operations. These include:

- bleeding
- damage to adjacent organs (spleen, pancreas)
- loss of bowel function
- blood clots in the lungs
- lung problems
- surgical infections
- pain
- scarring

Normal results

The outcome of an adrenalectomy depends on the condition for which it was performed. For example, in the case of hyperaldosteronism, the surgical removal of the adrenal glands provides excellent results, with the

QUESTIONS TO ASK THE DOCTOR

- What procedure do you intend to use for my adrenalectomy?
- What do I need to know about my adrenalectomy?
- How long is the procedure?
- How long will it take to recover from the surgery?
- What are the major risks of the surgery?
- Why must my adrenal gland(s) be removed?
- What restrictions can I expect on my physical activity after the surgery?
- How many adrenalectomies do you perform each year?

majority of patients being cured. In the case of patients diagnosed with pheochromocytoma, long-term cures are rare in cases of malignant pheochromocytomas. In cases of metastatic disease, five-year survival rates as high as 36% have been reported.

Morbidity and mortality rates

There is wide agreement that laparoscopic approaches decrease operative morbidity. The laparoscopic approach is commonly used to treat smaller adrenal tumors. At many laparoscopic centers, the laparoscopic adrenalectomy has become the standard practice. Several centers recommend a particular approach or laparoscopic method, but regardless of which approach is preferred, the cure and morbidity rates are similar for laparoscopic and open adrenalectomy (in the case of small tumors). No method is suitable for all patients. In general, selecting the approach based on patient and tumor characteristics while considering the familiarity of the surgeon yields the best results.

Alternatives

Alternatives to adrenalectomy depend on the medical condition underlying the decision to perform the surgery. In some cases, drug therapy may be considered as an alternative when the condition being treated in benign.

Resources

BOOKS

Bradley, Edward L., III. *The Patient's Guide to Surgery.* Philadelphia: University of Pennsylvania Press, 1994.

KEY TERMS

Hyperaldosteronism—A disorder of excessive aldosterone secretion.

Laparoscope—An instrument that enables the surgeon to see inside the abdominal cavity by means of a thin tube that carries an image to a television monitor.

Pancreas—An organ that secretes a number of digestive hormones and also secretes insulin to regulate blood sugar.

Pheochromocytoma—A tumor of specialized cells of the adrenal gland.

Spleen—An organ that traps and breaks down red blood cells at the end of their useful life and manufactures some key substances used by the immune system.

Vena cava—The large vein that drains directly into the heart after gathering incoming blood from the entire body.

Fauci, Anthony S., et al., ed. *Harrison's Principles of Internal Medicine.* New York: McGraw-Hill, 1997.

Little, M., and D. C. Garrell. *The Endocrine System: The Healthy Body.* New York: Chelsea House, 1990.

PERIODICALS

Del Pizzo, J. J. "Transabdominal laparoscopic adrenalectomy." *Current Urology Reports* 4 (February 2003): 81–86.

Desai, M. M., I. S. Gill, J. H. Kaouk, S. F. Matin, G. T. Sung, and E. L. Bravo. "Robotic-assisted laparoscopic adrenalectomy." *Urology* 60 (December 2002): 1104–1107.

Hawn, M. T., D. Cook, C. Deveney, and B. C. Sheppard. "Quality of life after laparoscopic bilateral adrenalectomy for Cushing's disease." *Surgery* 132 (December 2002): 1068–1069.

Ikeda, Y., H. Takami, G. Tajima, Y. Sasaki, J. Takayama, H. Kurihara, M. Niimi. "Laparoscopic partial adrenalectomy." *Biomedical Pharmacotherapy* 56 (2002) suppl.1: 126s–131s.

Martinez, D. G. "Adrenalectomy for primary aldosteronism." *Annals of Internal Medicine* 138 (January 2003): 157–159.

Munver, R., J. J. Del Pizzo, and R. E. Sosa. "Adrenal-preserving Minimally Invasive Surgery: The Role of Laparoscopic Partial Adrenalectomy, Cryosurgery, and Radiofrequency Ablation of the Adrenal Gland." *Current Urology Reports* 4 (February 2003): 87–92.

ORGANIZATIONS

American Association of Clinical Endoctrinologists. 1000 Riverside Ave., Suite 205, Jacksonville, FL 32204. (904) 353-7878. <http://www.aace.com>.

American College of Surgeons. 633 N. Saint Clar St., Chicago, IL 60611-3211. (312) 202-5000. <http://www.facs.org>.

OTHER

"Adrenalectomy." <2000 [cited April 7, 2003]. http://www.dundee.ac.uk/medicine/tayendoweb/images/adrenalectomy.htm >

"Laparoscopic Adrenalectomy: The preferred operation for benign adrenal tumors." [cited April 7, 2003]. <http://www.endocrineweb.com/laparo.html>

"Laparoscopic Removal of the Adrenal Gland." 2001 [cited April 7, 2003]. <http://mininvasive.med.nyu.edu/urology/adrenalectomy.html >.

Richard H. Lampert
Monique Laberge, Ph.D.

Adrenergic drugs

Definition

Adrenergic amines are drugs that stimulate the sympathetic nervous system (also called the adrenergic nervous system). These compounds are also called sympathomimetic drugs. The sympathetic nervous system is the part of the autonomic nervous system that originates in the thoracic (chest) and lumbar (lower back) regions of the spinal cord and regulates involuntary reactions to stress. It stimulates the heartbeat, sweating, breathing rate, and other stress-related body processes.

Purpose

Adrenergic drugs have many uses. They are used to increase the output of the heart, to raise blood pressure, and to increase urine flow as part of the treatment of shock. Adrenergics are also used as heart stimulants. They may be given to a patient to reverse the drop in blood pressure that is sometimes caused by general anesthesia. They may be used to stop bleeding by causing the blood vessels to constrict, and to keep local anesthetics in a small area of the body by closing off the nearby blood vessels that would otherwise spread the anesthetic to other parts of the body. This ability to make blood vessels constrict makes adrenergics useful in reducing nasal stuffiness associated with colds and allergies. They may also be given to open the bronchi (the tubes leading to the lungs) for treatment of asthma and chronic obstructive pulmonary disease (COPD).

Description

There are several types of adrenergic receptors in the human body. Although all types of adrenergic receptors (nerve endings) respond to the same drugs, the effects depend on which specific receptors are stimulated. The alpha receptors make the heart beat faster, the pupils of the eyes dilate, and the muscles contract. The beta receptors have similar effects and also cause the bronchi in the lungs to open up. Both alpha and beta receptors are divided into subgroups—alpha-1, alpha-2, beta-1, and beta-2—each with its own specific effects. A hormone called norepinephrine that is secreted in the body affects all types of adrenergic receptors; the drugs used in medicine and surgery, however, have been developed to affect only specific types of receptors.

There are several adrenergic amines in common use:

• Albuterol (Alupent, Ventolin, others): given by mouth or as a nasal spray to improve breathing.

• Dobutamine (Dobutrex and generic forms): used to stimulate the heart during surgery or after a heart attack or cardiac arrest.

• Dopamine (Intropin): used to increase cardiac output, blood pressure, and urine flow in treating patients with shock.

• Epinephrine (Adrenalin): used locally to control bleeding from arterioles and capillaries during surgery. It is used to treat shock, as a heart stimulant, and as a decongestant. Epinephrine may be added to local anesthetics to keep the anesthetic in the area where it is applied. Epinephrine may also be applied to the eye to reduce the symptoms of conjunctivitis (red eye).

• Isoproteranol: most widely used to ease breathing problems in asthma and COPD, but also used to control several types of irregular heartbeat until a pacemaker can be implanted.

• Phenylephrine (Neo-Synephrine): used to treat shock and low blood pressure; also used in the form of nose drops or spray to relieve nasal congestion from colds and allergies.

• Metaraminol (Aramine): used to raise the blood pressure and stimulate the heart in treating patients with shock.

• Norepinephrine (Levophed): used to increase the output of the heart and raise blood pressure as part of the treatment of shock.

Recommended dosage

The recommended dosage of an adrenergic drug depends on the specific compound, the purpose for which it is given, and the route of administration (oral or intravenous).

People who use adrenergic amines to treat breathing problems or conjunctivitis (red eye) should not use over-the-counter preparations of these drugs as an alternative to seeking professional care. These medications may temporarily relieve the symptoms of some disorders but will not cure the underlying problems, which may be serious.

Precautions

When adrenergic amines are given during surgery, they will be administered by an anesthesiologist or other health care professional skilled in their use. It is the anesthesiologist's responsibility to exercise appropriate care when these drugs are used during an operation.

The following are some of the hazards associated with the use of adrenergic amines. Patients under anesthesia may not be aware of these side effects:

• nervousness

• rapid heart beat

• high blood pressure

• irregular heart beat

• rapid heartbeat

• chest pain

• dizziness

• dry mouth

• headache

• flushing

• nausea

• vomiting

• weakness

Before undergoing procedures that may involve the use of an adrenergic amine, people with any of these medical problems should make sure their physicians know about them:

• narrow-angle glaucoma

• liver disease

• enlarged heart

• disorders affecting the arteries and veins

• diseases and disorders affecting the blood supply to the brain

Side effects

The most common side effects of adrenergic amines are nervousness, agitation, and wakefulness. These side effects do not usually cause problems when the drugs are given during surgery or in combination with local anesthetics.

KEY TERMS

Adrenergic—Characteristic of or releasing epinephrine or related substances. The term often refers to the nerve fibers in the sympathetic nervous system that release norepinephrine as a neurotransmitter.

Amine—A chemical compound that contains NH_3 (a nitrogen-hydrogen combination) as part of its structure.

Autonomic nervous system—The part of the nervous system that regulates the activity of heart muscle, smooth muscle, and glands.

Bronchi—The large air tubes leading from the trachea to the lungs that convey air to and from the lungs.

Conjunctivitis—Inflammation of the conjunctiva, the membrane on the inner part of the eyelids and the covering of the white of the eye.

Norepinephrine—A naturally occurring hormone that acts as a neurotransmitter and affects both alpha- and beta-adrenergic receptors. It is also known as noradrenaline.

Receptor—A sensory nerve ending that responds to chemical or other stimuli of various kinds.

Shock—A serious condition in which the body's blood circulation and metabolism is severely impaired by injury, pain, blood loss, or certain diseases. The symptoms of shock include a pale complexion, very low blood pressure, and a weak pulse.

Sympathetic nervous system—The part of the nervous system stimulated by adrenergic drugs. It regulates such involuntary reactions to stress as changes in the heartbeat and breathing rate, sweating, and changes in digestive secretions.

Sympathomimetic drugs—Another name for adrenergic drugs.

The following side effects sometimes occur when adrenergic amines are used to treat nasal congestion due to allergies or infections:

• rapid heartbeat

• increased sweating

• nervousness

• hallucinations

• sleep disturbances

• paleness

Other rare side effects may occur. Anyone who has unusual symptoms after taking adrenergic amines should contact his or her physician right away.

Interactions

Adrenergic amines may interact with many different types of drugs. People should discuss the use of these drugs with their pharmacist or physician before using over-the-counter preparations that contain them for colds or allergies. Patients scheduled for surgery should be sure to give the surgeon and anesthesiologist a list of all the drugs they take, including nonprescription, herbal, and alternative preparations. Some drugs that interact with adrenergic amines should be discontinued several days before surgery, since they last for a long time after the last dose.

Drugs that may interact with adrenergic amines include:

• furazolidone (Furoxone)

• tricyclic antidepressants (Adapin, Asendin, Aventyl, Elavil, Endep, Norpramin, Pamelor, Sinequan, Surmontil, Tofranil, Vivactil)

• guanethidine (Ismelin)

• methyldopa (Aldomet)

Herbs that have been reported to interact with adrenergic amines include ephedra (ma huang), often sold in over-the-counter weight loss formulas; St. John's wort, a popular remedy for anxiety or depression; alfalfa; hibiscus; ginseng; angelica (dong quai); and yohimbe.

The list above does not include every drug or herb that may interact with adrenergic amines. People should consult their physician or pharmacist before combining adrenergic amines with any other prescription or nonprescription (over-the-counter) medicine.

Resources

BOOKS

Brody, T. M., J. Larner, K. P. Minneman, and H. C. Neu. *Human Pharmacology: Molecular to Clinical*, 2nd ed. St. Louis, MO: Mosby Year-Book, 1995.

"Drug Interactions." Section 22, Chapter 301 in *The Merck Manual of Diagnosis and Therapy*, edited by Mark H. Beers, MD, and Robert Berkow, MD. Whitehouse Station, NJ: Merck Research Laboratories, 1999.

Reynolds, J. E. F., ed. *Martindale: The Extra Pharmacopoeia*, 31st ed. London, UK: The Pharmaceutical Press, 1996.

PERIODICALS

Brumley, Cindy, RN. "Herbs and the Perioperative Patient." *AORN Journal* 72 (November 2000): 785-794.

ORGANIZATIONS

American Herbal Products Association (AHPA). 8484 Georgia Avenue, Suite 370, Silver Spring, MD 20910. (301) 588-1171. <www.ahpa.org>.

American Society of Health-System Pharmacists (ASHP). 7272 Wisconsin Avenue, Bethesda, MD 20814. (301) 657-3000. <www.ashp.org>.

United States Food and Drug Administration (FDA). 5600 Fishers Lane, Rockville, MD 20857-0001. (888) INFO-FDA. <www.fda.gov>.

OTHER

"Adrenergic Drugs." Lutherans Online. <www.lutheranson line.com/servlet/lo_ProcServ/dbpage=page&GID=01158 00136098606436561961&PG=0126800136101640472 0815396>.

"Bronchodilators, Adrenergic." Medline Plus Drug Information. <www.nlm.nih.gov/medlineplus/druginfo/uspdi/202096. html>.

Samuel Uretsky, PharmD

Adult day care

Definition

Adult day care includes programs, services, and facilities designed to assist physically or mentally impaired adults remain in their communities. These are persons who might otherwise require institutional or long-term care and rehabilitation.

Purpose

There are two general purposes for adult day-care. The first is to provide an alternative to placement in a residential institution. The second is to create a respite for care-givers, often the children of the persons for whom the care is being provided.

Description

There are two general types of adult day care programs. One is based on a medical model and the other on a social model. The medical model provides comprehensive medical, therapeutic, and rehabilitation day treatment. The social model offers supervised activities, peer support, companionship, and recreation. Both models assist older adults and those with chronic conditions to remain as independent as possible, for as long as possible.

Programs organized along the medical model lines are often called adult day health care to distinguish them from social programs. Adult day health care programs offer health services such as physician visits, nursing care, and podiatry, as well as rehabilitation services such as physical, occupational, and speech therapy in a secure environment. This model of adult day care is offered to persons with a variety of chronic medical conditions including the following:

- adults with Alzheimer's disease, other forms of dementia, or depression
- persons recovering from stroke or head or spinal cord injuries
- people with chronic conditions such as diabetes or cardiovascular disease
- adults with developmental disabilities such as Down syndrome
- adults suffering from mental illnesses
- weak or frail older adults requiring nursing care or assistance with daily living activities

The social model of adult day care emphasizes supervised group activities such as crafts, gardening, music, and **exercise**. Participants in this model may require some assistance with the activities of daily living (e.g., eating, bathing, dressing) but they generally do not require skilled nursing care. Like adult day health care facilities, these social programs generally provide transportation and a midday meal for participants, as well as caregiver support groups, information and referral services, and community outreach programs.

In 2005, an estimated 36 million Americans will be aged 65 or older. According to statistics from the U.S. Department of Labor, the fastest growing segment of older adults is the population aged 85 and older. Historically, approximately 80% of the frail elderly remain in the community and are cared for by relatives, most commonly by adult daughters. Today, however, an increasing number of women aged 35–54 are in the workforce and unable to care for aging parents or disabled adult children living at home.

Although the participants of adult day care are adults who attend the programs daily or several times each week, adult day care also meets the needs of families and other caregivers. Before women entered the workforce, they were available to care for relatives at home. Today, adult day care provides a secure, alternative source of care for women who work outside the home. It also offers respite, or much needed breaks, for caregivers. Older adults caring for spouses, or children caring for aging parents find that adult day care helps ease the burden of caring for ill, confused, or disabled family members.

The first adult day care centers opened in England during the 1940s and 1950s. Established by psychiatric hospitals, these centers were designed to reduce the frequency of hospital admissions. The first adult day care centers in the United States appeared during the early 1970s. Today, there are more than 4,000 services and centers. Most centers and programs operate during normal business hours, Monday through Friday, but some offer weekend and evening care.

As of 2003, 34 states offer licensure of adult day care, but only 25 require such licensure. Adult day care services or programs may be affiliated with hospitals, **nursing homes**, home health agencies, or senior centers, but many are unaffiliated, independent programs. They may be located in storefronts, senior centers, community health and medical centers, and nursing homes.

Among centers responding to a 1997 National Adult Day Services Association (NADSA) survey, the average number of persons in an adult day care facility was approximately 40 and the average age of persons served was 76. About three out of four persons receiving adult day care services lived with family. Nearly 80% of adult day centers offered nursing services, and approximately 90% were not-for-profit. Fees ranged from $1 to $200 per day, with an average of $28 to $43 dollars per day. As of 2003, **Medicare** does not pay for any type of adult day care. However, in 35 states, **Medicaid** can be used to pay for adult day care services.

Though fees for adult day care vary widely, the service is generally considered to be cost effective when compared with the cost of institutional care, such as skilled nursing facilities or even home health care. More importantly, adult day care enables older adults, persons with physical disabilities, and those with cognitive impairments to maintain their independence. Research has demonstrated that adult day care also reduces the risks and frequency of hospitalization for older adults. Adult day care satisfies two requirements of care. It provides a secure, protected environment and is often the least restrictive setting in which care may be delivered.

Quality and standards of care vary from state to state and from one center or program to another. NADSA and the National Council on the Aging have developed standards and benchmarks for care, but adherence to these standards is voluntary. NADSA is currently developing a certification program for adult day center administrators and directors. A certification process for program assistants also exists. Since no uniform national standards exist, it is difficult for consumers to know whether a program or center is staffed by qualified personnel or provides appropriate services.

Generally, quality adult day care centers or programs conduct thorough assessments of each person and develop individualized plans of care and activities to meet the needs of impaired, disabled, or frail older adults. The plans for each individual describe objectives in terms of improvement or maintenance of health status, functional capabilities, and emotional well being. Centers must have sufficient staff to ensure safety, supervision, and close attention. Further, all personnel and volunteers should be qualified, trained, and sensitive to the special needs of older adults. For example, centers and services for persons with Alzheimer's disease or other dementias must take special precautions to ensure that people do not wander away from the facility.

Results

The aging population in the United States, the increasing incidence of Alzheimer's disease, and rising popularity of adult day care have created new and additional opportunities for health professionals and other care-giving and service personnel.

See also Nursing homes.

Resources

BOOKS

Arnold, Dorothy T. *Better Elder Care: A Nurse's Guide to Caring for Older Adults.* Philadelphia: Lippincott Williams & Wilkins, 2001.

Beisgen, B. A., M. C. Kraitchman, and A. C. Ellis. *Senior Centers: Opportunities for Successful Aging.* New York: Springer Publishing Company, 2003.

Clark, Chris L. *Adult Day Services and Social Inclusion: Better Days.* London: Jessica Kingsley Publishers, 2001.

Harris, Phyllis J. *The National Directory of Adult Day Care Centers, 3rd edition.* Silver Spring, MD: Health Resources Publisher, 2002.

PERIODICALS

Nieves, E. J. "The Effectiveness of the Assertive Community Treatment Model." *Administration and Policy in Mental Health* 29, no. 6 (2002): 461–480.

Powell, J., and H. Roberts. "Identifying 'Value' in Day Care Provision for Older People." *Journal of the Royal Society of Health* 122, no. 3 (2002): 158–164.

Ritchie, L. "Adult Day Care: Northern Perspectives." *Public Health Nursing* 20, no. 2 (2003): 120–131.

Sanfilippo, J. G., and J. E. Forker. "Creating Family: A Holistic Milieu at a Geriatric Adult Day Center." *Holistic Nursing Practice* 17, no. 1 (2003): 19–21.

ORGANIZATIONS

Adult Day Care Group. 3 Ramsgate Ct., Blue Bell, PA 19422. Telephone(610) 941-0340, FAX (610) 834-0459. <http://www.libertynet.org/adcg>.

Alzheimer's Association. 919 North Michigan Avenue, Suite 100, Chicago, IL 60611-1676. 800-272-3900 or 312-375-8700, FAX 312-335-1110. <http://www.alz.org>.

KEY TERMS

Alzheimer's disease—Progressive dementia characterized by worsening memory and other cognitive impairment.

Geriatrician—Physician specializing in the care and treatment of older adults.

California Association for Adult Day Services. 921 11th Street Suite 701, Sacramento, CA 95814. (916) 552-7400, Fax: (916) 552-7404. caads@caads.org.

National Adult Day Services Association. 8201 Greensboro Drive, Suite 300, McLean, VA 22102. (866) 890-7357 or (703) 610-9035, Fax: (703) 610-9005. info@nadsa.org.

U.S. Administration on Aging. 200 Independence Avenue, SW, Washington, DC 20201. 202-619-0724. AoA Info@aoa.gov.

OTHER

Administration on Aging. *1998 State Performance Reports.* 1998 [cited March 21, 2003]. <http://www.aoa.gov/napis/98spr/tables/table4a.html>.

"Adult Day Care Checklist." *Care Guide.* [cited March 21, 2003]. <http://www.careguide.com/Careguide/livingalternatives contentview.jsp?ContentKey=1060>.

"Nursing Homes: Alternatives for Care." *Medicare.* [cited March 21, 2003]. <http://www.medicare.gov/Nursing/Alternatives/Pace.asp>.

L. Fleming Fallon, Jr., M.D., Dr.PH

AICD *see* **Implantable cardioverter-defibrillator**

Alanine aminotransferase test *see* **Liver function tests**

Albumin test *see* **Liver function tests**

Allogenic transplant *see* **Bone marrow transplantation**

Ambulatory surgery centers

Definition

Ambulatory surgery centers (ASCs) are medical facilities that specialize in elective same-day or outpatient surgical procedures. They do not offer emergency care.

The word ambulatory comes from the Latin verb *ambulare*, which means "to walk." It means that the patients treated in these surgical centers do not require admission to a hospital and are well enough to go home after the procedure. Ambulatory surgical centers are also known as surgicenters.

Demographics

As of 2003, there are about 3,700 ambulatory surgical centers in the United States, compared with 275 in 1980 and 1,450 in 1990. This rapid increase reflects a general trend toward surgeries performed on an outpatient basis. According to *American Medical News*, 70% of all surgical procedures performed in the United States in 2000 were done in outpatient facilities, compared to 15% in 1980. As of 2003, over seven million surgeries are performed annually in American ASCs. Between 1990 and 2000, the number of operations performed annually in these centers rose 191%, from 2.3 million procedures in 1990 to 6.7 million in 2000.

The types of surgical procedures performed in ASCs have also undergone significant changes in recent years. Many of the early ASCs were outpatient centers for plastic surgery. Advances in minimally invasive surgical techniques in other specialties, however, led to the establishment of ASCs for orthopedic, dental, and ophthalmologic procedures. According to the Federated Ambulatory Surgery Association (FASA), gastroenterology accounted for only 10% of all procedures performed in ASCs in 1995, while plastic surgery still represented 20%. These proportions changed rapidly. By 1998, only three years later, ophthalmology accounted for more procedures performed in ASCs than any other surgical specialty (26.8%), followed by gastroenterology (18.8%), **orthopedic surgery** (9.8%), gynecology (9.5%), plastic surgery (7.7%), and otolaryngology (6.9%). The remaining 20.6% included dental, urological, neurological, podiatric, and pain block procedures.

As of 2003, ASCs are not distributed evenly across the United States; they tend to be concentrated in urban areas, particularly those with a high ratio of physicians to the general population.

Description

Ambulatory surgical centers are sometimes classified as either hospital-associated or freestanding. The term freestanding is somewhat confusing because some hospital-associated ASCs are located in buildings that may be several blocks away from the main hospital. As a result, some states have defined an ASC for legal purposes as "a facility primarily organized or established for the purpose of performing surgery for outpatients and… a separate identifiable legal entity from any other health care facility." More recently, some ASCs have sought institutional relationships with academic medical centers, hoping to benefit from the prestige associated with teaching and research.

Ambulatory surgery centers should not be confused with office-based surgery practices or with other outpatient centers that provide diagnostic services or primary health care, such as urgent care centers, community health centers, mobile diagnostic units, or rural health clinics. ASCs are distinguished from these other health care facilities by their use of a referral system for accepting patients and their maintenance of a dedicated **operating room**. The first characteristic means that any patient who wants to be treated in an ambulatory surgery center must first consult their primary health care provider, or PCP, and choose to have their condition treated by surgery rather than an alternative approach. The second feature means that the surgical facility must have at least one room that is used only for operations.

Accreditation and ownership

The Joint Commission on Accreditation of Healthcare Organizations (JCAHO) lists nine types of ASCs that it presently accredits:

• cosmetic and facial surgery centers

• endoscopy centers

• ophthalmology practices

• laser eye surgery centers

• centers for oral and maxillofacial surgery

• orthopedic surgery centers

• plastic surgery centers

• podiatry clinics

• multi-specialty surgery centers

Medicare inspection and certification of ambulatory surgery centers is a separate process from professional accreditation. An ASC does not have to be certified by Medicare in order to be accredited by JCAHO. Office-based surgical practices are accredited by JCAHO under a specialized Office-Based Surgery Accreditation program.

ASCs are sometimes categorized on the basis of ownership. Some are owned by hospitals and others are owned by the physicians who treat patients in them; about half, however, are operated by investor-owned businesses. The rapid growth of ASCs is in part a reflection of the general commercialization of health care in the United States over the past two decades.

Patient care

A patient in an ambulatory surgical center is asked to observe some of the same precautions and preparations that hospital patients undergo, including routine blood tests and a thorough medical history to make certain that they will not have an adverse reaction to anesthesia. In most cases the patient will be told to avoid eating and drinking before the procedure. Patients are asked to have a friend or family member drive them home after surgery; some ASCs request that the friend or relative come with the patient in the morning and stay at the center in a waiting area until the patient feels well enough to leave.

On average, patients leave the ASC within two hours after their surgery. If the patient needs overnight care or has a serious complication, he or she is transferred to an acute care hospital. Most ASCs that are not hospital-owned have arrangements with nearby hospitals to cover emergency situations.

Historical background

The first ambulatory surgical center was opened in 1970 by a group of anesthesiologists in Phoenix, Arizona. Relatively few ASCs were built, however, until the mid-1980s. Two factors that encouraged the rapid spread of ASCs after that point were the development of accreditation programs and standards on the one hand and government approval on the other. In 1980 the American Society of Plastic and Reconstructive Surgeons (ASPRS) established the American Association for Accreditation of Ambulatory Plastic Surgery Facilities, or AAAAPSF, in order to guarantee the quality of outpatient surgical facilities. The AAAAPSF then formed the American Association for Accreditation of Ambulatory Surgical Facilities, or AAAASF, to establish standards for single-specialty and multi-specialty ASCs owned or operated by surgeons who are board-certified in other types of surgery. In 1982 procedures performed at ASCs were made eligible for Medicare payments on the grounds that they were low-risk surgeries provided in less expensive settings. As of 2003, 85% of the ASCs in the United States are certified by Medicare.

Other factors involved in the expansion of ASCs include:

• Advances in medical technology. The development of instruments that made minimally invasive procedures possible made certain types of surgery less complicated to perform and less painful for the patient. The most important single development that made **outpatient surgery** increasingly safe, however, is the discovery of new anesthetic agents combined with better techniques for administering anesthesia. The number of anesthesia-related deaths has dropped sharply since the 1980s, from 1:10,000 operations in 1982 to 1:400,000 in 2002.

• Demographic changes. Instead of a shortage, by the late 1990s there was an oversupply of physicians as well as hospital beds in the United States. This situation has led to increasing competition for patients among both doctors and hospital managers.

• The increasing commercialization of health care. The rise of investor-owned hospitals and ambulatory surgery centers encouraged many doctors to invest money in these facilities, particularly the ASCs. Since ambulatory surgery centers accept patients only on a referral basis, questions have been raised about the legitimacy of doctors referring patients to facilities in which they have a financial interest. The former editor of the *New England Journal of Medicine* cites a Florida study revealing that almost 40% of the doctors practicing in that state had money invested in the ASCs to which they sent their patients.

Advantages of ASCs

Surgeons as well as patients tend to prefer ambulatory surgery centers for outpatient procedures for several reasons:

• Cost. In many cases, an outpatient procedure done in an ASC costs between one-half and one-third as much as the same procedure done in a hospital. It is important, however, for patients to compare costs carefully, because some ASC procedures may cost as much as or even more than hospital-based procedures. For example, the Medicare Payment Advisory Commission found that whereas a cataract operation cost only $942 at an ambulatory surgery center in 2001 as opposed to $1334 at a hospital, after-cataract **laser surgery** cost $429 at the ASC versus $246 at a hospital. Figures for an endoscopy and biopsy of the upper digestive tract were $429 and $359 respectively; for a diagnostic **colonoscopy**, $429 and $401; and for epidural anesthesia, $320 and $183.

• Convenience. There is much less administrative paperwork and "red tape" at an ambulatory surgical center compared to the admissions process at most hospitals. Patients also like the fact that they can leave an ASC relatively quickly after their surgery, which translates into less time lost from work.

• Presence of family and friends. Whereas most hospitals keep patients recovering from a surgical procedure in separate rooms, in an ASC the patient can usually spend the recovery period after surgery with their loved ones.

• Greater efficiency. This advantage is particularly important to surgeons. It takes much less time to prepare an operating room in a specialized ASC for the next patient than in a standard hospital. Improved efficiency allows the surgeon to treat more patients in the same

amount of time than he or she would be able to do in a hospital; some surgeons maintain that they can do three times the number of procedures in an ASC as they could in a hospital setting.

• Greater control over procedures and standards. Many doctors prefer working in an ASC because they can set the standards for staffing, safety precautions, **postoperative care**, etc., rather than having these things decided for them by a hospital manager.

ASCs within the American health care system

As of 2003, there are several areas of tension in the health care system related to ambulatory surgical centers. One is opposition from hospitals. Most hospitals have relied on income from surgical procedures to make up for losses incurred by treating other patients who cannot afford to pay. The movement toward freestanding ambulatory surgery centers means a considerable loss of income for many hospitals.

On the other hand, there is also increasing competition between ASCs and office-based surgical practices. The same improvements in anesthesia and surgical equipment that made outpatient surgery in an ASC safe to perform have also made it safe to do a growing number of fairly complex procedures in a doctor's office. Such procedures as hernia repair, arthroscopic joint repair, and **liposuction** are now being performed in office-based facilities. It is estimated that by 2005, 10 million surgical procedures will be performed annually in American doctors' offices, or twice as many as were done in 1995. The American Society of Anesthesiologists predicts that office-based surgical procedures will account for a steadily growing proportion of outpatient surgeries. The ASA has stated that ".... the trend toward office-based surgery is growing at least as fast [as of 2003] as the trend toward ambulatory surgery grew a few years ago."

Legal and regulatory issues

The growing number of for-profit ASCs as well as government involvement with outpatient facilities through the Medicare program has led to a number of legal and regulatory questions. One issue concerns the level of Medicare reimbursement for procedures performed in ASCs. The present Medicare fee schedule is based on data from 1986, when the operating costs of many ambulatory surgical centers were higher than they are in 2003, due to advances in technology. As a result, some observers think that ASCs are being overpaid for services to Medicare patients. Another issue is a proposal to add more procedures to the list approved by Medicare

KEY TERMS

Ambulatory—Referring to a condition that is treatable without admission to a hospital, or to a surgical procedure performed on an outpatient basis.

Dedicated—Reserved for a specific purpose. An ambulatory surgical center must have at least one dedicated operating room in order to qualify for accreditation.

Elective—Referring to a surgical procedure that is a matter of choice; an elective operation may be beneficial to the patient but is not urgently needed.

Podiatry—The surgical specialty that treats disorders of the foot.

Surgicenter—Another term for ambulatory surgical center.

for ASC patients. The present list has not been updated since 1995. The proposed additions would increase ASC services available to Medicare patients by 20%.

The major legal question facing surgeons who own or have investments in ambulatory surgical centers is whether they are breaking the law by referring patients to ASCs in which they have invested or in which they perform surgery. The existing laws are not entirely clear on this point, but experts in health law do not expect the confusion to be resolved in the near future.

See also Hospital services; Medicare; Outpatient surgery.

Resources

PERIODICALS

Aker, J. "Safety of Ambulatory Surgery." *Journal of Perianesthesia Nursing* 16 (December 2001): 353–358.

Baker, J. J. "Medicare Payment System for Ambulatory Surgical Centers." *Journal of Health Care Finance* 28 (Spring 2002): 76–87.

Becker, S. and M. Biala. "Ambulatory Surgery Centers—Current Business and Legal Issues." *Journal of Health Care Finance* 27 (Winter 2000): 1–7.

Becker, S. and N. Harned. "The Fraud and Abuse Statute and Investor-Owned Ambulatory Surgery Centers." *Health Care Law Monthly* (April 2002): 13–23.

Hawryluk, Markian. "Ambulatory Surgery Centers' Medicare Pay Rate Questioned." *American Medical News* November 25, 2002 [cited March 12, 2003]. <http://www.ama-assn.org/sci-pubs/amnews/pick_02/gvsa1125.htm>.

Jackson, Cheryl. "Cutting Into the Market: Rise of Ambulatory Surgical Centers." *American Medical News*, April 15, 2002. [cited March 12, 2003]. <http://www.ama-assn.org/sci-pubs/amnews/pick_02/bisa0415.htm>.

Lynk, W. J. and C. S. Longley. "The Effect of Physician-Owned Surgicenters on Hospital Outpatient Surgery." *Health Affairs (Millwood)* 21 (July-August 2002): 215–221.

Mamel, J. J. and H. J. Nord. "Endoscopic Ambulatory Surgery Centers in the Academic Medical Center. We Can Do It Too!" *Gastrointestinal Endoscopy Clinics of North America* 12 (April 2002): 275–284.

O'Brien, D. "Acute Postoperative Delirium: Definitions, Incidence, Recognition, and Interventions." *Journal of Perianesthesia Nursing* 17 (December 2002): 384–392.

Relman, Arnold S., MD. "Canada's Romance with Market Medicine." *American Prospect* 13 (October 21, 2002) [cited March 12, 2003]. <http://www.prospect.org/print_friendly/print/V13/19/relman-a.html>.

Relman, Arnold S., MD. "What Market Values Are Doing to Medicine." *Atlantic Monthly* 269 (March 1992): 99–106.

ORGANIZATIONS

Accreditation Association for Ambulatory Health Care (AAAHC). 3201 Old Glenview Road, Suite 300, Wilmette, IL 60091-2992. (847) 853-6060. <http://www.aahc.org>.

American Association for Accreditation of Ambulatory Surgery Facilities (AAAASF). 1202 Allanson Road, Mundelein, IL 60060. (888) 545-5222.

American Association of Ambulatory Surgical Centers (AAASC). P. O. Box 23220, San Diego, CA 92193. (800) 237-3768. <http://www.aaasc.org>.

American Health Lawyers Association. Suite 600, 1025 Connecticut Avenue NW, Washington, DC 20036-5405. (202) 833-1100. <http://www.healthlawyers.org>.

American Society of Anesthesiologists (ASA). 520 N. Northwest Highway, Park Ridge, IL 60068-2573. (847) 825-5586. <http://www.asahq.org>.

Federated Ambulatory Surgery Association (FASA). 700 North Fairfax Street, #306, Alexandria, VA 22314. (703) 836-8808. <http://www.fasa.org>.

Joint Commission on Accreditation of Healthcare Organizations (JCAHO). One Renaissance Boulevard, Oakbrook Terrace, IL 60181. (630) 792-5000. <http://www.jcaho.org>.

OTHER

American Society of Anesthesiologists. *Office-Based Anesthesia and Surgery*. [cited March 13, 2003]. <http://www.asahq.org/patientEducation/officebased.htm>.

Rebecca Frey, Ph.D.

Ammonia (blood) test *see* **Liver function tests**

Amniocentesis

Definition

Amniocentesis is a procedure used to diagnose fetal defects in the early second trimester of pregnancy. A sample of the amniotic fluid, which surrounds a fetus in the womb, is collected through a pregnant woman's abdomen using a needle and syringe. Tests performed on fetal cells found in the amniotic fluid can reveal the presence of many types of genetic disorders. Early diagnosis allows doctors and prospective parents to make important decisions about treatment and intervention prior to birth.

Purpose

Since the mid-1970s, amniocentesis has been used routinely to test for Down syndrome, by far the most common, nonhereditary, genetic birth defect, afflicting about one in every 1,000 babies. By 1997, approximately 800 different diagnostic tests were available, most of them for hereditary genetic disorders such as Tay-Sachs disease, sickle cell disease, hemophilia, muscular dystrophy, and cystic fibrosis.

Amniocentesis, often called amnio, is recommended for women who will be older than 35 on their due-date. It is also recommended for women who have already borne children with birth defects, or when either of the parents has a family history of a birth defect for which a diagnostic test is available. Another reason for the procedure is to confirm indications of Down syndrome and certain other defects that may have shown up previously during routine maternal blood screening.

The risk of bearing a child with a nonhereditary genetic defect such as Down syndrome is directly related to a woman's age—the older the woman, the greater the risk. Thirty-five is the recommended age to begin amnio testing because that is the age at which the risk of carrying a fetus with such a defect roughly equals the risk of miscarriage caused by the procedure—about one in 200. At age 25, the risk of giving birth to a child with this type of defect is about one in 1,400; by age 45 it increases to about one in 20. Nearly half of all pregnant women over 35 in the United States undergo amniocentesis and many younger women also decide to have the procedure. Notably, some 75% of all Down syndrome infants born in the United States each year are to women younger than 35.

One of the most common reasons for performing amniocentesis is an abnormal alpha-fetoprotein (AFP) test. Alpha-fetoprotein is a protein produced by the fetus and present in the mother's blood. A simple blood screening, usually conducted around the fifteenth week of pregnancy, can determine the AFP levels in the mother's blood. Levels that are too high or too low may signal possible fetal defects. Because this test has a high false-positive rate, another test such as amniocentesis is recommended whenever the AFP levels fall outside the normal range.

Amniocentesis is generally performed during the sixteenth week of pregnancy, with results usually available within three weeks. It is possible to perform an amnio as early as the eleventh week but this is not usually recommended because there appears to be an increased risk of miscarriage when done at this time. The advantage of early amnio and speedy results lies in the extra time for decision making if a problem is detected. Potential treatment of the fetus can begin earlier. Important, also, is the fact that elective abortions are safer and less controversial the earlier they are performed.

Precautions

As an invasive surgical procedure, amniocentesis poses a real, although small, risk to the health of a fetus. Parents must weigh the potential value of the knowledge gained, or indeed the reassurance that all is well, against the small risk of miscarriage. The serious emotional and ethical dilemmas that adverse test results can bring must also be considered. The decision to undergo amnio is always a matter of personal choice.

Description

The word amniocentesis literally means "puncture of the amnion," the thin-walled sac of fluid in which a developing fetus is suspended during pregnancy. During the procedure, the obstetrician inserts a very fine needle through the woman's abdomen into the uterus and amniotic sac and withdraws approximately 1 oz (28.3 g) of amniotic fluid for testing. The relatively painless procedure is performed on an outpatient basis, sometimes using local anesthesia.

The physician uses ultrasound images to guide needle placement and collect the sample, thereby minimizing the risk of fetal injury and the need for repeated needle insertions. Once the sample is collected, the woman can return home after a brief observation period. She may be instructed to rest for the first 24 hours and to avoid heavy lifting for two days.

The sample of amniotic fluid is sent to a laboratory where fetal cells contained in the fluid are isolated and grown in order to provide enough genetic material for testing. This takes about seven to 14 days. The material is then extracted and treated so that visual examination for defects can be made. For some disorders, like Tay-Sachs, the simple presence of a telltale chemical compound in the amniotic fluid is enough to confirm a diagnosis. Depending on the specific tests ordered, and the skill of the lab conducting them, all the results are available one to four weeks after the sample is taken.

KEY TERMS

Alpha-fetoprotein (AFP)—A protein normally produced by the liver of a fetus and detectable in maternal blood samples. AFP screening measures the amount of alpha-fetoprotein in the blood. Levels outside the norm may indicate fetal defects.

Anencephaly—A hereditary defect resulting in the partial to complete absence of a brain and spinal cord. It is fatal.

Chorionic villus sampling (CVS)—A procedure similar to amniocentesis, except that cells are taken from the chorionic membrane for testing. These cells, called chorionic villus cells, eventually become the placenta. The samples are collected either through the abdomen, as in amnio, or through the vagina. CVS can be done earlier in the pregnancy than amnio, but carries a somewhat higher risk.

Chromosome—Chromosomes are the strands of genetic material in a cell that occur in nearly identical pairs. Normal human cells contain 23 chromosome pairs—one in each pair inherited from the mother, and one from the father. Every human cell contains the exact same set of chromosomes.

Down syndrome—The most prevalent of a class of genetic defects known as trisomies, in which cells contain three copies of certain chromosomes rather than the usual two. Down syndrome, or tri-

somy 21, usually results from three copies of chromosome 21.

Genetic—The term refers to genes, the basic units of biological heredity, which are contained on the chromosomes, and contain chemical instructions which direct the development and functioning of an individual.

Hereditary—Something which is inherited or passed down from parents to offspring. In biology and medicine, the word pertains to inherited genetic characteristics.

Maternal blood screening—Maternal blood screening is normally done early in pregnancy to test for a variety of conditions. Abnormal amounts of certain proteins in a pregnant woman's blood raise the probability of fetal defects. Amniocentesis is recommended if such a probability occurs.

Tay-Sachs disease—An inherited disease prevalent among the Ashkenazi Jewish population of the United States. Infants with the disease are unable to process a certain type of fat that accumulates in nerve and brain cells, causing mental and physical retardation, and death by age four.

Ultrasound—A technique that uses high-frequency sound waves to create a visual image (a sonogram) of soft tissues. The technique is routinely used in prenatal care and diagnosis.

Cost of the procedure depends on the doctor, the lab, and the tests ordered. Most insurers provide coverage for women over 35, as a follow-up to positive maternal blood screening results, and when genetic disorders run in the family.

An alternative to amnio, now in general use, is chorionic villus sampling (CVS), which can be performed as early as the eighth week of pregnancy. While this allows for the possibility of a first trimester abortion, if warranted, CVS is apparently also riskier and is more expensive. The most promising area of new research in prenatal testing involves expanding the scope and accuracy of maternal blood screening as this poses no risk to the fetus.

Preparation

It is important for a woman to fully understand the procedure and to feel confident in the obstetrician performing it. Evidence suggests that a physician's experience with the procedure reduces the chance of mishap.

Almost all obstetricians are experienced in performing amniocentesis. The patient should feel free to ask questions and seek emotional support before, during, and after amniocentesis is performed.

Aftercare

Necessary aftercare falls into two categories, physical and emotional.

Physical aftercare

During and immediately following the sampling procedure, a woman may experience dizziness, nausea, a rapid heartbeat, and cramping. Once past these immediate hurdles, the physician will send the woman home with instructions to rest and to report any complications requiring immediate treatment, including:

• Vaginal bleeding. The appearance of blood could signal a problem.

• Premature labor. Unusual abdominal pain and/or cramping may indicate the onset of premature labor. Mild cramping for the first day or two following the procedure is normal.

• Signs of infection. Leaking of amniotic fluid or unusual vaginal discharge, and fever could signal the onset of infection.

Emotional aftercare

Once the procedure has been safely completed, the anxiety of waiting for the test results can prove to be the worst part of the process. A woman should seek and receive emotional support from family and friends, as well as from her obstetrician and family doctor. Professional counseling may also prove necessary, particularly if a fetal defect is detected.

Risks

Most of the risks and short-term side effects associated with amniocentesis relate to the sampling procedure. A successful amnio sampling results in no long-term side effects. Risks include:

• Maternal/fetal hemorrhaging. While spotting in pregnancy is fairly common, bleeding following amnio should always be investigated.

• Infection. Infection, although rare, can occur after amniocentesis. An unchecked infection can lead to severe complications.

• Fetal injury. A very slight risk of injury to the fetus resulting from contact with the amnio needle does exist.

• Miscarriage. The rate of miscarriage occurring during standard, second trimester amnio is approximately 0.5%. This compares to a miscarriage rate of 1% for CVS. Many fetuses with severe genetic defects miscarry naturally during the first trimester.

• The trauma of difficult family-planning decisions. The threat posed to parental and family mental health from the trauma accompanying an abnormal test result can not be underestimated.

Normal results

Negative results from an amnio analysis indicate that everything about the fetus appears normal and the pregnancy can continue without undue concern. A negative result for Down syndrome means that it is 99% certain that the disease does not exist.

An overall "normal" result does not, however, guarantee that the pregnancy will come to term, or that the fetus does not suffer from some other defect. Laboratory tests are not 100% accurate at detecting targeted conditions, nor can every possible fetal condition be tested for.

Abnormal results

Positive results on an amnio analysis indicate the presence of a fetal defect, with an accuracy approaching 100%. With such a diagnosis, prospective parents face emotionally and ethically difficult choices regarding prenatal treatment options, the prospect of treating the defect at birth, and the option of elective abortion. At this point, the parents need expert medical advice and counseling.

Resources

BOOKS

Hassold, Terry and Stuart Schwartz. "Chromosome Disorders." In *Harrison's Principles of Internal Medicine*, edited by Eugene Braunwald, et al. Philadelphia: McGraw-Hill, 2001.

Miesfeldt, Susan and J. Larry Jameson. "Screening, Counseling, and Prevention of Genetic Disorders." In *Harrison's Principles of Internal Medicine*, edited by Eugene Braunwald, et al. Philadelphia: McGraw-Hill, 2001.

Wallach, Jacques. *Interpretation of Diagnostic Tests*. 7th ed. Philadelphia, PA: Lippincott Williams & Wilkens, 2000.

ORGANIZATIONS

American College of Obstetricians and Gynecologists. 409 12th St., S.W., P.O. Box 96920, Washington, DC 20090-6920. <http://www.acog.org>.

OTHER

National Institutes of Health. [cited April 4, 2003]. <http://www.nlm.nih.gov/medlineplus/encyclopedia.html>.

Kurt Richard Sternlof
Mark A. Best

Amniotic fluid analysis *see* **Amniocentesis**

Amputation

Definition

Amputation is the surgical removal of a limb or body part. It is performed to remove diseased tissue or relieve pain.

Purpose

Arms, legs, hands, feet, fingers, and toes can all be amputated. In the United States, there are approximately

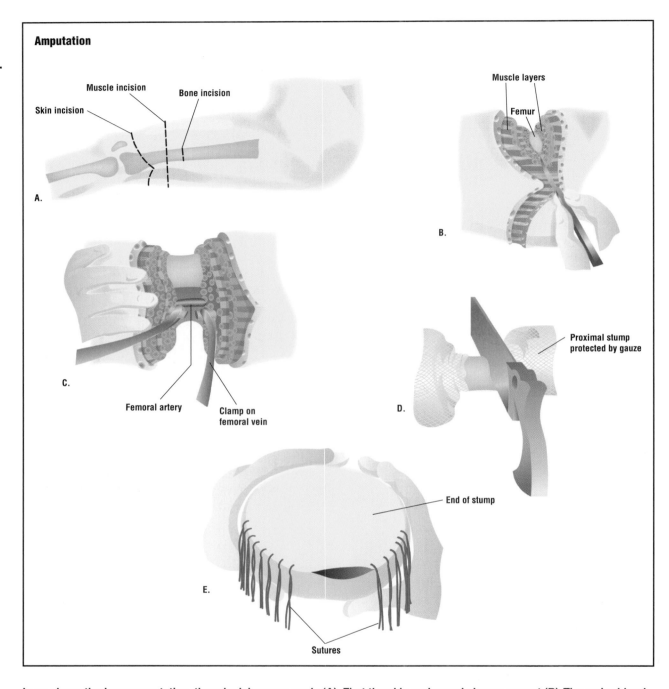

Amputation

In an above-the-knee amputation, three incisions are made (A). First the skin and muscle layers are cut (B). The major blood vessels are clamped and severed (C). The bone is cut with a special saw (D). Finally, the muscles are stitched over the bone, and the skin is closed over the wound (E). *(Illustration by GGS Inc.)*

350,000 amputees, with some 135,000 new amputations occurring each year. The number of amputees worldwide is not currently known.

Here in the United States, the most common causes of amputation of the lower extremity are: disease (70%),

trauma (22%), congenital or birth defects (4%), and tumors (4%). As for upper extremity amputation, it is usually performed because of trauma or birth defect. Seldom is disease as great a contributing factor. The causes of amputation differ significantly in various countries. For example, countries with a recent history of warfare and civil unrest will have a higher incidence of amputations, due to war itself or its technology (landmines, uncontrolled ordnance, etc).

Among the diseases and conditions that may lead to amputation of an extremity, the most prevalent are:

• hardening of the arteries

• arterial embolism

• impaired circulation as a complication of diabetes mellitus

• gangrene

• severe frostbite

• Raynaud's disease

• Buerger's disease

More than 90% of amputations performed in the United States are due to circulatory complications of diabetes. Sixty to eighty percent of these operations involve the legs.

Demographics

Most amputations involve small body parts such as a finger, rather than an entire limb. About 65,000 amputations are performed in the United States each year.

In the United States, there are approximately 350,000 amputees, with some 135,000 new amputations occurring each year. The number of amputees worldwide is not currently known.

Description

Amputations can be either planned or emergency procedures. Injury and arterial embolisms are the main reasons for emergency amputations. The operation is performed under regional or general anesthesia by a general or orthopedic surgeon in a hospital **operating room**.

Details of the operation vary slightly depending on what part is to be removed. All amputations consist of a two-fold surgical procedure: to remove diseased tissue so that the wound will heal cleanly, and to construct a stump that will allow the attachment of a prosthesis or artificial replacement part.

The surgeon makes an incision around the part to be amputated. The part is removed, and the bone is smoothed. A flap is constructed of muscle, connective tissue, and skin to cover the raw end of the bone. The flap is closed over the bone with sutures (surgical stitches) that remain in place for about one month. Often, a rigid dressing or cast is applied that stays in place for about two weeks.

WHO PERFORMS THE PROCEDURE AND WHERE IS IT PERFORMED?

Amputations are performed in a hospital, usually by an orthopaedic surgeon. Orthopedics is a medical specialty that focuses on the diagnosis, care and treatment of patients with disorders of the bones, joints, muscles, ligaments, tendons, nerves, and skin. These elements make up the musculoskeletal system. The physicians who specialize in this area are called orthopedic surgeons or orthopedists. Orthopedic surgery is a specialty of immense variety, and includes amputation surgery.

Diagnosis/Preparation

Before an amputation is performed, extensive testing is done to determine the proper level of amputation. The goal of the surgeon is to find the place where healing is most likely to be complete, while allowing the maximum amount of limb to remain for effective rehabilitation.

The greater the blood flow through an area, the more likely healing is to occur. These tests are designed to measure blood flow through the limb. Several or all of them can be done to help choose the proper level of amputation.

• measurement of blood pressure in different parts of the limb

• xenon 133 studies, which use a radiopharmaceutical to measure blood flow

• oxygen tension measurements in which an oxygen electrode is used to measure oxygen pressure under the skin (If the pressure is 0, the healing will not occur. If the pressure reads higher than 40mm Hg [40 milliliters of mercury], healing of the area is likely to be satisfactory.)

• laser doppler measurements of the microcirculation of the skin

• skin fluorescent studies that also measure skin microcirculation

• skin perfusion measurements using a blood pressure cuff and photoelectric detector

• infrared measurements of skin temperature

No one test is highly predictive of healing, but taken together, the results give the surgeon an excellent idea of the best place to amputate.

Aftercare

After amputation, medication is prescribed for pain, and patients are treated with **antibiotics** to discourage infection. The stump is moved often to encourage good circulation. Physical therapy and rehabilitation are started as soon as possible, usually within 48 hours. Studies have shown that there is a positive relationship between early rehabilitation and effective functioning of the stump and prosthesis. Length of stay in the hospital depends on the severity of the amputation and the general health of the amputee, but ranges from several days to two weeks.

Rehabilitation is a long, arduous process, especially for above the knee amputees. Twice daily physical therapy is not uncommon. In addition, psychological counseling is an important part of rehabilitation. Many people feel a sense of loss and grief when they lose a body part. Others are bothered by phantom limb syndrome, where they feel as if the amputated part is still in place. They may even feel pain in this limb that does not exist. Many amputees benefit from joining self-help groups and meeting others who are also living with amputation. Addressing the emotional aspects of amputation often speeds the physical rehabilitation process.

Risks

Amputation is major surgery. All the risks associated with the administration of anesthesia exist, along with the possibility of heavy blood loss and the development of blood clots. Infection is of special concern to amputees. Infection rates in amputations average 15%. If the stump becomes infected, it is necessary to remove the prosthesis and sometimes to amputate a second time at a higher level.

Failure of the stump to heal is another major complication. Nonhealing is usually due to an inadequate blood supply. The rate of nonhealing varies from 5–30% depending on the facility. Centers that specialize in amputation usually have the lowest rates of complication.

Persistent pain in the stump or pain in the phantom limb is experienced by most amputees to some degree. Treatment of phantom limb pain is difficult. One final complication is that many amputees give up on the rehabilitation process and discard their prosthesis. Better fitting prosthetics and earlier rehabilitation have decreased the incidence of this problem.

Normal results

The five year survival rate for all lower extremity amputees is less than 50%. For diabetic amputees, the rate is less than 40%. Up to 50% of people who have one leg amputated because of diabetes will lose the other within five years. Amputees who walk using a prosthesis have a less stable gait. Three to five percent of these people fall and break bones because of this instability. Although the fractures can be treated, about half the amputees who suffer them then remain wheelchair bound.

Alternatives

Alternatives to amputation depend on the medical cause underlying the decision to amputate and the degree of medical urgency. In some cases, drug therapy may be considered as an alternative.

For example, one serious complication of diabetes is the development of foot ulcers that often lead to amputation. Some studies have suggested non-surgical treatment of diabetic foot ulcers with a new, recombinant drug (Becaplermin/Regranex). Combined with competent ulcer nursing, the drug leads to fewer amputations compared to the alternative of ulcer nursing on its own.

Resources

BOOKS

Meier, R. H. *Functional Restoration of Adults and Children With Upper Extremity Amputation.* New York: Demos Medical Publishing, 2003.

Murdoch, G. and A. Bennett Wilson. *A Primer on Amputations and Artificial Limbs.* Springfield: Charles C. Thomas Pub. Ltd., 1998.

Watts, H. and M. Williams. *Who Is Amelia?: Caring for Children With Limb Difference.* Rosemont, IL: American Academy of Orthopaedic Surgeons, 1998.

PERIODICALS

Buzato, M. A., E. C. Tribulatto, S. M. Costa, W G. Zorn, and B. van Bellen. "Major amputations of the lower leg. The

KEY TERMS

Arterial embolism—A blood clot arising from another location that blocks an artery.

Buerger's disease—An episodic disease that causes inflammation and blockage of the veins and arteries of the limbs. It tends to be present almost exclusively in men under age 40 who smoke, and may require amputation of the hand or foot.

Diabetes mellitus—A disease in which insufficient insulin is made by the body to metabolize sugars.

Raynaud's disease—A disease found mainly in young women that causes decreased circulation to the hands and feet. Its cause is unknown.

patients two years later." *Acta Chirurgica Belgica* 102 (August 2002): 248–252.

Cull, D. L., S. M. Taylor, S. E. Hamontree, E. M. Langan, B. A. Snyder, T. M. Sullivan, and J. R. Youkey. "A reappraisal of a modified through-knee amputation in patients with peripheral vascular disease." *American Journal of Surgery* 182 (July 2001): 44–48.

Gerstein, H. and D. Hunt. "Foot ulcers and amputations in diabetes." *Clinical Evidence* 7 (June 2002): 521–528.

Hagberg, K. and R. Branemark. "Consequences of non-vascular trans-femoral amputation: a survey of quality of life, prosthetic use and problems." *Prosthetic Orthotherapy International* 25 (December 2001): 186–194.

Kazmers, A., A. J. Perkins and L. A. Jacobs. "Major lower extremity amputation in Veterans Affairs medical centers." *Annals of Vascular Surgery* 14 (May 2000): 216–222.

Oyibo, S. O., E. B. Jude, I. Tarawneh, H. C. Nguyen, D. G. Armstrong, L. B. Harkless, and A. J. Boulton. "The effects of ulcer size and site, patient's age, sex and type and duration of diabetes on the outcome of diabetic foot ulcers." *Diabetic Medicine* 18 (February 2001): 133–138.

ORGANIZATIONS

American Academy of Orthopaedic Surgeons. 6300 North River Road, Rosemont, Illinois 60018-4262. Phone (847) 823-7186. <www.aaos.org>.

American College of Surgeons. 633 N. Saint Clar st., Chicago, IL 60611-3211. (312) 202-5000. <www.facs.org>.

American Diabetes Association. 1701 North Beauregard Street, Alexandria, VA 22311. (800) 342-2383. <www.diabetes.org>.

National Amputation Foundation. 40 Church Street, Malverne, NY 11565. (516) 887-3600. <www.nationalamputation.org/>.

OTHER

The Amputee Newswire. <http://www.amputee-online.com/amputation/>.

Amputation Prevention Global Resource Center Page. <www.diabetesresource.com>.

Cripworld Guide to Amputation. <http://www.cripworld.com/amputee/ampinfo.htm>.

Tish Davidson, A.M.
Monique Laberge, Ph.D.

Anaerobic bacteria culture

Definition

An anaerobic bacteria culture is a method used to grow anaerobes from a clinical specimen. Obligate anaerobes are bacteria that can live only in the absence of oxygen. Obligate anaerobes are destroyed when exposed to the atmosphere for as briefly as 10 minutes. Some anaerobes are tolerant to small amounts of oxygen. Facultative anaerobes are those organisms that will grow with or without oxygen. The methods of obtaining specimens for anaerobic culture and the culturing procedure are performed to ensure that the organisms are protected from oxygen.

Purpose

Anaerobic bacterial cultures are performed to identify bacteria that grow only in the absence of oxygen and which may cause human infection. If overlooked or killed by exposure to oxygen, anaerobic infections result in such serious consequences as **amputation**, organ failure, sepsis, meningitis, and death. Culture is required to correctly identify anaerobic pathogens and institute effective antibiotic treatment.

Precautions

It is crucial that the health care provider obtain the sample for culture via **aseptic technique**. Anaerobes are commonly found on mucous membranes and other sites such as the vagina and oral cavity. Therefore, specimens likely to be contaminated with these organisms should not be submitted for culture (e.g., a throat or vaginal swab). Some types of specimens should always be cultured for anaerobes if an infection is suspected. These include abscesses, bites, blood, cerebrospinal fluid and exudative body fluids, deep wounds, and dead tissues. The specimen must be protected from oxygen during collection and transport and must be transported to the laboratory immediately.

Description

Anaerobes are normally found within certain areas of the body but result in serious infection when they have access to a normally sterile body fluid or deep tissue that is poorly oxygenated. Some anaerobes normally live in the crevices of the skin, in the nose, mouth, throat, intestine, and vagina. Injury to these tissues (i.e., cuts, puncture wounds, or trauma) especially at or adjacent to the mucous membranes allows anaerobes entry into otherwise sterile areas of the body and is the primary cause of anaerobic infection. A second source of anaerobic infection occurs from the introduction of spores into a normally sterile site. Spore-producing anaerobes live in the soil and water, and spores may be introduced via wounds, especially punctures. Anaerobic infections are most likely to be found in persons who are immunosuppressed, those treated recently with broad-spectrum **antibiotics**, and persons who have a decaying tissue injury on or near a mucous membrane, especially if the site is foul-smelling.

Some specimens from which anaerobes are likely to be isolated are:

• blood

• bile

• bone marrow

• cerebrospinal fluid

• direct lung aspirate

• tissue biopsy from a normally sterile site

• fluid from a normally sterile site (like a joint)

• dental abscess

• abdominal or pelvic abscess

• knife, gunshot, or surgical wound

• severe burn

Some of the specimens that are not suitable for anaerobic cultures include:

• coughed throat discharge (sputum)

• rectal swab

• nasal or throat swab

• urethral swab

• voided urine

Specimen collection

The keys to effective anaerobic bacteria cultures include collecting a contamination-free specimen and protecting it from oxygen exposure. Anaerobic bacteria cultures should be obtained from an appropriate site without the health care professional contaminating the sample with bacteria from the adjacent skin, mucus membrane, or tissue. Swabs should be avoided when collecting specimens for anaerobic culture because cotton fibers may be detrimental to anaerobes. Abscesses or fluids can be aspirated using a sterile syringe that is then tightly capped to prevent entry of air. Tissue samples should be placed into a degassed bag and sealed, or into a gassed out screw top vial that may contain oxygen-free prereduced culture medium and tightly capped. The specimens should be plated as rapidly as possible onto culture media that has been prepared.

Culture

Cultures should be placed in an environment that is free of oxygen, at 95°F (35°C) for at least 48 hours before the plates are examined for growth.

Gram staining is performed on the specimen at the time of culture. While infections can be caused by aerobic or anaerobic bacteria or a mixture of both, some infections have a high probability of being caused by anaerobic bacteria. These infections include brain abscesses, lung abscesses, aspiration pneumonia, and dental infections. Anaerobic organisms can often be suspected because many anaerobes have characteristic microscopic morphology (appearance). For example, *Bacteroides* spp. are gram-negative rods that are pleomorphic (variable in size and shape) and exhibit irregular bipolar staining. *Fusobacterium* spp. are often pale gram-negative spindle-shaped rods having pointed ends. *Clostridium* spp. are large gram-positive rods that form spores. The location of the spore (central, subterminal, terminal, or absent) is a useful differential characteristic. The presence of growth, oxygen tolerance, and Gram stain results are sufficient to establish a diagnosis of an anaerobic infection and begin antibiotic treatment with a drug appropriate for most anaerobes such as clindamycin, metronidazole, or vancomycin.

Gram-negative anaerobes and some of the infections they produce include the following genera:

• *Bacteroides* (the most commonly found anaerobes in cultures; intra-abdominal infections, rectal abscesses, soft tissue infections, liver infection)

• *Fusobacterium* (abscesses, wound infections, pulmonary and intracranial infections)

• *Porphyromonas* (aspiration pneumonia, periodontitis)

• *Prevotella* (intra-abdominal infections, soft tissue infections)

Gram-positive anaerobes include the following:

• *Actinomyces* (head, neck, pelvic infections; aspiration pneumonia)

• *Bifidobacterium* (ear infections, abdominal infections)

• *Clostridium* (gas, gangrene, food poisoning, tetanus, pseudomembranous colitis)

Anaerobic bacteria culture

- *Peptostreptococcus* (oral, respiratory, and intra-abdominal infections)
- *Propionibacterium* (shunt infections)

The identification of anaerobes is highly complex, and laboratories may use different identification systems. Partial identification is often the goal. For example, there are six species of the *Bacteroides* genus that may be identified as the *Bacteroides fragilis* group rather than identified individually. Organisms are identified by their colonial and microscopic morphology, growth on selective media, oxygen tolerance, and biochemical characteristics. These include sugar fermentation, bile solubility, esculin, starch, and gelatin hydrolysis, casein and gelatin digestion, catalase, lipase, lecithinase, and indole production, nitrate reduction, volatile fatty acids as determined by gas chromatography, and susceptibility to antibiotics. The antibiotic susceptibility profile is determined by the microtube broth dilution method. Many species of anaerobes are resistant to penicillin, and some are resistant to clindamycin and other commonly used antibiotics.

Diagnosis/Preparation

The health care provider should take special care to collect a contamination-free specimen. All procedures must be performed aseptically. The health care professional who collects the specimen should be prepared to take two samples, one for anaerobic culture and one for aerobic culture, since it is unknown whether the pathogen can grow with or without oxygen. In addition, health care professionals should document any antibiotics that the patient is currently taking and any medical conditions that could influence growth of bacteria.

Aftercare

In the case of vein puncture for anaerobic blood cultures, direct pressure should be applied to the vein puncture site for several minutes or until the bleeding has stopped. An adhesive bandage may be applied, if appropriate. If swelling or bruising occurs, ice can be applied to the site. For collection of specimens other than blood, the patient and the collection site should be monitored for any complications after the procedure.

Risks

Special care must be taken by the health care team obtaining, transporting, and preparing the specimen for anaerobic culture. Poor methodology may delay the identification of the bacterium, may allow the patient's condition to deteriorate, and may require the patient to provide more samples than would otherwise be required. Patients may

---

KEY TERMS

Aerobic bacteria—Bacteria that can grow freely in oxygen-rich environments.

Aseptic—Free from living disease-causing organisms; sterile and without contamination.

Gram staining—Use of a purple dye to identify pathogens, usually bacteria

Pathogen—An organism capable of causing disease.

Sepsis—The systemic inflammatory response due to an infectious organism circulating throughout the body. Sepsis can progress to severe sepsis and septic shock, where blood pressure drops (hypotension), the blood supply to tissues decreases, and organs fail.

Venipuncture—Puncture of a vein with a needle for the purpose of withdrawing a blood sample for analysis.

---

experience bruising, discomfort, or swelling at the collection site when tissue, blood, or other fluids are obtained.

Results

Negative results will show no pathogenic growth in the sample. Positive results will show growth, the identification of each specific bacterium, and its antibiotic susceptibility profile.

Patient education

A health care team member should explain the specimen collection procedure to the patient. If the patient is seriously ill, the team member should explain the procedure to the patient's family members. The patient and his or her family should understand that because bacteria need time to grow in the laboratory, several days may be required for bacterium identification.

Resources

BOOKS

Anel, Ramon L. and R. Phillip Dellinger. "Sepsis and Bacteremia." In *Conn's Current Therapy 2001,* edited by Robert E. Rakel and Edward T. Bope. Philadelphia: W.B. Saunders Company, 2001, pp.56–62.

Fischbach, Frances. "Blood Cultures." In *A Manual of Laboratory & Diagnostic Tests.* 6th ed. Philadelphia: Lippincott Williams & Wilkins, 2000, pp.542–545.

Henry, J.B. *Clinical Diagnosis and Management by Laboratory Methods.* 20th ed. New York: W.B.Saunders Company, 2001.

GALE ENCYCLOPEDIA OF SURGERY

49

Wallach, Jacques. *Interpretation of Diagnostic Tests.* 7th ed. Philadelphia, PA: Lippincott Williams & Wilkens, 2000.

PERIODICALS

Brook, Itzhak. "Anaerobic Infections in Children." *Advances in Pediatrics* 47 (2000): 395–437.

ORGANIZATIONS

The American Society for Microbiology. 1752 N St. N.W., Washington, DC 20036. (202) 737-3600. <http://www.asmusa.org>.

National Center for Infectious Disease, Centers for Disease Control and Prevention. 1600 Clifton Road NE, Atlanta, GA 30333. (800) 311-3435. <http://www.cdc.gov>.

OTHER

National Institutes of Health. [cited April 5, 2003] <http://www.nlm.nih.gov/medlineplus/encyclopedia.html>.

Linda D. Jones, BA, PBT (ASCP)
Mark A. Best, M.D., MPH, MBA

Analgesia, patient-controlled *see* **Patient-controlled analgesia**

Analgesics

Definition

Analgesics are medicines that relieve pain.

Purpose

The primary classes of analgesics are the narcotics, including additional agents that are chemically based on the morphine molecule but have minimal abuse potential; **nonsteroidal anti-inflammatory drugs** (NSAIDs) including the salicylates; and **acetaminophen**. Other drugs, notably the tricyclic antidepressants and anti-epileptic agents such as gabapentin, have been used to relieve pain, particularly neurologic pain, but are not routinely classified as analgesics. Analgesics provide symptomatic relief, but generally have no effect on causation.

Description

Pain has been classified as "productive" pain and "non-productive" pain. While this distinction has no physiologic meaning, it may serve as a guide to treatment. "Productive" pain has been described as a warning of injury, and so may be both an indication of need for treatment and a guide to diagnosis. "Non-productive" pain by definition serves no purpose either as a warning or diagnostic tool.

Although pain syndromes may be dissimilar, the common factor is a sensory pathway from the affected organ to the brain. Analgesics work at the level of the nerves, either by blocking the signal from the peripheral nervous system, or by distorting the interpretation by the central nervous system. Selection of an appropriate analgesic is based on consideration of the risk-benefit factors of each class of drugs, based on type of pain, severity of pain, and risk of adverse effects. Traditionally, pain has been divided into two classes, acute and chronic, although severity and projected patient survival are other factors that must be considered in drug selection.

Acute pain

Acute pain is self limiting in duration, and includes post-operative pain, pain of injury, and childbirth. Because pain of these types is expected to be short term, the long-term side effects of analgesic therapy may routinely be ignored. Thus, these patients may safely be treated with narcotic analgesics without concern for their addictive potential, or NSAIDs with only limited concern for their ulcerogenic risks. Drugs and doses should be adjusted based on observation of healing rate, switching patients from high to low doses, and from narcotic analgesics to non-narcotics when circumstances permit.

An important consideration of **pain management** in severe pain is that patients should not be subject to the return of pain. Analgesics should be dosed adequately to assure that the pain is at least tolerable, and frequently enough to avoid the anxiety that accompanies the anticipated return of pain. Analgesics should never be dosed on a "prn" (as needed) basis, but should be administered often enough to assure constant blood levels of analgesic. This applies to both the narcotic and non-narcotic analgesics.

Chronic pain

Chronic pain, pain lasting over three months and severe enough to impair function, is more difficult to treat, since the anticipated side effects of the analgesics are more difficult to manage. In the case of narcotic analgesics this means the addiction potential, as well as respiratory depression and constipation. For the NSAIDs, the risk of gastric ulcers may be dose limiting. While some classes of drugs, such as the narcotic agonist/antagonist drugs bupronophine, nalbuphine and pentazocine, and the selective COX-2 inhibitors celecoxib and rofecoxib represent advances in reduction of adverse effects, they are still not fully suitable for long-term management of severe pain. Generally, chronic pain management requires a combination of drug therapy, life-style modification, and other treatment modalities.

Narcotic analgesics

The narcotic analgesics, also termed opioids, are all derived from opium. The class includes morphine, codeine, and a number of semi-synthetics including meperidine (Demerol), propoxyphen (Darvon), and others. The narcotic analgesics vary in potency, but all are effective in treatment of pain when used in adequate doses. Adverse effects are dose related. Because these drugs are all addictive, they are controlled under federal and state laws. A variety of dosage forms are available, including oral solids, liquids, intravenous and intrathecal injections, and transcutaneous patches.

NSAIDs, non-steroidal anti-inflammatory drugs, are effective analgesics even at doses too low to have any anti-inflammatory effects. There are a number of chemical classes, but all have similar therapeutic effects and side effects. Most are appropriate only for oral administration; however ketorolac (Toradol) is appropriate for injection and may be used for moderate to severe pain for short periods.

Acetaminophen is a non-narcotic analgesic with no anti-inflammatory properties. It is appropriate for mild to moderate pain. Although the drug is well tolerated in normal doses, it may have significant toxicity at high doses. Because acetaminophen is largely free of side effects at therapeutic doses, it has been considered the first choice for mild pain, including that of osteoarthritis.

Recommended dosage

Appropriate dosage varies by drug, and should consider the type of pain, as well as other risks associated with patient age and condition. For example, narcotic analgesics should usually be avoided in patients with a history of substance abuse, but may be fully appropriate in patients with cancer pain. Similarly, because narcotics are more rapidly metabolized in patients who have used these drugs for a long period, higher than normal doses may be needed to provide adequate pain management. NSAIDs, although comparatively safe in adults, represent an increased risk of gastrointestinal bleeding in patients over the age of 60.

Precautions

Narcotic analgesics may be contraindicated in patients with respiratory depression. NSAIDs may be hazardous to patients with ulcers or an ulcer history. They should be used with care for patients with renal insufficiency or coagulation disorders. NSAIDs are contraindicated in patients allergic to **aspirin**.

KEY TERMS

Acute pain—Pain that is usually temporary and results from something specific, such as a surgery, an injury, or an infection.

Analgesic—Medicine used to relieve pain.

Chronic pain—Pain that lasts more than three months and threatens to disrupt daily life.

Dose limiting—Case in which the side effects of a drug prevent an increase in dose

Inflammation—Pain, redness, swelling, and heat that usually develops in response to injury or illness.

Side effects

Adverse effects of each drug vary individually. Drugs within a class may vary in their frequency and severity of adverse effects.

The primary adverse effects of the narcotic analgesics are addiction, constipation, and respiratory depression. Because narcotic analgesics stimulate the production of enzymes that cause the metabolism of these drugs, patients on narcotics for a prolonged period may require increasing doses. This is not the same thing as addiction, and is not a reason for withholding medication from patients in severe pain.

NSAIDs are ulcerogenic and may cause kidney problems. Gastrointestinal discomfort is common, although in some cases, these drugs may cause ulcers without the prior warning of gastrointestinal distress. Platelet aggregation problems may occur, although not to the same extent as if seen with aspirin.

Interactions

Interactions depend on the specific type of analgesic. See specific references or ask a physician.

Resources

BOOKS

Brody, T. M., J. Larner, K. P. Minneman, and H. C. Neu. *Human Pharmacology: Molecular to Clinical, 2nd ed.* St. Louis: Mosby Year-Book, 1998.

Griffith, H. W. and S. Moore. *2001 Complete Guide to Prescription and Nonprescription Drugs.* New York: Berkely Publishing Group, 2001.

OTHER

"Acetaminophen." Federal Drug Administration. Center for Drug Evaluation and Research [cited May 2003]. <http://

---

www.fda.gov/cder/foi/nda/2000/75077_Acetaminophen. pdf>.

"Acetaminophen." Medline Plus Drug Information [cited May 2003]. <http://www.nlm.nih.gov/medlineplus/druginfo/medmaster/a681004.html>.

"Anti-inflammatories, nonsteroidal." Medline Plus Drug Information [cited June 25 2003]. <http://www.nlm.nih.gov/medlineplus/druginfo/uspdi/202743.html>.

"Narcotic analgesics for pain relief." Medline Plus Drug Information [cited June 25 2003]. <http://www.nlm.nih.gov/medlineplus/druginfo/uspdi/202390.html>.

Samuel Uretsky, PharmD

Analgesics, opioid

Definition

Opioid **analgesics**, also known as narcotic analgesics, are pain relievers that act on the central nervous system. Like all narcotics, they may become habit-forming if used over long periods.

Purpose

Opioid analgesics are used to relieve pain from a variety of conditions. Some are used before or during surgery (including dental surgery), both to relieve pain and to make anesthetics work more effectively. They may also be used for the same purposes during labor and delivery.

Description

Opioid analgesics relieve pain by acting directly on the central nervous system. However, this can also lead to unwanted side effects, such as drowsiness, dizziness, breathing problems, and physical or mental dependence.

Among the drugs in this category are codeine; propoxyphene (Darvon); propoxyphene and **acetaminophen** (Darvocet N); meperidine (Demerol); hydromorphone (Dilaudid); morphine; oxycodone; oxycodone and acetaminophen (Percocet, Roxicet); and hydrocodone and acetaminophen (Lortab, Anexsia). These drugs come in many forms—tablets, syrups, suppositories, and injections—and are sold only by prescription. For some, a new prescription is required for each new supply; refills are prohibited, according to federal regulations.

Recommended dosage

Recommended doses vary, depending on the type of opioid analgesic and the form in which it is being used.

Doses may be different for different patients. The person should check with the physician who prescribed the drug or the pharmacist who filled the prescription for correct dosages, and to understand how to take the drug.

A patient should always take opioid analgesics exactly as directed. Larger or more frequent doses should never be taken, and the drug should not be taken for longer than directed. The person should not stop taking the drug suddenly without checking with the physician or dentist who prescribed it. Gradually tapering the dose may reduce the risk of withdrawal symptoms.

For pain following major surgery, it is common practice to give narcotic analgesics by intravenous injection for the first 24–48 hours. This may be followed by oral narcotics for the next 24–48 hours, and then nonnarcotic analgesics.

Many hospitals use **patient-controlled analgesia** (PCA), a system in which the analgesics are given intravenously (by vein), and the patient can control the dose by pushing a button on a pump. This system lets the patient have more control over the amount of medication needed to relieve pain, and eliminates the anxiety that comes from expecting the return of pain when the dose wears off.

Precautions

Anyone who uses opioid analgesics—or any narcotic—over a long time may become physically or mentally dependent on the drug. Physical dependence may lead to withdrawal symptoms when the person stops taking the medicine. Building tolerance to these drugs is also possible when they are used for a long period. The need for larger and more frequent doses is due to enzyme induction, in which narcotics are metabolized by the liver and changed to a form that can be eliminated from the body. The metabolism of narcotics relies on enzymes that are produced by the liver. As narcotics are used, the liver produces more and more of these enzymes, so that a dose of pain medication is removed from the body more rapidly. This is not a problem when narcotics are used for surgical pain, since this type of pain only lasts for a short time.

Opiod analgesics should be taken exactly as directed. It is not advised to take more than the recommended dose, or more often than directed. If the drugs do not seem to be working, the physician should be consulted. These drugs (or any other prescription drugs) should never be shared with others because the drug may have a completely different effect on different people.

Children and older people are especially sensitive to opioid analgesics and may have serious breathing problems after taking them. Children may also become un-

Opioid analgesics

Drug	Route of administration	Onset of action (min)	Time to peak effect (min)	Duration of action (h)
Strong agonists				
Fentanyl (Sublimaze)	IM	7–15	20–30	1–2
	IV	1–2	3–5	0.5–1
Hydromorphone (Dilaudid)	Oral	30	90–120	4
	IM	15		
	IV	10–15	30–60	2–3
	Sub-Q	30		15–30
Levorphanol (Levo-Dromoran)	Oral	10–60	90–120	4–5
	IM			
	IV	—	60	4–5
	Sub-Q	10–60	within 20	
Meperidine (Demerol)	Oral	15	60–90	2–4
	IM	10–15		
	IV		30–50	2–4
	Sub-Q	1		
Methadone (Dolophine)	Oral	30–60	90–120	4–6
	IM			
	IV	10–20	60–120	4–5
Morphine (many trade names)	Oral	—	60–120	4–5
	IM	10–30		
	IV		30–60	4–5
	Sub-Q	—		
	Epidural	10–30	20	4–5
Oxymorphone (Numorphan)	IM	10–15	30–90	3–6
	IV			
	Sub-Q	5–10	15–30	3–4
	Rectal			
Mild-to-moderate agonists				
Codiene (many trade names)	Oral	30–40	60–120	4
	Im	10–30	30–60	4
	Sub-Q	10–30		4
Hydrocodone (Hycodan)	Oral	10–30	30–60	4–6
Oxycodone (Percodan)	Oral	—	60	3–4
Propoxyphene (Darvon, Dolene)	Oral	15–60	120	4–6
Butophanol (Stadol)	IM	10–30	30–60	3–4
	IV	2–3	30	2–4
Nalbuphine (Nubian)	IM	within 15	60	3–6
	IV	2–3	30	3–4
	Sub-Q	within 15	—	3–6
Pentazocine (Talwin)	Oral	15–30	60–90	3
	IM	15–20	30–60	2–3
	IV	2–3	15–30	2–3
	Sub-Q	15–20	30–60	2–3

usually restless or agitated when given these drugs. These problems can be controlled by adjusting the dose of medication to a safer level.

Opioid analgesics increase the effects of alcohol. Anyone taking these drugs should not drink alcoholic beverages. Some of these drugs may also contain **aspirin**, caffeine, or acetaminophen. A person should refer to the entries on each of these drugs for additional precautions.

Special conditions

People with certain medical conditions or who are taking certain other medicines can have problems if they take opioid analgesics. Before prescribing these drugs, the physician should be informed of any of these conditions.

ALLERGIES. The patient should let the physician know about any allergies to foods, dyes, preservatives, or other substances, and about any previous reactions to opioid analgesics.

PREGNANCY. Women who are pregnant or plan to become pregnant while taking opioid analgesics should let their physicians know. No evidence exists that these drugs cause birth defects in people, but some do cause birth defects and other problems when given to pregnant animals in experiments. Babies can become dependent on opioid analgesics if their mothers use too much during pregnancy. This can cause the baby to go through withdrawal symptoms after birth. If taken just before delivery, some opioid analgesics may cause serious breathing problems in the newborn.

BREASTFEEDING. Some opioid analgesics can pass into breast milk. Women who are breastfeeding should check with their physicians about the safety of taking these drugs.

OTHER MEDICAL CONDITIONS. These conditions may influence the effects of opioid analgesics:

- head injury (The effects of some opioid analgesics may be stronger and may interfere with recovery in people with head injuries.)

- history of convulsions (Some of these drugs may trigger convulsions.)

- asthma, emphysema, or any chronic lung disease

- heart disease

- kidney disease

- liver disease

- underactive thyroid (The chance of side effects may be greater.)

- Addison's disease (a disease of the adrenal glands)

- colitis

- gallbladder disease or gallstones (Side effects can be dangerous in people with these conditions.)

- enlarged prostate or other urinary problems

- current or past alcohol abuse

- current or past drug abuse, especially narcotic abuse

- current or past emotional problems (The chance of side effects may be greater.)

USE OF CERTAIN MEDICINES. Taking opioid narcotics with certain other drugs may increase the chances of serious side effects. In some cases, the physician may combine narcotic analgesics with other drugs that increase the activity of the analgesic. These include some sedatives, tranquilizers, and antihistamines. When these drugs are used together with narcotic analgesics, it may be possible to get the same pain relief with a lower dose of narcotic.

Side effects

Some people experience drowsiness, dizziness, lightheadedness, or a false sense of well-being after taking opioid analgesics. Anyone who takes these drugs should not drive, use machinery, or do anything else that might be dangerous until they know how the drug affects them. Nausea and vomiting are common side effects, especially when first beginning to take the medicine. If these symptoms do not go away after the first few doses, the person should check with the physician or dentist who prescribed the medicine.

Dry mouth is another common side effect, which can be relieved by sucking on sugarless hard candy or ice chips or by chewing sugarless gum. Saliva substitutes, which come in liquid or tablet forms, may also help. Patients who must use opioid analgesics over long periods and who have dry mouth should see their dentists, as the problem can lead to tooth decay and other dental problems.

The following side effects are less common. They usually do not need medical attention and will go away after the first few doses. If they continue or interfere with normal activity, the patient should check with the physician who prescribed the medicine for:

- headache

- loss of appetite

- restlessness or nervousness

- nightmares, unusual dreams, or problems sleeping

- weakness or tiredness

- mental sluggishness

- stomach pain or cramps

- blurred or double vision or other vision problems

- problems urinating such as pain, difficulty urinating, frequent urge to urinate, or decreased amount of urine

- constipation

Other side effects may be more serious and may require quick medical attention. These symptoms could be signs of an overdose. The person should get emergency medical care immediately:

- cold, clammy skin

- bluish discoloration of the skin

- extremely small pupils

- serious difficulty breathing or extremely slow breathing

- extreme sleepiness or unresponsiveness

- severe weakness

- confusion

- severe dizziness

- severe drowsiness

- slow heartbeat

- low blood pressure

- severe nervousness or restlessness

In addition, the following less-common side effects do not require emergency medical care, but should have medical attention as soon as possible, and include:

- hallucinations, or a sense of unreality

- depression or other mood changes

KEY TERMS

Analgesic—Medicine used to relieve pain.

Central nervous system—The brain, spinal cord, and nerves throughout the body.

Colitis—Inflammation of the colon (large bowel).

Enzyme—A protein, produced by cells, that causes chemical changes in other substances.

Hallucination—A false or distorted perception of objects, sounds, or events that seem real. Hallucinations usually result from drugs or mental disorders.

Inflammation—Pain, redness, swelling, and heat that usually develop in response to injury or illness.

Metabolize—The chemical changes that occur in the body, including the changes that occur in the liver, converting molecules to forms that are more easily removed from the body.

Narcotic—A drug derived from opium or compounds similar to opium. Such drugs are potent pain relievers and can affect mood and behavior. Long-term use of narcotics can lead to dependence and tolerance.

Tolerance—A decrease in sensitivity to a drug. When tolerance occurs, a person must take more and more of the drug to get the same effect.

Withdrawal symptoms—A group of physical or mental symptoms that may occur when a person suddenly stops using a drug to which he or she has become dependent.

- ringing or buzzing in the ears

- pounding or unusually fast heartbeat

- itching, hives, or rash

- facial swelling

- trembling or twitching

- dark urine, pale stools, or yellow eyes or skin (after taking propoxyphene)

- increased sweating, red or flushed face (more common after taking hydrocodone and meperidine)

Interactions

Anyone taking the following drugs should notify his or her physician before taking opioid analgesics:

- central nervous system (CNS) depressants such as antihistamines and other medicines for allergies, hay fever, or colds; tranquilizers; some other prescription pain relievers; seizure medicines; sleeping pills; some anesthetics (including dental anesthetics)

- monoamine oxidase (MAO) inhibitors such as phenelzine (Nardil) and tranylcypromine (Parnate) (The combination of the opioid analgesic meperidine [Demerol] and MAO inhibitors is especially dangerous.)

- tricyclic antidepressants such as amitriptyline (Elavil)

- anti-seizure medicines such as carbamazepine (Tegretol) (They may lead to serious side effects, including coma, when combined with propoxyphene and acetaminophen [Darvocet-N] or propoxyphene [Darvon].)

- muscle relaxants such as cyclobenzaprine (Flexeril)

- sleeping pills such as triazolam (Halcion)

- blood-thinning drugs such as warfarin (Coumadin)

- Naltrexone (Trexan, Revia) (It cancels the effects of opioid analgesics.)

- Rifampin (Rifadin)

- Zidovudine (AZT, Retrovir) (It causes serious side effects when combined with morphine.)

Resources

BOOKS

AHFS: Drug Information. Washington, DC: American Society Healthsystems Pharmaceuticals, 2002.

Drug Facts and Comparisons. St. Louis: Facts & Comparisons, 2003.

Reynolds, J.E.F., ed. *Martindale: The Extra Pharmacopeia*, 31st ed. London: The Pharmaceutical Press, 1993.

OTHER

"Narcotic Analgesics for Surgery and Obstetrics (Systemic)." Medline Plus Drug Information. [cited May 2003] <http://www.nlm.nih.gov/medlineplus/druginfo/uspdi/202391.html>.

Nancy Ross-Flanigan
Sam Uretsky, PharmD

Anesthesia evaluation

Definition

Anesthesia evaluation refers to the series of interviews, physical examinations, and laboratory tests that are generally used in North America and western Europe to assess the general fitness of patients scheduled for surgery and to determine the need for special precautions or additional testing. There is no universally accepted definition of anesthesia evaluation as of 2003; however, the Task Force on Preanesthesia Evaluation of the American Society of Anesthesiologists (ASA) has tentatively defined it as "....the process of clinical assessment that precedes the delivery of anesthesia care for surgery and for non-surgical procedures." Anesthesia evaluation is usually discussed in the context of elective or scheduled surgical procedures rather than **emergency surgery**.

Anesthesia evaluation is a relatively recent development in preoperative patient care. Prior to the 1970s, anesthesiologists were often given only brief notes or outlines of the patient's history and **physical examination** written by the operating surgeon or the patient's internist. This approach became increasingly unsatisfactory as the practice of anesthesiology became more complex. In the last four decades, the introduction of new anesthetics and other medications, laser-assisted surgical procedures, increasingly sophisticated monitoring equipment, and new discoveries in molecular biochemistry and genetics have made the **anesthesiologist's role** more demanding. During the 1980s and 1990s, some departments of anesthesiology in large urban medical centers and major university teaching hospitals began to set up separate clinics for anesthesia evaluation in order to improve the assessment of patients before surgery.

Purpose

Anesthesia evaluation has several different purposes. The information that is obtained during the evaluation may be used to:

- Guide the selection of anesthetics and other medications to be used during surgery.

- Plan for the patient's postoperative recovery and pain management.

- Educate the patient about the operation itself, the possible outcomes, and self-care during recovery at home.

- Determine the need for additional staff during or after surgery.

- Minimize confusion caused by rescheduling operations because of last-minute discoveries about patients' health.

- Improve patient safety and quality of care by collecting data for later review and analysis. The ASA has noted that few controlled trials of different approaches to anesthesia evaluation have been conducted as of 2003, and that further research is needed.

Description

There are several parts or stages in a typical anesthesia evaluation. The evaluation itself may be done in the hospital where the operation is scheduled, or in a separate facility attached to the hospital. The timing of the evaluation is affected by two major variables: the invasiveness of the operation to be performed and the patient's overall physical condition. An invasive operation or procedure is one that requires the surgeon to insert a needle, catheter, or instrument into the body or a part of the body. Surgical procedures are classified as high, medium, or low in invasiveness. Procedures that involve opening the chest, abdomen, or skull are usually considered highly invasive. Examples of less invasive procedures would include **tooth extraction**, most forms of cosmetic surgery, and operations on the hands and feet.

The patient's physical condition is classified according to the ASA's six-point system as follows:

- P1. Normal healthy patient.
- P2. Patient with mild systemic disease.
- P3. Patient with severe systemic disease.
- P4. Patient with severe systemic disease that is life-threatening.
- P5. Moribund (dying) patient who is not expected to survive without an operation.
- P6. Brain-dead patient whose organs are being removed for donation.

As of 2003, the ASA recommends that patients with severe disease be interviewed and have their physical examination before the day of surgery. Patients in good health or with mild systemic disease who are scheduled for a highly invasive procedure should also be interviewed and examined before the day of surgery. Patients in categories P1 and P2 who are scheduled for low- or medium-invasive procedures may be evaluated on the day of surgery or before it.

Patient history and records

The first part of an anesthesia evaluation is the anesthesiologist's review of the patient's medical history and records. This review allows the anesthesiologist to evaluate the patient for risk factors that may increase the patient's sensitivity to the sedatives or other medications given before and during the operation; increase the danger of complications related to heart function and breathing; and increase the difficulty of treating such complications.

These risk factors may include:

- Heart or lung disease. These diseases often require the anesthesiologist to lower the dosages of sedatives and pain-control medications.

- Liver or kidney disease. Disorders of these organs often slow down the rate of medication clearance from the patient's body.

- Present prescription medications. These may interact with the sedatives given before the operation or with the anesthetic agent.

- Herbal preparations and other alternative medicines. Some herbal preparations, particularly those taken for insomnia or anxiety (St. John's wort, valerian, kava kava) may intensify the effects of anesthetics. Others, like ginseng or gingko biloba, may affect blood pressure or blood clotting. It is important for patients to include alternative health products in the list of medications that they give the doctor.

- Allergies, particularly allergies to medications.

- Alcohol or substance abuse. Substance use typically affects patients' responses to sedatives and anesthetics in one of two ways. If the patient has developed a tolerance for alcohol or another drug of abuse, he or she may require an increased dose of sedatives or pain medications. On the other hand, if the patient has recently consumed a large amount of alcohol or other mood-altering substance, it may interact with the anesthetic by intensifying its effects.

- Smoking. Smoking increases the risk of coughing, bronchospasm, or other airway problems during the operation.

- Previous adverse reactions to sedatives or anesthetics. A family history of anesthesia problems should be included because some adverse reactions are genetically determined.

- Age. The elderly and children below the age of puberty do not respond to medications in the same way as adults, and the anesthesiologist must often adjust dosages. In addition, elderly patients often take a number of different prescription medications, each of which may interact with anesthetics in a different way.

Patient interview

The anesthesiologist is responsible for interviewing the patient during the anesthesia evaluation. The interview serves in part as additional verification of the patient's identity; cases have been reported in which patients have been scheduled for the wrong procedure because of administrative errors. The anesthesiologist will check the patient's name, date of birth, medical record number, and type or location of scheduled surgery for any inconsistencies. Although the anesthesiologist will ask for some of the same information that is included in the patient's written medical records, he or she may have additional questions. Moreover, it is not unusual for pa-

tients to recall significant events or details during the interview that were left out of the written records. The anesthesiologist will explain what will happen during the operation and give instructions about fasting, discontinuing medications, and other precautions that the patient should take before the procedure. The patient will have an opportunity to ask questions about choice of anesthetic and other concerns during the interview.

Physical examination

The physical examination will focus on three primary areas of concern: the heart and circulatory system; the respiratory system; and the patient's airway. Heart and lung function are evaluated because surgery under general anesthesia puts these organ systems under considerable stress. The usual tests performed to evaluate heart and lung fitness are an electrocardiogram (ECG) and chest x-ray (CXR). These tests may be omitted if the patient was tested within the previous six months and the results were normal. If the patient has an ECG and CXR as part of the anesthesia evaluation and the findings are abnormal, the doctor may order additional tests of heart and lung function. These may include stress or **exercise** tests; **echocardiography**; **angiography**; pulmonary function tests (PFTs); and a computed tomography (CT) scan of the lungs.

Assessment of the airway includes an examination of the patient's teeth, nasal passages, mouth, and throat to check for any signs of disease or structural abnormalities. Certain physical features, such as an abnormally shaped windpipe, prominent upper incisor teeth, an abnormally small mouth opening, a short or inflexible neck, a throat infection, large or swollen tonsils, and a protruding or receding chin can all increase the risk of airway problems during the operation. A commonly used classification scheme rates patients on a four-point scale, with Class I being the least likely to have airway problems under anesthesia and Class IV the most likely.

Laboratory tests

Laboratory tests are categorized as either routine, meaning that they are given to all patients as part of the anesthesia evaluation, or indicated, which means that the test is ordered for a specific reason for a particular patient. Routine preoperative laboratory tests include blood tests and urine tests. Blood samples are taken for white and red blood cell counts and coagulation studies; tests of kidney function, most commonly measurements of blood urea nitrogen (BUN) and creatinine; and measurements of blood glucose and electrolyte levels. Urine samples are taken to evaluate the patient's nutritional status, to test for diabetes or the presence of a urinary tract infection, and to determine whether the patient is dehydrated. Some hospitals will accept blood and urine tests performed within six weeks of the operation if the results were within normal ranges. Some facilities also routinely test urine samples from women of childbearing age for pregnancy.

Indicated laboratory tests include platelet counts, certain blood chemistry measurements, and measurements of blood hemoglobin levels. These tests are usually performed for patients with blood or endocrine disorders; persons taking blood-thinning medications; persons who have been treated with some types of alternative therapy; and persons who are known to have kidney or liver disorders.

Consultations

The anesthesiologist may consult other doctors as part of the anesthesia evaluation in order to obtain additional information about the patient's condition. Consultations are often necessary if the patient is very young or very old; is being treated for cancer; or has a rare disease or disorder.

Preparation

Patients can prepare for an anesthesia evaluation by gathering information beforehand to give the hospital or clinic staff. This information includes such matters as insurance cards and documentation; a list of medications presently taken and their dosages; a list of previous operations or hospitalizations, if any; the names and telephone numbers of other physicians who have been consulted within the past two years; information about allergies to medications, if any; the name and telephone number of a designated family member or primary contact; and similar matters.

See also Anesthesiologist's role; Preoperative care.

Resources

BOOKS

Catania, Robert M., MD. *A Patient Guide to Surgery.* 1999. Available for download without charge at <www.preopguide.com>.

PERIODICALS

American Society of Anesthesiologists Task Force on Preanesthesia Evaluation. "Practice Advisory for Preanesthesia Evaluation." *Anesthesiology* 96 (February 2002): 485–496.

Karim, A. and M. Esteve. "Specific Aspects of the Pre-Anesthetic Consultation in Patients with Cancer." [in French] *Bulletin du Cancer* 89 (June 2002): 612–618.

Larson, Merlin, MD. "Waters, Guedel, and the Pre-Anesthetic Evaluation." *California Society of Anesthesiologists Bulletin* 51 (January-March 2002): 69–75.

Lignau, W. and H. U. Strohmenger. "Responsibility of the Anaesthesiologist in the Preoperative Risk Evaluation."

KEY TERMS

Anesthesiologist—A doctor of medicine (MD) or osteopathy (DO) who has completed advanced training in administering anesthesia and monitoring patients' well-being during surgery. Many anesthesiologists have completed additional training in critical care medicine or pain management.

Bronchospasm—A spasmodic contraction of the muscles that line the two branches of the trachea that lead into the lungs, causing difficulty in breathing. Bronchospasm is a common complication in heavy smokers under anesthesia.

Clearance—The rate at which a drug or other substance is removed from the blood by the liver or kidneys.

Indicated test—A test that is given for a specific clinical reason.

Invasiveness—A term that refers to the extent of surgical intrusion into the body or a part of the body. An invasive procedure is one that requires the insertion of a needle, catheter, or surgical instrument.

Nurse anesthetist—A registered nurse who has obtained advanced training in anesthesia delivery and patient care.

Routine test—A medical test performed on all patients without regard to specific medical conditions.

Sedative—A type of medication given to calm or relax patients before surgery.

[in German] *Der Anaesthesist* 51 (September 2002): 704–715.

Michota, F. A. and F. D. Frost. "Perioperative Management of the Hospitalized Patient." *Medical Clinics of North America* 86 (July 2002): 731–748.

Tobias, J. D. "Anesthesia for Minimally Invasive Surgery in Children." *Best Practice and Research: Clinical Anesthesiology* 16 (March 2002): 115–130.

ORGANIZATIONS

American Association of Nurse Anesthetists (AANA). 222 South Prospect Avenue, Park Ridge, IL 60068-4001. (847) 692-7050. <www.aana.com>.

American Society of Anesthesiologists (ASA). 520 N. Northwest Highway, Park Ridge, IL 60068-2573. (847) 825-5586. <www.asahq.org>.

Anesthesia Patient Safety Foundation (APSF). 4246 Colonial Park Drive, Pittsburgh, PA 15227-2621. (412) 882-8040. <www.gasnet.org/societies/apsf>.

OTHER

American Society of Anesthesiologists. *Guidelines for Patient Care in Anesthesiology.* Approved by ASA House of Delegates on October 3, 1967; last amended, October 17, 2001 [cited February 20, 2003]. <www.asahq.org/publicationsAndServices/standards/13.html>.

Hata, Tara, MD, Ellen J. Nickel, Pharm. D., Bradley Hinman, MD, and Douglas Morgan, RPh. *Guidelines, Education, and Testing for Procedural Sedation and Analgesia.* Iowa City, IA: University of Iowa Hospitals and Clinics, 2001.

Phillips, Chester, MD. "Pre-Anesthesia Evaluation and Data Capture." *Anesthesia Patient Safety Foundation Newsletter* 16 (Summer, 2001) [cited February 16, 2003]. <www.gasnet.org/societies/apsf/newsletter/>.

Rooke, G. Alec, MD, PhD, editor. *Syllabus on Geriatric Anesthesiology.* Park Ridge, IL: American Society of Anesthesiologists, 2001.

Rebecca Frey, Ph.D.

Anesthesia, general

Definition

General anesthesia is the induction of a balanced state of unconsciousness, accompanied by the absence of pain sensation and the paralysis of skeletal muscle over the entire body. It is induced through the administration of anesthetic drugs and is used during major surgery and other invasive surgical procedures.

Purpose

General anesthesia is intended to bring about five distinct states during surgery:

• analgesia, or pain relief

• amnesia, or loss of memory of the procedure

• loss of consciousness

• motionlessness

• weakening of autonomic responses

Precautions

A complete medical history, including a history of allergies in family members, is an important precaution. Patients may have a potentially fatal allergic response to anesthesia known as malignant hyperthermia, even if there is no previous personal history of reaction.

General anesthetics should be administered only by board-certified medical professionals. Anesthesia providers consider many factors, including a patient's age, weight, allergies to medications, medical history, and general health when deciding which anesthetic or combination of anesthetics to use. The American Society of Anesthesiologists has compiled guidelines for classifying patients according to risk levels as follows:

• I: healthy patient

• II: patient with mild systemic disease without functional limitations

• III: patient with severe systemic disease with definite functional limitations

• IV: patient with severe systemic disease that is life-threatening

• V: dying patient not expected to survive for 24 hours without an operation

Equipment for general anesthesia should be thoroughly checked before the operation; all items that might be needed, such as extra tubes or laryngoscope blades, should be available. Staff members should be knowledgeable about the problems that might arise with the specific anesthetic being used, and be able to recognize them and respond appropriately. General anesthetics cause a lowering of the blood pressure (hypotension), a response that requires close monitoring and special drugs to reverse it in emergency situations.

Description

General anesthetics may be gases or volatile liquids that evaporate as they are inhaled through a mask along with oxygen. Other general anesthetics are given intravenously. The amount of anesthesia produced by inhaling a general anesthetic can be adjusted rapidly, if necessary, by adjusting the anesthetic-to-oxygen ratio that is inhaled by the patient. The degree of anesthesia produced by an intravenously injected anesthetic cannot be changed as rapidly and must be reversed by administration of another drug.

The precise mechanism of general anesthesia is not yet fully understood. There are, however, several hypotheses that have been advanced to explain why general anesthesia occurs. The first, the so-called Meyer-Overton theory, suggests that anesthesia occurs when a sufficient number of molecules of an inhalation anesthetic dissolve in the lipid cell membrane. The second theory maintains that protein receptors in the central nervous system are involved, in that inhalation anesthetics inhibit the enzyme activity of proteins. A third hypothesis, proposed by Linus Pauling in 1961, suggests that anesthetic molecules interact with water molecules to form clathrates (hydrated microcrystals), which in turn inhibit receptor function.

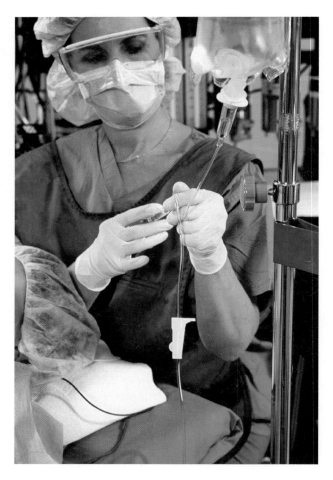

A nurse anesthetist injecting medication into the intra-venous tube of a patient during surgery. *(Photo Researchers Inc. Reproduced by permission.)*

Stages of anesthesia

There are four stages of general anesthesia that help providers to better predict the course of events, from anesthesia induction to emergence.

• Stage I begins with the induction of anesthesia and ends with the patient's loss of consciousness. The patient still feels pain in Stage I.

• Stage II, or REM stage, includes uninhibited and sometimes dangerous responses to stimuli, including vomiting and uncontrolled movement. This stage is typically shortened by administering a barbiturate, such as sodium pentothal, before the anesthetic agent.

• Stage III, or surgical anesthesia, is the stage in which the patient's pupillary gaze is central and the pupils are constricted. This is the target depth of surgical anesthesia. During this stage, the skeletal muscles relax, the patient's breathing becomes regular, and eye movements stop.

• Stage IV, or overdose, is marked by hypotension or circulatory failure. Death may result if the patient cannot be revived quickly.

Types of anesthetic agents

There are two major types of anesthetics used for general anesthesia, inhalation and intravenous anesthetics. Inhalation anesthetics, which are sometimes called volatile anesthetics, are compounds that enter the body through the lungs and are carried by the blood to body tissues. Inhalation anesthetics are less often used alone in recent clinical practice; they are usually used together with intravenous anesthetics. A combination of inhalation and intravenous anesthetics, often with opioids added for pain relief and neuromuscular blockers for muscle paralysis, is called balanced anesthesia.

INHALATION ANESTHETICS. The following are the most commonly used inhalation anesthetics:

• Halothane causes unconsciousness but provides little pain relief; often administered with **analgesics**. It may be toxic to the liver in adults. Halothane, however, has a pleasant smell and is therefore often the anesthetic of choice when mask induction is used with children.

• Enflurane is less potent, but produces a rapid onset of anesthesia and possibly a faster recovery. Enflurane is not used in patients with kidney failure.

• Isoflurane is not toxic to the liver but can induce irregular heart rhythms.

• Nitrous oxide (laughing gas) is used with other such drugs as thiopental to produce surgical anesthesia. It has the fastest induction and recovery time. It is regarded as the safest inhalation anesthetic because it does not slow respiration or blood flow to the brain. However, because nitrous oxide is a relatively weak anesthetic, it is not suited for use in major surgery. Although it may be used alone for dental anesthesia, it should not be used as a primary agent in more extensive procedures.

• Sevoflurane works quickly and can be administered through a mask since it does not irritate the airway. On the other hand, one of the breakdown products of sevoflurane can cause renal damage.

• Desflurane, a second-generation version of isoflurane, is irritating to the airway and therefore cannot be used for mask (inhalation) inductions, especially not in children. Desflurane causes an increase in heart rate, and so should be avoided for patients with heart problems. Its advantage is that it provides a rapid awakening with few adverse effects.

INTRAVENOUS ANESTHETICS. Commonly administered intravenous general anesthetics include ketamine, thiopental (a barbiturate), methohexital (Brevital), etomidate, and propofol (Diprivan). Ketamine produces a different set of reactions from other intravenous anesthetics. It resembles phencyclidine, which is a street drug that may cause hallucinations. Because patients who have been anesthetized with ketamine often have sensory illusions and vivid dreams during post-operative recovery, ketamine is not often given to adult patients. It is, however, useful in anesthetizing children, patients in shock, and trauma casualties in war zones where anesthesia equipment may be difficult to obtain.

General anesthesia in dental procedures

The use of general anesthesia in dental and oral surgery patients differs from its use in major surgery because the patient's level of fear is usually a more important factor than the nature of the procedure. In 1985, an NIH Consensus Statement reported that high levels of preoperative anxiety, lengthy and complex procedures, and the need for a pain-free operative period may be indications for general anesthesia in healthy adults and very young children. The NIH statement specified that at least three professionals are required when general anesthesia is used during dental procedures: one is the operating dentist; the second is a professional responsible for observing and monitoring the patient; the third person assists the operating dentist.

Although the United States allows general anesthesia for dental procedures to be administered outside hospitals (provided that the facility has the appropriate equipment and emergency drugs), Scotland banned the use of general anesthesia outside hospitals in 2000, after a ten-year-old boy died during a procedure to have a tooth removed.

Preparation

Preparation for general anesthesia includes the taking of a complete medical history and the evaluation of all factors—especially a family history of allergic responses to anesthetics—that might influence the patient's response to specific anesthetic agents.

Patients should not eat or drink before general anesthesia because of the risk of regurgitating food and liquid or aspirating vomitus into the lungs.

Informed consent

Patients should be informed of the risks associated with general anesthesia as part of their **informed consent**. These risks include possible dental injuries from intubation as well as such serious complications as stroke, liver damage, or massive hemorrhage. If local anesthesia is an option for some procedures, the patient should be informed of this alternative. In all cases, pa-

tients should be given the opportunity to ask questions about the risks and benefits of the procedure requiring anesthesia as well as questions about the anesthesia itself.

Premedication

Depending on the patient's level of anxiety and the procedure to be performed, the patient may be premedicated. Most medications given before general anesthesia are either anxiolytics, usually benzodiazepines; or analgesics. Patients in severe pain prior to surgery may be given morphine or fentanyl. Anticholinergics (drugs that block impulses from the parasympathetic nervous system) may be given to patients with a known history of bronchospasm or heavy airway secretions.

Aftercare

The anesthetist and medical personnel provide supplemental oxygen and monitor patients for **vital signs** and monitor their airways. Vital signs include an EKG (unless the patient is hooked up to a monitor), blood pressure, pulse rate, oxygen saturation, respiratory rate, and temperature. The staff also monitors the patient's level of consciousness as well as signs of excess bleeding from the incision.

Risks

Although the risk of serious complications from general anesthesia are low, they can include heart attack, stroke, brain damage, and death. The risk of complications depends in part on the patient's age, sex, weight, allergies, general health, and history of smoking, alcohol or drug use.

The overall risk of mortality from general anesthesia is difficult to evaluate, because so many different factors are involved, ranging from the patient's overall health and the circumstances preceding surgery to the type of procedure and the skill of the physicians involved. The risk appears to be somewhere between 1:1,000 and 1:100,000, with infants younger than age one and patients older than 70 being at greater risk.

Awareness during surgery

One possible complication is the patient's "waking up" during the operation. It is estimated that about 30,000 patients per year in the United States "come to" during surgery. This development is in part the result of the widespread use of short-acting general anesthetics combined with blanket use of neuromuscular blockade. The patients are paralyzed with regard to motion, but otherwise "awake and aware." At present, special devices that measure brain wave activity are used to monitor the patient's state of consciousness. The **bispectral index**

KEY TERMS

Analgesia—Relief from pain.

Anticholinergics—Drugs that interfere with impulses from the parasympathetic nervous system. They may be given before general anesthesia to reduce airway secretions or the risk of bronchospasm.

Anxiolytics—Medications given to reduce anxiety; tranquilizers. Benzodiazepines are the anxiolytics most commonly used to premedicate patients before general anesthesia.

Balanced anesthesia—The use of a combination of inhalation and intravenous anesthetics, often with opioids for pain relief and neuromuscular blockers for muscle paralysis.

Clathrates—Substances in which a molecule from one compound fills a space within the crystal lattice of another compound. One theory of general anesthesia proposes that water molecules interact with anesthetic molecules to form clathrates that decrease receptor function.

Laryngoscope—An endoscope equipped for viewing a patient's larynx through the mouth.

Malignant hyperthermia—A type of allergic reaction (probably with a genetic basis) that can occur during general anesthesia in which the patient experiences a high fever, the muscles become rigid, and the heart rate and blood pressure fluctuate.

Volatile anesthetics—Another name for inhalation anesthetics.

monitor was approved by the FDA in 1996 and the patient state analyzer in 1999.

Nausea and vomiting

Post-operative nausea and vomiting is a common problem during recovery from general anesthesia. In addition, patients may feel drowsy, weak, or tired for several days after the operation, a combination of symptoms sometimes called the hangover effect. Fuzzy thinking, blurred vision, and coordination problems are also possible. For these reasons, anyone who has had general anesthesia should not drive, operate machinery, or perform other activities that could endanger themselves or others for at least 24 hours, or longer if necessary.

Anesthetic toxicity

Inhalation anesthetics are sometimes toxic to the liver, the kidney, or to blood cells. Halothane may cause

hepatic necrosis or hepatitis. Sevoflurane may react with the carbon dioxide absorbents in anesthesia machines to form compound A, a haloalkene that is toxic to the kidneys. The danger to red blood cells comes from carbon monoxide formed by the breakdown products of inhalation anesthetics in the circuits of anesthesia machines.

Malignant hyperthermia

Malignant hyperthermia is a rare condition caused by an allergic response to a general anesthetic. The signs of malignant hyperthermia include rapid, irregular heartbeat; breathing problems; very high fever; and muscle tightness or spasms. These symptoms can occur following the administration of general anesthetics, especially halothane.

Normal results

General anesthesia is much safer today than it was in the past, thanks to faster-acting anesthetics; improved safety standards in the equipment used to deliver the drugs; and better devices to monitor breathing, heart rate, blood pressure, and brain activity during surgery. Unpleasant side effects are also less common, in part because of recent developments in equipment that reduces the problems of anesthetizing patients who are difficult to intubate. These developments include the laryngeal mask airway and the McCoy laryngoscope, which has a hinged tip on its blade that allows a better view of the patient's larynx.

Resources

BOOKS

U.S. Pharmacopeia Staff. *Consumer Reports Complete Drug Reference.* Yonkers, NY: Consumer Reports Books, 2002.

PERIODICALS

Christie, Bryan. "Scotland to Ban General Anaesthesia in Dental Surgeries." *British Medical Journal* 320 (March 4, 2000): 55–59.

Fox, Andrew J. and David J. Rowbotham. "Recent Advances in Anaesthesia." *British Medical Journal* 319 (August 28, 1999): 557–560.

Marcus, Mary Brophy. "How Does Anesthesia Work? A State That Is Nothing Like Sleep: No Memory, No Fight-or-Flight Response, No Pain." *U.S. News & World Report* 123 (August 18, 1997): 66.

Preboth, Monica. "Waking Up Under the Surgeon's Knife." *American Family Physician* (February 15, 1999).

Wenker, Olivier C., MD. "Review of Currently Used Inhalation Anesthetics: Parts I and II." *The Internet Journal of Anesthesiology* 3, nos. 2 and 3 (1999).

ORGANIZATIONS

American Academy of Anesthesiologist Assistants. PO Box 81362, Wellesley, MA 02481-0004. (800) 757-5858. <http://www.anesthetist.org>.

American Association of Nurse Anesthetists. 222 South Prospect Avenue, Park Ridge, IL 60068-4001 (847) 692-7050. <http://www.aana.com>.

American Society of Anesthesiologists. 520 N. Northwest Highway, Park Ridge, IL 60068-2573. (847) 825-5586. <http://www.asahq.org>.

OTHER

American Medical Association, Office of the General Counsel, Division of Health Law. *Informed Consent.* Chicago, IL: AMA Press, 1998.

Interview with Harvey Plosker, MD, board-certified anesthesiologist. The Pain Center, 501 Glades Road, Boca Raton, FL 33431.

NIH Consensus Statement. *Anesthesia and Sedation in the Dental Office.* 5, no. 10 (April 22–24, 1985): 1–18.

Lisette Hilton
Sam Uretsky, PharmD

Anesthesia, local

Definition

Local, or regional, anesthesia involves the injection or application of an anesthetic drug to a specific area of the body. This is in contrast to general anesthesia, which provides anesthesia to the entire body and brain.

Purpose

Local anesthetics are used to prevent patients from feeling pain during medical, surgical, or dental procedures. Over-the-counter local anesthetics are also available to provide temporary relief from pain, irritation, and itching caused by various conditions such as cold sores, canker sores, sore throats, sunburn, insect bites, poison ivy, and minor cuts and scratches.

Precautions

People who feel strongly that they do not want to be awake and alert during certain procedures may not be good candidates for local or regional anesthesia. However, other medications that have systemic effects may be given in addition to an anesthetic to relieve anxiety and help the patient relax.

Local anesthetics should be used only for the conditions for which they are intended. For example, a topical anesthetic meant to relieve sunburn pain should not be used on cold sores. Anyone who has had an unusual reaction to any local anesthetic in the past should check with a doctor before using any type of local anesthetic

again. The doctor should also be told about any allergies to foods, dyes, preservatives, or other substances.

Older people may be more sensitive to the effects of local anesthetics, especially lidocaine. Children may also be especially sensitive to some local anesthetics, and certain types should not be used at all on young children. People caring for these groups need to be aware that they are at increased risk of more severe side effects. Packages should be followed carefully so that the recommended dosage is not exceeded. A doctor or pharmacist should be consulted about any concerns.

Regional anesthetics

Serious and possibly life-threatening side effects may occur when injectable or inhaled anesthetics are given to people who use street drugs. Doctors and nurses should inform patients about the dangers of mixing anesthetics with cocaine, marijuana, amphetamines, **barbiturates**, phencyclidine (PCP, or angel dust), heroin, or other street drugs. Some anesthetic drugs may interact with other medicines. When this happens, the effects of one or both of the drugs may change, or the risk of side effects may be greater. In select cases, a **urinalysis** can help identify drug use.

Patients who have a personal or family history of malignant hyperthermia after receiving a general anesthetic must also be cautious when receiving regional or local anesthetics. Malignant hyperthermia is a serious reaction that involves a fast or irregular heartbeat, high fever, breathing problems, and muscle spasms. All patients should be asked if they are aware of such a risk in their family before receiving any kind of anesthetic.

Although problems are rare, some side effects may occur when regional anesthetics are used during labor and delivery. Anesthetics can prolong labor and increase the risk of requiring a **cesarean section**. Doctors should discuss the risks and benefits associated with epidural or spinal anesthesia with pregnant patients.

Regional anesthetics should be used only by an experienced anesthesiologist in a properly equipped environment with suitable resuscitative equipment. Although these anesthetics are generally safe when properly selected and administered, severe adverse reactions are still possible. If inadvertent subarachnoid injection occurs, the patient is likely to require resuscitation with oxygen and drug therapy. Careful positioning of the patient is essential to prevent leaking of cerebrospinal fluid.

Patients should not drive or operate machinery immediately following a procedure involving regional anesthesia because numbness or weakness may cause impairment. Doctors and nurses should also warn patients who have had local anesthesia, especially when combined with drugs to make patients sleep or to reduce pain, about operating any type of machinery.

Injectable local anesthetics

Until the anesthetic wears off, patients should be careful not to inadvertently injure the numbed area. If the anesthetic was used in the mouth, patients should not eat or chew gum until feeling returns.

Topical anesthetics

Unless advised by a doctor, topical anesthetics should not be used on or near any part of the body with large sores, broken or scraped skin, severe injury, or infection. They should also not be used on large areas of skin. Some topical anesthetics contain alcohol and should not be used near an open flame or while smoking.

Patients should be careful not to get topical anesthetics in the eyes, nose, or mouth. If a spray-type anesthetic is to be used on the face, it can be applied with a cotton swab or sterile gauze pad. After using a topical anesthetic on a child, the caregiver should make sure the child does not get the medicine in his or her mouth or eyes.

Topical anesthetics are intended for the temporary relief of pain and itching. They should not be used for more than a few days at a time. A doctor should be consulted if:

• Discomfort continues for more than seven days.

• The problem gets worse.

• The treated area becomes infected.

• New signs of irritation such as skin rash, burning, stinging, or swelling appear.

Dental anesthetics

Dental anesthetics should not be used if certain kinds of infections are present. Package directions should be checked or a dentist, pharmacist, or doctor should be consulted if there is any uncertainty. Dental anesthetics should be used only for temporary pain relief. Consult the dentist if problems such as toothache, mouth sores, or pain from dentures or braces continue or if signs of general illness such as fever, rash, or vomiting develop.

Patients should not eat or chew gum while the mouth is numb from a dental anesthetic to avoid accidentally biting the tongue or the inside of the mouth. In addition, nothing should be eaten or drunk for one hour after applying a dental anesthetic to the back of the mouth or throat, because the medicine may interfere with swallowing and may cause choking. If normal feeling does not return to the mouth within a few hours after receiving a dental anesthetic or if it is difficult to open the mouth, the dentist should be consulted.

Ophthalmic anesthetics

When anesthetics are used in the eye, it is important not to rub or wipe the eye until the effect of the anesthetic has worn off and feeling has returned. Rubbing the eye while it is numb could cause injury.

Description

Medical procedures and situations that regularly make use of local or regional anesthesia include the following:

• biopsies, in which skin or tissue samples are taken for diagnostic procedures

• childbirth

• scar repair

• surgery on the face (including plastic surgery), skin, arms, hands, legs, and feet

• eye surgery

• surgery involving the urinary tract or reproductive organs

Surgery involving the chest or abdomen is usually performed under general anesthesia. **Laparoscopy** and hernia repair, however, may be performed under local or regional anesthesia.

Local and regional anesthesia have many advantages over general anesthesia. Most importantly, the risk of unusual and sometimes fatal reactions to general anesthesia is lessened. More minor, but significant, risks of general anesthesia include longer recovery time and the psychological discomfort of losing consciousness.

Regional anesthesia typically affects a larger area than local anesthesia. As a result, regional anesthesia is typically used for more involved or complicated procedures. The duration of action of an anesthetic depends on the type and amount of anesthetic administered.

Regional anesthetics are injected. Local anesthesia involves the injection into the skin or application to the skin surface of an anesthetic directly where pain will occur. Local anesthesia can be divided into four groups: injectable, topical, dental (non-injectable), and regional blockade injection.

Local and regional anesthesia work by altering the flow of sodium molecules into nerve cells (neurons) through the cell membrane. The exact mechanism is not understood, since the drug apparently does not bind to any receptor on the cell surface and does not seem to affect the release of chemicals that transmit nerve impulses (neurotransmitters) from the nerve cells. Experts believe, however, that when the sodium molecules do not get into the neurons, nerve impulses are not generated and pain impulses are not transmitted to the brain.

Regional anesthesia

Types of regional anesthesia include:

- Spinal anesthesia, which involves the injection of a small amount of local anesthetic into the cerebrospinal fluid surrounding the spinal cord (the subarachnoid space). A drop in blood pressure is a common but easily treated side effect.

- Epidural anesthesia, which involves the injection of a large volume of local anesthetic into the space surrounding the spinal fluid sac (the epidural space), not directly into the spinal fluid. Pain relief occurs more slowly, but is less likely to produce a drop in blood pressure. The block can be maintained for long periods, even for days if necessary.

- Nerve blockades, which involve the injection of an anesthetic into the area around a sensory or motor nerve that supplies a particular region of the body, preventing the nerve from carrying nerve impulses to and from the brain.

Local and regional anesthetics may be administered with other drugs to enhance their action. Examples include vasoconstrictors such as epinephrine (adrenaline) to decrease bleeding, or sodium bicarbonate to lower acidity, which may make a drug work faster. In addition, medications may be administered to help a patient remain calm and more comfortable or to make them sleepy.

Local anesthesia

INJECTABLE LOCAL ANESTHETICS. Injectable local anesthetics provide pain relief for some part of the body during surgery, dental procedures, or other medical procedures. They are given only by a trained health care professional and only in a doctor's office or a hospital. Some commonly used injectable local anesthetics are lidocaine (Xylocaine), bupivacaine (Marcaine), and mepivacaine (Carbocaine).

TOPICAL ANESTHETICS. Topical anesthetics such as benzocaine, lidocaine (in smaller quantities or doses), dibucaine, and tetracaine relieve pain and itching by blocking the sensory nerve endings in the skin. They are ingredients in a variety of nonprescription products that are applied to the skin to relieve the discomfort of sunburn, insect bites or stings, poison ivy, and minor cuts, scratches, and burns. These products are sold as creams, ointments, sprays, lotions, and gels.

Topical dental anesthetics are intended for pain relief in the mouth or throat. They may be used to relieve throat pain, teething pain, painful canker sores, toothaches, or discomfort from dentures, braces, or bridgework. Some dental anesthetics are available only with a doctor's prescription. Others may be purchased over the counter, including products such as Num-Zit, Orajel, Chloraseptic lozenges, and Xylocaine.

Ophthalmic anesthetics are designed for use in the eye. Lidocaine and tetracaine are used to numb the eye before certain eye examinations. Eye doctors may also use these medicines before measuring eye pressure or removing stitches or foreign objects from the eye. These drugs are to be given only by a trained health care professional.

The recommended dosage of a topical anesthetic depends on the type of local anesthetic and the purpose for which it is being used. When using a nonprescription local anesthetic, patients are advised to follow the directions on the package. Questions concerning how to use a product should be referred to a doctor, dentist, or pharmacist.

Aftercare

Most patients can return home immediately after a local anesthetic, but some patients might require limited observation. The degree of aftercare needed depends on where the anesthetic was given, how much was given, and other individual circumstances. Patients who have had their eyes numbed should wear a patch after surgery or treatment until full feeling in the eye area has returned. If the throat was anesthetized, the patient cannot drink until the gag reflex returns. If a major extremity was anesthetized, the patient may have to wait until function returns before being discharged. Some local anesthetics can cause cardiac arrhythmias and therefore require monitoring for a time with an EKG. Patients who have had regional anesthesia or larger amounts of local anesthesia usually recover in a post-anesthesia care unit before being discharged. There, medical personnel watch for immediate postoperative problems. These patients need to be driven home after discharge.

Risks

Side effects of regional or local anesthetics vary depending on the type of anesthetic used and the way it is administered. Any unusual symptoms following the use of an anesthetic requires the immediate attention of a doctor.

Paralysis after a regional anesthetic such as an epidural, spinal, or ganglionic blockade is extremely rare, but can occur. Paralysis reportedly occurs even less frequently than deaths due to general anesthesia.

There is also a small risk of developing a severe headache called a spinal headache following a spinal or epidural block. This headache is severe when the patient is upright, even when only elevated 30°, and is hardly felt when the patient lies down. It is treated by increasing fluids to help clear the anesthetic and enhance the flow of spinal fluid.

Finally, blood clots or abscess can form at the site where an anesthetic is injected. Although they can usually be treated, antibiotic resistance is becoming increasingly common. Such infections must be regarded as potentially dangerous, particularly if they develop at the site of a spinal injection.

A physician should be notified immediately if any of the following occur:

- symptoms of an allergic reaction such as hives (urticaria), which are itchy swellings on the skin, or swelling in the mouth or throat
- severe headache
- blurred or double vision or photophobia (sensitivity to light)
- dizziness or lightheadedness
- drowsiness
- confusion
- an irregular, too slow, or rapid heartbeat
- anxiety, excitement, nervousness, or restlessness
- convulsions (seizures)
- feeling hot, cold, or numb anywhere other than the anesthetized area
- ringing or buzzing in the ears
- shivering or trembling
- sweating
- pale skin
- breathing problems
- unusual weakness or tiredness

Normal results

Local and regional anesthetics help to make many conditions and procedures more comfortable and tolerable for patients.

Resources

BOOKS

Nettina, Sandra. *Lippincott Manual of Nursing Practice,* 7th edition. Philadelphia: Lippincott, 2001, pp. 115-117.

ORGANIZATIONS

American Academy of Anesthesiologist Assistants. PO Box 81362, Wellesley, MA 02481-0004. (800) 757-5858. <http://www.anesthetist.org>.

KEY TERMS

Canker sore—A painful sore inside the mouth.

Cerebrospinal fluid—A clear fluid that fills the hollow cavity inside the brain and spinal cord. The cerebrospinal fluid has several functions, including providing a cushion for the brain against shock or impact, and removing waste products from the brain.

Cold sore—A small blister on the lips or face, caused by a virus. Also called a fever blister.

Epidural space—The space surrounding the spinal fluid sac.

Malignant hyperthermia—A type of reaction (probably with a genetic basis) that can occur during general anesthesia in which the patient experiences a high fever, the muscles become rigid, and the heart rate and blood pressure fluctuate.

Subarachnoid space—The space surrounding the spinal cord that is filled with cerebrospinal fluid.

Topical—Not ingested; applied to the outside of the body, for example to the skin, eye, or mouth.

American Society of Anesthesiologists. 520 N. Northwest Highway, Park Ridge, IL 60068-2573. (847) 825-5586. <http://www.asahq.org>.

OTHER

Interview with Harvey Plosker, MD. The Pain Center. 501 Glades Road, Boca Raton, FL 33431.

Lisette Hilton
Sam Uretsky, PharmD

Anesthesiologist's role

Definition

The anesthesiologist's role is the practice of medicine dedicated to the relief of pain and total care of the surgical patient before, during, and after surgery.

Training

Anesthesiologists are fully trained physicians. After completing a four-year college program and four years of medical school, anesthesiologists undergo four additional years of specialized residency training. Some will spend one to two more years training in such anesthesiology subspecialty areas as obstetrics, neurosurgery, cardiac surgery, pediatrics, or critically ill patients, or to learn more about the treatment of pain. Others may select to work in research laboratories, investigating, for example, how anesthetics work and how they influence disease or recovery.

In the United States, the education of anesthesiologists takes into account their ever-expanding role in offering the best-quality health care available anywhere in the world.

Description

The medical expertise of recent generations of anesthesiologists has significantly expanded the role of the anesthesiologist. Historically, the anesthesiologist's role was limited to that of the physician who administers anesthesia to suppress pain and consciousness in a patient undergoing surgery. Now, anesthesiologists also provide medical care in settings other than the **operating room**. The American Society of Anesthesiologists defines the anesthesiologist as the perioperative physician—the "all-around" physician responsible for providing medical care to each patient undergoing surgery at all stages. This includes providing the medical evaluation of the patient before surgery (preoperative), holding consultations with the **surgical team**, providing pain control and support of life functions during surgery (intraoperative), supervising care after surgery (postoperative), and discharging the patient from the recovery unit.

Specifically, the anesthesiologist's role has moved beyond just the operating room and into other areas of care.

- Ninety percent of the approximately 40 million anesthetics used annually in the United States is administered by anesthesiologists. During a surgical procedure, the anesthesiologist continually assesses the medical status of the patient, monitoring and controlling vital life functions, as well as managing pain.

- Postoperatively the anesthesiologist determines when a patient can return home following an outpatient procedure and when a patient can be moved to another ward following a procedure that requires hospitalization.

- The anesthesiologist is also involved in postoperative **pain management**, prescribing the appropriate pain-relieving medication and therapies.

- The anesthesiologist also prescribes individualized drug therapies to patients suffering from acute, chronic, and cancer pain.

- During childbirth, the anesthesiologist must provide pain relief with epidural or spinal blocks for the mother while managing the life functions of both the mother and the baby.

KEY TERMS

Anesthetic—A drug that causes unconsciousness or a loss of general sensation.

Anesthesia—Loss of normal sensation or feeling.

Angioplasty—The surgical repair of a blood vessel.

Catheterization—Placement of a flow-directed catheter for measuring pulmonary arterial pressures.

Endoscopy—The visual inspection of any cavity of the body by means of an endoscope.

Intraoperative—During surgery.

Postoperative—After surgery.

Preoperative—Before surgery.

- In critical care and trauma medicine, the anesthesiologist makes immediate diagnoses while supporting respiratory and cardiovascular functions, controlling infection, providing airway management, cardiac and pulmonary resuscitation, advanced life support, and pain control.

- The anesthesiologist is also present during cardiac catheterizations, angioplasties, radiological imaging, gastrointestinal endoscopies, **in vitro fertilization**, electroshock therapy, and respiratory therapy.

- The anesthesiologist participates in research and clinical studies, as well as medical education programs and legislative activities.

In the past, complications caused by the use of anesthesia were a medical issue; however during the past 25 years, complications have significantly declined. Despite the growing need for anesthesia and the doubling of the total number of anesthesiologists practicing within the United States since 1970, patient outcomes have improved. During the past 10 years, the number of deaths resulting from anesthesia have dropped from an estimated one in 10,000 to one in 250,000.

Resources

BOOKS

Jaffe, R. A. and S. I. Samuels, eds. *Anesthesiologist's Manual of Surgical Procedures*. Philadelphia: Lippincott Williams and Wilkins Publishers, 1999.

Morgan, G. E., M. S. Mikhail, M. J. Murray, and P. C. Larson. *Clinical Anesthesiology*. New York: McGraw-Hill, 2001.

Stoelting, R. K. and R. D. Miller. *Basics of Anesthesia*. New York: Churchill Livingstone, 2000.

PERIODICALS

Guzzi, L. M. "The Anesthesiologist's Role in Nuclear, Biological and Chemical Warfare: A Response." *ASA Newsletter* 66, no. 3 (March 2002).

ORGANIZATIONS

American Board of Anesthesiology. 4101 Lake Boone Trail, Suite 510, Raleigh, North Carolina 27607-7506. (919) 881-2570. <http://www.abanes.org/>.

American Society of Anesthesiologists. 520 N. Northwest Highway, Park Ridge, IL 60068-2573. (847) 825-5586. <http://www.asahq.org/>.

OTHER

"Anesthesiology." [cited April 24, 2003]. <http://jhhs.client. web-health.com/web-health/topics/GeneralHealth/gener alhealthsub/generalhealth/surgicalpro/anesthesiology. html >.

Florida Society of Anesthesiologists. "The role of an anesthesiologist." [cited April 24, 2003]. <http://www.fsahq.org/role. htm>.

Monique Laberge, Ph.D.

Aneurysm repair, aortic *see* **Aortic aneurysm repair**

Aneurysm repair, cerebral *see* **Cerebral aneurysm repair**

Angiography

Definition

Angiography is the x-ray (radiographic) study of the blood vessels. An angiogram uses a radiopaque substance, or contrast medium, to make the blood vessels visible under x ray. The key ingredient in most radiographic contrast media is iodine. Arteriography is a type of radiographic examination that involves the study of the arteries.

Purpose

Angiography is used to detect abnormalities, including narrowing (stenosis) or blockages in the blood vessels (called occlusions) throughout the circulatory system and in some organs. The procedure is commonly used to identify atherosclerosis; to diagnose heart disease; to evaluate kidney function and detect kidney cysts or tumors; to map renal anatomy in transplant donors; to detect an aneurysm (an abnormal bulge of an artery that can rupture leading to hemorrhage), tumor, blood clot, or arteriovenous malformations (abnormal tangles of arteries and veins) in the brain; and to diagnose problems with the retina of the eye. It is also used to provide surgeons with an accurate vascular "map" of the heart prior to open-heart surgery, or of the brain prior to **neurosurgery**. Angiography may be used after penetrating trauma, like a gunshot or knife wound, to detect blood vessel injury; it may be used to check the position of shunts and stents placed by physicians into blood vessels.

Precautions

Patients with kidney disease or injury may suffer further kidney damage from the contrast media used for angiography. Patients who have blood-clotting problems, have a known allergy to contrast media, or are allergic to iodine may also not be suitable candidates for an angiography procedure. Newer types of contrast media classified as non-ionic are less toxic and cause fewer side effects than traditional ionic agents. Because x rays carry risks of ionizing radiation exposure to the fetus, pregnant women are also advised to avoid this procedure.

Description

Angiography requires the injection of a contrast medium that makes the blood vessels visible to x ray. The contrast medium is injected through a procedure known as arterial puncture. The puncture is usually made in the groin area, armpit, inside elbow, or neck.

Patients undergoing an angiogram are advised to stop eating and drinking eight hours prior to the procedure. They must remove all jewelry before the procedure and change into a hospital gown. If the arterial puncture is to be made in the armpit or groin area, shaving may be required. A sedative may be administered to relax the patient for the procedure. An IV (intravenous) line is also inserted into a vein in the patient's arm before the procedure begins, in case medication or blood products are required during the angiogram or complications arise.

Prior to the angiographic procedure, patients are briefed on the details of the test, the benefits and risks, and the possible complications involved, and asked to sign an **informed consent** form.

The site is cleaned with an antiseptic agent and injected with a local anesthetic. Then, a small incision is made in the skin to help the needle pass. A needle containing a solid inner core called a stylet is inserted through the incision and into the artery. When the radiologist has punctured the artery with the needle, the stylet is removed and replaced with another long wire called a guide wire. It is normal for blood to spurt out of the needle before the guide wire is inserted.

The guide wire is fed through the outer needle into the artery to the area that requires angiographic study. A fluoroscope displays a view of the patient's vascular system and is used to direct the guide wire to the correct location. Once it is in position, the needle is then removed, and a catheter is threaded over the length of the guide wire until it to reaches the area of study. The guide wire is then removed, and the catheter is left in place in preparation for the injection of the contrast medium.

Depending on the type of angiographic procedure being performed, the contrast medium is either injected by hand with a syringe or is mechanically injected with an automatic injector, sometimes called a power injector, connected to the catheter. An automatic injector is used frequently because it is able to deliver a large volume of contrast medium very quickly to the angiographic site. Usually a small test injection is made by hand to confirm that the catheter is in the correct position. The patient is told that the injection will start, and is instructed to remain very still. The injection causes some mild to moderate discomfort. Possible side effects or reactions include headache, dizziness, irregular heartbeat, nausea, warmth, burning sensation, and chest pain, but they usually last only momentarily. To view the area of study from different angles or perspectives, the patient may be asked to change positions several times, and subsequent contrast medium injections may be administered. During any injection, the patient or the imaging equipment may move.

Throughout the injection procedure, radiographs (x-ray pictures) or fluoroscopic images are obtained. Because of the high pressure of arterial blood flow, the contrast medium dissipates through the patient's system quickly and becomes diluted, so images must be obtained in rapid succession. One or more automatic film changers may be used to capture the required radiographic images. In many imaging departments, angiographic images are captured digitally, obviating the need for film changers. The ability to capture digital images also makes it possible to manipulate the information electronically allowing for a procedure known as digital subtraction angiography (DSA). Because every image captured is comprised of tiny picture elements called pixels, computers can be used to manipulate the information in ways that enhance diagnostic information. One common approach is to electronically remove or (subtract) bony structures that otherwise would be superimposed over the vessels being studied, hence the name digital subtraction angiography.

Once the x rays are complete, the catheter is slowly and carefully removed from the patient. Manual pressure is applied to the site with a sandbag or other weight for 10 to 20 minutes to allow for clotting to take place and the arterial puncture to reseal itself. A pressure bandage is then applied.

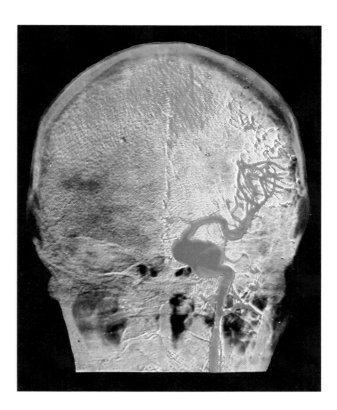

X ray showing a brain aneurism (to the right of the midline). *(CNRI/National Audubon Society Collection/Photo Researchers, Inc. Reproduced by permission.)*

Most angiograms follow the general procedures outlined above, but vary slightly depending on the area of the vascular system being studied. A variety of common angiographic procedures are outlined below:

Cerebral angiography

Cerebral angiography is used to detect aneurysms, stenosis, blood clots, and other vascular irregularities in the brain. The catheter is inserted into the femoral or carotid artery, and the injected contrast medium travels through the blood vessels in the brain. Patients frequently experience headache, warmth, or a burning sensation in the head or neck during the injection portion of the procedure. A cerebral angiogram takes two to four hours to complete.

Coronary angiography

Coronary angiography is administered by a cardiologist with training in radiology or, occasionally, by a radiologist. The arterial puncture is typically made in the femoral artery, and the cardiologist uses a guide wire and catheter to perform a contrast injection and x-ray series on the coronary arteries. The catheter may also be placed in the left ventricle to examine the mitral and aortic valves of the heart. If the cardiologist requires a view of the right ventricle of the heart or of the tricuspid or pulmonic valves, the catheter is inserted through a large vein and guided into the right ventricle. The catheter also serves the purpose of monitoring blood pressures in these different locations inside the heart. The angiographic procedure takes several hours, depending on the complexity of the procedure.

Pulmonary angiography

Pulmonary, or lung, angiography is performed to evaluate blood circulation to the lungs. It is also considered the most accurate diagnostic test for detecting a pulmonary embolism. The procedure differs from cerebral and coronary angiography in that the guide wire and catheter are inserted into a vein instead of an artery, and are guided up through the chambers of the heart and into the pulmonary artery. Throughout the procedure, the patient's **vital signs** are monitored to ensure that the catheter doesn't cause arrhythmias, or irregular heartbeats. The contrast medium is then injected into the pulmonary artery where it circulates through the lungs' capillaries. The test typically takes up to 90 minutes and carries more risk than other angiography procedures.

Kidney (renal) angiography

Patients with chronic renal disease or injury can suffer further damage to their kidneys from the contrast medium used in a renal angiogram, yet they often require the test to evaluate kidney function. These patients should be well hydrated with an intravenous saline drip before the procedure, and may benefit from available medications (e.g., dopamine) that help to protect the kidney from further injury associated with contrast agents. During a renal angiogram, the guide wire and catheter are inserted into the femoral artery in the groin area and advanced through the abdominal aorta, the main artery in the abdomen, and into the renal arteries. The procedure takes approximately one hour.

Fluorescein angiography

Fluorescein angiography is used to diagnose retinal problems and circulatory disorders. It is typically conducted as an outpatient procedure. The patient's pupils are dilated with eye drops, and he or she rests the chin and forehead against a bracing apparatus to keep it still. Sodium fluorescein dye is then injected with a syringe into a vein in the patient's arm. The dye travels through the patient's body and into the blood vessels of the eye. The procedure does not require x rays. Instead, a rapid series of close-up photographs of the patient's eyes are

taken, one set immediately after the dye is injected, and a second set approximately 20 minutes later once the dye has moved through the patient's vascular system. The entire procedure takes up to one hour.

Celiac and mesenteric angiography

Celiac and mesenteric angiography involves radiographic exploration of the celiac and mesenteric arteries, arterial branches of the abdominal aorta that supply blood to the abdomen and digestive system. The test is commonly used to detect aneurysm, thrombosis, and signs of ischemia in the celiac and mesenteric arteries, and to locate the source of gastrointestinal bleeding. It is also used in the diagnosis of a number of conditions, including portal hypertension and cirrhosis. The procedure can take up to three hours, depending on the number of blood vessels studied.

Splenoportography

A splenoportograph is a variation of an angiogram that involves the injection of contrast medium directly into the spleen to view the splenic and portal veins. It is used to diagnose blockages in the splenic vein and portal-vein thrombosis and to assess the patency and location of the vascular system prior to **liver transplantation**.

Most angiographic procedures are typically paid for by major medical insurance. Patients should check with their individual insurance plans to determine their coverage.

Computerized tomographic angiography (CTA), a new technique, is used in the evaluation of patients with intracranial aneurysms. CTA is particularly useful in delineating the relationship of vascular lesions with bony anatomy close to the skull base. While such lesions can be demonstrated with standard angiography, it often requires studying several projections of the two-dimensional films rendered with standard angiography. CTA is ideal for more anatomically complex skull-base lesions because it clearly demonstrates the exact relationship of the bony anatomy with the vascular pathology. This is not possible using standard angiographic techniques. Once the information has been captured a workstation is used to process and reconstruct images. The approach yields shaded surface displays of the actual vascular anatomy that are three dimensional and clearly show the relationship of the bony anatomy with the vascular pathology.

Angiography can also be performed using MRI (**magnetic resonance imaging**) scanners. The technique is called MRA (magnetic resonance angiography). A contrast medium is not usually used, but may be used in some body applications. The active ingredient in the contrast medium used for MRA is one of the rare earth elements, gadolinium. The contrast agent is injected into

KEY TERMS

Arteriosclerosis—A chronic condition characterized by thickening and hardening of the arteries and the build-up of plaque on the arterial walls. Arteriosclerosis can slow or impair blood circulation.

Carotid artery—An artery located in the neck.

Catheter—A long, thin, flexible tube used in angiography to inject contrast material into the arteries.

Cirrhosis—A condition characterized by the destruction of healthy liver tissue. A cirrhotic liver is scarred and cannot break down the proteins in the bloodstream. Cirrhosis is associated with portal hypertension.

Embolism—A blood clot, air bubble, or clot of foreign material that travels and blocks the flow of blood in an artery. When blood supply to a tissue or organ is blocked by an embolism, infarction (death of the tissue the artery feeds) occurs. Without immediate and appropriate treatment, an embolism can be fatal.

Femoral artery—An artery located in the groin area that is the most frequently accessed site for arterial puncture in angiography.

Fluorescein dye—An orange dye used to illuminate the blood vessels of the retina in fluorescein angiography.

Fluoroscope—An imaging device that displays "moving x rays" of the body. Fluoroscopy allows the radiologist to visualize the guide wire and catheter he or she is moving through the patient's artery.

Guide wire—A wire that is inserted into an artery to guide a catheter to a certain location in the body.

Ischemia—A lack of normal blood supply to a organ or body part because of blockages or constriction of the blood vessels.

Necrosis—Cellular or tissue death; skin necrosis may be caused by multiple, consecutive doses of radiation from fluoroscopic or x-ray procedures.

Plaque—Fatty material that is deposited on the inside of the arterial wall.

Portal hypertension—A condition caused by cirrhosis of the liver. It is characterized by impaired or reversed blood flow from the portal vein to the liver, an enlarged spleen, and dilated veins in the esophagus and stomach.

Portal vein thrombosis—The development of a blood clot in the vein that brings blood into the liver. Untreated portal vein thrombosis causes portal hypertension.

an arm vein, and images are acquired with careful attention being paid to the timing of the injection and selection of MRI specific imaging parameters. Once the information has been captured, a workstation is used to process and reconstruct the images. The post-processing capabilities associated with CTA and MRA yield three-dimensional representations of the vascular pathology being studied and can also be used to either enhance or subtract adjacent anatomical structures.

Aftercare

Because life-threatening internal bleeding is a possible complication of an arterial puncture, an overnight stay in the hospital is sometimes recommended following an angiographic procedure, particularly with cerebral and coronary angiography. If the procedure is performed on an outpatient basis, the patient is typically kept under close observation for a period of at six to 12 hours before being released. If the arterial puncture was performed in the femoral artery, the patient is instructed to keep his or her leg straight and relatively immobile during the obser-

vation period. The patient's blood pressure and vital signs are monitored, and the puncture site observed closely. Pain medication may be prescribed if the patient is experiencing discomfort from the puncture, and a cold pack is often applied to the site to reduce swelling. It is normal for the puncture site to be sore and bruised for several weeks. The patient may also develop a hematoma at the puncture site, a hard mass created by the blood vessels broken during the procedure. Hematomas should be watched carefully, as they may indicate continued bleeding of the arterial puncture site.

Angiography patients are also advised to have two to three days of rest after the procedure in order to avoid placing any undue stress on the arterial puncture site. Patients who experience continued bleeding or abnormal swelling of the puncture site, sudden dizziness, or chest pain in the days following an angiographic procedure should seek medical attention immediately.

Patients undergoing a fluorescein angiography should not drive or expose their eyes to direct sunlight for 12 hours following the procedure.

Risks

Because angiography involves puncturing an artery, internal bleeding or hemorrhage are possible complications of the test. As with any invasive procedure, infection of the puncture site or bloodstream is also a risk, but this is rare.

A stroke or heart attack may be triggered by an angiogram if blood clots or plaque on the inside of the arterial wall are dislodged by the catheter and form a blockage in the blood vessels, or if the vessel undergoes temporary narrowing or spasm from irritation by the catheter. The heart may also become irritated by the movement of the catheter through its chambers during pulmonary and coronary angiographic procedures, and arrhythmias may develop.

Patients who develop an allergic reaction to the contrast medium used in angiography may experience a variety of symptoms, including swelling, difficulty breathing, heart failure, or a sudden drop in blood pressure. If the patient is aware of the allergy before the test is administered, certain medications can be administered at that time to counteract the reaction.

Angiography involves minor exposure to radiation through the x rays and fluoroscopic guidance used in the procedure. Unless the patient is pregnant, or multiple radiological or fluoroscopic studies are required, the dose of radiation incurred during a single procedure poses little risk. However, multiple studies requiring fluoroscopic exposure that are conducted in a short time period have been known to cause skin necrosis in some individuals. This risk can be minimized by careful monitoring and documentation of cumulative radiation doses administered to these patients, particularly in those who have therapeutic procedures performed along with the diagnostic angiography.

Normal results

The results of an angiogram or arteriogram depend on the artery or organ system being examined. Generally, test results should display a normal and unimpeded flow of blood through the vascular system. Fluorescein angiography should result in no leakage of fluorescein dye through the retinal blood vessels.

Abnormal results of an angiogram may display a narrowed blood vessel with decreased arterial blood flow (ischemia) or an irregular arrangement or location of blood vessels. The results of an angiogram vary widely by the type of procedure performed, and should be interpreted by and explained to the patient by a trained radiologist.

Resources

BOOKS

Baum, Stanley and Michael J. Pentecost, eds. *Abrams' Angiography.* 4th ed. Philadelphia: Lippincott-Raven, 1996.

LaBergem Jeanne, ed. *Interventional Radiology Essentials.* 1st ed. Philadelphia: Lippincott Williams & Wilkins, 2000.
Ziessman, Harvey, ed. *The Radiologic Clinics of North America, Update on Nuclear Medicine* Philadelphia: W. B. Saunders Company, September 2001.

OTHER

Food and Drug Administration. *Public Health Advisory: Avoidance of Serious X-Ray-Induced Skin Injuries to Patients During Fluoroscopically Guided Procedures. September 30, 1994.* Rockville, MD: Center for Devices and Radiological Health, FDA, 1994.
Radiological Society of North America CMEJ. *Renal MR Angiography.* April 1, 1999 [cited June 27, 2003]. <http://ej.rsna.org/ej3/0091-98.fin/mainright.html>.

Stephen John Hage, AAAS, RT(R), FAHRA
Lee Alan Shratter, MD

Angioplasty

Definition

Angioplasty is a term describing a procedure used to widen vessels narrowed by stenoses or occlusions. There are various types of angioplasty. The specific names of these procedures are derived from the type of equipment used and the path of entry to the blood vessel. For example, percutaneous transluminal angioplasty (PTA) means that the vessel is entered through the skin (percutaneous) and that the catheter is moved into the blood vessel of interest through the same vessel or one that communicates with it (transluminal). In the case of an angioplasty involving the coronary arteries, the point of entry might be the femoral artery in the groin, with the catheter/guidewire system passed through the aorta to the heart and the origin of the coronary arteries at the base of the aorta just outside the aortic valve.

Purpose

An angioplasty is done to reopen a partially blocked blood vessel so that blood can flow through it again at a normal rate. In patients with an occlusive vascular disease such as atherosclerosis, the flow of blood to other organs or remote parts of the body is limited by the narrowing of the vessel's lumen due to fatty deposits or patches known as plaque. Once the vessel has been widened, an adequate blood flow is restored. The vessel may narrow again over time at the same location, however, and the procedure may need to be repeated.

For some patients, **thrombolytic therapy** (treatment with drugs that dissolve blood clots) is an alterna-

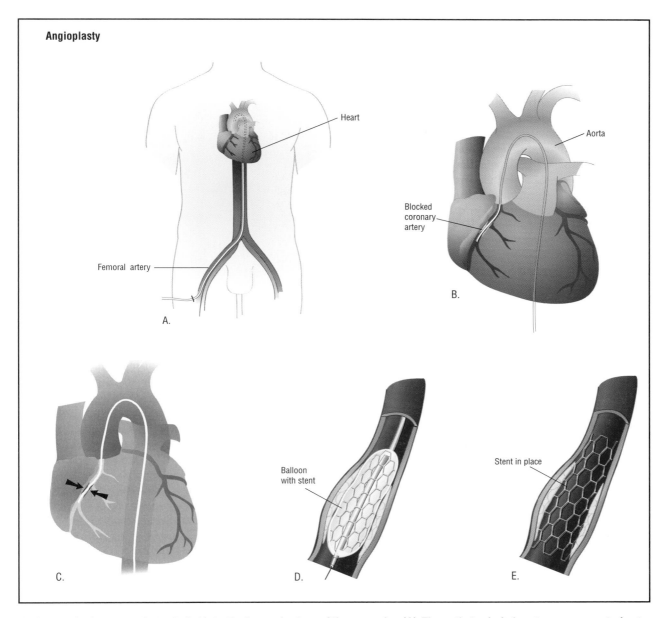

Angioplasty

During angioplasty, a catheter is fed into the femoral artery of the upper leg (A). The catheter is fed up to coronary arteries to an area of blockage (B). A dye is released, allowing visualization of the blockage (C). A stent is placed on the balloon-tipped catheter. The balloon is inflated, opening the artery (D). The stent holds the artery open after the catheter is removed (E). *(Illustration by Argosy.)*

tive to angioplasty. Many medical centers, in fact, restrict the use of angioplasty to patients who cannot be treated with thrombolytic therapy.

Description

Angioplasties were originally performed by dilating the blood vessel with the introduction of larger and larger stiff catheters through the narrowed space. The complications that resulted from this approach led researchers to develop ways to open the vessel with smaller devices. As of 2003, the catheters used to perform angioplasties contain balloons that are inflated to widen the vessel, and stents (thin collapsed tubes made of wire mesh) to provide structural support for the vessel. Lasers may be used to help break up the plaque or fat deposits. Some catheters are equipped with spinning wires or drill tips to clean out the plaque.

Angioplasty may be performed while the patient is sedated or anesthetized, depending on which vessels are

KEY TERMS

Anticoagulant—A type of medication given to prevent the formation of blood clots. Anticoagulants are also known as blood thinners.

Cardiac catheterization—A procedure to pass a catheter to the heart and its vessels for the purpose of diagnosing coronary artery disease, assessing injury or disease of the aorta, or evaluating cardiac function.

Contrast medium—A substance that is swallowed or injected into the body for radiographic studies of internal structures.

Electrocardiogram (EKG)—A graphic tracing of the electrical activity of the heart.

Embolus—A gas or air bubble, bit of tissue, blood clot, or foreign object that circulates in the bloodstream until it lodges in a vessel. A large embolus can narrow or block the vessel, which leads to decreased blood flow in the organ supplied by that vessel.

Fluoroscopy—A radiologic technique that creates x-ray images of internal body structures for immediate projection on a fluorescent screen.

Hematoma—A localized collection of blood in an organ or tissue due to broken blood vessels.

Lumen—The cavity or channel inside a blood vessel or tube-shaped organ.

Occlusion—An obstruction or blockage in a blood vessel.

Patency—Being widely open. A blood vessel that has been widened or reopened is said to be patent.

Plaque—In atherosclerosis, a swollen area in the lining of an artery formed by fatty deposits.

Stenosis (plural, stenoses)—The narrowing or constriction of an opening or passageway in the body.

Stent—A thin rodlike or tubelike device made of wire mesh, inserted into a vein or artery to keep the vessel open.

---

involved. If a percutaneous transluminal coronary angioplasty (PTCA) is to be performed, the patient is sedated so that he or she can report discomfort and cough if asked to do so. PTCA procedures are performed in **cardiac catheterization** laboratories with sophisticated monitoring devices. If angioplasty is performed in the radiology department's angiographic suite, the patient may be sedated for the procedure while a nurse monitors the patient's **vital signs**. Angioplasties performed by vascular surgeons are done in an **operating room** or specially designed vascular procedure suite.

Typically, patients are given anticoagulant (blood thinning) medications prior to the procedure to assist in the prevention of thromboses (blood clots), even though these drugs may slow down the sealing of the entry point into the vein. Patients may also be given calcium blockers and nitrates to reduce the risk of vascular spasm. The procedure is performed using fluoroscopic guidance and contrast media. Since the decision to perform angioplasty may have been made following a diagnostic angiogram, the patient's sensitivity to iodinated contrast media is likely to be known. The procedure may then require the use of non-ionic contrast agents.

The patient's skin is cleansed with an antiseptic solution at the site where the surgeon will insert the catheter and other equipment, and the area is protected with a sterile drape. Although many angioplasties are performed by puncturing the vessel through the skin, others are done by surgically exposing the site of entry. Direct view of the vessel's puncture site aids in monitoring damage to the vessel or excessive bleeding at the site. After the vessel has been punctured and the guidewire introduced, a fluoroscope is used to monitor the small amounts of contrast media that have been injected. This technique allows the surgeon to see the guidewire's movement through the vessel. If the fluoroscope has a feature called "roadmap," the amount of contrast media injected is greater in order to define the full route the guidewire will take. The fluoroscopy system then superimposes subsequent images over the roadmap while the physician moves the guidewire along the roadmap to the destination.

When the surgeon reaches the location of the stenosis, he or she inflates the balloon on the catheter that has been passed along the guidewire. The size of the balloon and the duration of its inflation depend on the size and location of the vessel. In some cases, the surgeon may also use a stent, which is opened or expanded inside the blood vessel after it has been guided to the proper location. The blood vessel may be widened before, during, or after the stent has been opened up. In cases where the vessel is tortuous (twisted) or at intersections of vessels, a graft may be necessary to strengthen the walls of the blood vessel. Stents, grafts, and balloon dilation may all be used together or separately. Sometimes radiation is used when a stent is placed.

After the surgeon has widened the blood vessel, he or she verifies its patency by using fluoroscopy and contrast media to produce an angiogram, by using intravascular ultrasound, or by using both techniques. After the imaging studies have been completed, the surgeon removes the equipment from the blood vessel and closes the puncture site.

Risks

There is a danger of puncturing the vessel with the guidewire during an angioplasty, although the risk is very small. Patients must be monitored for hematoma or hemorrhage at the puncture site. There is also a small risk of heart attack, stroke, and, although unlikely, death—all related to vessel spasm (transient vessel narrowing from irritation by the catheter), or from emboli (as plaque can be dislodged by the catheter or and travel to the heart or brain). Abrupt closure of the coronary artery occurs in about 4% of patients.

Recurrence of stenosis is an additional potential complication. The risk of recurrence is highest in the first six months after angioplasty, with rates as high as 35% reported in some studies.

The length of the patient's hospital stay following an angioplasty depends on his or her overall condition, the occurrence of complications, and the availability of **home care**.

Health care team roles

Physicians often have specially trained assistants for vascular procedures. These assistants may be nurses, surgical technicians, or x ray specialists. Cardiac catheterization laboratories will include someone specially trained in monitoring EKG equipment and vital signs. Either a nurse, nurse anesthetist, or anesthesiologist will administer sedation or anesthesia for the procedure.

Resources

BOOKS

"Diagnostic Cardiovascular Procedures: Invasive Procedures." Section 16, Chapter 198 in *The Merck Manual of Diagnosis and Therapy*, edited by Mark H. Beers, MD, and Robert Berkow, MD. Whitehouse Station, NJ: Merck Research Laboratories, 1999.

Schneider, Peter A. *Endovascular Skills: Guidewires, Catheters, Arteriography, Balloon Angioplasty, Stents*. St. Louis, MO: Quality Medical Publishing, Inc., 1998.

PERIODICALS

Carnall, Douglas. "Angioplasty." *Western Journal of Medicine* 173 (September 2000): 201.

"New Imaging Technique Could Improve Outcome of Popular Heart Procedure." *Heart Disease Weekly* (May 13, 2001): 3.

Schiele, F. "The 'Angioplastically Correct' Follow Up Strategy After Stent Implantation." *Heart* 85 (April, 2001): 363-364.

"Success Clearing Clogged Arteries." *Science News* 159 (February 3, 2001): 72.

ORGANIZATIONS

American Heart Association (AHA), National Center. 7272 Greenville Avenue, Dallas, TX 75231. (800) 242-8721. <www.americanheart.org>.

OTHER

American Heart Association. *Heart & Stroke Guide: Laser Angioplasty*. [cited July 5, 2001]. <www.americanheart.org/Heart_and_Stroke_A_Z_Guide/angiol.html>.

MayoClinic.com. *Coronary Angioplasty: Opening Clogged Arteries*. [cited July 5, 2001]. <www.mayoclinic.com>.

Miami Heart Research Institute. *Cardiovascular System*, 2001. [cited July 5, 2001]. <www.miamiheartresearch.org/LearningCenter/YourCardiovascular../Cardiovascular.htm>.

Elaine R. Proseus MBA/TM, BSRT, RT(R)
Lee A. Shratter, M.D.

Anterior temporal lobectomy

Definition

An anterior temporal lobectomy (ATL) is the complete removal of the anterior portion of the temporal lobe of the brain.

Purpose

ATL surgery has been recognized as an efficient treatment option for certain types of seizures in patients diagnosed with temporal lobe epilepsy (TLE). Characterized by transient disturbances of brain function and seizures, TLE is the most common form of epilepsy. ATL is optimal for patients with seizures that do not respond to medications, patients who are unable to tolerate medication side effects, or patients with seizures caused by structural abnormalities in the brain.

Demographics

Epilepsy is the most common serious neurological condition in the United States. Its incidence is greatest in young chidren and in the elderly, with five to 10 cases diagnosed per 1,000. The lifetime prevalence amounts to 2–5% of the population. Epilepsy is slightly more common in males than females. The frequency of seizure activity in the epileptic population is as follows.

- 33% have less than one seizure per year
- 33% have one to 12 seizures per year
- 33% have more than one seizure per month
- 60% also have other neuropsychiatric problems

Description

ATL surgical procedures:

- Anesthesia. The patient is anesthetized with a combination of drugs that achieves a state of unconsciousness.

- Preparation of the surgical field. An antiseptic solution is applied to the patient's scalp, face, and neck. Surgical drapes are placed around the surgical region to maintain a sterile surgical field.

- Temporal incision. Using a scalpel blade, the neurosurgeon makes an incision in the skin and muscle of the temporal region of the head located on the side of the head above the ear, and pulls away the flap of scalp.

- Control of bleeding. Blood obstructing the surgeon's view of the surgical field is irrigated and suctioned away as surgery proceeds.

- Craniotomy. Using a high-speed drill, the neurosurgeon removes a section of bone (bone flap) from the skull and makes an incision through the protective membranes of the brain (dura) in order to expose the temporal lobe.

- Removal of the anterior lobe. Using an operating microscope to enlarge the features of the surgical area, the neurosurgeon removes the temporal anterior lobe.

- Closure. Once bleeding is under control, every layer of tissue cut or divided to reach the surgical site is closed. The cavity is irrigated completely and the dura is closed in a watertight manner using tack-up sutures. The bone flap is returned into place. Muscle and tissues are closed with sutures, while the skin is closed with staples. No drain is needed.

Diagnosis/Preparation

An ATL pre-surgical diagnosis requires reliable diagnostic levels classified as (1) seizure, (2) epilepsy, and (3) syndrome. The epilepsy and syndromic diagnoses are usually combined. The seizure diagnosis is determined from the physical and neurological manifestations of the condition recorded in the patient's history and from electroencephalogram (EEG) evaluations. Because seizures commonly result from cortical damage, neuroimaging techniques are used to identify and localize the damaged area. They include:

- **Magnetic resonance imaging** (MRI). Brain MRI is the best structural imaging technique available. Every ATL surgical evaluation usually includes a complete MRI study.

- **Positron emission tomography (PET)**. Unlike MRI, PET provides information on brain metabolism rather than on structure. Typically, the epileptic region's metabolism is lowered unless the scan is obtained during a seizure.

- Single photon emission tomography (SPECT). SPECT scans visualize blood flow through the brain and are used as another method for localizing the epileptic site.

Routinely, all ATL candidates also undergo neuropsychological testing.

To prepare for ATL, the patient discontinues any medication being taken and that has been associated with bleeding disorders at least three weeks prior to ATL surgery. **Antibiotics** may be administered intravenously one hour before surgery. Minimal hair is shaved over the temporal area of the head.

Aftercare

After ATL surgery, the neurosurgeon provides instructions for the nurses, pharmacists, therapists, and other physicians caring for the patient postoperatively. Once the anesthesiologist determines that the patient is stable, the surgeon authorizes transport to the **postoperative care** area. Most patients go to the recovery area, but some critical patients may be taken to an **intensive care unit** (ICU) for close monitoring. As is the case for almost all types of brain surgery, the patient is initially nursed with the head of the bed elevated to 30 degrees.

Risks

All surgical procedures are associated with risks and complications that vary depending on the location of the procedure (the approach and dissection required), the pathology (what has to be done to accomplish the surgical objective), and patient factors (such as age, general medical condition, etc.).

A specific risk associated with ATL is possible injury to the cerebral cortex, the outer portion of the brain that consists of layers of nerve cells and their connections, during the lobectomy procedure.

Normal results

ATL offers a high chance of seizure-free outcome in patients suffering from drug-resistant seizures originating in the temporal lobe of the brain. The procedure is considered to be the most common and rewarding of all the surgeries for epilepsy.

Morbidity and mortality rates

ATL is the most common surgery performed to treat medically refractory epilepsy and, in most cases, will diminish or abolish seizures.

In 1997, Sperling et al. reported in the *Epilepsy Quarterly* the five-year outcomes of 89 patients with uncontrolled seizures who underwent ATL at the Graduate Hospital in Philadelphia, Pennsylvania. The patients in this study underwent ATL as a result of no response (or allergy) to at least three medications. Five years postoperatively, 80 of 89 patients (90%) no longer had seizures or experienced more than 80% seizure reduction. Only five patients (6%) exhibited no worthwhile improvement, although a modest reduction in seizure frequency may have been noted. Among the seizure-free patients, 49 were cured of their epilepsy (i.e., they had no seizures after temporal lobectomy).

Alternatives

Anti-convulsant drug development programs

Once the diagnosis of epilepsy is established, a course of medication is usually prescribed for the control of seizures. ATL only becomes the preferred approach when a patient does not respond to medication. As an alternative to surgery, a patient may elect to become an active participant in an anti-convulsant drug development program that may offer an opportunity to participate in studies of experimental medications.

Other surgical techniques

Other surgical techniques such as corpus callosotomy can be performed in selected patients who are ineligible for ATL. In this procedure, the white matter tract connecting the two halves of the brain is cut to halt the spread of seizures and to limit their severity.

QUESTIONS TO ASK THE DOCTOR

- What are the possible complications involved in ATL surgery?
- If the cortex is injured during the surgery, what will the consequences be?
- How long will it take to recover from the surgery?
- What procedures do you follow?
- How many ATL surgeries do you perform each year?

Resources

BOOKS

Chilton, L. *Seizure Free: From Epilepsy to Brain Surgery, I Survived, and You Can, Too!* Dallas: English Press Publications, 2000.

Freeman, J. M., E. P. G. Vining, and D. J. Pillas. *Seizures and Epilepsy in Childhood: A Guide.* Baltimore: Johns Hopkins University Press, 2002.

Hauser, W. A. and D. C. Hesdorffer. *Epilepsy: Frequency, Causes, and Consequences.* New York: Demos Publications, 1990.

Waltz, M. *Partial Seizure Disorders: Help for Patients and Families.* Sebastopol, CA: Patient-Centered Guides, 2001.

PERIODICALS

Clusmann, H., J. Schramm, T. Kral, C. Helmstaedter, B. Ostertun, R. Fimmers, D. Haun, and C. E. Elger. "Prognostic factors and outcome after different types of resection for temporal lobe epilepsy." *Journal of Neurosurgery* 97 (November 2002): 1131–1141.

Crino, P. B. "Outcome Assessment of Anterior Temporal Lobectomy." *Epilepsy Quarterly* 5 (Spring 1997): 1–4.

Elwes, R. D., G. Dunn, C. D. Binnie, and C. E. Polkey. "Outcome following resective surgery for temporal lobe epilepsy: a prospective follow up study of 102 consecutive cases." *Journal of Neurology, Neurosurgery and Psychiatry* 54 (1991): 949–952.

Jarrar, R. G., J. R. Buchhalter, F. B. Meyer, F. W. Sharbrough, and E. Laws. "Long-term follow-up of temporal lobectomy in children." *Neurology* 59 (November 2002): 1635–1637.

Jones, J. E., N. L. Berven, L. Ramirez, A. Woodard, B. P. Hermann. "Long-term psychosocial outcomes of anterior temporal lobectomy." *Epilepsia* 43 (August 2002): 896–903.

Radhakrishnan, K., E. L. So, P. L. Silbert, G. D. Cascino, W. R. Marsh, R. H. Cha, and P. C. O'Brien. "Prognostic implications of seizure recurrence in the first year after anterior temporal lobectomy." *Epilepsia* 44 (January 2003): 77–80.

Sperling, M. R., M. J. O'Connor, A. J. Saykin, and C. Plummer. "Temporal lobectomy for refractory epilepsy." *Journal of the American Medical Association* 276 (1996): 470–475.

KEY TERMS

Anesthesia—A combination of drugs administered by a variety of techniques by trained professionals that provide sedation, amnesia, analgesia, and immobility adequate for the accomplishment of the surgical procedure with minimal discomfort, and without injury, to the patient.

Cerebral cortex—The outer portion of the brain, consisting of layers of nerve cells and their connections. The cerebral cortex is the part of the brain in which thought processes take place.

Craniotomy—A surgical incision into the skull.

Electroencephalogram (EEG)—A diagnostic test that measures the electrical activity of the brain (brain waves) using highly sensitive recording equipment attached to the scalp by electrodes.

Epilepsy—Chronic medical condition produced by temporary changes in the electrical function of the brain, causing seizures that affect awareness, movement, and/or sensation.

Seizures—Attacks consisting of sudden and abnormal muscle, sensory, or psychic events resulting from transient dysfunction of the brain.

Temporal lobe epilepsy (TLE)—The most common type of epilepsy, with elaborate and multiple sensory, motor, and psychic symptoms. A common feature is the loss of consciousness and amnesia during seizures. Other manifestations may include more complex behaviors like bursts of anger, emotional outbursts, fear, or automatisms.

Zimmerman, R. S. and J. I. Sirven. "An overview of surgery for chronic seizures." *Mayo Clinic Proceedings* 78 (January 2003): 109–117.

ORGANIZATIONS

The American Academy of Neurology. 1080 Montreal Avenue, Saint Paul, MN 55116. (800) 879-1960. <http://www.aan.com/>.

The American Epilepsy Society. 342 North Main Street, West Hartford, CT 06117-2507. (860) 586-7505. <http://www.aesnet.org/>.

The Epilepsy Foundation. 4351 Garden City Drive Landover, MD 20785-7223. (800) 332-1000. <http://www.epilepsyfoundation.org/>.

OTHER

Gruen, John Peter M.D. *Temporal lobectomy.* 2000 [cited April 7, 2003]. <http:// uscneurosurgery.com/operating%20room/procedures/temporal%20lobectomy/temporal%20lobectomy.htm >.

Monique Laberge, Ph.D.

Antianxiety drugs

Definition

Antianxiety drugs are medicines that calm and relax people with excessive anxiety, nervousness, or tension, or for short-term control of social phobia disorder or specific phobia disorder.

Purpose

Antianxiety agents, or anxiolytics, may be used to treat mild transient bouts of anxiety as well as more pronounced episodes of social phobia and specific phobia. Clinically significant anxiety is marked by several symptoms. The patient experiences marked or persistent fear of one or more social or performance situations in which he or she is exposed to unfamiliar people or possible scrutiny by others, and may react in a humiliating or embarrassing way. The exposure to the feared situation produces an anxiety attack. Fear of these episodes of anxiety leads to avoidance behavior, which impairs normal social functioning, including working or attending classes. The patient is aware that these fears are unjustified.

Antianxiety drugs, particularly the injectable benzodiazepines lorazepam (Ativan) and midazolam (Versed), are also used for preoperative sedation in surgery. Used for this purpose, they may induce relaxation, provide sedation, and also reduce memory of an unpleasant experience. They offer the combined benefits of relaxing the patient, and reducing the need for other agents including **analgesics**, anesthetics, and **muscle relaxants**.

Description

In psychiatric practice, treatment of anxiety has largely turned from traditional antianxiety agents, anxiolytics, to antidepressant therapies. In current use, the benzodiazepines, the best-known class of anxiolytics, have been largely supplanted by serotonin-specific reuptake inhibitors (SSRIs, including citalopram, fluoxetine, fluvoxamine, and others), which have a milder side effect profile and less risk of dependency. However, traditional anxiolytics remain useful for patients who need a rapid onset of action, or whose frequency of exposure to anxiety-provoking stimuli is low enough to eliminate the need for continued treatment. While SSRIs may require three to five weeks to show any effects, and must be taken continuously, benzodiazepines may produce a response within 30 minutes, and may be dosed on an as-needed basis.

The intermediate-action benzodiazepines, alprazolam (Xanax), and lorazepam (Ativan), are the appropriate choice for treatment of mild anxiety and social phobia. Diazepam (Valium) is still widely used for anxiety,

Antianxiety Drugs

Brand Name (Generic Name)	Possible Common Side Effects Include:
Atarax (hydroxyzine hydrochloride)	Drowsiness, dry mouth
Ativan (lorazepam)	Dizziness, excessive calm, weakness
BuSpar, Buspirone (buspirone hydrochloride)	Dry mouth, dizziness, headache, fatigue, nausea
Centrax (pazepam)	Decreased coordination, dizziness, drowsiness, fatigue, weakness
Librium, Libritabs (chlordiazepoxide)	Constipation, drowsiness, nausea, swelling
Miltown, Equanil (meprobamate)	Diarrhea, bruising, fever, headache, nausea, rash, slurred speech
Serax (oxazepam)	Dizziness, fainting, headache, liver problems, decreased coordination, nausea, swelling, vertigo
Stelazine (trifluoperazine hydrochloride)	Abnormal glucose in urine, allergic reactions, blurred vision, constipation, eye spasms, fluid retention and swelling
Tranxene, Tranxene-SD (clorazepate dipotassium)	Drowsiness
Valium (diazepam)	Decreased coordination, drowsiness, light-headedness

but its active metabolite, desmethyldiazepam, which has a long half-life, may make this a poorer choice than other drugs in its class. There is considerable variation between individuals in the metabolism of benzodiazepines, so patient response may not be predictable. As a class, benzodiazepines are used not only as anxiolytics, but also as sedatives, muscle relaxants, and in treatment of epilepsy and alcoholism. The distinctions between these uses are largely determined by onset and duration of action, and route of administration.

Buspirone (BuSpar), which is not chemically related to other classes of central nervous system drugs, is also a traditional anxiolytic, although it is now considered either a third-line or adjunctive agent for use after trials of SSRIs and benzodiazepines. It is appropriate for use in patients who have either failed trials of other treatments, or who should not receive benzodiazepines because of a history of substance abuse problems. Buspirone, in common with antidepressants, requires a two- to three-week period before there is clinical evidence of improvement, and must be continuously dosed to maintain its effects.

In surgery, antianxiety drugs may be used to provide relaxation and reduce fear of surgery. They may reduce the need for anesthetics and muscle relaxants. In addition, some antianxiety drugs may impair memory, which is a benefit since it reduces concern about an unpleasant experience. Short-acting benzodiazepines such as midazolam (Versed) and lorazepam (Ativan) are most often used for this purpose.

Benzodiazepines are controlled drugs under federal law. Buspirone is not a controlled substance and has no established abuse potential.

Recommended dosage

Pre-surgical dosing of midazolam varies with the route of administration, the age and physical condition of the patient, and the other drugs to be used. For patients under the age of 60, who have not received narcotic analgesics, a dose of 2–3 mg is normally adequate, but some elderly patients may respond to a dose as low as 1 mg. The usual dose of lorazepam is up to 4 mg, administered by intramuscular injection at least two hours prior to surgery. If the drug is given intravenously, a dose of up to 2 mg may be given 15–20 minutes before surgery.

Benzodiazepines should be administered 30–60 minutes before exposure to the anticipated stress. Dosage should be individualized to minimize sedation. The normal dose of alprazolam is 0.25–0.5 mg. The usual dose of lorazepam is 2–3 mg. Doses may be repeated if necessary.

Buspirone is initially dosed at 5 mg three times a day. The dosage should be increased 5 mg/day, at intervals of two to three days, as needed. A dosage of 60 mg/day should not be exceeded. Two to three weeks may be required before a satisfactory response is observed.

Precautions

Precautions and warnings apply to the use of antianxiety agents for use over long periods of time. They are unlikely to occur in patients who have only received a single dose prior to surgery.

Benzodiazepines should not be used in patients with psychosis, acute narrow-angle glaucoma, or liver disease. The drugs can act as respiratory depressants and should be avoided in patients with respiratory conditions. Benzodiazepines are potentially addictive and should not be administered to patients with substance abuse disorders. Because benzodiazepines are sedatives, they should be avoided in patients who must remain alert. Their use for periods over four months has not been documented. These drugs should not be used during the second and third trimester of pregnancy, although

KEY TERMS

Anxiety—Worry or tension in response to real or imagined stress, danger, or dreaded situations. Physical reactions such as fast pulse, sweating, trembling, fatigue, and weakness may accompany anxiety.

Epilepsy—A brain disorder with symptoms that include seizures.

Panic disorder—An disorder in which people have sudden and intense attacks of anxiety in certain situations.

Phobia—An intense, abnormal, or illogical fear of something specific such as heights or open spaces.

Pregnancy category B—Animal studies indicate no fetal risk, but no human studies; or adverse effects in animals, but not in well-controlled human studies.

Pregnancy category C—No adequate human or animal studies; or adverse fetal effects in animal studies, but no available human data.

Seizure—A sudden attack, spasm, or convulsion.

use during the first trimester appears to be safe. They should not be taken while breastfeeding. Specialized references for use in children should be consulted.

Buspirone is metabolized by the liver and excreted by the kidney, and should be used with care in patients with hepatic or renal disease. The drug is classified as schedule B during pregnancy, but should not be taken during breastfeeding. Its use in children under the age of 18 years has not been studied.

Interactions

The metabolism of alprazolam may be increased by cimetidine, oral contraceptives, disulfiram, fluoxetine, isoniazid, ketoconazole, metoprolol, propoxyphene, propranolol, and valproic acid. The absorption of all benzodiazepines is inhibited by concomitant use of antacids. Benzodiazepines may increase blood levels of digoxin, and reduce the efficacy of levodopa. Other drug interactions have been reported.

Buspirone levels will be increased by concomitant use of erythromycin, itraconazole, and nefazadone. Doses should be adjusted based on clinical response. Use of buspirone at the same time as monoamine oxidase inhibitors (MAOIs, including phenelzine and tranycypromine) may cause severe blood pressure elevations. Use of buspirone with MAOIs should be avoided.

Side effects

The most common side effects of benzodiazepines are secondary to their central nervous system (CNS) effects and include sedation and sleepiness; depression; lethargy; apathy; fatigue; hypoactivity; lightheadedness; memory impairment; disorientation; anterograde amnesia; restlessness; confusion; crying or sobbing; delirium; headache; slurred speech; aphonia; dysarthria; stupor; seizures; coma; syncope; rigidity; tremor; dystonia; vertigo; dizziness; euphoria; nervousness; irritability; difficulty in concentration; agitation; inability to perform complex mental functions; akathisia; hemiparesis; hypotonia; unsteadiness; ataxia; incoordination; weakness; vivid dreams; psychomotor retardation; "glassy-eyed" appearance; extrapyramidal symptoms; and paradoxical reactions. Other reactions include changes in heart rate and blood pressure, changes in bowel function, severe skin rash, and changes in genitourinary function. Other adverse effects have been reported.

Buspirone has a low incidence of side effects. Dizziness and drowsiness are the most commonly reported adverse effects. Other CNS effects include dream disturbances; depersonalization, dysphoria, noise intolerance, euphoria, akathisia, fearfulness, loss of interest, disassociative reaction, hallucinations, suicidal ideation, seizures; feelings of claustrophobia, cold intolerance, stupor and slurred speech, and psychosis. Rarely, heart problems, including congestive heart failure and myocardial infarction, have been reported. Other adverse effects have been reported.

Resources

BOOKS

AHFS: Drug Information. Washington, DC: American Society of Healthsystems Pharmaceuticals, 2003.

Brody, T.M., J. Larner, K.P. Minneman, and H.C. Neu. *Human Pharmacology: Molecular to Clinical, 2nd ed.* St. Louis: Mosby Year-Book, 1998.

Karch, A.M. *Lippincott's Nursing Drug Guide.* Springhouse, PA: Lippincott Williams & Wilkins, 2003.

Racagni, G, C. Massotto, and L. Steardo. *Pharmacology of Anxiolytic Drugs. Who Expert Series on Neuroscience.* Vol. 3. Cambridge, MA: Hogrefe and Huber, 1997.

Reynolds, J.E.F., ed. *Martindale: The Extra Pharmacopoeia,* 31st ed. London: The Pharmaceutical Press, 1993.

OTHER

"Anxiolytic Drugs." West Virginia University Health Sciences College. [cited May 2003]. <http://www.hsc.wvu.edu/som/physio/P&P%20750/Woodfork/Anxiolytics%20PP%2002.pdf>.

"Benzodiazepines (Systemic)." Medline Plus Drug Information. [cited May 2003]. <http://www.nlm.nih.gov/medlineplus/druginfo/uspdi/202084.html>.

Samuel Uretsky, PharmD

Antibiotic prophylaxis *see* **Prophylaxis, antibiotic**

Antibiotics

Definition

Antibiotics may be informally defined as the subgroup of anti-infectives derived from bacterial sources and used to treat bacterial infections.

Purpose

Antibiotics are used for treatment or prevention of bacterial infection. Other classes of drugs, most notably the **sulfonamides**, may be effective antibacterials. Similarly, some antibiotics may have secondary uses, such as the use of demeclocycline (Declomycin, a tetracycline derivative) to treat the syndrome of inappropriate antidiuretic hormone (SIADH) secretion. Other antibiotics may be useful in treating protozoal infections.

Description

Although there are several classification schemes for antibiotics, based on bacterial spectrum (broad versus narrow), route of administration (injectable versus oral versus topical), or type of activity (bactericidal versus bacteriostatic), the most useful is based on chemical structure. Antibiotics within a structural class will generally show similar patterns of effectiveness, toxicity, and allergic potential.

Penicillins

The penicillins are the oldest class of antibiotics and have a common chemical structure that they share with the **cephalosporins**. The two groups are classed as the beta-lactam antibiotics, and are generally bacteriocidal—that is, they kill bacteria rather than inhibit growth. The penicillins can be further subdivided. The natural penicillins are based on the original penicillin G structure; penicillinase-resistant penicillins, notably methicillin and oxacillin, are active even in the presence of the bacterial enzyme that inactivates most natural penicillins. Aminopenicillins such as ampicillin and amoxicillin have an extended spectrum of action compared with the natural penicillins; extended spectrum penicillins are effective against a wider range of bacteria. These generally include coverage for *Pseudomonas aeruginosa* and may provide the penicillin in combination with a penicillinase inhibitor.

Cephalosporins

Cephalosporins and the closely related cephamycins and carbapenems, like the penicillins, contain a beta-lactam chemical structure. Consequently, there are patterns of cross-resistance and cross-allergenicity among the drugs in these classes. The "cepha" drugs are among the most diverse classes of antibiotics, and are themselves subgrouped into first, second, and third generations. Each generation has a broader spectrum of activity than the one before. In addition, cefoxitin (Mefoxin), a cephamycin, is highly active against anaerobic bacteria, which makes it useful in prevention and treatment of infections of the intestines. The third generation drugs, cefotaxime, ceftizoxime, ceftriaxone, and others, cross the blood-brain barrier and may be used to treat meningitis and encephalitis. Cephalosporins are the usually preferred agents for prevention of infection during surgery.

Fluroquinolones

The fluroquinolones are synthetic antibacterial agents, and are not derived from bacteria. They are included here because they can be readily interchanged with traditional antibiotics. An earlier, related class of antibacterial agents, the quinolones, were not well absorbed, and could be used only to treat urinary tract infections. The fluroquinolones, which are based on the older group, are broad-spectrum bactericidal drugs that are chemically unrelated to the penicillins or the cephalosporins. They are well distributed into bone tissue, and so well absorbed that in general they are as effective by the oral route as by intravenous infusion.

Tetracyclines

Tetracyclines got their name because they share a chemical structure having four rings. They are derived from a species of *Streptomyces* bacteria. Broad-spectrum bacteriostatic agents, the tetracyclines may be effective against a wide variety of microorganisms, including rickettsia and amebic parasites.

Macrolides

The macrolide antibiotics are derived from *Streptomyces* bacteria, and got their name because they all have a macrocyclic lactone chemical structure. Erythromycin, the prototype of this class, has a spectrum and use similar to penicillin. Newer members of the group, azithromycin and clarithyromycin, are particularly useful for their high level of lung penetration. Clarithromycin has been widely used to treat *Helicobacter pylori* infections, the cause of stomach ulcers. For people who are allergic to penicillin, erythromycin is a valuable alternative. But, unlike penicillin, erythromycin can be very irritating

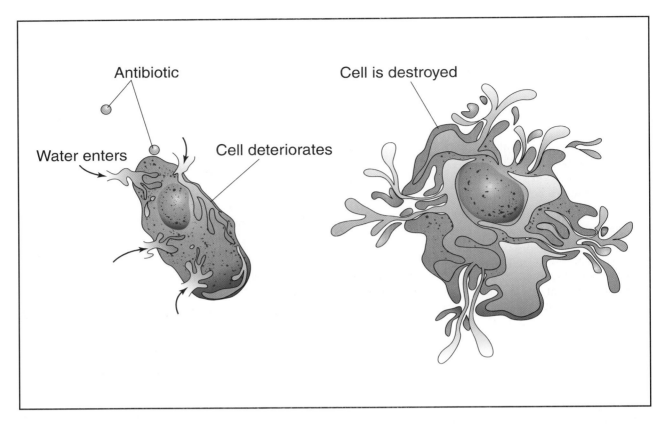

Antibiotic

Cell is destroyed

Water enters

Cell deteriorates

Different antibiotics destroy bacteria in different ways. Some short-circuit the processes by which bacteria receive energy. Others disturb the structure of the bacterial cell wall, as shown in the illustration above. Still others interfere with the production of essential proteins. *(Illustration by Electronic Illustrators Group.)*

both to the stomach when given by mouth, or to veins when given by injection.

Other classes

Other classes of antibiotics include the aminoglycosides, which are particularly useful for their effectiveness in treating *Pseudomonas aeruginosa* infections, and the lincosamindes, clindamycin and lincomycin, which are highly active against anaerobic pathogens. In addition, other individual drugs are available that may have utility in specific infections.

Recommended dosage

Dosage varies with drug, route of administration, pathogen, site of infection, and severity. Additional considerations include renal (kidney) function, age of patient, and other factors. Patients should consult manufacturers' recommendations or ask their doctors.

Side effects

All antibiotics cause risk of overgrowth by non-susceptible bacteria. Manufacturers list other major hazards

by class; however, the health care provider should review each drug individually to assess the degree of risk. Generally, breastfeeding is not recommended while taking antibiotics because of risk of alteration to infant's intestinal flora, and risk of masking infection in the infant. Excessive or inappropriate use may promote growth of resistant pathogens.

- *Penicillins.* Hypersensitivity may be common, and cross allergenicity with cephalosporins has been reported. Penicillins are classed as category B during pregnancy.

- *Cephalosporins.* Several cephalosporins and related compounds have been associated with seizures. Cefmetazole, cefoperazone, cefotetan and ceftriaxone may be associated with a fall in prothrombin activity and coagulation abnormalities. Pseudomembranous colitis (inflammation of the colon) has been reported with cephalosporins and other broad spectrum antibiotics. Some drugs in this class may cause renal toxicity. Pregnancy category B.

- *Fluoroquinolones.* Lomefloxacin has been associated with increased photosensitivity. All drugs in this class have been associated with convulsions. Pregnancy category C.

- *Tetracyclines*. Demeclocycline may cause increased photosensitivity. Minocycline may cause dizziness. Children under the age of eight should not use tetracyclines, and specifically during periods of tooth development. Oral tetracyclines bind to anions such as calcium and iron. Although doxycycline and minocycline may be taken with meals, patients are advised to take other tetracycline antibiotics on an empty stomach, and not to take the drugs with milk or other calcium-rich foods. Expired tetracycline should never be administered. Pregnancy category D; use during pregnancy may cause alterations in bone development.

- *Macrolides*. Erythromycin may aggravate the weakness of patients with myasthenia gravis. Azithromycin has, rarely, been associated with allergic reactions, including angioedema, anaphylaxis, and dermatologic reactions, including Stevens-Johnson syndrome and toxic epidermal necrolysis. Oral erythromycin may be highly irritating to the stomach and may cause severe phlebitis (inflammation of the vein) when given by injection. These drugs should be used with caution in patients with liver dysfunction. Pregnancy category B: Azithromycin, erythromycin. Pregnancy category C: Clarithromycin, dirithromycin, troleandomycin.

- *Aminoglycosides*. This class of drugs causes kidney and hearing problems. These problems can occur even with normal doses. Dosing should be based on renal function, with periodic testing of both kidney function and hearing. Pregnancy category D.

Interactions

Use of all antibiotics may temporarily reduce the effectiveness of birth control pills; alternative birth control methods should be used while taking these medications. Antacids should be avoided while on tetracyclines as the calcium can impair absorption of this antibiotic class. For this reason, tetracyclines should not be taken just before or after consuming foods rich in calcium or iron. Consult specialized references for additional interactions to specific antibiotics.

Recommended usage

To minimize risk of adverse reactions and development of resistant strains of bacteria, antibiotics should be restricted to use in cases where there is either known or a reasonable presumption of bacterial infection. The use of antibiotics in viral infections is to be avoided. Avoid use of fluroquinolones for trivial infections.

In severe infections, presumptive therapy with a broad-spectrum antibiotic such as a third generation cephalosporin may be appropriate. Treatment should be

> **KEY TERMS**
>
> **Anaerobic**—An organism that lives without oxygen. Anaerobic bacteria are commonly found in the mouth and the intestines.
>
> **Bacteria**—Tiny, one-celled forms of life that cause many diseases and infections.
>
> **Bactericidal**—An agent that kills bacteria.
>
> **Bacteriostatic**—An agent that stops the multiplication of bacteria.
>
> **Inflammation**—Pain, redness, swelling, and heat that usually develop in response to injury or illness.
>
> **Meningitis**—Inflammation of tissues that surround the brain and spinal cord.
>
> **Microorganism**—An independent unit of life that is too small to be seen with the naked eye.
>
> **Pregnancy category**—A system of classifying drugs according to their established risks for use during pregnancy. Category A: Controlled human studies have demonstrated no fetal risk. Category B: Animal studies indicate no fetal risk, but no human studies; or adverse effects in animals, but not in well-controlled human studies. Category C: No adequate human or animal studies; or adverse fetal effects in animal studies, but no available human data. Category D: Evidence of fetal risk, but benefits outweigh risks. Category X: Evidence of fetal risk. Risks outweigh any benefits.

changed to a narrow spectrum agent as soon as the pathogen has been identified. After 48 hours of treatment, if there is clinical improvement, an oral antibiotic should be considered.

When the pathogen is known or suspected to be *Pseudomonas*, a suitable beta-lactam drug is often prescribed in combination with an aminoglycoside. A single agent cannot be relied upon for treatment of *Pseudomonas*. When the patient has renal insufficiency, azactam should be considered in place of the aminoglycoside.

In treatment of children with antibiotic suspensions, caregivers should be instructed in use of oral syringes or measuring teaspoons. Household teaspoons are not standardized and will give unreliable doses.

Resources

PERIODICALS

Moellering, R. C., Jr. "Linezolid." Summaries for Patients. *Annals of Internal Medicine* 138 (January 21, 2003): I-44.

OTHER

Alliance for the Prudent Use of Antibiotics. Consumer Information. <http://www.tufts.edu/med/apua/Patients/patient.html>.

"Using antibiotics sensibly." *MayoClinic.com.* February 6, 2002 [cited June 25, 2003]. <http://www.mayoclinic.com/invoke.cfm?id=FL00075>.

Samuel Uretsky, PharmD

Antibiotics, topical

Definition

Topical **antibiotics** are medicines applied to the skin to kill or stop the growth of bacteria.

Purpose

Topical antibiotics help prevent infections caused by bacteria that get into minor cuts, scrapes, and burns. Treating minor wounds with antibiotics allows quicker healing. If the wounds are left untreated, the bacteria will multiply, causing pain, redness, swelling, itching, and oozing. Untreated infections can eventually spread and become much more serious.

Topical antibiotics may also be applied to surgical incision sites to prevent infection. However, when antibiotics are given intravenously (by vein) or during surgery and intravenously or by mouth following surgery, this may be enough to prevent infection, and antibiotic ointments may not be needed.

Different kinds of topical antibiotics kill different kinds of bacteria. Many antibiotic first-aid products contain combinations of antibiotics to make them effective against a broad range of bacteria.

When treating a wound, it is not enough to simply apply a topical antibiotic. The wound must first be cleaned with soap and water and patted dry. After the antibiotic is applied, the wound should be covered with a dressing such as a bandage or a protective gel or spray. For many years, it was thought that wounds heal best when exposed to the air. But now most experts say it is best to keep wounds clean and moist while they heal. The covering should still allow some air to reach the wound, however.

Description

Some topical antibiotics are available without a prescription and are sold in many forms, including creams, ointments, powders, and sprays. Some widely used topical antibiotics are bacitracin, neomycin, mupirocin, and polymyxin B. Among the products that contain one or more of these ingredients are Bactroban (a prescription item), Neosporin, Polysporin, and Triple Antibiotic Ointment or Cream.

Recommended dosage

The recommended dosage depends on the type of topical antibiotic. The patient is advised to follow the directions on the package label or ask a pharmacist for directions.

Because only the ointment or cream that actually touches the skin has any benefit, a thin layer of topical antibiotic ointment or cream will usually work just as well as a thick layer.

In general, topical antibiotics should be applied within four hours after injury. It is advised not to use more than the recommended amount and do not apply it more often than three times a day; the medicine should not be applied over large areas of skin or on open wounds.

When topical antibiotics are used for surgical incision sites, a surgeon or nurse should be consulted for instructions.

Precautions

Many public health experts are concerned about antibiotic resistance, a problem that can develop when antibiotics are overused. Over time, bacteria develop new defenses against the antibiotics that once were effective against them. Because bacteria reproduce so quickly, these defenses can be rapidly passed on through generations of bacteria until almost all are immune to the effects of a particular antibiotic. The process happens faster than new antibiotics can be developed. To help control the problem, many experts advise people to use topical antibiotics only for short periods, that is, until the wound heals, and only as directed. For the topical antibiotic to work best, it should be used only to prevent infection in a fresh wound, not to treat an infection that has already started. Wounds that are not fresh may need the attention of a physician to prevent complications such as blood poisoning.

Topical antibiotics are meant to be used only on the skin and for only a few days at a time. If the wound has not healed in five days, the patient is advised to stop using the antibiotic and call a doctor.

It is advised not to use topical antibiotics on large areas of skin or on open wounds. These products should not be used to treat diaper rash in infants or incontinence rash in adults.

Only minor cuts, scrapes, and burns should be treated with topical antibiotics. Certain kinds of injuries may need medical care and should not be self-treated with topical antibiotics. These include:

- large wounds
- deep cuts
- cuts that continue bleeding
- cuts that may need stitches
- burns any larger than a few inches in diameter
- scrapes imbedded with particles that will not wash away
- animal bites
- deep puncture wounds
- eye injuries

Regular topical antibiotics should never be used in the eyes. Special antibiotic products are available for treating eye infections.

Although topical antibiotics control infections caused by bacteria, they may allow fungal infections to develop. The use of other medicines to treat the fungal infections may be necessary. It is recommended to check with the physician.

Some people may be allergic to one or more ingredients in a topical antibiotic product. If an allergic reaction develops, the person should stop using the product immediately and call a physician.

No harmful or abnormal effects have been reported in babies whose mothers used topical antibiotics while pregnant or nursing. However, pregnant women generally are advised not to use any drugs during the first three months after conception. A woman who is pregnant or breastfeeding or who plans to become pregnant should check with her physician before using a topical antibiotic.

Unless a physician says to do so, topical antibiotics should not be used on children under two years of age.

Side effects

The most common minor side effects are itching or burning. These problems usually do not require medical treatment unless they do not go away or they interfere with normal activities.

If any of the following side effects occur, a doctor should be consulted as soon as possible:

- rash
- swelling of the lips and face

KEY TERMS

Bacteria—Tiny, one-celled forms of life that cause many diseases and infections.

Conception—The union of egg and sperm to form a fetus.

Fungal—Caused by a fungus.

Fungus—A member of a group of simple organisms that are related to yeast and molds.

Incision—A cut, usually made by a surgeon during a surgical procedure.

Incontinence—The inability to control the bladder or bowel.

Inflammation—Pain, redness, swelling, and heat that usually develop in response to injury or illness.

- sweating
- tightness or discomfort in the chest
- breathing problems
- fainting or dizziness
- low blood pressure
- nausea
- diarrhea
- hearing loss or ringing in the ears

Other rare side effects may occur. Anyone who has unusual symptoms after using a topical antibiotic should get in touch with the physician who prescribed it or the pharmacist who recommended the medication.

Interactions

Using certain topical antibiotics at the same time as hydrocortisone (a topical corticosteroid used to treat inflammation) may hide signs of infection or allergic reaction. These two medicines should not be used at the same time unless recommended by a health care provider.

Anyone who is using any other type of prescription or nonprescription (over-the-counter) medicine on the skin should check with a doctor before using a topical antibiotic.

Resources

PERIODICALS

Farley, Dixie. "Help for Cuts, Scrapes and Burns." *FDA Consumer* (May 1996): 12.

O'Connor, L.T. Jr., and M. Goldstein. "Topical Perioperative Antibiotic Prophylaxis for Minor Clean Inguinal Surgery." *Journal of the American College of Surgeons* 194, no. 4 (April 2002): 407–10.

Nancy Ross-Flanigan
Sam Uretsky

Antibody screening *see* **Type and screen**

Anticlotting drugs *see* **Anticoagulant and antiplatelet drugs**

Anticoagulant and antiplatelet drugs

Definition

Anticoagulants are drugs used to prevent clot formation or to prevent a clot that has formed from enlarging. They inhibit clot formation by blocking the action of clotting factors or platelets. Anticoagulant drugs fall into one of three categories: inhibitors of clotting factor synthesis, inhibitors of thrombin, and antiplatelet drugs.

Purpose

Anticoagulant drugs reduce the ability of the blood to form clots. Although blood clotting is essential to prevent serious bleeding in the case of skin cuts, clots inside the blood vessels block the flow of blood to major organs and cause heart attacks and strokes. Although these drugs are sometimes called blood thinners, they do not actually thin the blood. Furthermore, this type of medication will not dissolve clots that already have formed, although the drug stops an existing clot from worsening. However, another type of drug, used in **thrombolytic therapy**, will dissolve existing clots.

Anticoagulant drugs are used for a number of conditions. For example, they may be given to prevent blood clots from forming after the replacement of a heart valve or to reduce the risk of a stroke or another heart attack after a first heart attack. They are also used to reduce the chance of blood clots forming during open-heart surgery or bypass surgery. Low doses of these drugs may be given to prevent blood clots in patients who must stay in bed for a long time after certain types of surgery. They may also be used to prevent the formation of clots in needles or tubes that are inserted into veins, such as indwelling catheters.

Anticoagulants may be given after major surgery to prevent the formation of clots due to lack of physical activity. Patients who are unable to move around may be at risk of developing clots, particularly in the legs. Anticoagulants are given to prevent this. At the same time, compression stockings may be used to reduce the risk of clots in the legs. Compression stocks are worn on the lower legs, and act by increasing the pressure on the veins of the leg, then relaxing. The compression-relaxation keeps the blood in the veins moving, and reduces the risk of clots following surgery.

Because anticoagulants affect the blood's ability to clot, they can increase the risk of severe bleeding and heavy blood loss. It is thus essential to take these drugs exactly as directed and to see a physician regularly as long as they are prescribed. With some of these drugs, regular blood tests, as often as once a day, may be required.

Description

Most anticoagulant drugs are available only with a physician's prescription. They come in tablet and injectable forms. They fall into three groups:

- Inhibitors of clotting factor synthesis. These anticoagulants inhibit the production of certain clotting factors in the liver. One example is warfarin (brand name: Coumadin).

- Inhibitors of thrombin. These drugs interfere with blood clotting by blocking the activity of thrombin. They include heparin and lepirudin (Refludan).

- Antiplatelet drugs. These drugs interact with platelets, which is a type of blood cell, to block platelets from aggregating into harmful clots. They include **aspirin**, ticlopidine (Ticlid), clopidogrel (Plavix), tirofiban (Aggrastat), and eptifibatide (Integrilin).

Recommended dosage

The recommended dosage depends on the type of anticoagulant drug and the medical condition for which it is prescribed. The prescribing physician or the pharmacist who fills the prescription can provide information concerning the correct dosage. Usually, the physician will adjust the dose after checking the patient's clotting time.

Anticoagulant drugs must be taken exactly as directed by the physician. Larger or more frequent doses should not be taken, and the drug should also not be taken for longer than prescribed. Taking too much of this medication can cause easy bruising or severe bleeding. Anticoagulants should also be taken on schedule. A record of each dose should be kept as it is taken. If a dose is missed, it should be taken as soon as possible followed by the regular dose schedule. However, a patient who forgets to take a missed dose until the next day should not take the missed dose at all and should not double the next dose, as this could lead to bleeding. A record of all missed doses should be kept for the prescribing physician who should be informed at the scheduled visits.

Precautions

Persons who take anticoagulants should see a physician regularly while taking these drugs, particularly at the beginning of therapy. The physician will order periodic blood tests to check the blood's clotting ability. The results of these tests will help the physician determine the proper amount of medication to be taken each day.

Time is required for normal clotting ability to return after anticoagulant treatment. During this period, patients must observe the same precautions they observed while taking the drug. The length of time needed for the blood to return to normal depends on the type of anticoagulant drug that was taken. The prescribing physician will advise as to how long the precautions should be observed.

People who are taking anticoagulant drugs should tell all physicians, dentists, pharmacists, and other medical professionals who provide them with medical treatments or services that they are taking such a medication. They should also carry identification stating that they are using an anticoagulant drug.

Other prescription drugs or over-the-counter medicine—especially aspirin—should be not be taken without the prescribing physician being informed.

Because of the risk of heavy bleeding, anyone who takes an anticoagulant drug must take care to avoid injuries. Sports and other potentially hazardous activities should be avoided. Any falls, blows to the body or head, or other injuries should be reported to a physician, as internal bleeding may occur without any obvious symptoms. Special care should be taken in shaving and in brushing and flossing the teeth. Soft toothbrushes should be used and the flossing should be very gentle. Electric razors should be used instead of a blade.

Alcohol can change the way anticoagulant drugs affect the body. Anyone who takes this medicine should not have more than one to two alcoholic drinks at any one time, and should not drink alcohol every day.

Special conditions

People with specific medical conditions or who are taking certain other medicines can have problems if they take anticoagulant drugs. Before taking these drugs, the prescribing physician should be informed about any of these conditions.

ALLERGIES. Anyone who has had unusual reactions to anticoagulants in the past should let the physician know before taking the drugs again. The physician should also be told about any allergies to beef, pork, or other foods; dyes; preservatives; or other substances.

PREGNANCY. Anticoagulants may cause many serious problems if taken during pregnancy. Birth defects, severe bleeding in the fetus, and other problems that affect the physical or mental development of the fetus or newborn are possible. The mother may also experience severe bleeding if she takes anticoagulants during pregnancy, during delivery, or even shortly after delivery. Women should not start taking anticoagulants during pregnancy and should not become pregnant while taking the drug. Any woman who becomes pregnant or suspects that she has become pregnant while taking an anticoagulant should check with her physician immediately.

BREASTFEEDING. Some anticoagulant drugs may pass into breast milk. Blood tests can be done on nursing babies to see whether the drug is causing any problems. If it is, other medication may be prescribed to counteract the effects of the anticoagulant drug.

OTHER MEDICAL CONDITIONS. Before using anticoagulant drugs, people should inform their physician about any medical problems they have. They should also let the physician who prescribed the medicine know if they are being treated by any other medical physician or dentist. In addition, people who will be taking anticoagulant drugs should let their physician know if they have recently had any of the following:

- fever lasting more than one to two days
- severe or continuing diarrhea
- childbirth
- heavy or unusual menstrual bleeding
- insertion of an intrauterine contraceptive device (i.e., IUD)
- falls, injuries, or blows to the body or head
- any type of surgery, including dental surgery
- spinal anesthesia
- radiation treatment
- any intestinal condition

Side effects

The most common minor side effects are bloating or gas. These problems usually go away as the body adjusts to the drug and do not require medical treatment.

More serious side effects may occur, especially if excessive anticoagulant is taken. If any of the following side effects occur, a physician should be notified immediately:

- bleeding gums
- sores or white spots in the mouth or throat
- unusual bruises or purplish areas on the skin
- unexplained nosebleeds
- unusually heavy bleeding or oozing from wounds
- unexpected or unusually heavy menstrual bleeding
- blood in the urine
- cloudy or dark urine
- painful or difficult urination or sudden decrease in amount of urine
- black, tarry, or bloody stools
- coughing up blood
- vomiting blood or something that looks like coffee grounds
- constipation
- pain or swelling in the stomach or abdomen
- back pain
- stiff, swollen, or painful joints
- painful, bluish or purplish fingers or toes
- puffy or swollen eyelids, face, feet, or lower legs
- changes in the color of the face
- skin rash, itching, or hives
- yellow eyes or skin
- severe or continuing headache
- sore throat and fever, with or without chills
- breathing problems or wheezing
- tightness in the chest
- dizziness
- unusual tiredness or weakness
- weight gain

In addition, patients taking anticoagulant drugs should check with their physicians as soon as possible if any of these side effects occur:

- nausea or vomiting
- diarrhea
- stomach pain or cramps

Other side effects may occur. Anyone who has unusual symptoms while taking anticoagulant drugs should get in touch with the prescribing physician.

KEY TERMS

Anticoagulant—Drug used to prevent clot formation or to prevent a clot that has formed from enlarging.

Antiplatelet drug—Drug that inhibits platelets from aggregating to form a plug.

Atherosclerosis—Condition characterized by deposits of fatty plaque in the arteries.

Catheter—A tube for passage of fluid into the body or into a body cavity.

Clot—A soft, semi-solid mass that forms when blood gels.

Platelet—A small, disk-shaped body in the blood that has an important role in blood clotting: they form the initial plug at the rupture site of a blood vessel.

Thrombin—A protein produced by the body that is a specific clotting factor that plays an important role in the blood-clotting process.

Thrombin inhibitor—One type of anticoagulant medication, used to help prevent formation of harmful blood clots in the body by blocking the activity of thrombin.

Interactions

Anticoagulants may interact with many other medications. When this happens, the effects of one or both of the drugs may change or the risk of side effects may be increased. Anyone who takes anticoagulants should inform the prescribing physician about other prescription or nonprescription (over-the-counter) medicines he or she is taking—even aspirin, **laxatives**, vitamins, and antacids.

Diet also affects the way anticoagulant drugs work in the body. A normal, balanced diet should be followed every day while taking such medication. No dietary changes should be made without informing first the prescribing physician, who should also be told of any illness or other condition interfering with the ability to eat normally. Diet is a very important consideration because the amount of vitamin K in the body affects how anticoagulant drugs work. Dicoumarol and warfarin act by reducing the effects of vitamin K, which is found in meats, dairy products, leafy, green vegetables, and some multiple vitamins and nutritional supplements. For the drugs to work properly, it is best to have the same amount of vitamin K in the body all the time. Foods containing vitamin K should not be increased or decreased without consulting with the prescribing physician. If the patient takes vitamin supplements, he or she should check the label to see if it contains vitamin K. Because vitamin K is also produced by intestinal bacteria, a severe case of diarrhea or the use of laxatives may also alter a person's vitamin K levels.

Resources

BOOKS

AHFS: Drug Information. Washington, DC: American Society Healthsystems Pharmaceuticals, 2002.

Brody, T.M., J. Larner, K.P. Minneman, H.C. Neu. *Human Pharmacology: Molecular to Clinical,* 2nd ed. St. Louis: Mosby Year-Book.

Reynolds, J.E.F., ed. *Martindale: The Extra Pharmacopoeia,* 31st ed. London: The Pharmaceutical Press, 1993.

OTHER

"Abciximab." Medline Plus Drug Information. [cited May 2003]/ <http://www.nlm.nih.gov/medlineplus/druginfo/uspdi/500417.html>.

"Heparin (Systemic)." Medline Plus Drug Information. [cited May 2003]. <http://www.nlm.nih.gov/medlineplus/drug info/uspdi/202280.html>.

"Salicylates (Systemic)." Medline Plus Drug Information. [cited May 2003]. <http://www.nlm.nih.gov/medlineplus/druginfo/uspdi/202515.html>.

"Warfarin." Medline Plus Drug Information. [cited May 2003]. <http://www.nlm.nih.gov/medlineplus/druginfo/med master/a682277.html>.

Nancy Ross-Flanigan
Sam Uretsky

Antiemetic drugs *see* **Antinausea drugs**

Antihypertensive drugs

Definition

Antihypertensive drugs are medicines that help lower blood pressure.

Purpose

All antihypertensive agents lower blood pressure, although the mechanisms of action vary greatly. Within this therapeutic class, there are several subgroups. There are a very large number of drugs used to control hypertension, and the drugs listed below are representatives, but not the only members of their classes.

Description

The calcium channel blocking agents, also called slow channel blockers or calcium antagonists, inhibit the movement of ionic calcium across the cell membrane. This reduces the force of contraction of heart muscles and arteries. Although the calcium channel blockers are treated as a group, there are four different chemical classes, leading to significant variations in the activity of individual drugs. Nifedipine (Adalat, Procardia) has the greatest effect on the blood vessels, while verapamil (Calan, Isoptin) and diltiazem (Cardizem) have a greater effect on the heart muscle itself.

Peripheral vasodilators such as hydralazine (Apresoline), isoxuprine (Vasodilan), and minoxidil (Loniten) act by relaxing blood vessels.

There are several groups of drugs that act by reducing adrenergic nerve stimulation, the excitatory nerve stimulation that causes contraction of the muscles in the arteries, veins, and heart. These drugs include the beta-adrenergic blockers and alpha/beta adrenergic blockers. There are also non-specific adrenergic blocking agents.

Beta-adrenergic blocking agents include propranolol (Inderal), atenolol (Tenormin), and pindolol (Visken). Propranolol acts on the beta-adrenergic receptors anywhere in the body, and has been used as a treatment for emotional anxiety and rapid heart beat. Atenolol and acebutolol (Sectral) act specifically on the nerves of the heart and circulation.

There are two alpha/beta adrenergic blockers, labetolol (Normodyne, Trandate) and carvedilol (Coreg). These work similarly to the beta blockers.

Angiotensin-converting enzyme inhibitors (ACE inhibitors) act by inhibiting the production of angiotensin II, a substance that induces both constriction of blood vessels and retention of sodium, which leads to water retention and increased blood volume. There are 10 ACE inhibitors currently marketed in the United States, including captopril (Capoten), benazepril (Lotensin), enalapril (Vasotec), and quinapril (Acupril). The primary difference between these drugs is their onset and duration of action.

The ACE II inhibitors, losartan (Cozaar), candesartan (Atacand), irbesartan (Avapro), telmisartan (Micardis), valsartan (Diovan), and eprosartan (Teveten) directly inhibit the effects of ACE II rather than blocking its production. Their actions are similar to the ACE inhibitors, but they appear to have a more favorable side effect and safety profile.

In addition to these drugs, other classes of drugs have been used to lower blood pressure, most notably the thiazide **diuretics**. There are 12 thiazide diuretics marketed in the United States, including hydrochlorothiazide (Hydrodiuril, Esidrex), indapamide (Lozol), polythiazide (Renese), and hydroflumethiazide (Diucardin). The drugs in this class appear to lower blood pressure through several

Antihypertensive Drugs

Brand Name (Generic Name)	Possible Common Side Effects Include:
Accupril (quinapril hydrochloride)	Headache, dizziness
Aldatazide	Diarrhea, fever, headache, decreased coordination
Aldactone (spironolactone)	Cramps, drowsiness, stomach disorders
Aldomet (methyldopa)	Fluid retention, headache, weak feeling
Altace (ramipril)	Headache, cough
Calan, Calan SR (verapamil hydrochloride)	Constipation, fatigue, decreased blood pressure
Capoten (captopril)	Decreased sense of taste, decreased blood pressure tiching, rash
Cardene (nicardipine Hydrochloride)	Dizziness, headache, indigestion and nausea, increased heartbeat
Cardizem (diltiazem hydrochloride)	Dizziness, fluid retention, headache, nausea, skin rash
Cardura (doxazosin mesylate)	Dizziness, fatigue, drowsiness, headache
Catapres	Dry mouth, drowsiness, dizziness, constipation
Corgard (nadolol)	Behaviorial changes, dizziness, decreased heartbeat, tiredness
Corzide	Dizziness, decreased heartbeat, fatigue, cold hands and feet
Diuril (chlorothiazide)	Cramps, constipation or diarrhea, dizziness, fever, increased glocose level in urine
Dyazide	Blurred vision, muscle and abdominal pain, fatigue
DynaCirc (isradipine)	Chest pain, fluid retention, headache, fatigue
HydroDIURIL (hydrochlorothiazide)	Upset stomach, headache, cramps, loss of appetite
Hygroton (chlorthalidone)	Anemia, constipation or diarrhea, cramps, itching
Hytrin (terazosin hydrochloride)	Dizziness, labored breathing, nausea, swelling
Inderal (propranolol hydrochloride)	Constipation or diarrhea, tingling sensation, nausea and vomiting
Inderide	Blurred vision, cramps, fatigue, loss of appetite
Lasix (furosemide)	Back and muscle pain, indigestion, nausea
Lopressor (metoprolol tartrate)	Diarrhea, itching/rash, tiredness
Lotensin (benazepril hydrochloride)	Nausea, dizziness, fatigue, headache
Alozol (indapamide)	Anxiety, headache, loss of energy, muscle cramps
Maxzide	Cramps, labored breathing, drowsiness, irritated stomach
Minipress (prazosin hdrochloride)	Headache, nausea, weakness, dizziness
Moduretic	Diarrhea, fatigue, itching, loss of appetite
Monopril (fosinopril sodium)	Nausea and vomiting, headache, cough
Normodyne (labetalol hydrochloride)	Fatigue, nausea, stuffy nose
Plendil (felodipine)	Pain in back, chest, muscles, joints, and abdomen, itching, dry mouth, respiratory problems
Procardia, Procardia X (nifedipine)	Swelling, constipation, decreased blood pressure, nausea, fatigue
Sectral (acebutolol hydrochloride)	Constipation or diarrhea, gas, chest and joint pain
Ser-Ap-Es	Blurred vision, cramps, muscle pain, dizziness
Tenex (guanfacine hydrochloride)	Headache, constipation, dry mouth, weakness
Tenoretic	Decreased heartbeat, fatigue, nausea
Tenormin (atenolol)	Nausea, fatigue, dizziness
Veseretic	Diarrhea, muscle cramps, rash
Vasotec (enalapril maleate)	Chest pain, blurred vision, constipation or diarrhea, hives, nausea
Visken (pindolol)	Muscle cramps, labored breathing, nausea, fluid retention
Wytensin (guanabenz acetate)	Headache, drowsiness, dizziness
Zaroxolyn (metolazone)	Constipation or diarrhea, chest pain, spasms, nausea
Zestoretic (lisinopril hydrochlorothiazide)	Fatigue, headache, dizziness
Zestril (lisinopril)	Labored breathing, abdominal and chest pain, nausea, decreased blood pressure

mechanisms. By promoting sodium loss they lower blood volume. At the same time, the pressure of the walls of blood vessels, the peripheral vascular resistance, is lowered. Thiazide diuretics are commonly used as the first choice for reduction of mild hypertension, and may be used in combination with other antihypertensive drugs.

Sodium nitroprusside (Nitropress) and diazoxide (Hyperstat) are used for rapid treatment of hypertensive emergencies. They are given by vein, often during surgery, to reduce blood pressure that suddenly becomes elevated.

Many classes of antihypertensive drugs have been used before surgery to maintain a low blood pressure during the procedure. There does not appear to be a significant difference between drugs when they are used for blood pressure reduction during surgery.

Recommended dosage

Recommended dosage varies with patient, drug, severity of hypertension, and whether the drug is being used alone or in combination with other drugs. Patients should consult specialized references or ask a physician for further information.

Precautions

The warnings and precautions given below apply to the use of antihypertensive drugs over a long period of time. These adverse effects are generally not a problem when the drugs are given as a single dose prior to surgery.

Because of the large number of classes and individual drugs in this group, patients should ask their physicians about specific drugs.

KEY TERMS

Adrenergic—Activated by adrenaline (norepinephrine), loosely applied to the sympathetic nervous system responses.

Angioedema—An allergic skin disease characterized by patches of circumscribed swelling involving the skin and its subcutaneous layers, the mucous membranes, and sometimes the viscera—also called angioneurotic edema, giant urticaria, Quincke's disease, or Quincke's edema.

Arteries—Blood vessels that carry blood away from the heart to the cells, tissues, and organs of the body.

Laryngospasm—Spasmodic closure of the larynx.

Pregnancy category—A system of classifying drugs according to their established risks for use during pregnancy. Category A: Controlled human studies have demonstrated no fetal risk. Category B: Animal studies indicate no fetal risk, but no human studies; or adverse effects in animals, but not in well-controlled human studies. Category C: No adequate human or animal studies; or adverse fetal effects in animal studies, but no available human data. Category D: Evidence of fetal risk, but benefits outweigh risks. Category X: Evidence of fetal risk. Risks outweigh any benefits.

Sympathetic nervous system—The part of the autonomic nervous system that is concerned with preparing the body to react to situations of stress or emergency; it contains chiefly adrenergic fibers and tends to depress secretion, decrease the tone and contractility of smooth muscle, and increase heart rate.

Peripheral vasodilators may cause dizziness and orthostatic hypotension—a rapid lowering of blood pressure when the patient stands up in the morning. Patients taking these drugs must be instructed to rise from bed slowly. Pregnancy risk factors for this group are generally category C, meaning they may result in adverse affects on the fetus. Hydralazine has been shown to cause cleft palate in animal studies, but there is no human data available. Breastfeeding is not recommended.

ACE inhibitors are generally well tolerated, but may rarely cause dangerous reactions including laryngospasm and angioedema. Persistent cough is a common side effect. ACE inhibitors should not be used in pregnancy. When used in pregnancy during the second and third trimesters, ACE inhibitors can cause injury to and even death in the developing fetus. When pregnancy is detected, discontinue the ACE inhibitor as soon as possible. Breastfeeding is not recommended.

ACE II inhibitors are generally well tolerated and do not cause cough. Pregnancy risk factor is category C during the first trimester and category D (known to cause adverse effects in the fetus) during the second and third trimesters. Drugs that act directly on the renin-angiotensin system can cause fetal and neonatal morbidity and death when administered to pregnant women. Several dozen cases have been reported in patients who were taking ACE inhibitors. When pregnancy is detected, discontinue ACE inhibitors as soon as possible. Breastfeeding is not recommended.

Thiazide diuretics commonly cause potassium depletion. Patients should have potassium supplementation either through diet, or potassium supplements. Pregnancy risk factor is category B (chlorothiazide, chlorthalidone, hydrochlorothiazide, indapamide, metolazone) or category C (bendroflumethiazide, benzthiazide, hydroflumethiazide, methyclothiazide, trichlormethiazide). Routine use during normal pregnancy is inappropriate. Thiazides are found in breast milk. Breastfeeding is not recommended.

Beta blockers may cause a large number of adverse reactions including dangerous heart rate abnormalities. Pregnancy risk factor is category B (acebutolol, pindolol, sotalol) or category C (atenolol, labetalol, esmolol, metoprolol, nadolol, timolol, propranolol, penbutolol, carteolol, bisoprolol). Breastfeeding is not recommended.

Interactions

Patients should ask their doctors and consult specific references for food and drug interactions.

Samuel Uretsky, PharmD

Antinausea drugs

Definition

Antinausea drugs are medicines that control nausea—a feeling of sickness or queasiness in the stomach with an urge to vomit. These drugs also prevent or stop vomiting. Drugs that control vomiting are called antiemetic drugs.

Antinausea Drugs

Brand Name (Generic Name)	Possible Common Side Effects Include:
Compazine (phochlorperazine)	Involuntary muscle spasms, dizziness, jitteriness, puckering of the mouth
Phenergan (promethazine hydrochloride)	Dizziness, dry mouth, nausea and vomiting, rash
Reglan (metoclopramide hydrochloride)	Fatigue, drowsiness, restlessness
Tigan (trimethobenzamide hydrochloride)	Blurred vision, diarrhea, cramps, headache
Zofan (ondansetron hydrochloride)	Constipation, headache, fatigue, abdominal pain

Purpose

Prochlorperazine (Compazine), the medication described in detail in this entry, controls both nausea and vomiting. Prochlorperazine is also sometimes prescribed for symptoms of mental disorders, such as schizophrenia. Prochlorperazine may be used to control the nausea and vomiting that occur during recovery from the general anesthetics used in surgery.

Some antihistamines such as dimenhydrinate (Dramamine) and meclizine (Antivert, Bonine) are useful for treatment of the nausea and vomiting associated with motion sickness.

A group of drugs called the 5HT3 inhibitors, ondansetron (Zofran) and granisetron (Kytril), are used to control the nausea and vomiting associated with anticancer drugs. Ondansetron and granisetron are also valuable for controlling nausea and vomiting following surgery.

Corticosteroid hormones such as dexamethasone (Decadron, Hexdrol) may also be used as antiemetics.

Description

Prochlorperazine is available only with a physician's prescription. It is sold in syrup, capsule, tablet, injection, and suppository forms.

Recommended dosage

To control nausea and vomiting in adults, the usual dose is:

- Tablets: one 5-mg or 10-mg tablet three to four times a day
- Extended-release capsules: one 15-mg capsule first thing in the morning or one 10-mg capsule every 12 hours
- Suppository: 25 mg, twice a day
- Syrup: 5–10 mg three to four times a day
- Injection: 5–10 mg injected into a muscle three to four times a day

Doses for children must be determined by a physician.

Precautions

Prochlorperazine may cause a movement disorder called tardive dyskinesia. Signs of this disorder are involuntary twitches and muscle spasms in the face and body and jutting or rolling movements of the tongue. The condition may be permanent. Older people, especially women, are particularly at risk of developing this problem when they take prochlorperazine.

Some people feel drowsy, dizzy, lightheaded, or less alert when using this medicine. The drug may also cause blurred vision, and movement problems. For these reasons, people who take this drug should not drive, use machines, or do anything else that might be dangerous until they have found out how the drug affects them.

Prochlorperazine makes some people sweat less, which can allow the body to overheat. The drug may also make the skin and eyes more sensitive to the sun. People who are taking prochlorperazine should try to avoid extreme heat and exposure to the sun. When going outdoors, they should wear protective clothing, a hat, a sunscreen with a skin protection factor (SPF) of at least 15, and sunglasses that block ultraviolet (UV) light. Saunas, sunlamps, tanning booths, tanning beds, hot baths, and hot tubs should be avoided while taking this medicine. Anyone who must be exposed to extreme heat while taking the drug should check with his or her physician.

This medicine adds to the effects of alcohol and other drugs that slow down the central nervous system, such as antihistamines, cold and flu medicines, tranquilizers, sleep aids, anesthetics, some pain medicines, and **muscle relaxants**. People taking prochlorperazine should not drink alcohol, and should check with the physician who prescribed the drug before combining it with any other medicines.

Patients should not stop taking this medicine without checking with the physician who prescribed it. Stopping the drug suddenly can dizziness, nausea, vomiting, tremors, and other side effects. When stopping the medicine, it may be necessary to taper the dose gradually.

Prochlorperazine may cause false pregnancy tests.

Women who are pregnant (or planning to become pregnant) or are breastfeeding should check with their physicians before using this medicine.

Before using prochlorperazine, people with any of these medical problems should make sure their physicians are aware of their conditions:

- previous sensitivity or allergic reaction to prochlorperazine
- heart disease
- glaucoma
- brain tumor
- intestinal blockage
- abnormal blood conditions, such as leukemia
- exposure to pesticides

Side effects

Many side effects are possible with this drug, including, but not limited to, constipation, dizziness, drowsiness, decreased sweating, dry mouth, stuffy nose, movement problems, changes in menstrual period, increased sensitivity to sun, and swelling or pain in breasts. Anyone who has unusual or troublesome symptoms after taking prochlorperazine should contact his or her physician.

Interactions

Prochlorperazine may interact with other medicines. When this happens, the effects of one or both of the drugs may change or the risk of side effects may be greater. Among the drugs that may interact with prochlorperazine are antiseizure drugs such as phenytoin (Dilantin) and carbamazepine (Tegretol), anticoagulants such as warfarin (Coumadin), and drugs that slow the central nervous system such as alprazolam (Xanax), diazepam (Valium), and secobarbital (Seconal). Not every drug that interacts with prochlorperazine is listed here, and all patients should consult with a physician or pharmacist before taking any other prescription or nonprescription (over-the-counter) drug with prochlorperazine.

Resources

BOOKS

Brody, T. M., J. Larner, K. P. Minneman, and H. C. Neu. *Human Pharmacology: Molecular to Clinical,* 2nd ed. St. Louis: Mosby Year-Book, 1998.

Griffith, H. W., and S. Moore. *2001 Complete Guide to Prescription and Nonprescription Drugs.* New York: Berkely Publishing Group, 2001.

OTHER

"Anticholinergics/Antispasmodics." Medline Plus Drug Information. [cited June 25 2003] < http://www.nlm.nih.gov/medlineplus/druginfo/uspdi/202049.html>.

KEY TERMS

Anesthetic—Medicine that causes a loss of feeling, especially pain. Some anesthetics also cause a loss of consciousness.

Antihistamine—Medicine that prevents or relieves allergy symptoms.

Central nervous system—The brain, spinal cord and the nerves throughout the body.

Corticosteroid—A steroid molecule, produced by the adrenal gland, used in medicine to reduce inflammation. May also apply to synthetic compounds which have structures and uses similar to the natural compounds.

Spasm—Sudden, involuntary tensing of a muscle or a group of muscles.

Tardive dyskinesia—A disorder brought on by certain medications that is characterized by uncontrollable muscle spasms.

Tranquilizer—Medicine that has a calming effect and is used to treat anxiety and mental tension.

"Antihistamines (Systemic)." Medline Plus Drug Information. [cited June 25 2003] <http://www.nlm.nih.gov/medlineplus/druginfo/uspdi/202060.html>.

"Ondansetron." Medline Plus Drug Information. [cited June 25 2003] <http://www.nlm.nih.gov/medlineplus/druginfo/medmaster/a601209.html>.

"Prochlorperazine." Medline Plus Drug Information. [cited June 25, 2003] < http://www.nlm.nih.gov/medlineplus/druginfo/medmaster/a682116.html>.

Nancy Ross-Flanigan
Sam Uretsky, PharmD

Antiplatelet drugs *see* **Anticoagulant and antiplatelet drugs**

Antiseptics

Definition

An antiseptic is a substance that inhibits the growth and development of microorganisms. For practical purposes, antiseptics are routinely thought of as topical agents, for application to skin, mucous membranes, and inanimate objects, although a formal definition includes agents that are used internally, such as the urinary tract antiseptics.

Purpose

Antiseptics are a diverse class of drugs that are applied to skin surfaces or mucous membranes for their anti-infective effects. This may be either bacteriocidal (kills bacteria) or bacteriostatic (stops the growth of bacteria). Their uses include cleansing of skin and wound surfaces after injury, preparation of skin surfaces prior to injections or surgical procedures, and routine disinfection of the oral cavity as part of a program of oral hygiene. Antiseptics are also used for disinfection of inanimate objects, including instruments and furniture surfaces.

Commonly used antiseptics for skin cleaning include benzalkonium chloride, chlorhexidine, hexachlorophine, iodine compounds, mercury compounds, alcohol, and hydrogen peroxide. Other agents that have been used for this purpose, but have largely been supplanted by more effective or safer agents, include boric acid and volatile oils such as methyl salicylate (oil of wintergreen).

Chlorhexidine shows a high margin of safety when applied to mucous membranes, and has been used in oral rinses and preoperative total body washes.

Benzalkonium chloride and hexachlorophine are used primarily as hand scrubs or face washes. Benzalkonium may also find application as a disinfecting agent for instruments, and in low concentration as a preservative for drugs including ophthalmic solutions. Benzalkonium chloride is inactivated by organic compounds, including soap, and must not be applied to areas that have not been fully rinsed.

Iodine compounds include tincture of iodine and povidone iodine compounds. Iodine compounds have the broadest spectrum of all topical anti-infectives, with action against bacteria, fungi, viruses, spores, protozoa, and yeasts. Iodine tincture is highly effective, but its alcoholic component is drying and extremely irritating when applied to abraded (scraped or rubbed) skin. Povidone iodine, an organic compound, is less irritating and less toxic, but not as effective. Povidone iodine has been used for hand scrubs and disinfection of surgical sites. Aqueous solutions of iodine have also been used as antiseptic agents, but are less effective than alcoholic solutions and less convenient to use that the povidone iodine compounds.

Hydrogen peroxide acts through the liberation of oxygen gas. Although the antibacterial activity of hydrogen peroxide is relatively weak, the liberation of oxygen bubbles produces an effervescent action, which may be useful for wound cleansing through removal of tissue debris. The activity of hydrogen peroxide may be reduced by the presence of blood and pus. The appropriate concentration of hydrogen peroxide for antiseptic use is 3%, although higher concentrations are available.

Thimerosol (Mersol) is a mercury compound with activity against bacteria and yeasts. Prolonged use may result in mercury toxicity.

Recommended dosage

Dosage varies with product and intended use. Patients should ask a physician.

Precautions

Precautions vary with individual product and use.

Hypersensitivity reactions should be considered with organic compounds such as chlorhexidine, benzalkonium and hexachlorophine.

Skin dryness and irritation should be considered with all products, but particularly with those containing alcohol.

Systemic toxicity may result from ingestion of iodine-containing compounds or mercury compounds.

Most antiseptics have not been rated according to pregnancy category under the pregnancy risk factor system. Hexachlorophene is schedule C during pregnancy, and should not be used on newborns due to risk of systemic absorption with potential central nervous system (CNS) effects, including convulsions. Application of hexachlorophene to open wounds, mucous membranes, or areas of thin skin, such as the genitalia, should be avoided, since this may promote systemic absorption.

Chlorhexidine should not be instilled into the ear. There is one anecdotal report of deafness following use of chlorhexidine in a patient with a perforated eardrum. Safety in pregnancy and breastfeeding have not been reported; however there is one anecdotal report of an infant developing slowed heartbeat apparently related to maternal use of chlorhexidine.

Iodine compounds should be used sparingly during pregnancy and lactation due to risk of infant absorption of iodine with alterations in thyroid function.

Interactions

Antiseptics are not known to interact with any other medicines. However, they should not be used together with any other topical cream, solution, or ointment.

Resources

PERIODICALS

Farley, Dixie. "Help for Cuts, Scrapes and Burns." *FDA Consumer* (May 1996): 12.

KEY TERMS

Antibiotic—A medicine used to treat infections.

Bacteria—Tiny, one-celled forms of life that cause many diseases and infections.

Mucous membrane—The moist lining of a body cavity or structure, such as the mouth or nose.

Pregnancy category—A system of classifying drugs according to their established risks for use during pregnancy. Category A: Controlled human studies have demonstrated no fetal risk. Category B: Animal studies indicate no fetal risk, but no human studies; or adverse effects in animals, but not in well-controlled human studies. Category C: No adequate human or animal studies; or adverse fetal effects in animal studies, but no available human data. Category D: Evidence of fetal risk, but benefits outweigh risks. Category X: Evidence of fetal risk. Risks outweigh any benefits.

McDonnell, Gerald and A. Denver Russell. "Antiseptics and Disinfectants: Activity, Action, and Resistance." *Clinical Microbiology Reviews* Vol. 12, No. 1 (January 1999): 147–179. Also available at <http://www.pubmedcentral. nih.gov/articlerender.fcgi?artid=88911>. [cited June 30, 2003].

Waldman, Hilary. "New ways to treat wounds; Doctors abandon failed conventions that focus on caring for bruises at the surface for methods that reach the source." *Los Angeles Times* (May 26, 2003).

Weber J. et al. "Efficacy of selected hand hygiene agents used to remove *Bacillus atrophaeus* (a surrogate of *Bacillus anthracis*) from contaminated hands." *Journal of the American Medical Association* (Mar 12, 2003).

OTHER

United States Department of Energy. "Antiseptics and Disinfectants." *Ask A Scientist: Molecular Biology Archive.* December 04, 2002 [cited June 29, 2003]. <http://newton. dep.anl.gov/askasci/mole00/mole00361.htm>.

Samuel Uretsky, PharmD

Antrectomy

Definition

An antrectomy is the resection, or surgical removal, of a part of the stomach known as the antrum. The antrum is the lower third of the stomach that lies between the body of the stomach and the pyloric canal, which empties into the first part of the small intestine. It is also known as the antrum pyloricum or the gastric antrum. Because an antrectomy is the removal of a portion of the stomach, it is sometimes called a partial or subtotal **gastrectomy**.

Purpose

An antrectomy may be performed to treat several different disorders that affect the digestive system:

• Peptic ulcer disease (PUD). An antrectomy may be done to treat complications from ulcers that have not responded to medical treatment. These complications include uncontrolled or recurrent bleeding and obstructions that prevent food from passing into the small intestine. Because the antrum produces gastrin, which is a hormone that stimulates the production of stomach acid, its removal lowers the level of acid secretions in the stomach.

• Cancers of the digestive tract and nearby organs. An antrectomy may be performed not only to remove a malignant gastric ulcer, but also to relieve pressure on the lower end of the stomach caused by cancers of the pancreas, gallbladder, or liver.

• Arteriovenous malformations (AVMs) of the stomach. AVMs are collections of small blood vessels that may develop in various parts of the digestive system. AVMs can cause bleeding into the gastrointestinal tract, resulting in hematemesis (vomiting blood) or melena (black or tarry stools containing blood). The type of AVM most likely to occur in the antrum is known as gastric antral vascular ectasia (GAVE) syndrome. The dilated blood vessels in GAVE produce reddish streaks on the wall of the antrum that look like the stripes on a watermelon.

• Gastric outlet obstruction (GOO). GOO is not a single disease or disorder but a condition in which the stomach cannot empty because the pylorus is blocked. In about 37% of cases, the cause of the obstruction is benign—most often PUD, gallstones, bezoars, or scarring caused by ingestion of hydrochloric acid or other caustic substance. The other 63% of cases are caused by pancreatic cancer, gastric cancer, or other malignancy that has spread to the digestive tract.

• Penetrating gunshot or stab wounds that have caused severe damage to the duodenum and pancreas. An antrectomy may be done as an emergency measure when the blood vessels supplying the duodenum have been destroyed.

Demographics

Peptic ulcer disease (PUD) is fairly common in the general United States population. According to the

Centers for Disease Control (CDC), about 10% of all Americans will develop an ulcer in the stomach or duodenum at some point in their life. About four million adults are diagnosed or treated each year for PUD; one million will be hospitalized for treatment; and 40,000 will have surgery for an ulcer-related condition. About 6,500 Americans die each year from complications related to PUD. The annual costs to the United States economy from peptic ulcer disease are estimated to be over $6 billion.

Peptic ulcers can develop at any age, but in the United States they are very unusual in children and uncommon in adolescents. Adults between the ages of 30 and 50 are most likely to develop duodenal ulcers, while gastric ulcers are most common in those over 60. Duodenal ulcers are more common in men, and gastric ulcers are more common in women. Other risk factors for PUD include heavy smoking and a family history of either duodenal or gastric ulcers.

GAVE, or watermelon stomach, is a very rare cause of gastrointestinal bleeding that was first identified in 1952. It has been associated with such disorders as scleroderma, cirrhosis of the liver, familial Mediterranean fever, and heart disease. GAVE affects women slightly more than twice as often as men. It is almost always found in the elderly; the average age at diagnosis is 73 in women and 68 in men.

Gastric cancer is the 14th most common type of malignant tumor in the United States; however, it occurs much more frequently in Japan and other parts of Asia than in western Europe and North America. About 24,000 people in the United States are diagnosed each year with gastric cancer. Risk factors for developing it include infection of the stomach lining by *Helicobacter pylori*; Asian American, Hispanic, or African American heritage; age 60 or older; heavy smoking; a history of pernicious anemia; and a diet heavy in dry salted foods. Men are more likely to develop gastric cancer than women. Some doctors think that exposure to certain toxic chemicals in the workplace is also a risk factor for gastric cancer.

Description

At present almost all antrectomies are performed as open procedures, which means that they are done through a large incision in the patient's abdomen with the patient under general anesthesia. After the patient is anesthetized, a urinary catheter is placed to monitor urinary output, and a nasogastric tube is inserted. After the patient's abdomen has been cleansed with an antiseptic, the surgeon makes a large incision from the patient's rib cage to the navel. After separating the overlying layers of tissue, the surgeon exposes the stomach. One clamp is placed at the lower end and another clamp somewhat higher, dividing off the lower third of the stomach. A cutting stapler may be used to remove the lower third (the antrum) and attach the upper portion of the stomach to the small intestine. After the stomach and intestine have been reattached, the area is rinsed with saline solution and the incision closed.

Most antrectomies are performed together with a **vagotomy**. This is a procedure in which the surgeon cuts various branches of the vagus nerve, which carries messages from the brain to the stomach to secrete more stomach acid. The surgeon may choose to perform a selective vagotomy in order to disable the branches of the nerve that govern gastric secretion without cutting the branches that control stomach emptying.

Some surgeons have performed antrectomies with a laparoscope, which is a less invasive type of surgery. However, as of 2003, this technique is still considered experimental.

Diagnosis/Preparation

Diagnosis

Diagnosis of PUD and other stomach disorders begins with taking the patient's history, including a family history. In many cases the patient's primary care physician will order tests in order to narrow the diagnosis. If the patient is older or has lost a large amount of weight recently, the doctor will consider the possibility of gastric cancer. If there is a history of duodenal or gastric ulcers in the patient's family, the doctor may ask questions about the type of discomfort the patient is experiencing. Pain associated with duodenal ulcers often occurs at night, is relieved at mealtimes, but reappears two to three hours after eating. Pain from gastric ulcers, on the other hand, may be made worse by eating and accompanied by nausea and vomiting. Vomiting that occurs repeatedly shortly after eating suggests a gastric obstruction.

The most common diagnostic tests for stomach disorders are:

- Endoscopy. An endoscope is a thin flexible tube with a light source and video camera on one end that can be passed through the mouth and throat in order to look at the inside of the upper digestive tract. The video camera attached to the endoscope projects images on a computer screen that allow the doctor to see ulcers, tissue growths, and other possible problems. The endoscope can be used to collect tissue cells for a cytology analysis, or a small tissue sample for a biopsy. A tissue biopsy can be used to test for the presence of *Helicobacter pylori*, a spiral bacterium that was discovered in 1982 to be the underlying cause of most gastric ulcers, as well as to test for cancer. Endoscopy is one of the most effective tests for diagnosing AVMs.

- Double-contrast barium x-ray study of the upper gastrointestinal tract. This test is sometimes called an upper GI series. The patient is given a liquid form of barium to take by mouth. The barium coats the tissues lining the esophagus, stomach, and small intestine, allowing them to be seen more clearly on an x ray. The radiologist can also watch the barium as it moves through the digestive system in order to pinpoint the location of blockages.

- Urease breath test. This test can be used to monitor the effects of ulcer treatment as well as to diagnose the presence of *H. pylori*. The patient is given urea labeled with either carbon 13-C or 14-C. *H. pylori* produces urease, which will break down the urea in the test dose to ammonia and carbon dioxide containing the labeled carbon. The carbon dioxide containing the labeled carbon can then be detected in the patient's breath.

Preparation

Preparation for an antrectomy requires tests to evaluate the patient's overall health and fitness for surgery. These tests include an EKG, x rays, blood tests, and a urine test. The patient is asked to discontinue **aspirin** and other blood-thinning medications about a week before surgery. No solid food or liquid should be taken after midnight of the evening before surgery.

In most hospitals the patient will be given a sedative before the operation either intravenously or by injection. The general anesthesia is given in the **operating room**.

Aftercare

Aftercare in the hospital for an antrectomy is similar to the aftercare given for other operations involving the abdomen, in terms of **incision care**, pain medication, and **antibiotics** to minimize the risk of infection. Recuperation at home usually takes several weeks. The patient is given an endoscopic check-up about six to eight weeks after surgery.

QUESTIONS TO ASK THE DOCTOR

- What are the alternatives to an antrectomy for my condition? Which would you recommend and why?
- How many antrectomies have you performed?
- How likely am I to develop dumping syndrome if I have the procedure?
- What is your opinion of laparoscopic antrectomies? Would I be eligible to participate in a clinical study of this procedure?

The most important aspect of aftercare following an antrectomy is careful attention to diet and eating habits. About 30% of patients who have had an antrectomy or a full gastrectomy develop what is known as dumping syndrome. Dumping syndrome results from food leaving the stomach too quickly after a meal and being "dumped" into the small intestine. There are two types of dumping syndrome, early and late. Early dumping occurs 10–20 minutes after meals and is characterized by feelings of nausea, lightheadedness, sweating, heart palpitations, rapid heartbeat, and abdominal cramps. Late dumping occurs one to three hours after meals high in carbohydrates and is accompanied by feelings of weakness, hunger, and mental confusion. Most patients are able to manage dumping syndrome by eating six small meals per day rather than three larger ones; by choosing foods that are high in protein and low in carbohydrate; by chewing the food thoroughly; and by drinking fluids between rather than with meals.

Risks

In addition to early or late dumping syndrome, other risks associated with antrectomies include:

- Diarrhea. This complication is more likely to occur in patients who had a vagotomy as well as an antrectomy.

- Weight loss. About 30–60% of patients who have had a combined antrectomy/vagotomy lose weight after surgery. The most common cause of weight loss is reduced food intake due to the smaller size of the stomach. In some cases, however, the patient loses weight because the nutrients in the food are not being absorbed by the body.

- Malabsorption/malnutrition. Iron-deficiency anemia, folate deficiency, and loss of calcium sometimes occur after an antrectomy because gastric acid is necessary for iron to be absorbed from food.

- Dysphagia. Dysphagia, or discomfort in swallowing, may occur after an antrectomy when digestive juices from the duodenum flow upward into the esophagus and irritate its lining.

- Recurrence of gastric ulcers.

- Bezoar formation. Bezoars are collections of foreign material (usually vegetable fibers or hair) in the stomach that can block the passage of food into the small intestine. They may develop after an antrectomy if the patient is eating foods high in plant fiber or is not chewing them thoroughly.

Normal results

Normal results of an antrectomy depend on the reasons for the surgery. Antrectomies performed to reduce acid secretion in PUD or to remove premalignant tissue to prevent gastric cancer are over 95% successful. The success rate is even higher in treating watermelon stomach. Antrectomies performed to treat gastric cancer or penetrating abdominal trauma are less successful, but this result is related to the severity of the patient's illness or injury rather than the surgical procedure itself.

Morbidity and mortality rates

The mortality rate for antrectomies related to ulcer treatment is about 1–2%; for antrectomies related to gastric cancer, 1%–3%.

The rates of complications associated with antrectomies for ulcer treatment are:

- Recurrence of ulcer: 0.5%–1%.

- Dumping syndromes: 25%–30%.

- Diarrhea: 10%.

Alternatives

As of 2003, antrectomy is no longer the first line of treatment for either peptic ulcer disease or GAVE. It is usually reserved for patients with recurrent bleeding or other conditions such as malignancy, perforation, or obstruction.

Although surgery, including antrectomy, is the most common treatment for stomach cancer, it is almost always necessary to combine it with chemotherapy, radiation treatment, or biological therapy (immunotherapy). The reason for a combination of treatments is that stomach cancer is rarely discovered early. Its first symptoms are often mild and easily mistaken for the symptoms of heartburn or a stomach virus. As a result, the cancer has often spread beyond the stomach by the time it is diagnosed.

Medication

Treatment of peptic ulcers caused by *H. pylori* has changed its focus in recent years from lowering the level of acidity in the stomach to eradicating the bacterium. Since no single antibiotic is effective in curing *H. pylori* infections, so-called triple therapy typically consists of a combination of one or two antibiotics to kill the bacterium plus a medication to lower acid production and a third medication (usually bismuth subsalicylate) to protect the stomach lining.

Specific types of medications that are used as part of triple therapy or for relief of discomfort include:

- H_2 blockers. These are used together with antibiotics in triple therapy to reduce stomach acid secretion. H_2 blockers include cimetidine, ranitidine, famotidine, and nizatidine. Some are available as over-the-counter (OTC) medications.

- Proton pump inhibitors. These medications include drugs such as omeprazole and lansoprazole. They are given to suppress production of stomach acid.

- Prostaglandins. These are given to treat ulcers produced by a group of pain medications known as NSAIDs. Prostaglandins protect the stomach lining as well as lower acid secretion. The best-known medication in this category is misoprostol.

- Sucralfate. Sucralfate is a compound of sucrose and aluminum that covers ulcers with a protective coating that allows eroded tissues to heal.

- Antacids. These compounds are available as OTC tablets or liquids.

- Bismuth subsalicylate. Sold as an OTC under the trade name Pepto-Bismol, this medication has some antibacterial effectiveness against *H. pylori* as well as protecting the stomach lining.

Endoscopy

Endoscopy can be used for treatment as well as diagnosis. About 10 different methods are in use as of 2003 for treating bleeding ulcers and AVMs with the help of an endoscope; the most common involve the injection of epinephrine or a sclerosing solution; the application of a thermal probe to the bleeding area; or the use of a Nd:YAG laser to coagulate the open blood vessels. Watermelon stomach is now treated more often with argon plasma coagulation than with an antrectomy. Recurrent bleeding, however, occurs in 15–20% of ulcers treated with endoscopic methods.

Complementary and alternative (CAM) approaches

Complementary and alternative approaches that have been used to treat gastric ulcers related to PUD in-

KEY TERMS

Antrum—The lower part of the stomach that lies between the pylorus and the body of the stomach. It is also called the gastric antrum or antrum pyloricum.

Bezoar—A collection of foreign material, usually hair or vegetable fibers or a mixture of both, that may occasionally occur in the stomach or intestines and block the passage of food.

Dumping syndrome—A complex physical reaction to food passing too quickly from the stomach into the small intestine, characterized by sweating, nausea, abdominal cramps, dizziness, and other symptoms.

Duodenum—The first portion of the small intestine, lying between the pylorus and the jejunum.

Dysphagia—Difficulty or discomfort in swallowing.

Endoscopy—A technique for looking inside the stomach or esophagus with the help of a flexible instrument containing a light and miniature video camera on one end.

Gastrin—A hormone produced by cells in the antrum that stimulates the production of gastric acid.

Gastroenterology—The branch of medicine that specializes in the diagnosis and treatment of disorders affecting the stomach and intestines.

Helicobacter pylori—A spiral-shaped bacterium that was discovered in 1982 to be the underlying cause of most ulcers in the stomach and duodenum.

Hematemesis—Vomiting blood.

Melena—The passing of blackish-colored stools containing blood pigments or partially digested blood.

Nonsteroidal anti-inflammatory drugs (NSAIDs)—A term used for a group of analgesics that are often given to arthritis patients. About 20% of peptic ulcers are thought to be caused by frequent use of NSAIDs.

Perforation—An opening or hole in the tissues of the stomach caused by a disease process.

Pylorus—The opening at the lower end of the stomach, encircled by a band of muscle. The contents of the stomach are pumped into the duodenum through the pylorus.

Resection—Removal of an organ or structure. An antrectomy is a resection of the antrum.

Vagotomy—Cutting or dividing various parts of the vagus nerve that supply the stomach. A vagotomy is done to reduce acid secretion.

Watermelon stomach—A type of arteriovenous malformation (AVM) that develops in the antrum. The dilated blood vessels in the AVM resemble the stripes of a watermelon. Watermelon stomach is also known as gastric antral vascular ectasia, or GAVE syndrome.

---

clude acupuncture, Ayurvedic medicine, and herbal preparations. Ayurvedic medicine, which is the traditional medical system of India, classifies people according to metabolic body type. People who belong to the type known as pitta are considered particularly prone to ulcers and treated with a diet that emphasizes "cooling" foods, including large quantities of vegetables. In Japanese medicine, ulcer remedies made from licorice or bupleurum are frequently prescribed. Western herbalists recommend preparations containing fennel, fenugreek, slippery elm, or marshmallow root in addition to licorice to relieve the pain of stomach ulcers.

See also Gastrectomy.

Resources

BOOKS

"Arteriovenous Malformations." In *The Merck Manual of Diagnosis and Therapy*, edited by Mark H. Beers, MD, and Robert Berkow, MD. Whitehouse Station, NJ: Merck Research Laboratories, 1999.

Pelletier, Kenneth R., MD. *The Best Alternative Medicine*, Part II, "CAM Therapies for Specific Conditions: Ulcers." New York: Simon & Schuster, 2002.

"Peptic Ulcer Disease." In *The Merck Manual of Diagnosis and Therapy*, edited by Mark H. Beers, MD, and Robert Berkow, MD. Whitehouse Station, NJ: Merck Research Laboratories, 1999.

Thomson, A. B. R. and E. A. Shaffer. *First Principles of Gastroenterology*, 3rd ed. Oakville, ON: Canadian Association of Gastroenterology, 2002.

PERIODICALS

Appleyard, M. N. and C. P. Swain. "Endoscopic Difficulties in the Diagnosis of Upper Gastrointestinal Bleeding." *World Journal of Gastroenterology* 7 (2001): 308-12.

Busteed, S., C. Silke, C. Molloy, et al. "Gastric Antral Vascular Ectasia—A Cause of Refractory Anaemia in Systemic Sclerosis." *Irish Medical Journal* 94 (November-December 2001): 310.

Castellanos, Andres, MD, Barry D. Mann, MD, and James de Caestecker, DO. "Gastric Outlet Obstruction." *eMedicine*,

February 12, 2002 [cited April 27, 2003]. <www.emedicine.com/med/topic2713.htm>.

De Caestecker, James, DO. "Upper Gastrointestinal Bleeding: Surgical Perspective." *eMedicine*, October 17, 2002 [cited April 27, 2003]. <www.emedicine.com/med/topic3566.htm>.

Fowler, Dennis, MD. "Laparoscopic Foregut Surgery: Less Commonly Performed Procedures." *Minimal Access Surgery Center Newsletter, New York-Presbyterian Hospital* 2 (Winter 2002): 7–10.

Komar, Aleksander R., MD and Prem Patel, MD. "Abdominal Trauma, Penetrating." *eMedicine*, April 25, 2002 [cited April 28, 2003]. <www.emedicine.com/med/topic2805.htm>.

Probst, A., R. Scheubel, and M. Wienbeck. "Treatment of Watermelon Stomach (GAVE Syndrome) by Means of Endoscopic Argon Plasma Coagulation (APC): Long-Term Outcome." *Zeitschrift für Gastroenterologie* 39 (June 2001): 447-52.

Stotzer, P. O., R. Willen, and A. F. Kilander. "Watermelon Stomach: Not Only an Antral Disease." *Gastrointestinal Endoscopy* 55 (June 2002): 897–900.

Tseng, Y. L., M. H. Wu, M. Y. Lin, and W. W. Lai. "Early Surgical Correction for Isolated Gastric Stricture Following Acid Corrosion Injury." *Digestive Surgery* 19 (2002): 276–80.

Yusoff, I., F. Brennan, D. Ormonde, and B. Laurence. "Argon Plasma Coagulation for Treatment of Watermelon Stomach." *Endoscopy* 34 (May 2002): 407–10.

Zarzaur, B. L., K. A. Kudsk, K. Carter, et al. "Stress Ulceration Requiring Definitive Surgery After Severe Trauma." *American Surgeon* 67 (September 2001): 875–79.

ORGANIZATIONS

American Gastroenterological Association (AGA). 4930 Del Ray Avenue, Bethesda, MD 20814. (301) 654-2055. <www.gastro.org>.

American Society for Gastrointestinal Endoscopy (ASGE). 1520 Kensington Road, Suite 202, Oak Brook, IL 60523 (630) 573-0600. <www.asge.org>.

Canadian Association of Gastroenterology (CAG). 2902 South Sheridan Way, Oakville, ON L6J 7L6 (888) 780-0007 or (905) 829-2504. <www.cag-acg.org>.

Centers for Disease Control and Prevention (CDC). 1600 Clifton Road, Atlanta, GA 30333. (888) MY-ULCER or (404) 639-3534. <www.cdc.gov>.

National Cancer Institute (NCI). NCI Public Inquiries Office, Suite 3036A, 6116 Executive Boulevard, MSC8332, Bethesda, MD 20892-8322. (800) 4-CANCER or (800) 332-8615 (TTY). <www.nci.nih.gov>.

National Digestive Diseases Information Clearinghouse (NDDIC). 2 Information Way, Bethesda, MD 20892-3570. <www.niddk.nih.gov/health/digest/pubs>.

OTHER

National Cancer Institute (NCI) Physician Data Query (PDQ). *Gastric Cancer: Treatment*, January 2, 2003 [cited April 28, 2003]. <www.nci.nih.gov/cancerinfo/pdq/treatment/gastric/healthprofessional>.

National Digestive Diseases Information Clearinghouse (NDDIC). *What I Need to Know About Peptic Ulcers*, August 2002 [cited April 28, 2003]. NIH Publication No. 02-5042. <www.niddk.nih.gov/health/digest/pubs/pepticulcers/pepticulcers.htm>.

Rebecca Frey, Ph.D.

Anxiolytics *see* **Antianxiety drugs**

Aortic aneurysm repair

Definition

Aortic aneurysm repair involves the removal of a dilated (enlarged) portion of the aorta replaced by a woven or knitted Dacron graft to continue uninterrupted blood flow through the aorta and all branch vessels.

Purpose

Aortic aneurysm repair is performed when a portion of the aorta has become dilated as a result of medionecrosis in the ascending aorta or atherosclerosis in the arch and descending segments. Congenital defects in connective tissue are also a risk factor. A history of blunt trauma may be associated with this disease propagation. Prior to 1950, patients exposed to syphilis were at risk of developing aortic aneurysm. Risk of clot formation and rupture of the aneurysm, seen in 50% of cases, as well as dilation to a size greater than 4 in (10 cm) promote repair of the aneurysm by surgical techniques.

Demographics

The patient population for this procedure is typically male with an average age of 65 and a history of medionecrosis or atherosclerosis of the aorta. Patients with a medical history significant for syphilis or blunt trauma are at risk. Congenital defects associated with Marfan syndrome or Ehlers-Danlos syndrome (congenital tissue disorders) need to be monitored.

All patients will be monitored until the aneurysm demonstrates consistent enlargement over time, or grows to greater than 2.2 in (5.5 cm) in diameter at which time surgery is suggested. At a diameter of 4 in (10 cm) surgery is the best option, as risk of rupture increases. Many patients live without symptoms, having the aneurysm identified during other medical procedures.

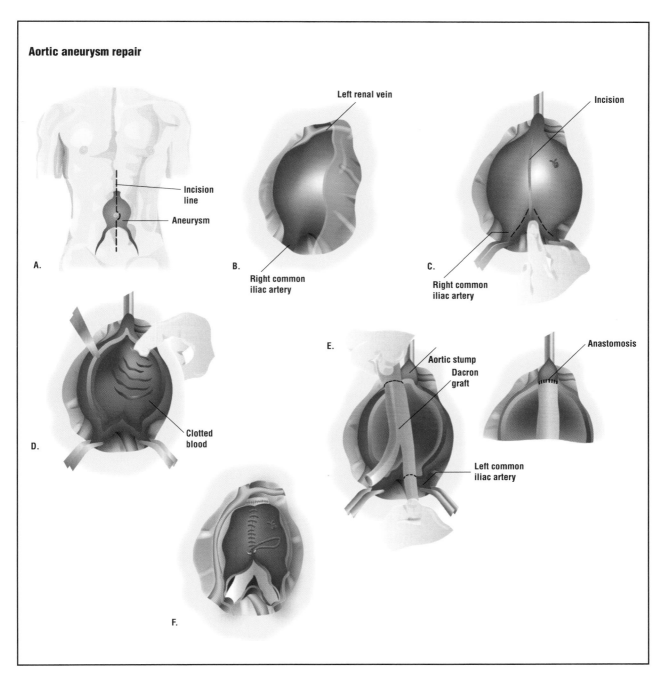

Aortic aneurysm repair

A. Incision line / Aneurysm

B. Left renal vein / Right common iliac artery

C. Incision / Right common iliac artery

D. Clotted blood

E. Aortic stump / Dacron graft / Left common iliac artery

Anastomosis

F.

An incision is made in the abdomen (A), and the aneurysm is visualized (B). The aorta is clamped above the aneurysm, and the aorta is cut open (C). The clotted blood is removed (D). A synthetic graft may be used to replace the part of the aorta that had the aneurysm, and it is stitched in place (E). The aorta is then closed over the graft (F). *(Illustration by GGS Inc.)*

Description

After general anesthesia is administered, the surgeon will make an incision through the length of the sternum to repair an ascending, arch, or thoracic aortic aneurysm. Abdominal aneurysms are approached through a vertical incision in the abdominal wall. Depending on the location of the aneurysm, cardiopulmonary bypass with deep hypothermic circulatory arrest (arch), cardiopulmonary bypass (ascending), or left heart bypass (thoracic) may be required. All procedures require some amount of anticoagulation, usually heparin, to be administered to prevent

WHO PERFORMS THE PROCEDURE AND WHERE IS IT PERFORMED?

Cardiothoracic or cardiovascular surgeons or vascular surgeons can perform these procedures. Abdominal and thoracic aortic aneurysm repairs require less sophisticated equipment during the surgical procedure, but do need extensive intensive care post-operatively. Anesthetic management plays a crucial role in the decrease in complications associated with these procedures. Facilities that can also provide cardiovascular surgery are best equipped to manage these patients, but this is not a limitation for all procedures.

QUESTIONS TO ASK THE DOCTOR

- How many of these procedures have been performed by the surgeon?
- What is the mortality rate for this procedure at the institution?
- What side effects are associated with this surgical procedure, and at what rate are they experienced by patients?
- What is the expected length of stay in the hospital?
- Are there any other suitable procedures, such as endovascular grafting?
- How long before normal activities, **exercise,** work, and driving can be resumed?

blood clot formation. Clamps will be applied across the aorta to prevent blood flow into the aneurysm. The aneurysm will be opened to an area where the tissue is healthy. The healthy tissue will be sutured to a synthetic fiber fabric graft. The fabric is knit or woven Dacron fibers and may be impregnated with collagen, gelatin, or other substances. Blood flow is reinstituted to check for a secure seal. Additional sutures will be added to prevent leaking. The incision is then closed at the completion of the procedure with blood drains penetrating the incision during healing.

Ascending aortic aneurysms may involve the aortic valve or coronary arteries. If the aortic valve is damaged, a graft with an integral aortic valve is used. The coronary arteries are reconnected to the graft.

Aortic arch aneurysms require the reattachment of the arch vessels, the innominate artery, the left common carotid artery, and the left subclavian artery. To decrease surgery time, these three vessels can be treated as a single vessel by using part of the patient's native aorta to create an island. This island is then connected to the graft.

Thoracic aneurysms require special care to protect the spinal vessels that supply blood to the spinal cord. Protecting the spinal cord during repair is still an area of intensive research. Some surgeons feel that rapid implant of the graft to restore blood flow is the best method to protect the spinal cord. A bypass graft called a Gott shunt can be used to redirect the blood flow around the area during surgical repair. Left-heart bypass provides the same benefit as a Gott shunt, with the addition of a mechanical pump for more controlled blood flow to the abdomen and lower extremities.

The abdominal aortic aneurysm is repaired by rapid anastomosis of the graft to return blood flow to the circulation. If the renal arteries are involved in the aneurysm, they will be reattached to the graft. Additionally, if the superior celiac, mesenteric, or inferior celiac arteries are involved, they will also be reattached to the graft. Finally, it is common for the bifurcation (separation into two) of the iliac arteries to be involved; this may require a Y-shaped graft to be used to reattach both lower limb vessels.

Diagnosis/Preparation

A simple x ray may provide the initial diagnosis of aortic aneurysm. Initial diagnosis can be made with non-invasive transesophageal **echocardiography** or ultrasound. Additional tests such as **magnetic resonance imaging** (MRI) or computed tomography (CT) will allow for additional visualization of the aneurysm. An **angiography** is the preferred method for determining the severity. Blood vessel and aortic valve health can be evaluated.

Aftercare

Following surgery the patient will be cared for in an **intensive care unit**. Cardiac monitoring will be continued for blood pressure and heart function. Intravenous fluids will continue to be given, and may include blood products. Additional medications will be continued to support cardiac function as needed. The ventilator will be removed after the patient is able to breathe on his/her own. The stay in the intensive care unit is approximately two to five days with hospital discharge following a week.

Risks

There are risks associated with general anesthesia, not associated with the aortic aneurysm repair. Additional risks of cardiopulmonary bypass are not associated with surgical repair. Depending on the type of aneurysm involved, the risks can differ significantly. Since blood flow to the spinal cord is jeopardized by the surgical repair, thoracic aorta aneurysm repair carries a relatively high rate of paralysis. Ascending arch aneurysms may jeopardize coronary blood flow and aortic valve function. Infection of the sternum can influence recovery time. Renal function can be impacted by abdominal aortic aneurysm repair. Renal function may improve or remain compromised. Long-term complications associated with the abdominal surgery include intra-abdominal adhesions, small bowel obstructions, and incisional hernia. Aortic arch aneurysms carry a risk of brain damage associated with deep hypothermic circulatory arrest.

Normal results

Repair of the aneurysm will provide normal blood flow to the systemic circulation. Pain associated with the aneurysm will be relieved by the repair. The risk of aneurysm rupture will be eliminated.

Morbidity and mortality rates

During 1999 over 15,000 deaths in the United States were attributed to aortic aneurysm as reported by the American Heart Association. Without treatment, the five-year survival rate is 13%. The Multicentre Aneurysm Screening Group studied non-emergent abdominal aortic aneurysm repair, showing a 2–6% mortality rate at 30 days post surgery. Emergency surgeries demonstrate 37% mortality. In another study, treatment of cardiac disease by open heart surgery, not **cardiac catheterization** intervention, demonstrated a better outcome prior to elective treatment for abdominal aortic aneurysm.

During treatment of thoracic aneurysm repair the incidence of paraplegia is 6–10%. Left vocal cord paralysis is recognized if the laryngeal nerve has been compromised by the procedure. Multiple organ failure is incident in death, with respiratory failure being among the most common. If the aneurysm is above or involves the renal arteries, renal failure can occur in 4–9% of patients.

Treatment of the ascending aorta and aortic arch repair carry many of the risks associated with cardiopulmonary bypass, including hemostatic difficulties, left ventricle dysfunction, or myocardial (heart muscle) dysfunction. Irreversible brain damage is also an additional risk.

Cardiac function can be compromised in all patients with thoracic or abdominal aortic aneurysms. Hemor-

rhage is of frequent concern and is more of a risk as the number of suture lines increases. Forty to seventy percent of all deaths can be contributed to cardiac malfunction and blood loss.

KEY TERMS

Abdominal aneurysm—Aneurysm that involves the descending aorta from the diaphragm to the point at which it separates into two iliac arteries.

Hemostatic—Relating to blood clotting and coagulation.

Medionecrosis—Death of the middle layer of tissues of the vessel.

Rupture—Severing of the aorta allowing blood to spill out into the body instead of being carried by the blood vessels.

Systemic circulation—Blood vessels not involved in carrying blood to and from the lungs between the right and left sides of the heart.

Thoracic aneurysm—Aneurysm that involves the ascending, arch, or descending thoracic aorta using the diaphragm as a landmark for transition to abdominal aorta.

Alternatives

Endovascular graft placement is being used as a suitable option to the open surgical procedure. The endovascular graft can be placed using minimally invasive techniques that reduce or eliminate the stay in the intensive care unit. Light sedation and epidural anesthetic are often adequate.

Resources

BOOKS

Hensley, Frederick A., Donald E. Martin, Glenn P. Gravlee, eds. *A Practical Approach to Cardiac Anesthesia.* 3rd Edition. Philadelphia: Lippincott Williams & Wilkins Philadelphia, 2003.

PERIODICALS

Busch, T., et al. "Importance of Cardiovascular Interventions Before Surgery for Abdominal Aortic Aneurysms." *Cardiovascular Surgery* 18 (2000):18–21.

Cooley, D. "Aortic Aneurysm Operations: Past, Present, and Future." *Ann Thorac Surg* 67 (1999):1959–62.

"The Multicentre Aneurysm Screening Study (MASS) into the Effect of Abdominal Aortic Aneurysm Screening on Mortality in Men: A Randomized Controlled Trial." *The Lancet* 360 (November 2002):1531–1539.

Porter J. M., et al. "Endovascular Aortic Grafting: Current Status." *Cardiovascular Surgery* 7 (1999):684–691.

OTHER

American Heart Association. *2002 Heart and Stroke Statistical Update*. Dallas, TX: American Heart Association, 2001.

Allison Joan Spiwak, MSBME

Aortic stenting *see* **Endovascular stent surgery**

Aortic valve replacement

Definition

Aortic valve replacement is the insertion of a mechanical or tissue valve in place of the diseased native aortic valve.

Purpose

Aortic valve replacement is necessary when the aortic valve has become diseased. The aortic valve can suffer from insufficiency (inability to perform adequately) or stenosis. An insufficient valve is leaky and allows blood flow retrograde from the aorta to the left ventricle during diastole. A stenotic valve prevents the flow of blood antegrade from the left ventricle to the aorta, during systole.

Either situation can result in heart failure and an enlarged left ventricle. With aortic stenosis (narrowing), angina pectoris, fainting, and congestive heart failure will develop with the severity of the narrowing. There is an increased rate of sudden death of patients with aortic stenosis. Dyspnea (labored breathing), fatigue, and palpitations are late symptoms of aortic insufficiency. Angina pectoris is associated with the latest stages of aortic insufficiency.

Demographics

Congenital birth defects involving a bicuspid aortic valve can develop stenosis. These patients may become symptomatic in mid-teen years through age 65. Patients with a history rheumatic fever have a disposition for aortic stenosis, but may live symptom free for more then four decades. Calcification of the aortic valve tends to effect an older population with 30% of patients over age 85 having stenosis at autopsy.

Patients with aortic stenosis who have angina, dyspnea, or fainting are candidates for aortic valve replacement. Asymptomatic patients undergoing coronary artery bypass grafting should be treated with aortic valve replacement, but otherwise are not candidates for preventive aortic valve replacement.

Patients with a history of rheumatic fever or syphilitic aortitis (inflammation of the aorta) face the possibility of developing aortic insufficiency. Successful treatment has decreased this causative relationship. Primary causes of aortic disease commonly include bacterial endocarditis, trauma, aortic dissection, and congenital diseases.

Patients showing acute symptoms, including pulmonary edema, heart rhythm problems, or circulatory collapse, are candidates for aortic valve replacement. Chronic pathologies are recommended for surgery when patients appear symptomatic, demonstrating angina and dyspnea. Asymptomatic patients must be monitored for heart dysfunction. Left ventricular dimensions greater then 2 in (50 mm) at diastole or 3 in (70 mm) at systole are indications for replacement when aortic insufficiency is diagnosed.

Description

While receiving general anesthesia in preparation for the surgery, the patient's cardiac function will be monitored. A sternotomy (incision in the sternum) or **thoracotomy** may be used to expose the heart, with the thoracotomy providing a smaller incision through the ribs. Anticoagulant is administered in preparation for cardiopulmonary bypass. Cardiopulmonary bypass is instituted by exposing and cannulating (putting tubes in) the great blood vessels of the heart, or by cannulating the

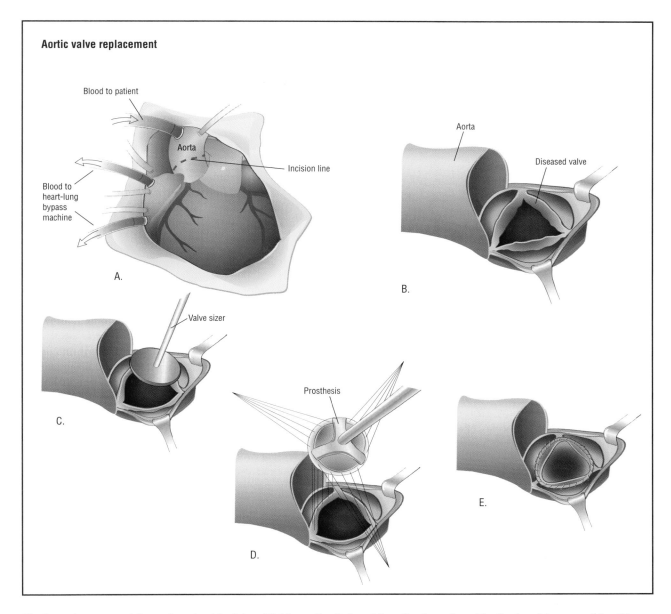

Aortic valve replacement

The heart is accessed through a chest incision (A). The patient's heart function is replaced by the heart-lung machine. The aorta is cut open to reveal a diseased aortic valve (B), which is then removed. A valve sizer is placed in the opening to determine the size of prosthesis needed (C). A prosthetic valve is sutured in place (D and E). *(Illustration by Argosy.)*

femoral artery and vein. A combination of cannulation sites may also be used. The heart is stopped after the aorta is clamped. The aortic root is opened and the diseased valve is removed. Sutures are placed in the aortic rim and into the replacement valve. The replacement valve can be either mechanical or biological tissue. The replacement valve will be sized prior to implant to ensure that it fits the patient based on the size of the aortic valve annulus. Once seated, the valve is secured by tying the individual sutures. The heart is then deaired. The cross clamp is removed and the heart is allowed to beat as deairing continues by manipulation of the left ventricle. Cardiopulmonary bypass is terminated, the tubes are removed and drugs to reverse anticoagulation are administered.

A heart valve is an orifice that blood passes through in systole, and it is also an occluding (blocking) mechanism necessary to prevent the flow of blood during diastole. Heart valves can be mechanical or biological tissue valves. For patients younger then 65 years of age, the mechanical valve offers superior longevity. Anticoagula-

QUESTIONS TO ASK THE DOCTOR

- What type of valve is best suited for me?
- What are the pros and cons associated with each type of valve for a person with my disease and/or associated diseases?
- Why am I a candidate for valve replacement?
- Are there any other more suitable alternative procedures?
- If I am a female interested in having children, or currently pregnant are there additional options?
- How often has the surgeon performed this procedure and what are the morbidity/mortality statistics for this surgeon and institution?
- If I have an associated disease or complicated scenario does the surgeon have experience with follow-up care?

tion is required for the life of the patient implanted with a mechanical valve. The biological tissue valve does not require anticoagulation but suffers from deterioration, leading to **reoperation** particularly in those under age 50. Women considering bearing children should be treated with biological tissue valves as the anticoagulant of choice with mechanical valves, warfarin, is associated with teterogenic effects in the fetus. **Aspirin** can be substituted in certain circumstances.

Diagnosis/Preparation

Initial diagnosis by auscultation (listening) is done with a **stethoscope**. Additional procedures associated with diagnosis to judge severity of the lesion include **chest x ray**, **echocardiography**, and **angiography** with **cardiac catheterization**. In the absence of angiography, **magnetic resonance imaging** (MRI) or computed tomographic (CT) imaging may be used.

Aftercare

The patient will have continuous cardiac monitoring performed in the **intensive care unit** (ICU) postoperatively. Medications or mechanical circulatory assist may be instituted during the surgery or postoperatively to help the heart provide the necessary cardiac output to sustain the pulmonary and systemic circulations. These will be discontinued as cardiac function improves. As the patient is able to breathe without assistance, ventila-

tory support will be discontinued. Drainage tubes allow blood to be collected from the chest cavity during healing and are removed as blood flow decreases. Prophylaxis **antibiotics** are given. Anticoagulation (warfarin, aspirin, or a combination) therapy is instituted and continued for patients who have received a mechanical valve. The ICU stay is approximately three days with a final hospital discharge occurring within a week after the procedure.

The patient receive **wound care** instructions prior to leaving the hospital. The instructions include how to recognize such adverse conditions as infection or valve malfunction, contact information for the surgeon, and guidelines on when to return to the emergency room.

Risks

There are unassociated risks with general anesthetic and cardiopulmonary bypass. Risks associated with aortic valve replacement include embolism, bleeding, and operative valvular endocarditis. Hemolysis is associated with certain types of mechanical valves, but is not a contraindication for implantation.

Normal results

Myocardial function typically improves rapidly, with decrease in left ventricle enlargement and dilation over several months, allowing the heart to return to normal dimensions. Anticoagulation therapy will be continued to elevate the INR to between 2.0 and 4.5, depending on the type of mechanical valve implanted. Implantation of biological tissue valves with maintenance of an INR of 2.0–3.0 for the initial three months post implant are associated with blood clot complications. If non-cardiac surgery or dental care is needed the antithrombotic therapy will be adjusted to prevent bleeding complications.

Morbidity and mortality rates

There is a 3–5% hospital mortality associated with aortic valve replacement. There is an average survival rate of five years in 85% of patients suffering from aortic stenosis that undergo aortic valve replacement. Structural valve deterioration can occur and is higher in mechanical valves during the first five years; however, biological tissue and mechanical valves have the same failure incidence at 10 years, with a 60% probability of death at 11 years as a result of a valve-related complications. Patients with a mechanical valve are more likely to experience bleeding complications. Reoperation is more likely for patients treated with a biological tissue valve, but not significantly different when compared to their mechani-

Apheres *see* **Transfusion**

Apicoectomy *see* **Root canal treatment**

KEY TERMS

Antithrombic—Preventing clot formation.

Biological tissue valve—An autograft is a valve that comes from the patient. Homograft (or allograft) valve that is harvested from a human cadaver.

Diastole—Period between contractions of te heart.

Hemolysis—Separation of hemoglobin from the red blood cells.

Mechanical valve—There are three types of mechanical valves: ball valve, disk valve, and bileaflet valve.

Systole—Contraction of the heart.

cal valve counterparts. This combines to an average rate of significant complications of 2–3% per year, with death rate of approximately 1% per year associated directly with the prosthesis.

Alternatives

Balloon valvotomy may provide short term relief of aortic stenosis, but is considered palliative until valve replacement can be accomplished. Aortic valve repair by direct commisurotomy may also be successful for some cases of aortic stenosis. Medical treatment for inoperable patients with severe aortic stenosis is used to relive pulmonary congestion and prevent atrial fibrillation.

Severe aortic insufficiency can be treated with medical therapy. Pharmaceuticals to decrease blood pressure, with **diuretics** and vasodilators, are helpful in patients with aortic insufficiency.

Resources

BOOKS

Hensley, Frederick A., Donald E. Martin, and Glenn P. Gravlee, eds. *A Practical Approach to Cardiac Anesthesia*. 3rd Edition. Philadelphia: Lippincott Williams & Wilkins Philadelphia, 2003.

PERIODICALS

Bonow R, et al. "ACC/AHA Guidelines for the Management of Patients with Valvular Heart Disease." *JACC* 32 (November 1998): 1486–588.

Allison Joan Spiwak, MSBME

Aortofemoral bypass *see* **Peripheral vascular bypass surgery**

Appendectomy

Definition

Appendectomy is the surgical removal of the appendix. The appendix is a worm-shaped hollow pouch attached to the cecum, the beginning of the large intestine.

Purpose

Appendectomies are performed to treat appendicitis, an inflamed and infected appendix.

Description

After the patient is anesthetized, the surgeon can remove the appendix either by using the traditional open procedure (in which a 2–3 in [5–7.6 cm] incision is made in the abdomen) or via **laparoscopy** (in which four 1-in [2.5-cm] incisions are made in the abdomen).

Traditional open appendectomy

When the surgeon uses the open approach, he makes an incision in the lower right section of the abdomen. Most incisions are less than 3 in (7.6 cm) in length. The surgeon then identifies all of the organs in the abdomen and examines them for other disease or abnormalities. The appendix is located and brought up into the wounds. The surgeon separates the appendix from all the surrounding tissue and its attachment to the cecum, and then removes it. The site where the appendix was previously attached, the cecum, is closed and returned to the abdomen. The muscle layers and then the skin are sewn together.

Laparoscopic appendectomy

When the surgeon performs a laparoscopic appendectomy, four incisions, each about 1 in (2.5 cm) in length, are made. One incision is near the umbilicus, or navel, and one is between the umbilicus and the pubis. Two other incisions are smaller and are on the right side of the lower abdomen. The surgeon then passes a camera and special instruments through these incisions. With the aid of this equipment, the surgeon visually examines the abdominal organs and identifies the appendix. The appendix is then freed from all of its attachments and removed. The place where the appendix was formerly attached, the cecum, is stitched. The appendix is removed through one of the incisions. The instruments are removed and then all of the incisions are closed.

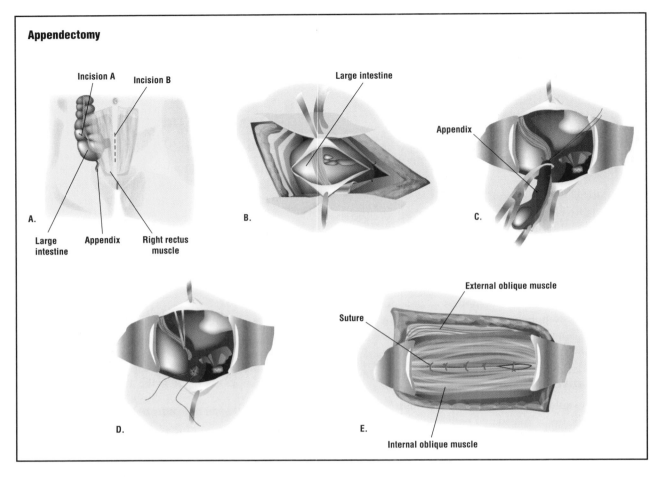

Appendectomy

Incision A   Incision B

Large intestine

Appendix

A.

Large intestine   Appendix   Right rectus muscle

B.

C.

External oblique muscle

Suture

D.

E.

Internal oblique muscle

To remove a diseased appendix, an incision is made in the patient's lower abdomen (A). Layers of muscle and tissue are cut, and large intestine, or colon, is visualized (B). The appendix is located (C), tied, and removed (D). The muscle and tissue layers are stitched (E). *(Illustration by GGS Inc.)*

Studies and opinions about the relative advantages and disadvantages of each method are divided. A skilled surgeon can perform either one of these procedures in less than one hour. However, laparoscopic appendectomy (LA) always takes longer than traditional appendectomy (TA). The increased time required to do a LA the greater the patient's exposure to anesthetics, which increases the risk of complications. The increased time requirement also increases the fees charged by the hospital for **operating room** time and by the anesthesiologist. Since LA also requires specialized equipment, the fees for its use also increase the hospital charges. Patients with either operation have similar pain medication needs, begin eating diets at comparable times, and stay in the hospital equivalent amounts of time. LA is of special benefit in women in whom the diagnosis is difficult and gynecological disease (such as endometriosis, pelvic inflammatory disease, ruptured ovarian follicles, ruptured ovarian cysts, and tubal pregnancies) may be the source of pain and not appendicitis. If LA is done in these patients, the pelvic or-

gans can be more thoroughly examined and a definitive diagnosis made prior to removal of the appendix. Most surgeons select either TA or LA based on the individual needs and circumstances of the patient.

Insurance plans do cover the costs of appendectomy. Fees are charged independently by the hospital and the physicians. Hospital charges include fees for operating and **recovery room** use, diagnostic and laboratory testing, as well as the normal hospital room charges. Surgical fees vary from region to region and range between $250–750. The anesthesiologist's fee depends on the health of the patient and the length of the operation.

Preparation

Once the diagnosis of appendicitis is made and the decision has been made to perform an appendectomy, the patient undergoes the standard preparation for an operation. This usually takes only one to two hours and includes signing the operative consents, patient identification procedures, evaluation by the anesthesiologist, and moving the patient to the operating area of the hospital. Occasionally, if the patient has been ill for a prolonged period of time or has had protracted vomiting, a delay of few to several hours may be necessary to give the patient fluids and **antibiotics**.

Aftercare

Recovery from an appendectomy is similar to other operations. Patients are allowed to eat when the stomach and intestines begin to function again. Usually the first meal is a clear liquid diet—broth, juice, soda pop, and gelatin. If patients tolerate this meal, the next meal usually is a regular diet. Patients are asked to walk and resume their normal physical activities as soon as possible. If TA was done, work and physical education classes may be restricted for a full three weeks after the operation. If a LA was done, most patients are able to return to work and strenuous activity within one to three weeks after the operation.

Risks

Certain risks are present when any operation is performed under general anesthesia and the abdominal cavity is opened. Pneumonia and collapse of the small airways (atelectasis) often occurs. Patients who smoke are at a greater risk for developing these complications. Thrombophlebitis, or inflammation of the veins, is rare but can occur if the patient requires prolonged bed rest. Bleeding can occur but rarely is a blood **transfusion** required. Adhesions (abnormal connections to abdominal organs by thin fibrous tissue) are a known complication of any abdominal surgery such as appendectomy. These adhesions can lead to intestinal obstruction that prevents the normal flow of intestinal contents. Hernia is a complication of any incision. However, they are rarely seen after appendectomy because the abdominal wall is very strong in the area of the standard appendectomy incision.

The overall complication rate of appendectomy depends upon the status of the appendix at the time it is removed. If the appendix has not ruptured, the complication rate is only about 3%. However, if the appendix has ruptured, the complication rate rises to almost 59%. Wound infections do occur and are more common if the appendicitis was severe, far advanced, or ruptured. An abscess may also form in the abdomen as a complication of appendicitis.

Occasionally, an appendix will rupture prior to its removal, spilling its contents into the abdominal cavity. Peritonitis or a generalized infection in the abdomen will occur. Treatment of peritonitis as a result of a ruptured appendix includes removal of what remains of the ap-

WHO PERFORMS THE PROCEDURE AND WHERE IS IT PERFORMED?

An appendectomy is performed by a fully trained surgeon who, after medical school, has gone through years of training in an accredited residency program to learn the specialized skills of a surgeon. A sign of a surgeon's competence is certification by a national surgical board approved by the American Board of Medical Specialties (ABMS). All board-certified surgeons have completed an approved training program and have passed a rigorous specialty examination. The letters F.A.C.S. (Fellow of the American College of Surgeons) after a surgeon's name are a further indication of a surgeon's qualifications.

Appendectomy is considered a major surgical operation. Therefore, the surgeon must perform this operation in the operating room of a hospital. An anesthesiologist is also present during the operation to administer an anesthetic.

pendix, insertion of drains (rubber tubes that promote the flow of infection inside the abdomen to outside of the body), and antibiotics. Fistula formation (an abnormal connection between the cecum and the skin) rarely occurs. It is only seen if the appendix has a broad attachment to the cecum and the appendicitis is far advanced, causing destruction of the cecum itself.

The complications associated with undiagnosed, misdiagnosised, or delayed diagnosis of appendicitis are very significant. This has led surgeons to perform an appendectomy any time that they feel appendicitis is the diagnosis. Most surgeons feel that in approximately 20% of their patients, a normal appendix will be removed. Rates much lower than this would seem to indicate that the diagnosis of appendicitis was being frequently missed.

Normal results

Most patients feel better immediately after an operation for appendicitis. Many patients are discharged from the hospital within 24 hours after the appendectomy. Others may require a longer stay, from three to five days. Almost all patients are back to their normal activities within three weeks.

Morbidity and mortality rates

The mortality rate of appendicitis has dramatically decreased over time. Currently, the mortality rate is esti-

QUESTIONS TO ASK THE DOCTOR

- What are the possible risks involved with this surgery?
- What are the expected results after having a laparoscopic appendectomy versus having an open abdominal appendectomy?
- Will I have a scar?
- Which procedure will you use to perform the appendectomy?
- Must I do anything special after the operation?
- How long does it take to recover?
- How many appendectomies do you perform each year?

mated at one to two per 1,000,000 cases of appendicitis. Death is usually due to peritonitis, intra abdominal abscess, or severe infection following rupture.

Alternatives

Appendectomies are usually carried out on an emergency basis to treat appendicitis. There are no alternatives, due to the serious consequence of not removing the inflamed appendix, which is a ruptured appendix and peritonitis, a life-threatening emergency.

See also Laparoscopy.

Resources

BOOKS

Schwartz, Seymour I. "Appendix." In *Principles of Surgery,* edited by Seymour Schwartz, et al. New York: McGraw-Hill, 1994.

Silen, William. "Acute Appendicitis." In *Harrison's Principles of Internal Medicine,* edited by Anthony S. Fauci, et al. New York: McGraw-Hill, 1997.

PERIODICALS

Eypasch, E., S. Sauerland, R. Lefering, and E. A. Neugebauer. "Laparoscopic versus Open Appendectomy: Between Evidence and Common Sense." *Digestive Surgery* 19 (2002): 518–522.

Peiser, J. G. and D. Greenberg. "Laparoscopic versus open appendectomy: results of a retrospective comparison in an Israeli hospital." *Israel Medical Association Journal* 4 (February, 2002): 91–94.

Piskun, G., D. Kozik, S. Rajpal, G. Shaftan, and R. Fogler. "Comparison of laparoscopic, open, and converted appendectomy for perforated appendicitis." *Surgery and Endoscopy* 15 (July 2001): 660–662.

KEY TERMS

Abscess—A collection of pus buried deep in the tissues or in a body cavity.

Anesthesia—A combination of drugs administered by a variety of techniques by trained professionals that provide sedation, amnesia, analgesia, and immobility adequate for the accomplishment of the surgical procedure with minimal discomfort to the patient.

Anesthesiologist—A physician who has special training and expertise in anesthesia techniques.

Anesthetics—Drugs used to make a body area free of sensation or pain.

Cecum—The beginning of the large intestine and the place where the appendix attaches to the intestinal tract.

General surgeon—A physician who has special training and expertise in performing a variety of operations.

Pelvic organs—The organs inside of the body that are located within the confines of the pelvis. This includes the bladder and rectum in both sexes and the uterus, ovaries, and fallopian tubes in females.

Pubis—The anterior portion of the pelvis located in the anterior abdomen.

Thrombophlebitis—Inflammation of the veins, usually in the legs, which causes swelling and tenderness in the affected area.

Umbilicus—The navel.

Long, K. H., M. P. Bannon, S. P. Zietlow, E. R. Helgeson, et al. "A prospective randomized comparison of laparoscopic appendectomy with open appendectomy: Clinical and economic analyses." *Pathology Case Reviews* 129 (April, 2001): 390–400.

Selby, W. S., S. Griffin, N. Abraham, and M. J. Solomon. "Appendectomy protects against the development of ulcerative colitis but does not affect its course." *American Journal of Gastroenterology* 97 (November, 2002): 2834–2838.

ORGANIZATIONS

American College of Surgeons. 633 N. Saint Clair St., Chicago, IL 60611-3211. (312) 202-5000. <www.facs.org>.

OTHER

"Appendectomy." MEDPLINE PLUS. [cited June 27, 2003]. <http://www.nlm.nih.gov/medlineplus>.

"The Appendix." Mayo Clinic Online. <http://www.mayo health.org>.

Mary Jeanne Krob, M.D., F.A.C.S.
Monique Laberge, Ph.D.

Appendix removal *see* **Appendectomy**

Arterial anastomasis *see* **Arteriovenous fistula**

Arteriography *see* **Angiography**

Arteriovenous fistula

Definition

An arteriovenous fistula (AV fistula) is the connection of a vein and an artery, usually in the forearm, to allow access to the vascular system for hemodialysis, a procedure that performs the functions of the kidneys in people whose kidneys have failed. Connecting the vein and artery is a surgical procedure. The fistula develops over a period of months after the surgery.

Purpose

The surgical creation of an AV fistula provides a long-lasting site through which blood can be removed and returned during hemodialysis. The fistula, which allows the person to be connected to a dialysis machine, must be prepared by a surgeon weeks or months before dialysis is started. When the vein and artery are joined, the vein gradually becomes larger and stronger, creating the fistula that provides vascular access years longer than other types of access and with fewer complications.

Sometimes dialysis is only needed temporarily, but some people need it for the rest of their lives or until a kidney is available for a transplant. When kidney failure is diagnosed, time is needed to prepare the patient's body with either an AV fistula or implantable devices that will connect the person to the dialysis machine.

Demographics

At any one time, the number of patients in the United States with kidney failure is approximately two million and rising. According to the National Kidney Foundation, by the year 2008, three million people will be expected to have what is known as end-stage renal (kidney) disease. These people can be of any age, from any background. They are typically suffering from another condition or disease that has led to kidney shutdown, and most will require dialysis. Among dialysis patients, over half will have an AV fistula as vascular access.

Description

Many advances in the treatment of kidney failure have been seen since the first attempts at dialysis treatments were made in the 1920s. At one time dialysis was only thought of as a way to keep people alive until kidney function could be restored. Often the treatment for kidney failure had to be discontinued within several days because patients' veins could not endure the trauma of frequent withdrawing and replacing blood. The first breakthrough came in 1960 with the introduction of an implantable Teflon tube, called a shunt, that was the first effective vascular access device. Since then, the development of the AV fistula has marked another important advance, allowing effective treatment for longer periods of time. The goal of researchers and medical institutions is to continue to improve treatment and improve the length and quality of life for people with chronic kidney failure.

The kidneys are two organs in the mid-abdomen, one on each side of the middle back. Their function is to clean the blood of wastes and regulate fluid and chemical balance in the body. Dialysis performs these functions in place of the failing kidneys. Dialysis cannot restore the kidneys, but it can prolong life, often for years, by preventing the build-up of waste products in the body. Acute kidney failure can happen in many conditions and diseases that place an extra burden on the renal system, such as in advanced kidney and liver diseases; in rapidly progressing terminal illnesses, such as cancer and certain severe anemias; after severe allergic reactions or reactions to drugs or medications; in diseases that involve the vascular system, such as heart and lung diseases or the formation of blood clots (embolism); and often following heart bypass surgery. Diabetes and vascular diseases, especially those with hypertension (high blood pressure), are the two most common underlying diseases contributing to chronic kidney failure.

Hemodialysis

Dialysis is performed as critical life support when someone suffers acute or chronic kidney failure. It is a mechanical way to cleanse the blood and balance body fluids and chemicals when the kidneys are not able to perform these essential functions. Because kidney function can be reversible in some cases, dialysis can provide temporary support until renal function is restored. Dialysis may also be used in irreversible or chronic kidney shutdown when transplantation is the medical goal and the patient is waiting for donated kidneys. Some critically ill patients, with life-threatening illnesses, such as cancer or severe heart disease, are not candidates for transplantation and dialysis may be the only option for treating what is called end-stage renal disease (ESRD).

There are two types of dialysis, hemodialysis and peritoneal dialysis. In hemodialysis, the blood circulates through a machine outside the body and is filtered as it circulates. In peritoneal dialysis, the blood is filtered through a membrane that has been placed in the abdomen. Blood remains in the body and waste material is filtered into an exchange fluid through an opening in the abdomen called a port. Only hemodialysis requires an AV fistula or other vascular access.

Hemodialysis circulates blood through a dialysis machine that contains a filter membrane. The blood is slowly pumped out of the body and into the machine for filtering. After being filtered, the blood is returned to the body through the same vascular access. About one cup of blood is outside the body at any given moment during the continuous circulation process.

Hemodialysis is usually done three times a week, taking between three and five hours each time. Healthcare professionals perform the procedure either at independent dialysis centers or in hospitals or medical centers. Dialysis patients must go to the hemodialysis center where they will sit to receive the treatment. Although they cannot walk around, they can watch television, read, or talk to other patients. The dialysis center offers patient education, including videos and brochures that describe treatment options and self-care. Patients can also be given advice and information about paying for this ongoing treatment through nationally sponsored programs that are available especially for dialysis patients. Often the dialysis center offers emotional support as well, letting people meet and talk with other people who have kidney problems. Some people prefer to perform their own dialysis by having a home dialysis machine. This requires that the dialysis patient and another person, usually a family member, take a three- to six-week training program to learn how to do the treatment.

Vascular access

An access or entry to the vascular system is needed to perform the blood-cleansing role of the kidneys through hemodialysis. There are three types of vascular access: arteriovenous fistula, grafts, and catheters.

ARTERIOVENOUS FISTULA. An AV fistula has proven to be the best kind of vascular access for people whose veins are large enough, not only because it lasts longer but it is also less likely than other types of access to form clots or become infected. If the veins are not large enough, or there is no time to wait for a fistula to develop, a graft or a catheter must be used.

GRAFT. Grafts are often the access of choice when a hemodialysis patient has small veins that will not likely develop properly into a fistula. This type of access uses a synthetic tube implanted under the skin of the arm that can be used repeatedly for needle placement. Unlike a fistula, which requires time to develop, a graft can be used as soon as two to three weeks after placement. Grafts are known to have more problems than fistulas, such as clots and infection, and will likely need replacement sooner.

CATHETER. A catheter may be used to provide temporary vascular access. When kidney disease has progressed quickly, there may not be time to prepare permanent vascular access before dialysis treatments are started. The catheter is a tube that is inserted into a vein in the neck, chest, or in the leg near the groin. Two chambers in the tube allow blood to flow in and out. Once the catheter is in place, needle insertion is not necessary. Catheters are effective for dialysis for several weeks or months while surgery is performed and an AV fistula develops. They are not selected for permanent access because they can clog, become infected, or can cause the veins to narrow. Long-term catheter access must be used in patients for whom fistula or graft surgery has not been successful. If more than three weeks' use is expected, catheters can be made to tunnel under the skin, which increases comfort and reduces complications

Diagnosis/Preparation

Diagnosis

The diagnosis of kidney disease and its progression to kidney failure is typically made by a nephrologist, a specialist in kidney structure and function. The nephrologist will determine whether the patient has acute or chronic kidney failure and if dialysis is appropriate for the patient. If dialysis is recommended, the nephrologist will determine if an AV fistula is the ideal vascular access for the patient. To make these determinations, the nephrologist will need to be aware of the patient's general condition, especially the presence of any underlying disease. Kidney function must be evaluated and determined to be seriously impaired before dialysis is recommended. It is typically started when kidney function is down to about 10% of its normal level. Among other tests that will be performed, such as **urinalysis** with microscopic examination of the urine, several blood and urine tests can be used to measure a person's kidney function when chronic or acute kidney failure is suspected. Some of the tests measure chemicals produced by the body that are normally excreted (passed in urine) by the kidneys; the tests can measure how much is passing through, and how much remains in the blood, and then determine how well the kidneys are functioning compared to normal. These tests include, but are not limited to:

• Serum creatinine, found in higher levels in the blood if kidneys fail.

• Urinary creatinine, lower in kidney failure.

• Urinary output, measuring both fluid intake and all urine produced.

• Urinary osmolality, measuring the concentration of the urine, an indicator of kidney filtering ability.

• Blood urea nitrogen (BUN), harmful nitrogen waste that increases in the blood as kidney function decreases.

• Electrolytes in blood and urine, minerals that result from the breakdown of salts (sodium, potassium, magnesium, and chloride), often out of balance when kidneys fail. Potassium, for example, increases in the blood during kidney failure and can cause heart irregularities.

Description

Surgery to create an arteriovenous fistula is usually conducted using a local anesthetic, injected at the site of the proposed fistula. The procedure is performed in a hospital or one-day surgery center and can usually be performed on an outpatient basis if the patient is not already hospitalized. After cleaning and sterilizing the site, the surgeon will make a small incision in the forearm sufficient to allow the permanent joining together of a vein and an artery in the arm. The blood vessels will be appropriately blocked to stop blood flow for the procedure and incisions will be made to join them. Silk sutures, just as those used in other types of surgical incisions, will be used to close incised areas as needed after the vein and artery have been joined. Once joined, blood flow will increase, the vein will become thicker, and over a period of months the connection will become strong and develop into the fistula that will allow permanent vascular access.

Aftercare

The hemodialysis patient should expect needle insertion in the AV fistula at every dialysis session. Patients who prefer to insert their own needles or who per-

form dialysis at home will need training, and all patients will have to learn how to avoid infection and to protect vascular access. Because vascular access problems can lead to treatment failure, the AV fistula requires regular care to make dialysis easier and to help avoid clots, infection, and other complications. Patients can help protect the access by:

• Making sure the access is checked before each treatment.

• Not allowing blood pressure to be taken on the access arm.

• Checking the pulse in the access every day.

• Keeping the access clean at all times.

• Using the access site only for dialysis.

• Being careful not to bump or cut the access.

• Not wearing tight jewelry or clothing near or over the access site.

• Not lifting heavy objects or putting pressure on the access arm.

• Sleeping with the access arm free, not under the head or body.

Risks

The most frequent complications in hemodialysis relate to the vascular access site where needles are inserted. This can include infection around the access area or the formation of clots in the fistula. Usually, because they are in the fistula itself and do not travel to other parts of the body, these clots are not life-threatening. The greatest danger is that clots may block the fistula and would have to be removed surgically. Frequent clotting may require creating a back-up fistula at another site, to allow dialysis when one access is blocked.

There are other complications from dialysis that are not directly related to the vascular access. For example, when the kidneys have shut down, they produce very little urine. Because dialysis is the only way people with kidney failure can balance fluid levels in their bodies, hemodialysis can cause bloating and fluid overload, indicating that too much fluid remains in the body. If fluid overload occurs, the patient will have swollen ankles, puffy eyes, weight gain, and shortness of breath. Fluid overload can cause heart and circulatory problems and fluctuations in blood pressure. Medications may be prescribed and changes in fluid intake or diet may be made to help balance fluids safely in conjunction with dialysis.

Other problems that can occur during or after hemodialysis include:

- Low blood pressure, if fluid and wastes are removed from the blood too quickly.

- Nausea, because of changes in blood pressure.

- Muscle cramps from the removal of too much fluid from the blood.

- Headaches near the end of a dialysis session, due to changes in the concentration of fluid and waste in the blood.

- Fatigue after treatment, lasting sometimes into the next day.

Normal results

An AV fistula can usually be created and can function well with no adverse affects in a person whose veins are large enough. The amount of time, usually a matter of months, it takes to develop the fistula after surgery will depend upon the size and strength of the patient's blood vessels and on the person's general condition and nutritional status. When the fistula develops, the thickened vein that has been joined to an artery can be seen in the arm and a pulse can be felt. The early development of an AV fistula as access for long-term dialysis has been shown to improve the survival of patients with chronic renal failure, and reduce the chances of being hospitalized with complications. It also gives them a better opportunity to choose self-dialysis as their treatment.

With good nutrition and a fully functioning AV fistula, dialysis patients can be relatively comfortable and free of complications. People may become tired and uncomfortable when it is nearly time for their next dialysis session. This is to be expected because wastes are building up in the blood, and the body senses that it is time to remove them.

KEY TERMS

Access—The point where a needle or catheter is inserted for dialysis.

Acute renal (kidney) failure—The sudden loss of kidney function, possibly temporary.

Artery—Blood vessel that carries blood away from the heart to the body.

Chronic renal (kidney) failure—Progressive loss of kidney function over several years, which can result in permanent kidney failure requiring dialysis.

Hypertension—High blood pressure caused by too much fluid in blood vessels or narrowing of blood vessels.

Morbidity and mortality rates

The earlier use of dialysis, especially with AV fistula access, has been shown to increase survival in patients with renal failure. The AV fistula is designed to improve the effectiveness of dialysis and is reported to present fewer risks and complications than other vascular access, such as reduced incidence of clotting and infection, and longer use overall.

Kidney failure is reported to account for 1% of hospital admissions in the United States. It occurs in 2–5% of patients hospitalized for other conditions, surgeries, or diseases. In patients undergoing cardiac bypass surgery, 15% are reported to require dialysis for kidney failure. Overall deaths in people undergoing dialysis are reported to be 50% because of the multi-organ dysfunction that has influenced kidney failure.

Resources

ORGANIZATIONS

National Kidney Foundation, Inc. 30 East 33rd Street, New York, NY 10016. (800)622-9010. <www.kidney.org>.

National Kidney and Urologic Diseases Information Clearinghouse. 31 Center Drive, MSC 2560 Building 31, Room 9A-04, Bethesda, MD 20892-2560. (800)891-5390. <www.niddk.nih.gov>.

OTHER

Getting the Most From Your Treatment: What You Need To Know About Hemodialysis Access. Booklet. New York: National Kidney Foundation, Inc. (800)622-9010. <www.kidney.org>.

NIDDK Kidney Failure Series. Booklet. Bethesda, MD: National Kidney and Urologic Diseases Information Clearinghouse. Email: nkudic@info.niddk.nih.gov.

Vascular Access to Hemodialysis. National Kidney and Urologic Diseases Information Clearinghouse, Home Health Information. December 1999. <www.niddk.nih.gov>.

L. Lee Culvert

Arthrography

Definition

Arthrograpy is a procedure involving multiple x rays of a joint using a fluoroscope, a special piece of x-ray equipment that shows an immediate x-ray image. A contrast medium (in this case, a contrast iodine solution) injected into the joint area helps highlight structures of the joint.

Purpose

Frequently, arthrography is ordered to determine the cause of unexplained joint pain. This fluoroscopic procedure can show the internal workings of specific joints and outline soft tissue structures. The procedure may also be conducted to identify problems with the ligaments, cartilage, tendons, or the joint capsule of the hip, shoulder, knee, ankle, wrist, or other joints. An arthrography procedure may locate cysts in the joint area, evaluate problems with the joint's arrangement and function, indicate the need for joint replacement, or show problems with existing joint replacement (prostheses). The most commonly studied joints are the knee and shoulder.

Description

Arthrograpy may be referred to as "joint radiography" or "x rays of the joint." The term arthrogram may be used interchangeably with arthrography. The joint area will be cleaned and a local anesthetic will be injected into the tissues around the joint to reduce pain. Next, if fluids are present in the joint, the physician may suction them out (aspirate) with a needle. These fluids may be sent to a laboratory for further study. Contrast agents are then injected into the joint through the same location by attaching the aspirating needle to a syringe containing the contrast medium. The purpose of contrast agents in x-ray procedures is to help highlight details of areas under study by making them opaque. Agents for arthrography are generally air- and water-soluble dyes, the most common containing iodine. Air and iodine may be used together or independently. After the contrast agent is administered, the site of injection will be sealed, and the patient may be asked to bend and flex the joint to distribute the contrast.

Before the contrast medium can be absorbed by the joint itself, several films will be quickly taken under the guidance of the fluoroscope. The patient will be asked to move the joint into a series of positions, keeping still between positioning. Sometimes, the patient will experience some tingling or discomfort during the procedure, which is normal and due to the contrast. Following fluoroscopic tracking of the contrast, standard x rays of the area may also be taken. The entire procedure will last about one hour.

Generally, a joint is evaluated first by MRI (**magnetic resonance imaging**) instead of an arthrogram, or by MRI combined with the arthrogram. Gadolinium, an MRI contrast agent, is injected if the arthrogram is performed as part of an MRI procedure. If the arthrogram is performed as part of a MRI arthrogram, the MRI scan will then be obtained immediately afterward.

Preparation

It is important to discuss any known sensitivity to local anesthetics or iodine prior to this procedure. A physician should explain the procedure and the risks associated with contrast agents and ask the patient to sign an **informed consent**. If iodine contrast will be administered, the patient may be instructed not to eat before the exam. The timeframe of fasting may range from only 90 minutes prior to the exam up to the night before. There is no other preparation necessary.

Aftercare

The affected joint should be rested for approximately 12 hours following the procedure. The joint may be wrapped in an elastic bandage, and the patient should receive instructions on the care and changing of the bandage. Noises in the joint such as cracking or clicking are normal for a few days following arthrography. These noises are the result of liquid in the joints. Swelling may also occur and can be treated with application of ice or cold packs. A mild pain reliever can be used to lessen pain in the first few days. However, if any of these symptoms persist for more than a few days, patients are advised to contact their physician.

Risks

In some patients iodine can cause allergic reactions, ranging from mild nausea to severe cardiovascular or nervous system complications. Since the contrast dye is put into a joint, rather than into a vein, allergic reactions are rare. Facilities licensed to perform contrast exams should meet requirements for equipment, supplies, and staff training to handle a possible severe reaction. Infection or joint damage are possible, although not frequent, complications of arthrography.

Normal results

A normal arthrography exam will show proper placement of the dye or contrast medium throughout the joint structures, joint space, cartilage, and ligaments.

Abnormal results

The abnormal placement of dye may indicate rheumatoid arthritis, cysts, joint dislocation, tear of the rotator cuff, tears in the ligament, and other conditions. The entire lining of the joint becomes opaque from the technique, which allows the radiologist to see abnormalities in the intricate workings of the joint. In the case of recurrent shoulder dislocations, arthrography results can be used to evaluate damage. Patients with hip prostheses may receive arthrography to evaluate proper placement or function of their prostheses.

Resources

BOOKS

Juhl, John H., and Andrew B. Crummy. *Paul and Juhl's Essentials of Radiologic Imaging.* Philadelphia: J. B. Lippincott Co., 1993.

ORGANIZATIONS

American College of Radiology. 1891 Preston White Drive, Reston, VA 22091. (800) 227-5463. <http://www.acr.org>.

Arthritis Foundation. 1300 W. Peachtree St., Atlanta, GA 30309. (800) 283-7800. <http://www.arthritis.org>.

Teresa Norris, RN
Lee A. Shratter, MD

Arthroplasty

Definition

Arthroplasty is surgery performed to relieve pain and restore range of motion by realigning or reconstructing a dysfunctional joint.

Purpose

The goal of arthroplasty is to restore the function of a stiffened synovial joint and relieve pain. As a surgical procedure, it is usually performed when medical treatment has not improved function in the affected joint. There are two types of arthroplastic surgery: joint resection and interpositional reconstruction. Joint resection involves removing a portion of the bone from a stiffened joint, increasing the space between the bone and the socket to improve the range of motion. Scar tissue eventually fills the gap, narrowing joint space again. Pain is relieved and motion is restored, but the joint is less stable.

Interpositional reconstruction is surgery to reshape the joint and add a prosthetic disk between the two bones forming the joint. The prosthesis can be made of plastic, metal, ceramic material, or formed from such body tissue as skin, muscle, or fascia. When interpositional reconstruction fails, total joint replacement may be necessary. Joint replacement is also called total joint arthroplasty.

In recent years, joint replacement has become the operation of choice for most chronic knee and hip problems, particularly because of advances in the type and quality of prostheses (articifical joints). Elbow, shoulder, ankle, and finger joints are more likely to be treated with joint resection or interpositional reconstruction.

Arthroplasty is performed on people suffering from severe pain and disabling joint stiffness. Osteoarthritis (OA), a degenerative joint disease, is the most common condition causing joint destruction with pain and impaired movement. Other causes include rheumatoid arthritis (RA), hemophilia, synovitis, and rare bone diseases, which are all known to destroy cartilage. Joint resection, rather than joint replacement, is more likely to be performed on people with rheumatoid arthritis, especially when the elbow joint is involved. Joint replacement is usually reserved for older patients, because of the limited longevity of benefits. The younger the patient, the greater the reliance on medical treatment.

Demographics

The American Academy of Orthopaedic Surgeons reports that approximately 713,000 arthroplasty surgeries are performed annually in the United States. Of

Arthroplasty

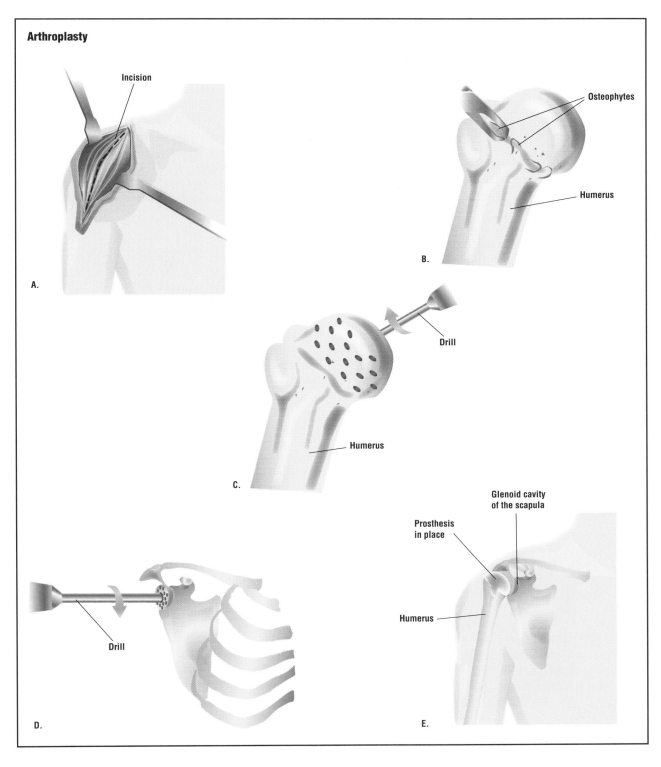

A.

Incision

B.

Osteophytes

Humerus

C.

Drill

Humerus

D.

Drill

E.

Prosthesis in place

Glenoid cavity of the scapula

Humerus

In this shoulder arthroplasty procedure, an incision is made into the shoulder (A). The head of the humerus (upper arm bone) is removed from the shoulder joint, and bone growths, or osteophytes, are removed (B). Small holes are drilled into the head to accept the prosthesis (C). Similar holes are drilled in the glenoid cavity (shoulder joint) (D). The final prosthesis improves shoulder function (E). *(Illustration by GGS Inc.)*

these, an average of about 362,000 are knee surgeries and 295,000 are hip surgeries. The remainder are ankle, shoulder, wrist, and hand surgeries. Joint replacement surgeries are increasing; for example, 259,000 total knee replacements were performed in 1997 and 299,000 were performed in 2000.

Because the primary underlying condition in patients undergoing arthroplasty is osteoarthritis, a common cause for disability among older adults, the majority of patients undergoing this surgery fit the demographic profile for osteoarthritis. Osteoarthritis is the most common type of arthritis, with over twenty million people in all parts of the United States. Both men and women have the disease; under age 45 men are more often affected, though more women than men are affected after age 45. Younger people can have the disease after a joint injury. Arthroplasty is reserved for the most severely afflicted—approximately 3% of all patients with osteoarthritis, women more often than men. Two and one-half million people in the United States have rheumatoid arthritis, which can strike people of all ages. Very few have arthroplasty because this chronic crippling disease affects not only multiple joints but other parts of the body as well, including the immune system. Patients weakened by this disease are more subject to infection and less likely to enjoy positive surgical results.

Description

Arthroplasty is performed under general (affecting the entire body) or regional (numbing a specific area of the body, such as spinal block) anesthesia in a hospital, by an orthopedic surgeon. Although many hospitals and medical centers perform common types of joint surgery, orthopedic hospitals that specialize in joint surgery tend to have higher success rates than less specialized centers.

In joint resection, the surgeon makes an incision at the joint, then carefully removes the minimum amount of bone necessary to allow free motion. The more bone that remains, the more stable the joint. Ligament attachments are preserved as much as possible. In interpositional reconstruction, both bones of the joint are reshaped, and a disk of material is placed between the bones to prevent their rubbing together. Length of hospital stay depends on the joint affected; in the absence of complications, a typical stay is only a few days.

Diagnosis/Preparation

Significant disabling pain, deformity, and reduced quality of life are the primary indications for arthroscopic procedures. Patients at this stage of discomfort and disability will most likely have already been diagnosed with a form of arthritis. Pain and stiffness on weight-bearing joints are the major symptoms that patients report, though some people experience night pain as well. Other symptoms may include stiffness, swelling, and locking of the joint; and even the joint giving way, particularly when the knees or hips are affected. To determine the extent of disabling, the referring physician and/or the surgeon will likely ask about walking distance, sporting ability, the need for walking aids, and the ability to perform self-care tasks such as dressing and bathing. Besides evaluation of the joint itself and level of mobility, the clinical examination will include evaluation of the patient's general health, the condition of the ligaments and muscles around the affected joint, and also assessment of the patient's mental outlook and social circumstances to help develop the most effective postoperative rehabilitation plan. Diagnostic testing will typically include:

- x rays of the affected joint (and other joints as well)to determine loss of joint space and to differentiate between OA and RA

- imaging studies, such as computed tomography (Cat scans), magnetic resonance (MRI), and bone densitometry to assess bone loss or bone infection

- cardiac tests, such as electrocardiogram, to evaluate the heart and circulatory system

- blood tests to rule out infection and possibly to confirm arthritis

Prior to arthroplasty, standard preoperative blood and urine tests are performed to rule out such conditions as anemia and infection. If a patient has a history of bleeding, the surgeon may ask that clotting tests be performed. The patient will meet with the anesthesiologist to discuss any special conditions that may affect the administration of anesthesia. Surgery will not be performed if infection is present anywhere in the body or if the patient has certain heart or lung diseases. Smokers will be asked to stop smoking. Weight loss may also be recommended for overweight patients. If surgery involves deep tissue and muscle, such as total hip arthroplasty, the surgeon may order units of blood to be prepared in case **transfusion** is needed to replace blood lost during the surgery. Healthy patients may be asked to donate their own blood, which will be returned to them at the time of surgery (autologous transfusion). Certain pain medications may have to be discontinued in the weeks just prior to surgery.

Aftercare

Immediately after surgery, while still in the hospital, patients will be given pain medications for the recovery period and **antibiotics** to prevent infection. When patients are discharged after joint surgery, they must be careful not to overstress or destabilize the joint, requiring rest at home for a period of weeks. Physical therapy will begin immediately to improve strength and range of motion; it is the most important aid to recovery and may continue for several months. Activity may be resumed gradually, using devices if necessary, such as walkers or crutches, as recommended by the physical therapist. Lifestyle changes may include the use of special seating or sleeping surfaces, and employing **home care** assistance for help with shopping, cooking, and household tasks.

Risks

Joint resection and interpositional reconstruction do not always produce successful results, especially in patients with rheumatoid arthritis, a chronic inflammatory disease that may continue to narrow the joint space and accelerate the formation of scar tissue. Repeat surgery or total joint replacement may be necessary. As with any major surgery, there is always a risk of an allergic reaction to anesthesia, post-operative infection, or the formation of blood clots (thrombophlebitis) that may cause pain and swelling near the surgery site and travel through the veins to other parts of the body. A joint that has undergone surgery is less stable than a healthy joint and dislocation or loosening of the resected joint may occur, especially with inappropriate physical activity.

Normal results

Most patients enjoy an improved range of motion in the joint and relief from pain. Younger people may actually return to some form of low-impact sports activity.

QUESTIONS TO ASK THE DOCTOR

- Is surgery my only option? What alternatives might work?
- How many surgeries like mine have you performed?
- What can I do after surgery to improve the result and avoid more surgery?
- Will joint replacement be inevitable in time even if I have resection or reconstruction?
- What changes can I make in my lifestyle to slow the progress of arthritis?

However, people who have degenerative or inflammatory diseases must understand that they will not suddenly have a normal joint, even while they will gain pain relief and improved function.

Morbidity and mortality rates

The number of deaths for all arthroplasty surgeries is less than 1%, with death more likely to occur among elderly patients and those with other serious medical conditions.

Alternatives

Pain management alone, particularly with the availability of more effective pain drugs that have fewer side effects, is the primary non-surgical option when the underlying diagnosis is a form of arthritis. Non-steroidal anti-inflammatory medications (NSAIDs) are commonly prescribed for arthritis sufferers, and people with RA are given certain drugs that suppress immune system activity, shown to be a factor in this type of arthritis. A range of nutritional supplements and vitamins are reported to offer health benefits to people with OA; among them, glucosamine and chondroitin sulfate have been shown to offer some relief for pain and stiffness. Weight loss is often recommended as well.

Because immobility of the affected joint can increase pain and stiffness, patients with joint disease are usually encouraged to continue some type of physical activity. Keeping the muscles strong through modest, non-weight-bearing **exercise**, such as stretching or swimming, is often recommended to help support the joint and maintain mobility. Various devices, such as braces or orthopedic shoes, may be recommended, as well as walking aids. Safety rails, special elevated toilet-

KEY TERMS

Cartilage—The slippery tissue that covers the ends of joint bones.

Fascia—Thin connective tissue covering or separating the muscles and internal organs of the body.

Osteoarthritis—A degenerative "wear-and-tear" joint disease related to aging.

Prosthesis—An artificial joint.

Rheumatoid arthritis—A chronic autoimmune disease characterized by inflammation of multiple joints and crippling effects.

Synovial fluid—A fluid that lubricates the joint and keeps cartilage smooth.

Synovitis—Inflammation of the synovium, the thin membrane in the joint.

Thrombophlebitis—A condition in which blood clots form in veins near surgery site, causing swelling and pain; clots may travel via veins to lungs.

seat extensions, bath and shower seats can make the patient more comfortable in daily life. Movement therapy, such as yoga, tai chi, and dance, may help maintain joint flexibility and slow chronic arthritis symptoms. Occupational therapy, massage therapy, and physiotherapy may help improve range of motion and overall comfort, as well as patient confidence.

Resources

BOOKS

"Joint Replacement." In *Everything You Need to Know About Medical Treatments*. Springhouse, PA: Springhouse Corp., 1996.

ORGANIZATIONS

American Academy of Orthopaedic Surgeons(AAOS). 6300 North River Rd. Rosemont, Illinois 60018. (847) 823-7186. (800) 346-AAOS. Fax: (847) 823-8125. <http://www.aaos.org>.

Tish Davidson, A.M.
L. Lee Culvert

Arthroplasty, shoulder *see* **Shoulder resection arthroplasty**

Arthroscopic knee surgery *see* **Knee arthroscopic surgery**

Arthroscopic surgery

Definition

Arthroscopic surgery is a procedure that allows surgeons to visualize, diagnose, and treat joint problems. The name is derived from the Greek words *arthron*, joint, and *skopein*, to look at. Arthroscopy is performed using an arthroscope, a small fiber-optic instrument that enables a close look at the inside of a joint through a small incision.

Purpose

Arthroscopic surgery is used to diagnose, treat, and monitor joint injuries and diseases that affect the joints. Diagnostic arthroscopic surgery is performed when the medical history, physical exam, x rays, and bone scanning examinations, such as MRI or CT, do not provide a definitive diagnosis. Corrective arthroscopic surgery is used primarily to remove bone or cartilage or repair tendons or ligaments.

Precautions

Diagnostic arthroscopic surgery is not recommended unless non-surgical treatment does not fix the problem.

Description

Arthroscopic surgery is performed most commonly on the knees, and also on ankles, shoulders, wrists, elbows, and hips. Knee joints are large enough to allow free movement of arthroscopic instruments and therefore are ideal for the benefits of this type of examination and treatment. The technique is valued because it allows surgeons to see inside the joint through incisions as tiny as a quarter of an inch (about 1 cm) rather than the large incisions that open surgery procedures require. The accuracy of arthroscopy is said to be 100% for diagnosis compared to diagnostic imaging such as MRI. Arthroscopic surgery may be used to relieve mechanical joint problems, such as buckling, stiffness, or locking, and can preclude or delay the need for more aggressive surgery such as a joint replacement.

In arthroscopic surgery, an orthopedic surgeon uses a pencil-sized arthroscope—a fiber-optic instrument fitted with a lens, a light source, and a miniature video camera—to see inside a joint. Advanced fiber optics allow even more detail to be seen than in open surgery, often identifying problems that may have been difficult to diagnose with other methods. The arthroscope transmits highlighted images of the structures to a television monitor in the **operating room**. The surgeon is able to view the entire examination, getting a full view of the joint, its cartilage, and surrounding tissue. The type and extent of the injury can be determined and repair or correction can be performed if necessary. Some of the most common joint problems diagnosed and treated with arthroscopic surgery are:

- synovitis (inflamed joint lining) of the knee, shoulder, elbow, wrist, or ankle

- injuries to the shoulder, such as rotator cuff tendon tears, impingement syndrome, and dislocations

- injuries to the knee, such as meniscal (cartilage) tears, wearing down of or injury to the cartilage cushion, and anterior cruciate ligament tears with instability

- injuries to the wrist, such as carpal tunnel syndrome

- loose bodies of bone and/or cartilage in the knee, shoulder, elbow, ankle, or wrist

- joint damage caused by rheumatoid arthritis or osteoarthritis

Arthroscopic procedures are performed in a hospital or outpatient surgical facility by an orthopedic surgeon. The type of anesthesia used (local, spinal, or general) varies, as does the length of the procedure; both depend on the joint that will be operated on, the type and extent of the suspected joint injury, and/or the complexity of the anticipated repair. Arthroscopic surgery rarely takes more than an hour. Most patients who have arthroscopic surgery, whether diagnostic or corrective, are discharged within the same day; some patients, depending on the complexity of the surgery or their post-operative condition, may stay in the hospital one or two days.

Considered the most important orthopedic development in the twentieth century, arthroscopic surgery is widely used. The American Association of Orthopedic Surgeons reports that it is performed by 80% of all orthopedic surgeons. The use of arthroscopic surgery on famous athletes has been well publicized. Although arthroscopic surgery was initially only a diagnostic tool used prior to open surgery, the availability of better instruments and techniques has encouraged its use to actually treat a variety of joint problems, often avoiding more complicated surgeries with longer recovery times. New techniques under development are likely to lead to other joints being treated with arthroscopic surgery in the future. Laser technology has been introduced as a treatment option in arthroscopic surgery and other advanced technologies are being explored.

Surgical procedure

After making two small incisions about the size of a buttonhole in the skin near the joint, the surgeon injects sterile sodium chloride solution through one incision into the joint to expand it for better viewing and movement of the instruments. The surgeon will also use this access to irrigate (flood with fluid) the joint area during surgery and to suction blood and debris away from the joint. This irrigation, or "washing" part of the procedure, is believed to be of value in itself, improving joint function. The arthroscope is then inserted into the second incision. While looking at the interior of the joint on the television monitor, the surgeon can determine the extent or type of injury and, if necessary, take a biopsy specimen or repair or treat the problem. A third tiny incision may be made in order to see other parts of the joint or to insert additional instruments, such as laser or tiny scalpels, when repairs or corrections need to be made. Arthroscopic surgery can be used to remove floating bits of cartilage, to debride (clean by removing tissue or bone), and to treat minor tears and other disorders. When the procedure is finished, the arthroscope is removed and the joint is once again irrigated. The site of the incision is dressed with compression bandages (ace bandages).

Diagnosis/Preparation

Prior to arthroscopy, the patient's medical history will be reviewed and the patient will have a complete **physical examination**. Standard pre-operative blood and urine tests will be done as well as scans of the affected joint, such as MRI (**magnetic resonance imaging**), CT (computed tomography), and arthrogram (an x ray using dye). In some cases, an **exercise** regimen or muscle stimulation treatment (TENS) may be recommended to strengthen muscles around the joint prior to surgery. Surgeons may recommend pre-operative guidelines, such as:

- Discontinue **aspirin** and anti-inflammatory medications two weeks before surgery.

- Stop smoking to encourage post-operative healing.

- Inform the surgeon if any fever or other illness occurs, or if cuts, scratches, or bruises appear near the surgical site before the scheduled surgery.

- Do not eat, drink, or chew gum for 12 hours prior to surgery.

WHO PERFORMS THE PROCEDURE AND WHERE IS IT PERFORMED?

Arthroscopic surgery is performed in a hospital operating room or an outpatient surgical facility by an orthopedic surgeon.

- Bring crutches or a walker if hip, knee, or ankle arthroscopy is being performed.
- Wear loose fitting clothing to allow for bulky dressings over the surgical site.

Aftercare

Immediately after the procedure, the patient will spend up to two hours in a recovery area before being discharged. Some patients may be transferred to a hospital room if the surgeon determines overnight care is necessary. The surgical site will be dressed with a compression bandage (ace bandage) or a tightly fitting stocking (support hose). An ice pack will be placed on the joint that was examined or treated by arthroscopy. This treatment may continue for up to 72 hours after surgery to keep swelling down and help prevent the formation of clots. Pain medication will be administered if needed, although most patients require little or no medicine for pain. Dressings can usually be removed on the morning after surgery and replaced by adhesive strips. The surgeon should be notified if the patient experiences any increase in pain, swelling, redness, drainage or bleeding at the site of the surgery, signs of infection (headache, muscle aches, dizziness, fever), and nausea or vomiting.

It takes several days for the puncture wounds to heal and several weeks for the joint to fully recover. Many patients can resume their daily activities, including going back to work, within a few days of the procedure. Muscle strength must be regained as soon as possible after surgery to help support the affected joint. A rehabilitation program, including physical therapy, may be suggested to speed recovery and improve the functioning of the joint. The surgeon's recommendations for recovery may include:

- Keep the surgical site and the dressings clean and dry.
- Use ice packs for up to 72 hours to reduce pain and swelling.
- Elevate the affected joint (wrist, elbow, ankle, knee) on pillows; exercise gently to encourage circulation.
- Use a knee brace or shoulder sling temporarily.
- Allow weight-bearing exercise as able.

Complications

Few complications are to be expected with arthroscopy. Those that may occur occasionally (fewer than 1% of all arthroscopies, according to the American Academy of Orthopedic Surgeons) are infection, blood clot formation, swelling or bleeding, or damage to blood vessels or nerves. Rare instrument breakage during procedures has also been reported.

Normal results

Most patients undergo arthroscopic surgery as an outpatient and are home with hours or at most a day or two. Pain and complications are rare and most patients will enjoy improved mobility as they recover over a period of days, possibly with the aid of physical therapy and gentle exercise.

Some people undergoing arthroscopy may have pre-existing conditions and diseases that will affect the surgical result. Recovery times will vary depending on each patient's overall condition. Certain problems may need to be treated with a combination of arthroscopic and open surgical procedures.

Alternatives

Alternatives to arthroscopic surgery include:

- changing activities to those less strenuous or demanding
- anti-inflammatory medications
- physical therapy and appropriate, gentle exercise such as yoga
- wearing a brace or using a walking aid
- glucosamine sulfate and chondroiten to reduce pain and stiffness
- therapeutic massage, acupuncture, or other body work

Resources

BOOKS

Andrews, James R. and Laura A. Timmerman. *Diagnostic and Operative Arthroscopy.* Philadelphia: W. B. Saunders Co., 1997.

Brillhart, Allen T., ed. *Arthroscopic Laser Surgery: Clinical Applications.* New York: Springer-Verlag, 1995.

Oxford Medical Publications. *Oxford Textbook of Sports Medicine.* New York: Oxford Medical Publications, 1994.

PERIODICALS

Wilkinson, Todd. "Pop, Crackle, Snap." *Women's Sports & Fitness* (April 1998): 68.

ORGANIZATIONS

American Academy of Orthopedic Surgeons(AAOS). 6300 North River Road, Rosemont, IL 60018. (800) 346-AAOS. <http://www.aaos.org>.

Institute for Bone and Joint Disorders. 2222 East Highland Avenue, Phoenix, AZ 85016; 602-553-3113. <http://www.ibjd. com>.

OTHER

American Academy of Orthopaedic Surgeons. *Arthroscopy.* April 15, 1998 [cited April 2003]. <http://www.aaos.org>.

The Arthritis Foundation. *About Arthroscopic Surgery.* [cited April 2003]. <http://www.arthritis.org>.

Cooke, K. V. "Arthroscopy for Rheumatoid Arthritis." *Laurushealth.com* September 5, 2002 [cited April 2003]. <http://www.laurushealth.com/library>.

"Joint Irrigation for Osteoarthritis." *Ivanhoe Newswire* 5(2003): 20–26 [cited April 2003]. <http://www.ivanhoe.com/newsalert>.

"Knee Arthroscopy." *The Center for Orthopaedics and Sports Medicine.* April 15, 1998 [cited April 2003]. <http://www.arthroscopy.com>.

Lori De Milto
L. Lee Culvert

Artificial sphincter insertion

Definition

Artificial sphincter insertion surgery is the implantation of an artificial valve in the genitourinary tract or in the anal canal to restore continence and psychological well being to individuals with urinary or anal sphincter insufficiency that leads to severe urinary or fecal incontinence.

Purpose

This procedure is useful for adults and children who have severe incontinence due to lack of muscle contraction by either the urethral sphincter or the bowel sphincter. The primary work of the lower urinary tract and the colon is the storage of urine and waste, respectively, until such time as the expulsion of urine or feces is appropriate. These holding and expelling functions in each system require a delicate balance of tension and relaxation of muscles, especially those related to conscious control of the act of urination or defecation through the valve-like sphincter in each system. Both types of incontinence have mechanical causes related to reservoir adequacy and sphincter, or "gatekeeper" control, as well as mixed etiologies in the chemistry, neurology, and psychology of human makeup. The simplest bases of incontinence lie in the mechanical components of reservoir mobility and sphincter muscle tone. These two factors receive the most surgical attention for both urinary and fecal incontinence.

Urinary sphincter surgery

There are four sources of urinary incontinence related primarily to issues of tone in pelvic, urethral, and sphincter muscles. Most urinary incontinence is caused by leakage when stress is applied to the abdominal muscles by coughing, sneezing, or exercising. Stress incontinence results from reduced sphincter adequacy in the ability to keep the bladder closed during movement. Stress incontinence can also be related to the mobility of the urethra and whether this reservoir for urine tilts, causing spilling of urine. The urethral cause of stress incontinence is treated with other surgical procedures. A second form of incontinence is urge incontinence. It relates to sphincter overactivity, or sphincter hyperflexia, in which the sphincter contracts uncontrollably, causing the patient to urinate, often many times a day. Finally, there is urinary incontinence due to an inadequately small urethra that causes urine overflow. This is known as overflow incontinence and can often be treated with augmentation to the urethra to increase its size.

Only severe stress incontinence related to sphincter adequacy can benefit from the artificial urinary sphinc-

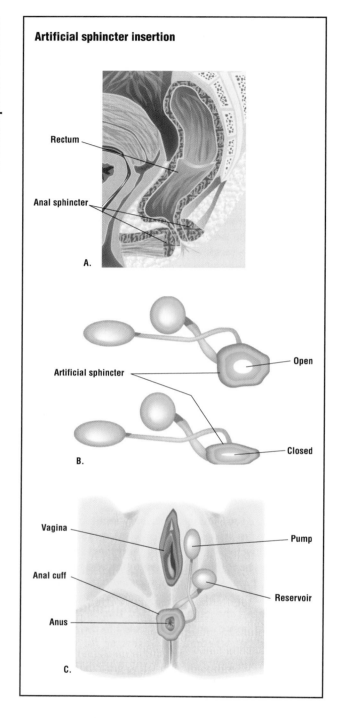

Artificial sphincter insertion

Rectum

Anal sphincter

A.

Artificial sphincter

Open

Closed

B.

Vagina

Pump

Anal cuff

Reservoir

Anus

C.

Normally, the anal sphincter muscles maintain fecal continence (A). In cases of incontinence, an artificial sphincter may be inserted, which can open and close to mimic the function of the natural sphincter (B). Once implanted, the patient uses a pump under the skin to inflate and deflate the anal cuff (C). *(Illustration by GGS Inc.)*

ter. This includes conditions that result in the removal of the sphincter. Sphincter deficiency can result directly from pelvic fracture; urethral reconstruction; prostate surgeries; spinal cord injury; neurogenic bladder conditions that include sphincter dysfunction; and some congential conditions. Each can warrant consideration for a sphincter implant.

Implantation surgery related to urinary sphincter incompetence is also called artificial sphincter insertion or inflatable sphincter insertion. The artificial urinary sphincter (AUS) is a small device placed under the skin that keeps pressure on the urethra until there is a decision to urinate, at which point a pump allows the urethra to open and urination commences. Since the 1990s, advances in prostate cancer diagnosis and surgery have resulted in radical prostatectomies being performed, with urinary incontinence rates ranging from 3–60%. The AUS has become a reliable treatment for this main source of urinary incontinence in men. Women with intrinsic sphincter deficiency, or weakened muscles of the sphincter, also benefit from the AUS. However, the use of AUS with women has declined with advances in the use of the sub-urethral sling due to its useful "hammock" effect on the sphincter and its high rates of continence success. Women with neurologenic incontinence can benefit from the AUS.

Artificial anal sphincter surgery

Fecal incontinence is the inability to control bowel function. The condition can be the result of a difficult childbirth, colorectal disease such as Crohn's disease, accidents involving neurological injuries, surgical resection for localized cancer, or by other neurological disorders. Severe fecal incontinence may, depending upon the underlying disease, require surgical intervention that can include repair of the anal sphincter, **colostomy**, or replacement of the anal sphincter. Artificial anal sphincter is a very easy-to-use device implanted under the skin that mimics the function of the anal sphincter.

Demographics

Artificial urinary sphincter surgery

According to the Agency for Health Care Policy and Research, urinary incontinence affects approximately 13 million adults. Men have incontinence rates that are much lower than women, with a range of 1.5–5%, compared to women over 65 with rates of almost 50%. In older men, prostate problems and their treatments are the most common sources of incontinence. Incontinence is a complication in nearly all male patients for the first three to six months after radical prostatectomy. A year after the procedure, most men regain continence. Stress incontinence occurs in 1–5% of men after the standard treatment for severe benign prostatic hyperplasia.

Artificial anal sphincter surgery

According to the National Institute of Diabetes & Digestive & Kidney Diseases (NIDDK), more than 6.5 million Americans have fecal incontinence. Fecal incontinence affects people of all ages. It is estimated that over 2% of the population is affected by fecal incontinence. Many cases are never reported. Community-based studies reveal that 30% of patients are over the age of 65, and 63% are female. According to one study published in the *American Journal of Gasteronology*, only 34% of incontinent patients have ever mentioned their problem to a physician, even though 23% wear absorbent pads, 12% are on medications, and 11% lead lives restricted by their incontinence. Women are more than five times as likely as men to have fecal incontinence, primarily due to obstetric injury, especially with forceps delivery and anal sphincter laceration. Fecal incontinence is frequent in men who have total and subtotal prostatectomies. Fecal incontinence is not a part of aging, even though it affects people over 65 in higher numbers than other populations.

Description

Artificial urinary sphincter surgery

The artificial urinary sphincter is an implantable device that has three components:

• an inflatable cuff

• a fluid reservoir (balloon)

• a semiautomatic pump that connects the cuff and balloon

Open surgery is the major form of surgery for the implant. Infections are minimized by sterilization of the urine preoperatively and preoperative bowel preparation. The pelvic space is entered from the abdomen or from the vagina, with general anesthesia for the patient. Broad-spectrum **antibiotics** are given intravenously and at the site of small incisions for the device. A urinary catheter is put into place. The cuff is implanted around the bladder neck and secured and passed through the rectus muscle and anterior fascia to be connected later to the pump. A space is fashioned to hold the balloon in the pubic region, and a pump is placed in a pouch below the abdomen. The artificial urinary sphincter is activated only after six to eight weeks to allow healing from the surgery. The patient is trained in the use of the device by understanding that the cuff remains inflated in its "resting state," and keeps the urethra closed by pressure, allowing continence. Upon the decision to urinate, the patient temporarily deflates the cuff by pressing the pump.

WHO PERFORMS THE PROCEDURE AND WHERE IS IT PERFORMED?

Implantation surgery is performed in a hospital **operating room** by urologic surgeons specially trained for implantation of the artificial sphincter in the urinary or anal tracts. Successful surgery depends upon very experienced surgeons.

The urethra opens and the bladder empties. The cuff closes automatically.

Artificial anal sphincter surgery

The artificial anal sphincter is an implantable device that has three components:

• an inflatable cuff

• a fluid reservoir (balloon)

• a semiautomatic pump that connects the cuff and balloon

In open abdominal surgery, the implant device is placed beneath the skin through small incisions within the pelvic space. One incision is placed between the anus and the vagina or scrotum, and the inflatable cuff is put around the neck of the anal sphincter. A second incision at the lower end of the abdomen is used to make a space behind the pubic bone for placement of the balloon. The pump is placed in a small pocket beneath the labia or scrotum, using two incisions. The artificial anal sphincter is activated only after six to eight weeks to allow healing from the surgery. The patient is trained in the use of the device by understanding that the anal cuff remains inflated in its "resting state," and keeps the anal canal closed by pressure, allowing continence. Upon the decision to have a bowel movement, the patient temporarily deflates the cuff by pressing the pump and fecal matter is released. The balloon re-inflates after the movement.

Diagnosis/Preparation

Artificial urinary sphincter surgery

Patients must be chosen carefully, exhibit isolated sphincter deficiency, and be motivated and able to work with the device and its exigencies. To characterize the condition to be treated and to determine outcomes, full clinical, urodynamic, and radiographic evaluations are necessary. The ability to distinguish mobility of the urethra as the cause of incontinence from sphincter insufficiency is difficult, but very important in the decision for surgery. A combination of pelvic examination for urethral hypermobility and a leak-point pressure as measured by coughing or other abdominal straining has been shown to be very effective in identifying the patient who needs the surgical implant. Visual examination of the bladder with a cystoscope is very important in the preoperative evaluation for placement of the sphincter. Urethral and bladder conditions found by the examination should be addressed before implantation. Previous reconstruction or repair of the urethra may prevent implantation of the cuff. In open abdominal surgery, the implant surgery uses preventive infection measures that are very important, including sterilization of the urine preoperatively with antibiotics, the cleansing of the intestines from fecal matter and secretions through **laxatives** immediately prior to surgery, and antibiotic treatment and vigorous irrigation of the wound sites.

Artificial anal sphincter surgery

Since only a limited number of patients with fecal incontinence would benefit from an artificial sphincter, it is very important that a thorough examination be performed to distinguish the causes of the incontinence. A medical history and physical, as well as documented entries or an incontinence diary are crucial to the diagnosis of fecal incontinence. The physical exam usually includes a visual inspection of the anus and the area lying between the anus and genitals for hemorrhoids, infections, and other conditions. The strength of the sphincter is tested by the doctor probing with a finger to test muscle strength.

Medical tests usually include:

- Anorectal manometry. This is a long tube with a balloon on the end that is inserted in the anus and rectum to measure the tightness of the anal sphincter and the ability to respond to nerve firings.

- Anorectal ultrasonography. This test also includes an insertion of a small instrument into the anus with a video screen that produces sound waves, picturing the rectum and anus.

- X rays. A substance called barium is used to make the rectum walls visible to x ray. This liquid is swallowed by the patient before the test.

- Anal electromyography. This test uses the insertion of tiny needle electrodes into muscles around the anus and tests for nerve damage.

Aftercare

Artificial urinary sphincter surgery

Surgery requires a few days of hospitalization. Oral and intravenous pain medications are administered, along with postoperative antibiotics. A general diet is available, usually on the evening of surgery. When the patient is able to walk, the urethral catheter is removed. Patients are discharged on the second day postoperatively, unless they have had other procedures and need extra recovery time. Patients may not lift heavy objects or engage in strenuous activity for approximately six weeks. After six to eight weeks, the patient returns to the physician for training in the use of the implant device.

Artificial anal sphincter surgery

Surgery hospitalization requires a few days with dietary restrictions and anti-diarrheal medicine to bind the bowels. Antibiotics are administered to lower the risk of infection, and skin incisions are cleaned frequently. Patients may not lift heavy objects or engage in strenuous activity for approximately six weeks. After the body has had time to heal over six to eight weeks, the patient returns to the physician for training in the use of the pump. Two or three sessions are required and after the training, the patient is encouraged to lead as normal a life as possible.

Normal results

Artificial urinary sphincter surgery

One problem with the urinary sphincter implant is failure. If the device fails, or the cuff erodes, the surgery must be repeated. In a study published in 2001, 37% of women had the implant after an average of seven years, but 70% had the original or a replacement and 82% were continent. Studies on men report similar findings. Malfunction has improved with advances in using a narrower cuff. In one large study encompassing one surgeon over 11 years, the re-operative rate of AUS related to malfunction in men was 21%. Over 90% of patients were alive with a properly functioning device.

Another problem with the surgery is urinary voiding. This may be difficult initially due to postoperative edema caused by bruising of the tissue. In the majority of cases, urination occurs after swelling has receded.

AUS is a good alternative for children. The results of AUS in children range from 62–90%, with similar rates for both girls and boys.

Artificial anal sphincter surgery

Anal sphincter implant surgery has been successfully performed for many years. The device most often used has a cumulative failure rate of 5% over 2.5 years. The long-term functional outcome of artificial anal sphincter implantation for severe fecal incontinence has not been determined. However, adequate sphincter function is recovered in most cases, and the removal rate of the device is low. Most of the good results are dependent upon careful patient selection and appropriate surgical and operative management with a highly experienced **surgical team**.

Morbidity and mortality rates

Artificial urinary sphincter surgery

Infection has been a frequent and serious complication of surgery, not only because of the infection per se, but also because infection can cause erosion of the urethra or bladder neck under the implant. The infection may actually worsen the incontinence. The overall infection rate with AUS implants is 1–3%. Because of interactions between the host and the foreign body represented by the implant, infections can occur soon after the surgery, or months and even years later. New techniques using antibiotics and skin preparations have improved infection rates considerably.

Artificial anal sphincter surgery

This surgery is for a limited number of patients who have isolated sphincter deficiency. Patients must be chosen who have little co-morbidity (serious illnesses) and can be trained in the use of the pump. Although it is a fairly simple operation, some researchers report a 30% infection rate.

Alternatives

Artificial urinary sphincter surgery

Milder forms of urinary incompetence can be treated with changes in diet, evaluation of medications, and the use of antidepressants and estrogen replacement, as well as bladder training and pelvic muscle strengthening. However, sphincter deficiency, unlike incontinence caused by urethral mobility, requires a substitute for the sphincter contraction by implant or by auxiliary tissue. If

---

AUS cannot treat sphincter deficiency, the sling or "hammock" procedure is a good second choice. It brings tightness to the sphincter by using tissue under the urethra to increase contractual function. The **sling procedure** is already preferred over the AUS for women.

Artificial anal sphincter surgery

Milder forms of fecal incontinence are being treated by changes in diet and the use of certain bowel-binding medications. For some forms of mild fecal incontinence, special forms of **exercise** can help to strengthen and tone the pelvic floor muscles, along with providing biofeedback to train the muscles to work with an appropriate schedule. Only after these measures have been tried, including the use of pads, is the patient counseled on the benefits of an anal sphincter implant.

Resources

BOOKS

Walsh, P., et al. *Campbell's Urology, 8th Edition.* St. Louis: Elsevier Science, 2000.

PERIODICALS

Michot, F. "Artificial Anal Sphincter in Severe Fecal Incontinence: Outcome of Prospective Experience with 37 Patients in One Institution." *Annals of Surgery,* Vol. 237, No. 1 (January 1, 2003): 52–56.

Rotholtz, N. A., and S. D. Wexner. "Surgical Treatment of Constipation and Fecal Incontinence." *Gastroenterology Clinics,* Vol. 30, No. 01 (March 2001).

ORGANIZATIONS

American Society of Colon and Rectal Surgeons. 85 W. Algonquin Rd., Suite 550, Arlington Heights, IL 60005. <www.fascrs.org.>.

National Institute of Diabetes and Digestive and Kidney Diseases. (800) 891-5390 (kidney); (800) 860-8747 (diabetes); (800) 891-5389 (digestive diseases). <www.niddk.nih.gov.>.

National Association of Incontinence. <www.nafc.org.>.

OTHER

Fecal Incontinence. National Institute of Diabetes & Digestive & Kidney Diseases (NIDDK). <www.niddk.nih.gov/health/digest/pubs/fecalincon/fecalincon.htm.>.

Incontinence in Men. Health and Age. <http://www.healthandage.com.>.

Urinary Incontinence. WebMD Patient Handout. <www.MDconsult.com.>.

Urinary Incontinence in Women. National Institute of Diabetes & Digestive & Kidney Diseases (NIDDK). <www.niddk.nih.gov/health/urolog/pubs/uiwomen/uiwomen.htm.>.

Nancy McKenzie, PhD

Ascending contrast phlebography *see*
Phlebography

Ascites shunt *see* **Peritoneovenous shunt**

Aseptic technique

Definition

Aseptic technique is a set of specific practices and procedures performed under carefully controlled conditions with the goal of minimizing contamination by pathogens.

Purpose

Aseptic technique is employed to maximize and maintain asepsis, the absence of pathogenic organisms, in the clinical setting. The goals of aseptic technique are to protect the patient from infection and to prevent the spread of pathogens. Often, practices that clean (remove dirt and other impurities), sanitize (reduce the number of microorganisms to safe levels), or disinfect (remove most microorganisms but not highly resistant ones) are not sufficient to prevent infection.

The Centers for Disease Control and Prevention (CDC) estimates that over 27 million surgical procedures are performed in the United States each year. Surgical site infections are the third most common nosocomial (hospital-acquired) infection and are responsible for longer hospital stays and increased costs to the patient and hospital. Aseptic technique is vital in reducing the morbidity and mortality associated with surgical infections.

Description

Aseptic technique can be applied in any clinical setting. Pathogens may introduce infection to the patient through contact with the environment, personnel, or equipment. All patients are potentially vulnerable to infection, although certain situations further increase vulnerability, such as extensive burns or immune disorders that disturb the body's natural defenses. Typical situations that call for aseptic measures include surgery and the insertion of intravenous lines, urinary catheters, and drains.

Asepsis in the operating room

Aseptic technique is most strictly applied in the **operating room** because of the direct and often extensive disruption of skin and underlying tissue. Aseptic technique helps to prevent or minimize postoperative infection.

PREOPERATIVE PRACTICES AND PROCEDURES. The most common source of pathogens that cause surgical site infections is the patient. While microorganisms normally colonize parts in or on the human body without causing disease, infection may result when this endogenous flora is introduced to tissues exposed during surgical procedures. In order to reduce this risk, the patient is prepared or prepped by shaving hair from the surgical site; cleansing with a disinfectant containing such chemicals as iodine, alcohol, or chlorhexidine gluconate; and applying sterile drapes around the surgical site.

In all clinical settings, handwashing is an important step in asepsis. The "2002 Standards, Recommended Practices, and Guidelines" of the Association of Perioperative Registered Nurses (AORN) states that proper handwashing can be "the single most important measure to reduce the spread of microorganisms." In general settings, hands are to be washed when visibly soiled, before and after contact with the patient, after contact with other potential sources of microorganisms, before invasive procedures, and after removal of gloves. Proper handwashing for most clinical settings involves removal of jewelry, avoidance of clothing contact with the sink, and a minimum of 10–15 seconds of hand scrubbing with soap, warm water, and vigorous friction.

A surgical scrub is performed by members of the **surgical team** who will come into contact with the sterile field or sterile instruments and equipment. This procedure requires use of a long-acting, powerful, antimicrobial soap on the hands and forearms for a longer period of time than used for typical handwashing. Institutional policy usually designates an acceptable minimum length of time required; the CDC recommends at least two to five minutes of scrubbing. Thorough drying is essential, as moist surfaces invite the presence of pathogens. Contact with the faucet or other potential contaminants should be avoided. The faucet can be turned off with a dry paper towel, or, in many cases, through use of a foot pedal. An important principle of aseptic technique is that fluid (a potential mode of pathogen transmission) flows in the direction of gravity. With this in mind, hands are held below elbows during the surgical scrub and above elbows following the surgical scrub. Despite this careful scrub, bare hands are always considered potential sources of infection.

Sterile surgical clothing or protective devices such as gloves, face masks, goggles, and transparent eye/face shields serve as barriers against microorganisms and are donned to maintain asepsis in the operating room. This practice includes covering facial hair, tucking hair out of sight, and removing jewelry or other dangling objects that may harbor unwanted organisms. This garb must be put on with deliberate care to avoid touching external, sterile surfaces with nonsterile objects including the skin. This ensures that potentially contaminated items such as hands and clothing remain behind protective barriers, thus prohibiting inadvertent entry of microorganisms into sterile areas. Personnel assist the surgeon to don gloves and garb and arrange equipment to minimize the risk of contamination.

Donning sterile gloves requires specific technique so that the outer glove is not touched by the hand. A large cuff exposing the inner glove is created so that the glove may be grasped during donning. It is essential to avoid touching nonsterile items once sterile gloves are applied; the hands may be kept interlaced to avoid inadvertent contamination. Any break in the glove or touching the glove to a nonsterile surface requires immediate removal and application of new gloves.

Asepsis in the operating room or for other invasive procedures is also maintained by creating sterile surgical fields with drapes. Sterile drapes are sterilized linens placed on the patient or around the field to delineate sterile areas. Drapes or wrapped kits of equipment are opened in such a way that the contents do not touch nonsterile items or surfaces. Aspects of this method include opening the furthest areas of a package first, avoiding leaning over the contents, and preventing opened flaps from falling back onto contents.

Equipment and supplies also need careful attention. Medical equipment such as **surgical instruments** can be sterilized by chemical treatment, radiation, gas, or heat. Personnel can take steps to ensure sterility by assessing that sterile packages are dry and intact and checking sterility indicators such as dates or colored tape that changes color when sterile.

INTRAOPERATIVE PRACTICES AND PROCEDURES. In the operating room, staff have assignments so that those

Proper removal of used gloves. (From Fundamentals of Nursing, Standards & Practice, 1st edition by DELAUNE. (c) 1998. Reprinted with permission of Delmar Learning, a division of Thomson Learning: www.thomsonrights.com. Fax: 800-730-2215.)

who have undergone surgical scrub and donning of sterile garb are positioned closer to the patient. Only scrubbed personnel are allowed into the sterile field. Arms of scrubbed staff are to remain within the field at all times, and reaching below the level of the patient or turning away from the sterile field are considered breaches in asepsis.

Other "unscrubbed" staff members are assigned to the perimeter and remain on hand to obtain supplies, acquire assistance, and facilitate communication with outside personnel. Unscrubbed personnel may relay equipment to scrubbed personnel only in a way that preserves the sterile field. For example, an unscrubbed nurse may open a package of forceps in a sterile fashion so that he or she never touches the sterilized inside portion, the scrubbed staff, or the sterile field. The uncontaminated item may either be picked up by a scrubbed staff member or carefully placed on to the sterile field.

The environment contains potential hazards that may spread pathogens through movement, touch, or proximity. Interventions such as restricting traffic in the operating room, maintaining positive-pressure airflow (to prevent air from contaminated areas from entering the operating room), or using low-particle generating garb help to minimize environmental hazards.

Other principles that are applied to maintain asepsis in the operating room include:

• All items in a sterile field must be sterile.

• Sterile packages or fields are opened or created as close as possible to time of actual use.

• Moist areas are not considered sterile.

- Contaminated items must be removed immediately from the sterile field.

- Only areas that can be seen by the clinician are considered sterile (i.e., the back of the clinician is not sterile).

- Gowns are considered sterile only in the front, from chest to waist and from the hands to slightly above the elbow.

- Tables are considered sterile only at or above the level of the table.

- Nonsterile items should not cross above a sterile field.

- There should be no talking, laughing, coughing, or sneezing across a sterile field.

- Personnel with colds should avoid working while ill or apply a double mask.

- Edges of sterile areas or fields (generally the outer inch) are not considered sterile.

- When in doubt about sterility, discard the potentially contaminated item and begin again.

- A safe space or margin of safety is maintained between sterile and nonsterile objects and areas.

- When pouring fluids, only the lip and inner cap of the pouring container is considered sterile; the pouring container should not touch the receiving container, and splashing should be avoided.

- Tears in barriers and expired sterilization dates are considered breaks in sterility.

Other clinical settings

A key difference between the operating room and other clinical environments is that the operating area has high standards of asepsis at all times, while most other settings are not designed to meet such standards. While clinical areas outside of the operating room generally do not allow for the same strict level of asepsis, avoiding potential infection remains the goal in every clinical setting. Observation of medical aseptic practices will help to avoid nosocomial infections. The application of aseptic technique in such settings is termed medical asepsis or clean technique (rather than surgical asepsis or sterile technique required in the operating room).

Specific situations outside of the operating room require a strict application of aseptic technique. Some of these situations include:

- wound care

- drain removal and drain care

- intravascular procedures

- vaginal exams during labor

- insertion of urinary catheters

- respiratory suction

For example, a surgical dressing change at the bedside, though in a much less controlled environment than the operating room, will still involve thorough handwashing, use of gloves and other protective garb, creation of a sterile field, opening and introducing packages and fluids in such a way as to avoid contamination, and constant avoidance of contact with nonsterile items.

General habits that help to preserve a clean medical environment include:

- safe removal of hazardous waste, i.e., prompt disposal of contaminated needles or blood-soaked bandages to containers reserved for such purposes

- prompt removal of wet or soiled dressings

- prevention of accumulation of bodily fluid drainage, i.e., regular checks and emptying of receptacles such as surgical drains or nasogastric suction containers

- avoidance of backward drainage flow toward patient, i.e., keeping drainage tubing below patient level at all times

- immediate clean-up of soiled or moist areas

- labeling of all fluid containers with date, time, and timely disposal per institutional policy

- maintaining seals on all fluids when not in use

The isolation unit is another clinical setting that requires a high level of attention to aseptic technique. Isolation is the use of physical separation and strict aseptic technique for a patient who either has a contagious disease or is immunocompromised. For the patient with a contagious disease, the goal of isolation is to prevent the spread of infection to others. In the case of respiratory infections (i.e., tuberculosis), the isolation room is especially designed with a negative pressure system that prevents airborne flow of pathogens outside the room. The severely immunocompromised patient is placed in reverse isolation, where the goal is to avoid introducing any microorganisms to the patient. In these cases, attention to aseptic technique is especially important to avoid spread of infection in the hospital or injury to the patient unprotected by sufficient immune defenses. Entry and exit from the isolation unit involves careful handwashing, use of protective barriers like gowns and gloves, and care not to introduce or remove potentially contaminated items. Institutions supply specific guidelines that direct practices for different types of isolation, i.e., respiratory versus body fluid isolation precautions.

In a multidisciplinary setting, all personnel must constantly monitor their own movements and practices, those of others, and the status of the overall field to prevent inadvertent breaks in sterile or clean technique. It is

KEY TERMS

Clean—To remove dirt and other impurities.

Contamination—A breach in the preservation of a clean or sterile object or environment.

Disinfect—To remove most microorganisms but not highly resistant ones.

Host—A living organism that harbors or potentially harbors infection.

Immunocompromised—Lacking or deficient in defenses provided by the immune system, usually due to disease state or a side effect of treatment.

Invasive—Involving entry into the body.

Nosocomial—Occurring in the hospital or clinical setting.

Pathogen—A disease-causing organism.

Resistant organisms—Organisms that are difficult to eradicate with antibiotics.

Sanitize—To reduce the number of microorganisms to safe levels.

Sterile—Completely free of pathogens.

expected that personnel will alert other staff when the field or objects are potentially contaminated. Health care workers can also promote asepsis by evaluating, creating, and periodically updating policies and procedures that relate to this principle.

Resources

PERIODICALS

Mangram, Alicia, Teresa Horan, Michele Pearson, Leah Christine Silver, and William Jarvis. "Guideline for Prevention of Surgical Site Infection, 1999." *Infection Control and Hospital Epidemiology* 20 (April 1999): 247–78.

Pittet, Didier. "Improving Adherence to Hand Hygiene Practice: A Multidisciplinary Approach." *Emerging Infectious Diseases* 7 (March/April 2001).

ORGANIZATIONS

Association of Perioperative Registered Nurses (AORN). 2170 South Parker Road, Suite 300, Denver, CO 80231-5711. (303) 755-6300 or (800) 755-2676. <http://www.aorn.org>.

Centers for Disease Control and Prevention (CDC). 1600 Clifton Road, Atlanta, GA 30333. (404) 639-3534 or (800) 311-3435. <http://www.cdc.gov>.

OTHER

Bjerke, Nancy. "Hand Hygiene in Healthcare: Playing by the New Rules." *Infection Control Today* February 2003 [cited February 2003]. <http://www.infectioncontroltoday.com/articles/321bpraaact.html>.

Dix, Kathy. "Observing Standard Precautions in the OR." *Infection Control Today* October 2002 [cited February 2003]. <http://www.infectioncontroltoday.com/articles/2a1topics.html>.

Osman, Cathy. "Asepsis and Aseptic Practices in the Operating Room." *Infection Control Today* July 2000 [cited February 2003]. <http://www.infectioncontroltoday.com/articles/071best.html>.

Katherine Hauswirth, APRN
Stephanie Dionne Sherk

Aspirin

Definition

Aspirin is a medication given to relieve pain and reduce fever. The name "aspirin" was originally a trademark, first used when the drug was introduced in Europe in 1899. Aspirin was developed by a German chemist named Felix Hoffman as a treatment for his father's arthritis.

Purpose

Aspirin is still used to relieve many kinds of minor aches and pains—headaches, toothaches, muscle pain, menstrual cramps, joint pains associated with arthritis, and the general achiness that many people experience with colds and flu. Some people take aspirin daily to reduce the risk of stroke, heart attack, or other heart problems.

Description

Aspirin, also known as acetylsalicylic acid, is not a prescription drug. It is sold over the counter in many forms, from the familiar white tablets to chewing gum and rectal suppositories. Coated, chewable, buffered, and extended-release forms are available. Many other over-the-counter medications contain aspirin. Alka-Seltzer Original Effervescent Antacid Pain Reliever (R), for example, contains aspirin for pain relief as well as sodium bicarbonate to relieve acid indigestion, heartburn, and sour stomach.

Aspirin belongs to a group of drugs called salicylates. Other members of this group include sodium salicylate, choline salicylate, and magnesium salicylate. These drugs are more expensive and no more effective than aspirin; however, they are a little easier on the patient's stomach. Aspirin is quickly absorbed into the bloodstream and provides rapid and relatively long-lasting pain relief. Aspirin in high doses also reduces inflammation. Researchers believe these effects are due to aspirin's ability to block the production of pain-producing chemicals called prostaglandins.

In addition to relieving pain and reducing inflammation, aspirin also lowers fever by acting on the hypothalamus, which is the part of the brain that regulates temperature. The brain then signals the blood vessels to dilate (widen), which allows heat to leave the body more quickly.

Recommended dosage

Adults

PAIN RELIEF OR FEVER REDUCTION. The usual dosage is one to two tablets every three to four hours, up to six times per day.

RISK REDUCTION FOR STROKE. One tablet four times a day or two tablets twice a day.

RISK REDUCTION FOR HEART ATTACK. Aspirin may be used as a first-line treatment for a heart attack. The patient should chew a single uncoated aspirin tablet, since chewing makes it easier for the body to absorb the medication rapidly. Aspirin will not stop a heart attack, and proper emergency care is essential; however, an aspirin tablet may reduce the amount of damage done by the heart attack.

Patients should check with a physician for the proper dose and number of times per week they should take aspirin to reduce the risk of a heart attack. The most common dose for this purpose is a single baby aspirin tablet taken daily. Enteric-coated aspirin is often used, since it reduces the risk of stomach irritation.

Children

Parents should consult the child's physician about the proper dosage for their child's condition.

Precautions

Aspirin—even children's aspirin—should never be given to children or teenagers with flu-like symptoms or chickenpox. Aspirin can cause Reye's syndrome, a life-threatening condition that affects the nervous system and liver. As many as 30% of children and teenagers who develop Reye's syndrome die. Those who survive may have permanent brain damage.

Parents should consult a physician before giving aspirin to a child under 12 years of age for arthritis, rheumatism, or any condition that requires long-term use of the drug.

No one should take aspirin for more than 10 days in a row unless instructed to do so by a physician. Anyone with fever should not take aspirin for more than three days without a physician's advice. In addition, no one should take more than the recommended daily dosage.

People in the following categories should not use aspirin without first checking with their physician:

- Pregnant women. Aspirin can cause bleeding problems in both the mother and the developing fetus. Aspirin can also cause the infant's weight to be too low at birth.
- Women who are breastfeeding. Aspirin can pass into breast milk and affect the baby.
- People with a history of bleeding problems.
- People who are taking such blood-thinning drugs as warfarin (Coumadin).
- People who have had recent surgery. Aspirin increases the risk of bleeding from an incompletely healed incision.
- People with a history of stomach ulcers.
- People with a history of asthma, nasal polyps, or both. Patients with these disorders are more likely to be allergic to aspirin.
- People who are allergic to fenoprofen, ibuprofen, indomethacin, ketoprofen, meclofenamate sodium, naproxen, sulindac, tolmetin, or an orange food coloring known as tartrazine. They may also be allergic to aspirin.
- People with AIDS or AIDS-related complex who are taking AZT (zidovudine). Aspirin can increase the risk of bleeding in these patients.
- People taking any of the drugs listed below under Interactions.
- People with liver damage or severe kidney failure.

Aspirin should not be taken before a surgical procedure, as it can increase the risk of excessive bleeding during surgery. People scheduled for an operation should check with their surgeon to find out when they should discontinue taking aspirin.

Aspirin can cause stomach irritation. Taking aspirin with food or milk, or drinking an eight-ounce glass of water with it may help to prevent damage to the stomach lining. Some patients find that using coated or buffered aspirin reduces the risk of stomach upset. Patients should be aware, however, that drinking alcoholic beverages can make the stomach irritation worse.

Patients with any of the following symptoms should stop taking aspirin immediately and call their physician:

- a sensation of ringing or buzzing in the ears
- hearing loss
- dizziness

KEY TERMS

Diuretic—A type of medication that increases the amount of urine produced and relieves excess fluid buildup in body tissues. Diuretics may be used in treating high blood pressure, lung disease, premenstrual syndrome, and other conditions.

Inflammation—A response to injury or illness characterized by pain, redness, swelling, and warmth.

Nonsteroidal anti-inflammatory drugs (NSAIDs)—Drugs that relieve pain and reduce inflammation but are not related chemically to cortisone. Common drugs in this class are aspirin, ibuprofen (Advil, Motrin), naproxen (Aleve, Naprosyn), ketoprofen (Orudis), and several others.

Polyp—Any mass of tissue that grows out of a mucous membrane in the digestive tract, uterus, or elsewhere in the body.

Prostaglandin—A hormonelike chemical produced in the body that has a variety of effects. Prosta-

glandins may be responsible for the production of some types of pain and inflammation.

Reye's syndrome—A life-threatening disease that affects the liver and the brain and sometimes occurs after a viral infection, such as flu or chickenpox. Children or teenagers who are given aspirin for flu or chickenpox are at increased risk of developing Reye's syndrome.

Rhinitis—Inflammation of the membranes inside the nose.

Salicylates—A group of drugs that includes aspirin and related compounds. Salicylates are used to relieve pain, reduce inflammation, and lower fever.

Stroke—An event that impairs the circulation of the brain. Ischemic stroke is caused by a blood clot in the brain. Hemorrhagic stroke is caused by bleeding into the brain.

• stomach pain that does not go away

Patients should discard any aspirin that has developed a vinegary smell. That is a sign that the medication is too old and ineffective.

Side effects

The most common side effects of aspirin include upset stomach, heartburn, loss of appetite, and small amounts of blood in the stool. Less common side effects are rashes, hives, fever, vision problems, liver damage, thirst, stomach ulcers, and bleeding. People with asthma, rhinitis, polyps in the nose, or allergies to aspirin may have trouble breathing after taking the drug.

Interactions

Aspirin may increase, decrease, or change the effects of many drugs. Aspirin can increase the toxicity of such drugs as methotrexate (Rheumatrex) and valproic acid (Depakote, Depakene). Taken with such blood-thinning drugs as warfarin (Coumadin) and dicumarol, aspirin can increase the risk of excessive bleeding. Aspirin counteracts the effects of certain other drugs, including angiotensin-converting enzyme (ACE) inhibitors and beta blockers, which lower blood pressure, and medicines used to treat gout (probenecid and sulfinpyrazone). Blood pressure may drop unexpectedly and cause faint-

ing or dizziness if aspirin is taken along with nitroglycerin tablets. Aspirin may also interact with **diuretics**, diabetes medications, other **nonsteroidal anti-inflammatory drugs** (NSAIDs), seizure medications, and steroids. Anyone who is taking these drugs should ask his or her physician whether they can safely take aspirin.

Resources

BOOKS

"Factors Affecting Drug Response: Drug Interactions." Section 22, Chapter 301 in *The Merck Manual of Diagnosis and Therapy*, edited by Mark H. Beers, MD, and Robert Berkow, MD. Whitehouse Station, NJ: Merck Research Laboratories, 1999.

Wilson, Billie Ann, RN, PhD, Carolyn L. Stang, PharmD, and Margaret T. Shannon, RN, PhD. *Nurses Drug Guide 2000*. Stamford, CT: Appleton and Lange, 1999.

PERIODICALS

Cryer, B. "Gastrointestinal Safety of Low-Dose Aspirin." *American Journal of Managed Care* 8 (December 2002) (22 Suppl): S701-S708.

Grattan. C. E. "Aspirin Sensitivity and Urticaria." *Clinical and Experimental Dermatology* 28 (March 2003): 123-127.

MacDonald, T. M., and L. Wei. "Effect of Ibuprofen on Cardioprotective Effect of Aspirin." *Lancet* 361 (February 15, 2003): 573-574.

Nordenberg, Tamar. "'An Aspirin a Day'— Just Another Cliché?" *FDA Consumer* (March-April 1999): 2-4.

ORGANIZATIONS

American Society of Health-System Pharmacists (ASHP). 7272 Wisconsin Avenue, Bethesda, MD 20814. (301) 657-3000. <www.ashp.org>.

Aspirin Foundation of America. (800) 432-3247; fax (202) 737-8406. <www.aspirin.org>.

United States Food and Drug Administration (FDA). 5600 Fishers Lane, Rockville, MD 20857-0001. (888) INFO-FDA. <www.fda.gov>.

Nancy Ross-Flanigan
Sam Uretsky, PharmD

Atrial fibrillation surgery *see* **Maze procedure for atrial fibrillation**

Atrial septal defect surgery *see* **Heart surgery for congenital defects**

Autograft *see* **Skin grafting**

Autologous blood donation

Definition

Autologous blood donation is the process of donating one's own blood prior to an elective surgical or medical procedure to avoid or reduce the need for an allogeneic blood **transfusion** (from a volunteer blood donor).

Purpose

Blood transfusions are given to restore lost blood, to improve clotting time, and to improve the ability of the blood to deliver oxygen to the body's tissues. There are some disadvantages to traditional allogeneic blood transfusions. Although strict regulations are in place to ensure correct matching by blood type, errors in this process can lead to the transfusion of mismatched blood, which can cause a serious and sometimes fatal adverse reaction called transfusion reaction. In addition, while donated blood is rigorously tested for infectious agents such as human immunodeficiency virus (HIV) and hepatitis, there is always a chance that an infectious disease may be transmitted via allogeneic transfusion.

The donation and transfusion of autologous blood has arisen as an alternative to allogeneic blood transfusion. Autologous donation is indicated for an elective surgical or medical procedure in which the likelihood of a blood transfusion is high. Such procedures include surgery on the heart, blood vessels, bones, and chest.

WHO PERFORMS THE PROCEDURE AND WHERE IS IT PERFORMED?

Blood may be donated at a hospital or a blood donor center. The procedure of blood donation is generally performed by a nurse or phlebotomist (a person trained to draw blood).

Some of the advantages of autologous blood donation include:

• The patient is assured that the blood is an exact match to his or her blood type, thereby avoiding transfusion reaction.

• There is no risk of inadvertently transmitting infectious agents.

• Autologous blood donations supplement the community blood supply.

• The process of donating blood promotes blood cell production by bone marrow.

• The patient is often reassured by the knowledge that his or her own blood will be used if a blood transfusion becomes necessary.

Some disadvantages to autologous blood donation do exist, which include:

• Contamination of autologous blood with infectious agents is possible during the donation process.

• There is a possibility that a patient's blood will be mislabeled or that allogeneic blood will be inadvertently transfused.

• Autologous blood donation costs more to process and store.

• Blood may be transfused unnecessarily because an autologous blood supply exists.

• Unused units of autologous blood are usually disposed of; approximately 44% of autologous donations remain unused after surgery.

Demographics

Autologous blood donations account for approximately 5% of all blood donated in the United States each year.

Description

The most common form of autologous donation is called preoperative autologous blood donation (PABD). PABD is generally indicated when there is a reasonable chance that a blood transfusion will become necessary, when the patient is in adequate health to donate blood, and when there is sufficient preoperative time for the patient to donate. As the shelf life of liquid blood is approximately 42 days, the patient may begin donating up to six weeks before the scheduled procedure. It is generally recommended that a patient donate no more than once or twice a week, and no later than 72 hours before surgery.

The PABD process is similar to the process of donating allogeneic blood. A tourniquet is placed on the upper arm to increase the pressure in the arm veins and make them swell and become more accessible. Once a suitable vein is identified, the area where the needle will be inserted is sterilized by washing with soap solution or an iodine-containing antiseptic. The donor lies on a bed or cot during the procedure, which takes about 10 minutes. Blood is collected in sterile plastic bags that hold one pint (450 ml). The bags contain an anticoagulant to prevent clotting and preservatives to keep the blood cells alive.

The collected blood may then be transfused during and/or after surgery in a similar manner to allogeneic blood. If the amount transfused is less than anticipated or if no blood was necessary, then the autologous blood is generally disposed of (since the restrictions placed on volunteer donors are stricter than those on autologous donors). If the patient's surgery is postponed, the donated blood may be frozen and stored until the procedure is rescheduled.

Acute normo-volemic hemodilution (ANH) is a variant of autologous donation in which a volume of the patient's blood is removed directly before surgery and replaced with fluids so that any blood lost during surgery has a lower red blood cell count (i.e., the red blood cells have been diluted). The removed blood is then reinfused after surgery. Advantages to ANH are that no processing and storage costs are necessary and the risk of contamination during processing is reduced.

Blood may also be collected during surgery (intra-operative **blood salvage**, or IBS) or after surgery (postoperative blood salvage, PBS). IBS is commonly used during cardiac, bone, transplant, and trauma surgery and involves the use of specialized equipment to collect and process the blood before reinfusion. PBS involves the collection of blood from drainage tubes, although generally this volume is small.

Diagnosis/Preparation

Patients must meet certain selection criteria before donating their own blood for future use. In the case of PABD, there must be sufficient time before the procedure to safely collect enough blood. A patient must be med-

ically stable, have no active infection, and have a close-to-normal red blood cell count to quality for PABD.

Aftercare

Individuals who donate blood are generally given fluids and/or light refreshments to prevent possible side effects such as dizziness and nausea. Iron supplements may be prescribed to prevent or treat anemia (low red blood cell count).

Risks

Complications associated with autologous blood donation are similar to those associated with allogeneic blood donation. These include dizziness, fainting, profuse sweating, hyperventilation, and/or low blood pressure. (This collection of symptoms is called a vasovagal response.) Among patients with heart disease, there is an increased risk of cardiac complications after donating blood.

Risks associated with autologous blood transfusion include transfusion reaction if an allogeneic blood transfusion was inadvertently given and transmission of infectious agents if the blood became contaminated. Symptoms of transfusion reaction include general discomfort, anxiety, breathing difficulties, dizziness, itching, fever, headache, rash, and swelling. Patients who are given too much blood can develop high blood pressure, which is a concern for people who have heart disease. Very rarely, an air embolism is created when air is introduced into a patient's veins through the tubing used for intravenous infusion.

Normal results

If a patient loses enough blood during a surgical or medical procedure to warrant a blood transfusion, a transfusion of autologous blood will under normal circum-

KEY TERMS

Allogeneic blood transfusion—Blood that has originated from volunteer blood donor (i.e., not the patient).

Directed donation—Blood donated by a patient's family member or friend, to be used by the patient.

Vasovagal reaction—A collection of symptoms that includes dizziness, fainting, profuse sweating, hyperventilation, and/or low blood pressure that occurs in a small percentage of individuals who donate blood.

stances confer the same benefits as a transfusion of allogeneic blood with none of the associated risks (i.e., transfusion reaction or transmission of infectious agents).

Morbidity and mortality rates

One study found the risk of a complication requiring hospitalization to be one in approximately 17,000 among autologous blood donors, and one in approximately 200,000 among volunteer blood donors. The most common complication is a vasovagal reaction, although approximately 12% of patients requiring hospitalization have angina (chest pain resulting from inadequate supply of oxygen to the heart). There is a higher chance of a vasovagal reaction with autologous blood donation than with allogeneic blood donation.

Alternatives

Allogeneic blood is a more commonly used alternative to autologous blood and accounts for 95% of all blood donations in the United States. Patients may also choose to have blood donated by family or friends, a process called directed donation. For patients who are interested in avoiding a blood transfusion, alternatives include:

- Volume expanders. Certain fluids (saline, Ringer's lactate solution, dextran, etc.) may be used to increase the volume of blood.

- Blood substitutes. Much research is currently being done into compounds that can replace some or all of the functions of blood components. One such compound, called HBOC-201, or Hemopure, is derived from bovine (cow) blood and is showing promise as a substitute for red blood cell transfusion.

- Bloodless surgery. It may be possible to avoid excessive blood loss through careful planning prior to surgery. Specialized instruments can minimize the amount of blood lost during a procedure.

Resources

PERIODICALS

Henry, D. A., et al. "Pre-operative Autologous Donation for Minimizing Perioperative Allogeneic Blood Transfusion." *Cochrane Review,* Issue 1 (January 20, 2003).

Vanderlinde, Elizabeth S., Joanna M. Heal, and Neil Blumberg. "Autologous Transfusion." *British Medical Journal,* 324 (March 30, 2002): 772–5.

ORGANIZATIONS

American Association of Blood Banks. 8101 Glenbrook Rd., Bethesda, MD 20814. (301) 907-6977. <http://www.aabb.org>.

American Red Cross. 431 18th St., NW, Washington, DC 20006. (202) 639-3520. <http://www.redcross.org>.

OTHER

"Autologous Blood as an Alternative to Allogeneic Blood Transfusion." *American Association of Blood Banks,* January 2002 [cited March 19, 2003]. <http://www.aabb.org/All_About_Blood/FAQs/4>.

"Preoperative Autologous Blood Donation (PABD)." *Health Technology Advisory Committee,* September 2000 [cited March 19, 2003]. <http://www.health.state.mn.us/htac/pabd.htm>.

"Transfusion Alert: Use of Autologous Blood." *National Heart, Lung, and Blood Institute,* [cited March 19, 2003]. <http://www.nhlbi.nih.gov/health/prof/blood/transfusion/logo.htm>.

Stephanie Dionne Sherk

Automatic implantable cardioverter-defibrillator *see* **Implantable cardioverter-defibrillator**

Axillary dissection

Definition

Axillary dissection is a surgical procedure that incises (opens) the armpit (axilla or axillary) to identify, examine, or remove lymph nodes (small glands, part of the lymphatic system, which filters cellular fluids).

Purpose

Axillary dissection is utilized to stage breast cancer in order to determine the necessity of further treatment based on cancer cell spread. Additionally, axillary dissection includes removal and pathological examination of axillary lymph nodes for persons having operable

Axillary dissection

Pectoralis major muscle

Incision

A.

Lymph nodes

B.

Scar tissue

C.

To determine the advancement of breast cancer, lymph nodes in the armpit are removed. An incision is made (A), and lymph nodes are removed and tested (B), leaving a small scar (C). *(Illustration by GGS Inc.)*

breast cancer. The anatomy of the axilla is complex and composed of several critical nerves, arteries, and muscles. Because of this complex anatomy and connection with the breast, the axilla is a common route for possible metastatic (cancer cell spread to distant areas within the body) involvement from breast cancer. The absence or presence of cancer cells in axillary lymph nodes is the most power prognostic (outcome) indicator for breast cancer. Axillary dissection is an accurate procedure for axillary node assessment (removal and pathological examination). Clinical examination of the breast (more specifically palpation, or feeling the affected area for lumps) for the axillary region is inaccurate and unreliable. The only method to identify whether or not a lymph node has cancer cells, is to surgically remove the node and perform examination with a microscope to detect abnormal cancer cells.

Demographics

If axillary dissection is not performed, recurrence of cancer in the armpit is common even after breast surgery. Recent evidence suggests that persons who underwent **lumpectomy** alone without axillary dissection had a 10-year average recurrence rate of 28% in the axilla. Generally, recent evidence also suggests that the more nodes and tissues removed in the axilla, the lower the risk of recurrence of cancer. Research also indicates that 10-year axillary cancer recurrence rates are low (10% for node negative and 3% for node positive) for women who have mastectomy and axillary node removal. The recurrence rate for breast cancer is approximately 17% for women who did not have axillary node removal.

Description

Lymph nodes (or lymph glands) are filtering centers for the lymphatic system (a system of vessels that collects fluids from cells for filtration and reentry into the blood). Additionally, there is a complex arrangement of muscles, tissues, nerves and blood vessels. Axillary dissection is surgically explained in terms of three levels. Level I axillary dissection is also called lower axillary dissection because it is the removal of all tissue below the axillary vein and extending to the side where the axillary vein crosses the tendon of a muscle called the latissimus dorsi. Level II dissection is continuous—it includes the removal of level tissues and further extensive removal of cancerous tissues. Level II dissection removes diseased tissues deeper in the middle (medial) area of another muscle called the pectoralis minor. Level III dissection is the most aggressive breast cancer axillary surgery, and it entails the removal of all nodal tissue (tissues related to the lymphatic system) from the axilla.

Diagnosis/Preparation

Operable breast cancer is the primary indication for axillary dissection. Persons receiving this surgery have been diagnosed with breast cancer and are undergoing surgical removal of the breast. Diagnosis of breast cancer typically involves palpation of a lump (mass), and other tests such as **mammography** (special type of x ray used to visualize deep into breast tissues) and biopsy. The specific diagnosis to estimate the extent of axillary (cancerous) involvement can be made by performing a sentinel node biopsy. The sentinel node is the first lymph node that drains fluid from the primary tumor site. If there is no presence of cancerous cells in the sentinel node, the likelihood that higher echelon lymph nodes have cancer is very small. Conversely, if cancerous cells are detected in the sentinel node, then axillary dissection is recommended.

Preparation for axillary dissection is the same as that for **modified radical mastectomy**. This includes but is not limited to preoperative assessments (special tests and blood analysis), patient education, **postoperative care**, and follow-up consultations with surgeon and cancer specialist (medical hematologist/oncologist). Psychotherapy and/or community-centered support group meetings may also be beneficial to treatment.

Aftercare

One of the major problems that can result from axillary lymph node removal is lymphedema (fluid accumulation in the arm). Postoperative aftercare should include the use of compression garments, pneumatic compression pumps, and massage to combat fluid retention. Additionally, persons may have pain and should discuss this with the attending surgeon. Other surgical measures for aftercare should be followed similar to persons receiving a modified radical mastectomy. Skin care is important and caution should be exercised to avoid cuts, bites, and skin infections in the affected area. Further measures to control lymphedema can include arm exercises and maintenance of normal weight.

Risks

There are several direct risks associated with axillary surgery. A recent study indicated that approximately 31% of persons may have numbness and tingling of the hand and 10% develop carpal tunnel syndrome. In females who have had a previous breast surgery before the axillary surgery, recurrent wound infections and progression of lymphedema can occur. Additionally, persons may also feel tightness and heaviness in the arm as a result of lymphedema.

QUESTIONS TO ASK
THE DOCTOR

- How do I prepare for the procedure?
- How long does it take to know the results?
- What postoperative care will be needed?
- What are the possible risks involved in this procedure?

Normal results

Normal results can include limited but controlled lymphedema and adequate wound healing. Persons receiving axillary dissection due to breast cancer require several weeks of postoperative recovery to regain full strength.

Morbidity and mortality rates

Sickness and/or death are not necessarily related to axillary surgery per se. Rather, breast cancer outcome is related to breast cancer staging. Staging determined by axillary surgery can yield valuable information concerning disease progression. Early stage (stage I) breast cancer usually has a better outcome, whereas advance stage cancer (stage 4) is correlated with a 10-year survival rate.

Alternatives

Currently research does not support other therapies. Further study is required but other therapies are currently not recommended. There are no adequate alternatives to axillary surgery in breast cancer persons. The most recent evidence suggests that removal of lymph nodes and tissues in the armpit is correlated with elevated survival rates.

Resources

BOOKS

Noble, John. *Textbook of Primary Care Medicine.* 3rd ed. St. Louis, MO: Mosby, Inc., 2001.

Townsend, Courtney. *Sabiston Textbook of Surgery.* 16th ed. St. Louis: W. B. Saunders Company, 2001.

PERIODICALS

Cantin, J., H. Scarth, M. Levine, and M. Hugi. "Clinical practice guidelines for the care and treatment of breast can-

KEY TERMS

Axillary vein—A blood vessel that takes blood from tissues back to the heart to receive oxygenated blood.

Latissimus dorsi—In Latin, this muscle literally means "widest of the back." This is a large fan-shaped muscle that covers a wide area of the back.

Lymph nodes—Small masses of lymphoid tissue that are connected to lymphatic vessels.

Lymphatic system—Part of the cardiovascular system, lymphatic vessels will bring fluids from cells (cellular debris) for filtration in lymph nodes. Filtered fluid is returned back to the blood circulation.

Lymphedema—Retention of lymph fluid in an affected (affected by surgery or disease) area.

Pectoralis minor—A triangular-shaped muscle in front of (anterior) the axilla.

Tendon—Attaches muscle to bone.

cer." *Canadian Medical Association Journal* 165 (July 24, 2001).

Fiorica, James. "Prevention and Treatment of Breast Cancer." *Obstetrics and Gynecology Clinics* 28 (December 2001).

Hugi,M. R., I. A. Olivotto, and S. R. Harris. "Clinical practice guidelines for the care and treatment of breat cancer:11.Lymphedema." *Canadian Medical Association Journal* 164 (January 23,2001).

ORGANIZATIONS

American Cancer Society. (800) ACS-2345. <http://www.cancer.org>.

Y-ME National Breast Cancer Organization. 212 W. Van Buren, Suite 500 Chicago, IL 60607. (312) 986-8338. Fax: (312) 294-8597. (800) 221-2141 (English). (800) 986-9505 (Español). <http:// www.y-me.org>.

OTHER

Cancernews. [cited May 15, 2003]. <http://www.cancernews.com>.

Laith Farid Gulli, MD, MS
Nicole Mallory, MS, PA-C
Bilal Nasser, MD, MS

B

Balloon angioplasty *see* **Angioplasty**

Balloon valvuloplasty

Definition

Balloon valvuloplasty, also called percutaneous balloon valvuloplasty, is a surgical procedure used to open a narrowed heart valve. The procedure is sometimes referred to as balloon enlargement of a narrowed heart valve.

Purpose

Balloon valvuloplasty is performed on children and adults who have a narrowed heart valve, a condition called stenosis. The goal of the procedure is to improve valve function and blood flow by enlarging the valve opening. It is sometimes used to avoid or delay open heart surgery and valve replacement.

There are four valves in the heart—the aortic valve, pulmonary valve, mitral valve, and tricuspid valve—each at the exit of one of the heart's four chambers. These valves open and close to regulate the blood flow from one chamber to the next and are vital to the efficient functioning of the heart and circulatory system. Balloon valvuloplasty is used primarily to treat pulmonary, mitral, and aortic valves when narrowing is present and medical treatment has not corrected or relieved the related problems. With mitral stenosis, for example, medical solutions are typically tried first, such as diuretic therapy (reducing excess fluid), anticoagulant therapy (thinning the blood and preventing blood clots), or blood pressure medications. Valvuloplasty is recommended for those patients whose symptoms continue to progress even after taking such medications for a period of time.

Valvular stenosis can be a congenital defect (develops in the fetus and is present at birth) or can be ac-quired, that is to stem from other conditions. Mitral valve stenosis in adults, for example, is rarely congenital and is usually acquired, either a result of having rheumatic fever as a child or developing calcium obstruction in the valve later in life. Pulmonary stenosis is almost entirely congenital. Aortic stenosis usually does not produce symptoms until the valve is 75% blocked; this occurs over time and is consequently found in people between the ages of 40 and 70. Tricuspid stenosis is usually the result of rheumatic fever; it occurs less frequently than other valve defects.

Childhood symptoms of valve narrowing may include heart dysfunction, heart failure, blood pressure abnormalities, or a murmur. Adult symptoms will likely mimic heart disease and may include blood pressure abnormalities, shortness of breath, chest pain (angina), irregular heart beat (arrhythmia), or fainting spells (syncope). Electrocardiogram (EKG), x ray, and **angiography** (a special x-ray examination using dye in the vascular system) may be performed to identify valvular heart problems. Depending on the severity of symptoms, **cardiac catheterization** may also be performed to examine heart valve function prior to recommending a surgical procedure. Valvular **angioplasty** is performed in children and adults to relieve stenosis. While it offers relief, it does not always cure the problem, particularly in adults, and often valvotomy (cutting the valve leaflets to correct the opening) or valve replacement is necessary at a later date.

Demographics

Congenital heart-valve disease occurs in one of every 1,000 newborns and is thought to be caused by inherited factors. In 2–4% of valve problems, health or environmental factors affecting the mother during pregnancy are believed to contribute to the defect. Pulmonary valve stenosis represents about 10% of all congenital heart problems. About 5% of all cardiac defects are stenosis of the aortic valve. Valve abnormalities are diagnosed in children and adults of both sexes; 80% of adult patients with stenosis are male, most adults with mitral stenosis are women who had rheumatic fever as a child. Tricuspid stenosis is rarely found in North America and Europe.

Description

In balloon valvuloplasty, a thin tube (catheter) with a small deflated balloon at its tip (balloon-tipped catheter) is inserted through the skin in the groin area into a blood vessel, and then is threaded up to the opening of the narrowed heart valve. The balloon is inflated to stretch the valve open and relieve the valve obstruction.

The procedure, which takes up to four hours, is performed in a cardiac catheterization laboratory that has a special x-ray machine and an x-ray monitor that looks like a regular TV screen. The patient will be placed on an x-ray table and covered with a sterile sheet. An area on the inside of the upper leg will be washed and treated with an antibacterial solution to prepare for the insertion of a catheter. The patient is given local anesthesia to numb the insertion site and will usually remain awake, able to watch the procedure on the monitor. After the insertion site is prepared and anesthetized, the cardiologist inserts a catheter into the appropriate blood vessel, then passes the smaller balloon-tipped catheter through the first catheter. Guided by the x-ray monitor that allows visualization of the catheter in the blood vessel, the physician slowly threads the catheter up into the coronary artery to the heart. The deflated balloon is carefully positioned in the opening of the valve that is being treated, and then is inflated repeatedly, which applies pressure to dilate the valve. The inflated balloon widens the valve opening by splitting the valve leaflets apart. Once the valve is widened, the balloon-tipped catheter is removed. The other catheter remains in place for six to 12 hours because, in some cases, the procedure must be repeated. A double-balloon valvuloplasty procedure is often performed on certain high-risk patients because it is considered more effective in restoring blood flow.

Preparation

For at least six hours before balloon valvuloplasty, the patient will have to avoid eating or drinking any-

thing. An intravenous line is inserted so that medications (anticoagulants to prevent clot formation and radioactive dye for x rays) can be administered. The patient's groin area is shaved and cleaned with an antiseptic. About an hour before the procedure, the patient is given an oral sedative such as diazepam (Valium) to ensure that he or she will relax sufficiently for the procedure.

Aftercare

After balloon valvuloplasty, the patient will spend several hours in the **recovery room** to be monitored for **vital signs** (such as heart rate and breathing) and heart sounds. During this time, electrical leads attached to an EKG machine will be placed on the patient's chest and limbs, and a monitor will display the electrical impulses of the heart continuously, alerting nurses quickly if any abnormality occurs. For at least 30 minutes after removal of the catheter, direct pressure is applied to the site of insertion; after this a pressure dressing will be applied. The skin condition is monitored. The insertion site will be observed for bleeding until the catheter is removed. The leg in which the catheter was inserted is temporarily prevented from moving. Intravenous fluids will be given to help eliminate the x-ray dye; intravenous anticoagulants or other medications may be administered to improve blood flow and to keep coronary arteries open. Pain medication is administered as-needed. Some patients will continue to take anticoagulant medications for months or years after the surgery and will have regular blood tests to monitor the effectiveness of the medication.

Following **discharge from the hospital**, the patient can usually resume normal activities. After balloon

KEY TERMS

Cardiac catheterization—A minimally invasive technique that runs a catheter through blood vessels into the heart to evaluate heart function. Fluoroscopy is used to observe the catheterization.

Dilate—To expand or open a valve or blood vessel.

Electrocardiography (EKG)—A method to measure the variations in the actions of the heart. An EKG machine is used, which produces a chart, either on paper or on a monitor, that shows the wave-like patterns and indicates any irregularities.

Stenosis—The narrowing of any valve, especially one of the heart valves, or the opening into the pulmonary artery from the right ventricle.

Valve—Flaps (leaflets) of tissue in the passageways between the heart's upper and lower chambers.

valvuloplasty, lifelong follow-up is necessary because valves sometimes degenerate or narrowing recurs, a condition called restenosis, which will likely require repeat valvulplasty, valvotomy, or valve replacement.

Risks

Balloon valvuloplasty can have serious complications. For example, the valve can become misshapen so that it does not close completely, which makes the condition worse. Embolism, where either clots or pieces of valve tissue break off and travel to the brain or the lungs causing blockage, is another possible risk. If the procedure causes severe damage to the valve leaflets, immediate valve replacement is required. Less frequent complications are bleeding and hematoma (a local collection of clotted blood) at the puncture site, abnormal heart rhythms, reduced blood flow, heart attack, heart puncture, infection, and circulatory problems. Because restenosis is frequent in adult patients with valvular disease, particularly when underlying heart disease or other conditions are present, the procedure is recommended only as an emergency rescue for high-risk patients who are not candidates for valve replacement.

Normal results

Balloon valvuloplasty is considered a safe, effective treatment in children with congenital stenosis, improving heart function and blood flow. In adults, balloon valvuloplasty may give temporary relief and improve heart function and blood flow, but underlying coronary artery disease or other disease conditions may encourage restenosis, making valve replacement eventually necessary. The

most successful valvuloplasty results are achieved in treating narrowed pulmonary valves, although the treatment of mitral valve stenosis is also generally good. The aortic valve procedure is more difficult to perform and is generally less successful.

Resources

BOOKS

Heart Owner's Handbook: Congenital Heart Disease and Diseases of the Heart Valves. Texas Heart Institute, New York: John Wiley & Sons, 1996.

Mayo Clinic Practice of Cardiology: Balloon Valvuloplasty. 3rd ed. Edited by Emilio R. Giuliani, et al. St. Louis: Mosby, 1996.

ORGANIZATIONS

American Heart Association. 7320 Greenville Ave. Dallas, TX 75231. (214) 373-6300. <http://www.americanheart.org>.

OTHER

"Heart Valve Problems." *Aetna Intelihealth.* [cited April 2003]. <http://www.intelihealth.com>.

Lori De Milto
L. Lee Culvert

Bandages and dressings

Definition

Bandages and dressings are both used in wound management. A bandage is a piece of cloth or other material used to bind or wrap a diseased or injured part of the body. Usually shaped as a strip or pad, bandages are either placed directly against the wound or used to bind a dressing to the wound. A dressing can consist of a wide range of materials, sometimes containing medication, placed directly against the wound.

Purpose

The purposes served by dressings include protecting wounds; promoting healing; and providing, retaining, or removing moisture. Bandages can be used to hold dressings in place, to relieve pain, and generally to make the patient comfortable. Elastic bandages are useful to provide ongoing pressure on wounds such as varicose veins, fractured ribs, and swollen joints.

Description

In recent years, there have been tremendous advances in the design and composition of bandages and dressings. The field is becoming increasingly complex, and there are numerous reports of health care workers applying inappropriate products. Wound-care materials come in a wide variety of product classes, including the following:

- Alginate dressings. These are derived from brown seaweed and contain calcium alginate, which turns into a sodium alginate gel when it comes in contact with wound fluid. They are available as pads or ropes.

- Biosynthetic dressings. These are composites of biological (often animal-derived) and synthetic materials such as polymers.

- Collagen dressings. These are made from collagen, a protein obtained from cowhide, cattle tendons, or birds. They are available as particles or gels.

- Composite dressings. These are similar to plastic adhesive strips and include an adhesive border, a non-adhesive or semi-adhesive surface that is applied to the wound, an absorbent layer, and a bacterial barrier.

- Contact layers. A low-adherent layer of perforated or woven polymer material designed to stop a secondary absorbent dressing from sticking to the surface of a wound.

- Gauze. This woven fabric of absorbent cotton is available in a number of formats and materials, including cotton or synthetic, non-impregnated, and impregnated with water, saline, or other substances. Gauze is sold as surgical swabs, sheets, rolls, pads, sponges, and ribbon.

- Growth factors. These short-chain proteins affect specific target cells. They exist naturally in humans, and can be transplanted from one part of the body to another or manufactured outside the body.

- Hydrocolloid dressings. Used for leg ulcers, minor burns, pressure sores and traumatic injuries, these self-adhesive dressings form a gel as they absorb fluid from the wound. They consist of materials such as sodium carboxymethylcellulose (an absorbent), pectin, and gelatin that are attached to a foam sheet or a thin polyurethane film.

- Hydrofibers. Similar in appearance to cotton, carboxymethylcellulose fibers turn into a gel when they come into contact with wound fluid. They are available as ribbons or pads and are highly absorbent.

- Hydrogels. These are sold as sheets and in gel form, and are primarily used to supply moisture to wounds. Depending on the state of the tissue, they can either absorb fluid or moisten the wound. An electrically conductive aloe vera gel is available to provide electrotherapy to wounds.

- Hydropolymers. These foamed-gel products consist of multiple layers. The surface layer is designed to expand to fill the contours of a wound and, at the same time, draw away fluids.

- Leg compression/wrapping products. These are designed to apply external pressure to improve blood flow and resolve chronic edema in the feet and legs. They are available in a broad range of formats, including stockings, compression bandages, or pneumatic pump.

- Polyurethane foam dressings. These are sheets of foamed polymer solutions with small open chambers that draw fluids away from the wound. Some of these foam products offer adhesive surfaces. They are available as sheets and rolls, as well as in various other formats suitable for packing wounds.

- Skin substitutes. Also known as allografts or skin equivalents, these are obtained from human cells cultured and expanded in vitro from neonatal foreskins.

- Superabsorbents. These are particles, hydropolymers, or foams that act like the material inside diapers, with a high capacity for rapid absorption.

- Transparent films. These consist of a thin, clear polyurethane sheet that, on one side, has a special adhesive that does not stick to moist surfaces like those found on a wound. They prevent bacteria and fluids from entering the wound through the dressing, but allow limited circulation of oxygen.

- Wound fillers. These can be bought as powders or pastes, or in strands or beads. They are used to fill wounds and also absorb wound fluid.

- Wound pouches. Equipped with a special collection system for wounds that have a high flow of secretion, they are designed to contain odors and to be easily drained.

- Other assorted wound-care products. These include adhesive bandages, surgical tapes, adhesive skin closures, surgical swabs, paste bandages, specialty absorptive dressings, support bandages, retention bandages, elasticized tubular bandages, lightweight elasticized tubular bandages, foam-padded elasticized tubular bandages, and plain stockinettes.

Just as there is a large selection of bandage and dressing products to choose from, there is also a broad range of applications for these products:

- Alginate dressings are used on wounds that exude moderate to heavy amounts of fluid. They are useful for packing wounds, although strip-packing gauze may be preferable for deeper wounds because it is easier to retrieve. Common applications of alginate dressings include treatment of acute surgical wounds, leg ulcers, sinuses, and pressure sores. These dressings should not be used on third-degree burns. Neither are they advisable for wounds that are dry or are secreting only small amounts of fluid, because their powerful absorbing capability may dry out the wound. These are primary dressings that need be covered by a secondary dressing.

- Biosynthetic dressings are used on burns and other wounds. Another application is as a temporary dressing for skin autograft sites. Some persons may be allergic to these dressing materials.

- Collagen dressings are believed to hasten wound repair and are often used on stubborn wounds. They are most effective on wounds that contain no dead tissue. Collagen dressings should not be used in dry wounds, third-degree burns, or on any patient who is sensitive to bovine (cow) products.

- Composite dressings are sometimes used alone, sometimes in combination with other dressings. Deep wounds should first be packed with wound-filler material. These dressings should not be cut, and are not recommended for use on third-degree burns.

- Contact layers are designed for use in clean wounds that contain no dead tissue. They are not recommended for infected, shallow, dry, or infected wounds, or on third-degree burns.

- Gauze is used to pack wounds, and also for **debridement** and wicking. It is especially desirable for packing deep wounds. When using gauze to pack wounds, a loose packing technique is preferred.

- Growth factors. These have highly specific applications against such conditions as diabetic foot ulcers involving disease of the peripheral nerves. Growth factors are heat sensitive and often require refrigeration. These are not recommended for persons with benign or malignant tumors.

- Hydrocolloid dressings are used for leg ulcers, minor burns, pressure sores, and traumatic injuries. Because they are not painful to remove, hydrocolloid dressings are often employed in pediatric wound management. Because of their absorbent capabilities, they are used on wounds that are secreting light to moderate amounts of fluid.

- Hydrofibers are highly absorbent, so they are particularly useful for wounds that are draining heavily. For this reason, they are not recommended for dry wounds or wounds with little secretion, because they may result in dehydration. Hydrofibers should not be used as surgical sponges or on third-degree burns.

- Hydrogels are often used on wounds that contain dead tissue, on infected surgical wounds, and on painful wounds. They should not be used on wounds with moderate to heavy secretions. As with all dressings, it is important to check and follow the directions of the manufacturer. In the case of hydrogels, directions on some products indicate they are not to be used on third-degree burns.

Dressings are used to protect wounds and promote healing. They are often held to the wound with bandages. This bandage allows the wound to have some exposure to the air. *(Custom Medical Stock Photo. Reproduced by permission.)*

- Hydropolymers are typically used on wounds with minimal to moderate drainage. They are not indicated for dry wounds or third-degree burns.

- Leg compression/wrapping products are used to increase blood flow and reduce edema in the lower extremities of the body. A medical doctor should be consulted before using these products on people with edema. In many cases, topical dressings are used under these products.

- Polyurethane foam dressings are very absorbent and are typically used on wounds with moderate to heavy secretions. They should not be used on third-degree burns or on wounds that are not draining or that have sinuses or tunneling.

- Skin substitutes are a relatively new product category, approved for treating venous leg ulcers. It is often advisable to cut slits in the artificial skin, so that wound secretions underneath do not lift the newly applied skin.

- Superabsorbents are employed on wounds that are secreting heavily, or in applications requiring extended wear. A packing material is commonly employed under this product. Superabsorbents should not be used on third-degree burns or wounds that are either dry or have minimal secretions.

- Transparent films are often employed as a secondary cover for another, primary dressing. They are used on superficial wounds and on intact skin at risk of infection. It is important to remove transparent films very carefully to avoid damaging fragile skin.

- Wound fillers are primary dressings that are usually used in conjunction with other, secondary dressings. Wound fillers are considered appropriate for shallow wounds with little or moderate secretions. They are not appropriate for use in third-degree burns or in dry wounds. They are similarly not recommended for wounds with tunnels or sinuses.

- Wound pouches are useful in treating wounds with high volumes of secretion. They are not suitable for dry wounds.

Recommended intervals between dressing changes vary widely among product classes. The materials used in some dressings require that they be changed several times a day. Others can remain in place for one week. Manufacturer's directions should be consulted and followed.

Preparation

Wounds require appropriate cleaning, debridement, closure, and medication before bandages and dressings are applied.

Determining the cause of wounds is often very important, especially the cause of chronic wounds such as skin ulcers. A physician should be advised of any signs of infection or other changes in a wound.

Wound-care nursing is a rapidly advancing field that requires considerable training, clinical experience, and judgment, causing some observers to predict that it will eventually develop into an advanced practice nursing or a specialty-based practice. Increasingly, the demands on wound-care nurses are expected to require that they undertake graduate studies. For all nurses working in the field, ongoing education is a must to keep up with new knowledge, technologies, and techniques. Numerous organizations and institutions offer continuing education courses in **wound care** management.

Results

Wounds that receive appropriate and timely care are most likely to heal in an acceptable manner.

See also Incision care; Wound care.

Resources

BOOKS

Brown, P., D. Oddo, and J. P. Maloy. *Quick Reference to Wound Care.* Boston: Jones & Bartlett Publishers, 2003.

Mani, Raj. *Chronic Wound Management: The Evidence for Change.* Boca Raton, FL: CRC Press, 2002.

Milne, C. T., L. Q. Corbett, and D. Duboc. *Wound, Ostomy, and Continence Nursing Secrets.* Philadelphia: Hanley & Belfus, 2002.

Peitzman, Andrew B. *The Trauma Manual, 2nd Edition.* Philadelphia: Lippincott Williams & Wilkins, 2002.

PERIODICALS

Atiyeh, B. S., K. A. El-Musa, and R. Dham. "Scar Quality and Physiologic Barrier Function Restoration after Moist and Moist-exposed Dressings of Partial-thickness Wounds." *Dermatolic Surgery* 29 no. 1 (2003): 14–20.

King, B. "Pain at First Dressing Change after Toenail Avulsion: The Experience of Nurses, Patients and an Observer: 1." *Journal of Wound Care* 12 no. 1 (2003): 5–10.

Ovington, Liza G., PhD. "Know Your Options for Secondary Dressings." *Wound Care Newsletter* 2, no. 4 July 1997 [cited March 24, 2003]. <http://www.woundcare.org/news vol2n4/prpt2.htm>.

Skelhorne, G., and H. Munro. "Hydrogel Adhesives for Wound-care Applications." *Medical Device Technology* 13 no. 9 (2002): 19–23.

St. Clair, K., and J. H. Larrabee. "Clean versus Sterile Gloves: Which to Use for Postoperative Dressing Changes?" *Outcomes Management* 6 no. 1 (2002): 17–21.

ORGANIZATIONS

American Academy of Family Physicians. 11400 Tomahawk Creek Parkway, Leawood, KS 66211-2672. (913) 906-6000. E-mail: <fp@aafp.org>. <http://www.aafp.org>.

American College of Physicians. 190 N. Independence Mall West, Philadelphia, PA 19106-1572. (800) 523-1546, x2600, or (215) 351-2600. <http://www.acponline.org>.

American Medical Association. 515 N. State Street, Chicago, IL 60610. (312) 464-5000. <http://www.ama-assn.org>.

American Nurses Association. 600 Maryland Avenue, SW, Suite 100 West, Washington, DC 20024. (800) 274-4262. <http://www.nursingworld.org>.

American Red Cross National Headquarters. 2025 E Street, NW, Washington DC 20006. (202)303-4498. <http://www.redcross.org>.

International Federation of Red Cross and Red Crescent Societies. PO Box 372, CH-1211 Geneva 19, Switzerland. +41 22 730 42 22. Email: secretariat@ifrc.org. <http://www.ifrc.org>.

Search and Rescue Society of British Columbia. PO Box 1146, Victoria, BC V8W 2T6. (250)384-6696. Email:sarbc.org. <http://www.sarbc.org>.

KEY TERMS

Debridement—Removing dead or non-viable tissue from a wound.

Edema—Swelling of body tissues, caused by collection of excess fluid.

Electrotherapy—The treatment of body tissues by passing electrical currents through them, stimulating the nerves and muscles.

Sinus—In the context of wound management, a narrow hollow in the body extending from an infected area to the surface of the skin.

Stockinette—A soft elastic material used for bandages and clothing for infants.

Wound, Ostomy, and Continence Nurses Society. 1550 South Coast Highway, Suite #201, Laguna Beach, CA 92651. (888) 224-9626. <http://www. wocn.org>.

OTHER

National Library of Medicine. <http://www.nlm.nih.gov/med lineplus/firstaidemergencies.html.> [cited March 24, 2003].

L. Fleming Fallon, Jr, MD, DrPH

Bankart procedure

Definition

A Bankart procedure, also known as a Broca-Perthes-Bankart procedure, is a surgical technique for the repair of recurrent shoulder joint dislocations. In the procedure, the torn ligaments are re-attached to the proper place in the shoulder joint, with the goal of restoring normal function.

Purpose

The shoulder is the junction of three bones: the upper arm bone (humerus), the collarbone (clavicle), and the shoulder blade (scapula). The shoulder joint (glenohumeral joint) is the result of the head of the humerus bone fitting in the cavity of the shoulder blade (glenoid cavity), the joint being held together by the labrum, a rim of soft tissue that surrounds the glenoid. As a result of excessive force being applied to the arm, the head of the humerus may be forced out of the glenoid cavity (dislocation), and the supporting ligaments of the shoulder joint may be torn. These ligaments may heal so that the shoulder regains its stability. However, sometimes the ligaments do not heal, making the shoulder unstable and painful. This condition is referred to as traumatic instability of the shoulder, traumatic glenohumeral instability, or a Bankart lesion.

The goal of a Bankart procedure for traumatic glenohumeral instability is the safe and secure re-attachment of the torn ligaments to the tip of the glenoid from which they were detached. The surgery has the advantage of allowing patients to resume many of their activities of daily living while the repair is healing. The surgery also minimizes the unwanted joint stiffness associated with such injuries.

Demographics

The shoulder is the most commonly dislocated major joint following severe trauma, such as an auto collision or a fall onto an outstretched arm. Some 96% of dislocations involve the front of the shoulder (anterior),

WHO PERFORMS THE PROCEDURE AND WHERE IS IT PERFORMED?

A Bankart procedure is performed in a hospital setting by an orthopedic surgeon specializing in shoulder instability problems.

with 1–3% occurring in the back (posterior). Falls and car accidents are common causes of first-time dislocations, but recurrent dislocations are often due to seemingly inoffensive activities such as raising the arm over the head, or combing hair. Shoulder dislocations are more common in males than females, and in young adults.

Description

In general, shoulder surgery can be performed in two fundamentally different ways: either using closed surgical techniques (**arthroscopic surgery**) or using open surgical techniques.

An open surgery Bankart procedure is performed under general anesthesia. The patient is placed in a 30-degree inclined chair position with the arm free over the edge of the operating table. A bag is placed under the center of the shoulder blade of the shoulder being operated on to support the shoulder and to push the shoulder blade forward. Prepping and draping allow the arm to be freely moveable and allow a good view of the surgical field.

The whole upper limb is prepared with antiseptic. An examination under anesthesia is performed to confirm the exact nature of the instability. The surgeon makes a long incision to gain access to the joint, often cutting through the deltoid muscle to operate on the internal structures of the shoulder, and proceeds to sew the joint capsule to the detached labrum tissues.

The arthroscopic Bankart procedure tries to imitate the open Bankart procedure. Arthroscopy is a microsurgical technique by which the surgeon can use an endoscope to look through a small hole into the shoulder joint. The endoscope is an instrument the size of a pen, consisting of a tube fitted with a light and a miniature video camera, which transmits an image of the joint interior to a television monitor. The detached part of the labrum and the associated ligaments are reattached to bone along the rim of the glenohumeral cavity through a small "keyhole" incision. This is done with little disruption to the other shoulder structures and without the need to detach and reattach the overlying shoulder muscle (subscapularis).

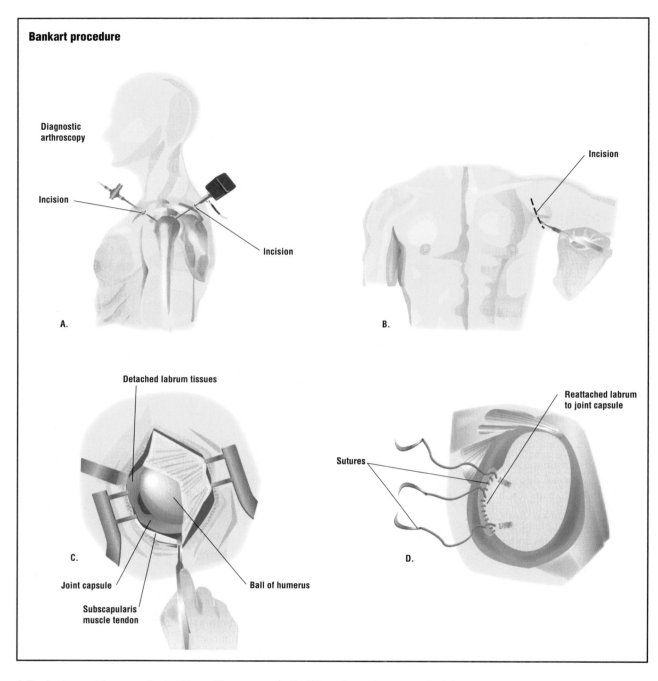

Bankart procedure

Diagnostic
arthroscopy

Incision

Incision

A.

Incision

B.

Detached labrum tissues

Reattached labrum
to joint capsule

Sutures

Joint capsule

Ball of humerus

Subscapularis
muscle tendon

C.

D.

A Bankart procedure may be performed laparoscopically (A), or through an open incision in the shoulder (B). In the open procedure, the surgeon exposes the joint capsule and labrum, a rim of soft tissue that surrounds the cavity, which has become detached (C). Sutures reattach the labrum to the joint capsule (D). *(Illustration by GGS Inc.)*

Diagnosis/Preparation

The physician diagnoses a Bankart lesion from the patient's history, by performing a thorough **physical examination** of the joint, and taking the proper x rays. The examination often reveals that the head of the humerus slips easily out of the joint socket, even when it is pressed into it. This is called the "load and shift test." X rays may also reveal that the bony lip of the glenoid socket is rounded or deficient, or that the head of the humerus is not centered in the glenoid cavity.

A diagnostic arthroscopy is also often used to confirm the presence and extent of the shoulder instability.

In this procedure, a thin fiberoptic scope is inserted into the shoulder joint space to allow direct visualization of its internal structures. An electromyogram may also be obtained if the treating physician suspects the possibility of nerve injury.

Patients should attend to any health problem so as to be in the best possible condition for this procedure. Smoking should be stopped a month before surgery and not resumed for at least three months afterwards. Any heart, lung, kidney, bladder, tooth, or gum problems should be managed before surgery. The orthopedic surgeon needs to be informed of all health issues, including allergies and the non-prescription and prescription medications being used by the patient.

Aftercare

Exercises are usually started on the day following surgery with instructions from a physical therapist, five times daily, including assisted flexion and external rotation of the arm. The other arm is used to support the arm that underwent surgery until it can perform the exercises alone. The patient is allowed to perform many activities of daily living as tolerated, but without lifting anything heavier than a glass or plate. If a patient can not comply with restricted use of the shoulder, the arm is kept in a sling for three weeks. Otherwise, a sling is used only for comfort between **exercise** sessions and to protect the arm when the patient is out in public and at night while sleeping. Driving is allowed as early as two weeks after surgery, if the shoulder can be used comfortably, especially if the patient's car has automatic transmission. At eight to 10 weeks, the patient can usually resume light, low-risk activities, such as swimming and jogging. If involved in sports, the patient may return to training at three months. Hospital physiotherapy is rarely prescribed and only in cases of delayed rehabilitation or shoulder stiffness.

Risks

The following risks are associated with a Bankart procedure:

• Perioperative: Nerve damage during surgery and poor placement of anchor sutures.

• Within six weeks after surgery: Wound infection and rupture of the repair.

• Between six weeks and six months: Shoulder stiffness, recurrence of instability, failure of the repair resulting in shoulder weakness, failure of the anchor sutures.

Normal results

Normal results for a Bankart procedure include:

QUESTIONS TO ASK THE DOCTOR

• How long will it take to recover from the surgery?

• What are the different types of surgery available for shoulder instability?

• Specifically, how will my shoulder be improved by a Bankart procedure?

• Will surgery cure my shoulder condition so that I may resume my activities?

• Can medications help?

• Are there any alternatives to surgery?

• How many Bankart procedures do you perform each year?

• good control of pain and inflammation

• normal upper arm strength and endurance

• normal shoulder range of motion

According to the American Academy of Family Physicians, the classic treatment of recurrent shoulder dislocations remains open surgical Bankart repair. This approach has a success rate as high as 95% in effectively removing shoulder instabilities. In a recent study of young athletes, Bankart repair was compared with three weeks of immobilization for the treatment of an initial anterior shoulder dislocation. The group treated surgically had fewer episodes of recurrent instability than the group managed with immobilization.

Morbidity and mortality rates

Surgery for anterior dislocation of the shoulder fails in one out of 10 to one out of 20 cases, with a higher incidence of failure in arthroscopic Bankart procedures when compared to the open surgical approach. There is also a higher incidence of failure in patients who smoke, those who start using their shoulder vigorously very early after the repair, and in those with very loose ligaments.

Alternatives

Surgical

The Bristow procedure is an alternative surgical procedure used to treat shoulder instability. In this technique, the coracoid process (a long, curved projection from the scapula) with its muscle attachments is trans-

KEY TERMS

Arthroscopy—The introduction of a thin fiberoptic scope (arthroscope) into a joint space to allow direct visualization of internal structures. In some cases, surgical repair can also be performed using the arthroscope.

Coracoid process—A long curved projection from the scapula overhanging the glenoid cavity; it provides attachment to muscles and ligaments of the shoulder and back region.

Electromyography—A test that measures muscle response to nerve stimulation. It is used to evaluate muscle weakness and to determine if the weakness is related to the muscles themselves or to a problem with the nerves that supply the muscles.

General anesthesia—A form of anesthesia that results in putting the patient to sleep.

Glenoid cavity—The hollow cavity in the head of the scapula that receives the head of the humerus to make the glenohumeral or shoulder joint.

Glenohumeral joint—A ball-and-socket synovial joint between the head of the humerus and the glenoid cavity of the scapula. Also called the glenohumeral articulation or shoulder joint.

Humerus—The bone of the upper part of the arm.

Scapula—A large, flat, triangular bone that forms the back portion of the shoulder. It articulates with the clavicle (at the acromion process) and the humerus (at the glenoid). Also called the shoulder blade.

ferred to the neck of the scapula and creates a muscle sling at the front of the glenohumeral joint.

Non-surgical

Shoulders can be stabilized and strengthened with special exercises. During the early phases of such physical therapy programs, the patient is taught to use the shoulder only in the most stable positions—those in which the humerus is elevated in the plane of the scapula. As coordination and confidence improve, progressively less stable positions are attempted.

See also Shoulder joint replacement; Shoulder resection arthroplasty.

Resources

BOOKS

Neumann, L., and W. A. Wallace. "Open Repair of Instability." In *Shoulder Surgery.* Ed. S. Copeland. London: WB Saunders, 1997.

Parker, J. N., ed. *The Official Patient's Sourcebook on Shoulder Dislocation.* San Diego: ICON Health Publications, 2002.

Warren, R. F., E. V. Craig, and D. W. Altcheck, eds. *The Unstable Shoulder.* Philadelphia: Lippincott Williams & Wilkins Publishers, 1999.

PERIODICALS

Itoi, E., S. B. Lee, K. K. Amrami, D. E. Wenger, and K. N. An. "Quantitative assessment of classic anteroinferior bony Bankart lesions by radiography and computed tomography." *American Journal of Sports Medicine* 31 (January-February 2003): 112–118.

Kim, S. H., K. I. Ha, and S. H. Kim. "Bankart repair in traumatic anterior shoulder instability: open versus arthroscopic technique." *Arthroscopy* 18 (September 2002): 755–763.

Magnusson, L., J. Kartus, L. Ejerhed, I. Hultenheim, N. Sernert, and J. Karlsson. "Revisiting the open Bankart experience: a four- to nine-year follow-up." *American Journal of Sports Medicine* 30 (November-December 2002): 778–782.

Massoud, S. N., O. Levy, and S. A. Copeland. " The vertical-apical suture Bankart lesion repair for anteroinferior glenohumeral instability." *Journal of Shoulder and Elbow Surgery* 11 (September-October 2002): 481–485.

Porcellini, G., F. Campi, and P. Paladini. "Arthroscopic approach to acute bony Bankart lesion." *Arthroscopy* 18 (September 2002): 764–769.

ORGANIZATIONS

American Academy of Orthopedic Surgeons. 6300 North River Road, Rosemont, Illinois, 60018-4262. (847) 823-7186; (800) 346-AAOS. <www.aaos.org>.

OTHER

McNeal, Melanie, and David Lintner, M.D. "Traumatic Instability: ACLR or Bankart Procedure." *Dr. Lintner.* Copyright 2003 [cited June 7, 2003]. <www.drlintner.com/aclr. htm>.

Monique Laberge, Ph. D.

Barbiturates

Definition

Barbiturates are medicines that act on the central nervous system. They cause drowsiness and can control seizures.

Purpose

Barbiturates are in the group of medicines known as central nervous system depressants (CNS). Also known as sedative-hypnotic drugs, barbiturates make people very relaxed, calm, and sleepy. These drugs are sometimes used to help patients relax before surgery. Some may also be used to control seizures (convulsions). Although barbiturates have been used to treat nervousness and sleep problems, they have generally been replaced by other medicines for these purposes.

Although barbiturates have largely been replaced by other classes of drugs, some are still used in anesthesiology to induce anesthsia and lower the dose of inhaled anesthetics required for surgical procedures.

Pentobarbital (Nembutal) has been used in **neurosurgery** to reduce blood flow to the brain. This reduces swelling and pressure in the brain, making brain surgery safer.

Secobarbital (Seconal) may be given by mouth or as a suppository to induce sleepiness and relaxation before local anesthesia or the insertion of a tube into the nose or throat.

These medicines may become habit-forming and should not be used to relieve everyday anxiety and tension or to treat sleeplessness over long periods.

Description

Barbiturates are available only with a physician's prescription and are sold in capsule, tablet, liquid, and injectable forms. Some commonly used barbiturates are phenobarbital (Barbita) and secobarbital (Seconal).

Recommended dosage

Recommended dosage depends on the type of barbiturate and other factors such as the patient's age and the condition for which the medicine is being taken. The patient should consult with the physician who prescribed the drug or the pharmacist who filled the prescription for the correct dosage.

The following recommendations do not apply when barbiturates are given as a single oral or intravenous dose prior to or during surgery. The recommendations should be considered if the drugs are used for treatment of anxiety or seizures.

Patients should always take barbiturates exactly as directed. Larger or more frequent doses should never be taken, and the drug should not be taken for longer than directed. If the medicine does not seem to be working, even after taking it for several weeks, the patient should

not increase the dosage. Instead, the physician who prescribed the medicine should be consulted.

People taking barbiturates should not stop taking them suddenly without first checking with the physician who prescribed the medication. It may be necessary to taper the dose gradually to reduce the chance of withdrawal symptoms. If it is necessary to stop taking the drug, the patient should check with the physician for instructions on how to stop.

Precautions

People taking barbiturates must see a physician regularly. The physician will check to make sure the medicine is working as it should and will note unwanted side effects.

Because barbiturates work on the central nervous system, they may add to the effects of alcohol and other drugs that slow the central nervous system, such as antihistamines, cold medicine, allergy medicine, sleep aids, medicine for seizures, tranquilizers, some pain relievers, and **muscle relaxants**. They may also add to the effects of anesthetics, including those used for dental procedures. The combined effects of barbiturates and alcohol or other CNS depressants (drugs that slow the central nervous system) can be very dangerous, leading to unconsciousness or even death. Anyone taking barbiturates should not drink alcohol and should check with his or her physician before taking any medicines classified as CNS depressants.

Taking an overdose of barbiturates or combining barbiturates with alcohol or other central nervous system depressants can cause unconsciousness and even death. Anyone who shows signs of an overdose or a reaction to combining barbiturates with alcohol or other drugs should get emergency medical help immediately. Signs include:

- severe drowsiness
- breathing problems
- slurred speech
- staggering
- slow heartbeat
- severe confusion
- severe weakness

Barbiturates may change the results of certain medical tests. Before having medical tests, anyone taking this medicine should alert the health care professional in charge.

People may feel drowsy, dizzy, lightheaded, or less alert when using these drugs. These effects may even occur the morning after taking a barbiturate at bedtime.

Because of these possible effects, anyone who takes these drugs should not drive, use machines or do anything else that might be dangerous until they have found out how the drugs affect him or her.

Barbiturates may cause physical or mental dependence when taken over long periods. Anyone who shows these signs of dependence should check with his or her physician right away:

- the need to take larger and larger doses of the medicine to get the same effect

- a strong desire to keep taking the medicine

- withdrawal symptoms, such as anxiety, nausea or vomiting, convulsions, trembling, or sleep problems, when the medicine is stopped

Children may be especially sensitive to barbiturates. This sensitivity may increase the chance of side effects such as unusual excitement.

Older people may also be more sensitive than others to the effects of this medicine. In older people, barbiturates may be more likely to cause confusion, depression, and unusual excitement. These effects are also more likely in people who are very ill.

Special conditions

People with certain medical conditions or who are taking certain other medicines can have problems if they take barbiturates. Before taking these drugs, be sure to let the physician know about any of these conditions:

ALLERGIES. Anyone who has had unusual reactions to barbiturates in the past should let his or her physician know before taking the drugs again. The physician should also be told about any allergies to foods, dyes, preservatives, or other substances.

PREGNANCY. Taking barbiturates during pregnancy increases the chance of birth defects and may cause other problems such as prolonged labor and withdrawal effects in the baby after birth. Pregnant women who must take barbiturates for serious or life-threatening conditions should thoroughly discuss with their physicians the benefits and risks of taking this medicine.

BREASTFEEDING. Barbiturates pass into breast milk and may cause problems such as drowsiness, breathing problems, or slow heartbeat in nursing babies whose mothers take the medicine. Women who are breast-feeding should check with their physicians before using barbiturates.

OTHER MEDICAL CONDITIONS. Before using barbiturates, people with any of these medical problems should make sure their physicians are aware of their conditions:

- alcohol or drug abuse
- depression
- hyperactivity (in children)
- pain
- kidney disease
- liver disease
- diabetes
- overactive thyroid
- underactive adrenal gland
- chronic lung diseases such as asthma or emphysema
- severe anemia
- porphyria

USE OF CERTAIN MEDICINES. Taking barbiturates with certain other drugs may affect the way the drugs work or may increase the chance of side effects.

Side effects

The most common side effects are dizziness, lightheadedness, drowsiness, and clumsiness or unsteadiness. These problems usually go away as the body adjusts to the drug and do not require medical treatment unless they persist or interfere with normal activities.

More serious side effects are not common, but may occur. If any of the following side effects occur, the physician who prescribed the medicine should be contacted immediately:

- fever
- muscle or joint pain
- sore throat
- chest pain or tightness in the chest
- wheezing
- skin problems, such as rash, hives, or red, thickened, or scaly skin
- bleeding sores on the lips
- sores or painful white spots in the mouth
- swollen eyelids, face, or lips

In addition, if confusion, depression, or unusual excitement occur after taking barbiturates, a physician should be contacted as soon as possible.

Patients who take barbiturates for a long time or at high doses may notice side effects for some time after they stop taking the drug. These effects usually appear within eight to 16 hours after the patient stops taking the medicine. If these or other troublesome symptoms occur after stopping treatment with barbiturates, a physician should be contacted:

- dizziness, lightheadedness or faintness
- anxiety or restlessness
- hallucinations
- vision problems
- nausea and vomiting
- seizures (convulsions)
- muscle twitches or trembling hands
- weakness
- sleep problems, nightmares, or increased dreaming

Other side effects may occur. Anyone who has unusual symptoms during or after treatment with barbiturates should consult with his or her physician.

Interactions

Birth control pills may not work properly when taken while barbiturates are being taken. To prevent pregnancy, additional methods of birth control are advised while taking barbiturates.

Barbiturates may also interact with other medicines. When this happens, the effects of one or both of the drugs may change or the risk of side effects may be greater. Anyone who takes barbiturates should let the physician know all other medicines he or she is taking. Among the drugs that may interact with barbiturates are:

- other central nervous system (CNS) depressants such as medicine for allergies, colds, hay fever, and asthma; sedatives; tranquilizers; prescription pain medicine; muscle relaxants; medicine for seizures; sleep aids; barbiturates; and anesthetics
- blood thinners
- adrenocorticoids (cortisone-like medicines)
- antiseizure medicines such as valproic acid (Depakote and Depakene), and carbamazepine (Tegretol)

The list above does not include every drug that may interact with barbiturates. A physician or pharmacist should be consulted before combining barbiturates with any other prescription or nonprescription (over-the-counter) medicine.

Resources

BOOKS

AHFS: Drug Information. Washington, DC: American Society of Healthsystems Pharmaceuticals, 2003.

Brody, T. M., J. Larner, K. P. Minneman, and H. C. Neu. *Human Pharmacology: Molecular to Clinical,* 2nd edition. St. Louis: Mosby Year-Book, 1998.

Karch, A. M. *Lippincott's Nursing Drug Guide.* Springhouse, Penn: Lippincott Williams & Wilkins, 2003.

> ## KEY TERMS
> . . . .
>
> **Adrenal glands**—Two glands located next to the kidneys. The adrenal glands produce the hormones epinephrine and norepinephrine and the corticosteroid (cortisone-like) hormones.
>
> **Anemia**—A lack of hemoglobin. Hemoglobin is the compound in blood that carries oxygen from the lungs throughout the body and brings waste carbon dioxide from the cells to the lungs, where it is released.
>
> **Central nervous system**—The brain, spinal cord, and nerves throughout the body.
>
> **Hallucination**—A false or distorted perception of objects, sounds, or events that seems real. Hallucinations usually result from drugs or mental disorders.
>
> **Hypnotic**—A medicine that causes sleep.
>
> **Porphyria**—A disorder in which porphyrins build up in the blood and urine.
>
> **Porphyrin**—A type of pigment found in living things, such as chlorophyll which makes plants green and hemoglobin which makes blood red.
>
> **Sedative**—Medicine that has a calming effect and may be used to treat nervousness or restlessness.
>
> **Seizure**—A sudden attack, spasm, or convulsion.
>
> **Withdrawal symptoms**—A group of physical or mental symptoms that may occur when a person suddenly stops using a drug on which he or she has become dependent.

Reynolds, J. E. F., ed. *Martindale The Extra Pharmacopoeia* 31st Ed. London: The Pharmaceutical Press, 1993.

PERIODICALS

Miller, Norman S. "Sedative-Hypnotics: Pharmacology and Use." *Journal of Family Practice* 29 (December 1989): 665.

Nancy Ross-Flanigan
Sam Uretsky

Barium enema

Definition

A barium enema, also known as a lower GI (gastrointestinal) exam, is a test that uses x-ray examination to view the large intestine. There are two types of tests: the single-contrast technique, where barium sulfate is injected into the rectum to gain a profile view of the large intestine, and the double-contrast (or "air contrast") technique, where air and barium are inserted into the rectum.

Purpose

A barium enema may be performed for a variety of reasons. One reason may be to help in the diagnosis of colon and rectal cancer (or colorectal cancer), and inflammatory disease. Detection of polyps (benign growths in the tissue lining the colon and rectum), diverticula (pouches pushing out from the colon), and structural changes in the large intestine can also be confirmed by the barium enema. The double-contrast barium enema is the best method for detecting small tumors (such as polyps), early inflammatory disease, and bleeding caused by ulcers.

A doctor's decision to perform a barium enema is based on a patient's history of altered bowel habits. These can include diarrhea, constipation, lower abdominal pain, or patient reports of blood, mucus, or pus in the stools. It is recommended that healthy people have a colorectal cancer screening **colonoscopy** every five to 10 years, because this form of cancer is the second most deadly type in the United States. Those who have a close relative with colorectal cancer, or who have had a precancerous polyp, are considered to be at an increased risk for the disease and should be screened more frequently by their doctor for possible abnormalities.

Description

To begin a barium enema, the doctor will have the patient lie with their back down on a tilting radiographic table so that x rays can of the abdomen can be taken. The film is then reviewed by a radiologist, who assesses if the colon has been adequately cleansed of stool during the prep process. After being assisted into a different position, a well-lubricated rectal tube is inserted through the anus. This tube allows the physician or the assisting health care provider to slowly administer the barium into the intestine. While this filling process is closely monitored, the patient must keep the anus tightly contracted against the rectal tube so that the position is maintained and the barium is prevented from leaking. This step is emphasized to the patient because inaccuracy may occur if the barium leaks. A rectal balloon may also be inflated to help the patient retain the barium. The table may be tilted or the patient may be moved to different positions to aid in the filling process.

As the barium fills the intestine, x rays of the abdomen are taken to distinguish significant findings.

There are many ways to perform a barium enema. One way is that shortly after filling, the rectal tube is removed and the patient expels as much of the barium as possible. Alternatively, the tube will remain in place, and the barium will move through that tube. A thin film of barium remains in the intestine, and air is then slowly injected through the rectum and to expand the bowel lumen. Usually no films will be taken until after the air is injected. Multiple films are generally obtained by a radiologist; then, additional films are made by a technologist.

Preparation

To conduct the most accurate barium enema test, the patient must follow a prescribed diet and bowel preparation instructions prior to the test. This preparation commonly includes restricted intake of diary products and a liquid diet for 24 hours prior to the test, in addition to drinking large amounts of water or clear liquids 12–24 hours before the test. Patients may also be given **laxatives**, and asked to give themselves a cleansing enema.

In addition to the prescribed diet and bowel preparation prior to the test, the patient can expect the following during a barium enema:

- They will be well draped with a gown as they are placed on a tilting x-ray table.
- As the barium or air is injected into the intestine, they may experience cramping pains or the urge to defecate.
- The patient will be instructed to take slow, deep breaths through the mouth to ease any discomfort.

Aftercare

Patients should follow several steps immediately after undergoing a barium enema, including:

- Drinking plenty of fluids to help counteract the dehydrating effects of bowel preparation and the test.
- Taking time to rest. A barium enema and the bowel preparation taken before it can be exhausting.
- A cleansing enema may be given to eliminate any remaining barium. Lightly colored stools will be prevalent for the next 24–72 hours following the test.

Risks

While a barium enema is considered a safe screening test used on a routine basis, it can cause complications in certain people. The following indications should be kept in mind before a barium enema is performed:

- Those who have a rapid heart rate, severe ulcerative colitis, toxic megacolon, or a presumed perforation in the intestine should not undergo a barium enema.

KEY TERMS

Barium sulfate—A barium compound used during a barium enema to block the passage of x rays during the exam.

Bowel lumen—The space within the intestine.

Colonoscopy—An examination of the colon performed with a colonoscope.

Diverticula—A diverticulum of the colon is a sac or pouch in the colon wall which is usually asymptomatic (without symptoms) but may cause difficulty if it becomes inflamed. Diverticula is the plural of diverticulum.

Diverticulitis—A condition of the diverticulum of the intestinal tract, especially in the colon, where inflammation may cause distended sacs extending from the colon and pain.

Diverticulosis—The development of diverticula.

Megacolon—Abnormally large colon associated with some chronic intestine disorders.

Proctosigmoidoscopy—A visual examination of the rectum and sigmoid colon using a sigmoidoscope, also known as sigmoidoscopy.

Sigmoidoscopy—Endoscopic examination of the lower colon.

Ulcerative colitis—An ulceration or erosion of the lining of the colon.

• The test can be performed cautiously if the patient has a blocked intestine, ulcerative colitis, diverticulitis, or severe bloody diarrhea.

• Complications that may be caused by the test include perforation of the colon, water intoxication, barium granulomas (inflamed nodules), and allergic reaction. However, these conditions are all very rare.

Normal results

When patients undergo single-contrast enemas, their intestines are steadily filled with barium to differentiate markings of the colon markings. Normal results display uniform filling of the colon.

As the barium is expelled, the intestinal walls collapse. A normal result on the x ray after defecation will show the intestinal lining as having a standard, feathery appearance.

The double-contrast enema expands the intestine, which is already lined with a thin layer of barium, using

air to display a detailed image of the mucosal pattern. Varying positions taken by the patient allow the barium to collect on the dependent walls of the intestine by way of gravity.

A barium enema allows abnormalities to appear on an x ray that may aid in the diagnosis of several different conditions. Most colon cancers occur in the rectosigmoid region, or on the upper part of the rectum and adjoining portion of the sigmoid colon. However, they can also be detected with a proctosigmoidoscopy (usually referred to as a **sigmoidoscopy**). Further, an enema can identify other early signs of cancer.

Identification of polyps, diverticulosis, and inflammatory disease (such as diverticulitis and ulcerative colitis) is attainable through a barium x ray. Some cases of acute appendicitis may also be apparent by viewing this x ray, though acute appendicitis is usually diagnosed clinically, or by CT scan.

Resources

BOOKS

PERIODICALS

Gazelle, G. "Screening for Colorectal Cancer." *Radiology* 327 (May 2000)

Rubesin, S. "Double Contrast Barium Enema Examination Technique." *Radiology* 642 (June 2000).

ORGANIZATIONS

American Cancer Society. 1599 Clifton Rd., NE, Atlanta, GA 30329-4251. (800) 227-2345. <http://www.cancer.org>.

Beth A. Kapes
Lee A. Shratter, M.D.

Barium swallow *see* **Upper GI exam**

Beating heart surgery *see* **Minimally invasive heart surgery**

Beclomethasone *see* **Corticosteroids**

Bedside monitors *see* **Cardiac monitor**

Bedsores

Definition

Bedsores, also called decubitus ulcers, pressure ulcers, or pressure sores, begin as tender, inflamed patches that develop when a person's weight rests against a hard surface, exerting pressure on the skin and soft tissue over bony parts of the body. For example, skin covering a weight-bearing part of the body, such as a knee or hip, is pressed between a bone and a bed, chair, another body part, splint, or other hard object. This is most likely to happen when the person is confined to a bed or wheelchair for long periods of time and is relatively immobile. Usually, mobile individuals, when either conscious or unconscious, will receive nerve signals from the compressed part of the body and will automatically move to relieve the pressure. Pressure sores do not usually develop in people with normal mobility and mental alertness. However, people compromised through acute illness, heavy sedation, unconsciousness, or diminished mental functioning, may not receive signals to move, and as a result of the constant pressure, tissue damage may progress to bedsores in these individuals.

Demographics

Each year, about one million people in the United States develop bedsores at a treatment cost of $1 billion. Pressure sores are most often found in elderly patients; records show that two thirds of all bedsores occur in people over age 70. People who are neurologically impaired, such as those with spinal injuries or paralysis, are also at high risk. Pressure sores have been noted as a direct cause of death in about 8% of paraplegics.

In 1992, the Federal Agency for Health Care Policy and Research reported that bedsores afflict:

• 10% of all hospital patients

• 25% of nursing home residents

• 60% of quadriplegics

Description

Bedsores range from mild inflammation to ulceration (breakdown of tissue) and deep wounds that involve muscle and bone. This painful condition usually starts with shiny red skin that quickly blisters and deteriorates into open sores. These sores become a target for bacterial contamination and will often harbor life-threatening infection. Bedsores are not contagious or cancerous, although the most serious complication of chronic bedsores is the development of malignant degeneration, which is a type of cancer.

Bedsores develop as a result of pressure that cuts off the flow of blood and oxygen to tissue. Constant pressure pinches off capillaries, the tiny blood vessels that deliver oxygen and nutrients to the skin. If the skin is deprived of essential oxygen and nutrients (a condition known as ischemia) for even as little as an hour, tissue cells can die (anoxia) and bedsores can form. Even the

slightest rubbing, called shear, or friction between a hard surface and skin stretched over bones, can cause minor pressure ulcers. They can also develop when a patient stretches or bends blood vessels by slipping into a different position in a bed or chair.

Since urine, feces, or other moisture increases the risk of skin infection, people who suffer from incontinence, as well as immobility, have a greater than average risk of developing bedsores.

Unfortunately, people who have been successfully treated for bedsores have a 90% chance of developing them again. While the pressure sores themselves can usually be cured, about 60,000 deaths per year are attributed to complications caused by bedsores. They can be slow to heal, particularly when the patient's overall status may be weakened. Without proper treatment, bedsores can lead to:

• gangrene (tissue death)

• osteomyelitis (infection of the bone beneath the bedsore)

• sepsis (a poisoning of tissue or the whole body from bacterial infection)

• other localized or systemic infections that slow the healing process, increase the cost of treatment, lengthen hospital or nursing home stays, or cause death

Bedsores are most apt to develop on bony parts of the body, including:

• ankles

• back of the head

• heels

• hips

• knees

• lower back

• shoulder blades

• spine

Although impaired mobility is a leading factor in the development of pressure sores, the risk is also increased by illnesses and conditions that weaken muscle and soft tissue, or that affect blood circulation and the delivery of oxygen to body tissue, leaving skin thinner and more vulnerable to breakdown and subsequent infection. These conditions include:

• atherosclerosis (hardening of arteries) that restricts blood flow

• diabetes

• diminished sensation or lack of feeling, unable to feel pain

- heart problems

- incontinence (inability to control bladder or bowel movements)

- malnutrition

- obesity

- paralysis

- poor circulation

- infection

- prolonged bed rest, especially in unsanitary conditions or with wet or wrinkled sheets

- spinal cord injury

Diagnosis/Preparation

Physical examination, medical history, and patient and caregiver observations are the basis of diagnosis. Special attention must be paid to physical or mental problems, such as an underlying disease, incontinence, or confusion that could complicate a patient's recovery. Nutritional status and smoking history should also be noted.

The National Pressure Ulcer Advisory Panel (NPUAP) recommends classification of bedsores in four stages of ulceration based primarily on the depth of a sore at the time of examination. This helps standardize the language and encourages effective communication of medical personnel caring for patients with bedsores. The NPUAP advises that not all bedsores follow the stages directly from I to IV. The four most widely accepted stages are described as:

- Stage I: intact skin with redness (erythema) and sometimes with warmth.

- Stage II: partial-thickness loss of skin, an abrasion, swelling, and possible blistering or peeling of skin.

- Stage III: full-thickness loss of skin, open wound (crater), and possible exposed under layer.

- Stage IV: full-thickness loss of skin and underlying tissue, extends into muscle, bone, tendon, or joint. Possible bone destruction, dislocations, or pathologic fractures (not caused by injury).

In addition to observing the depth of the wound, the presence or absence of wound drainage and foul odors, or any debris in the wound, such as pieces of dead skin tissue or other material, should also be noted. Any condition that could likely contaminate the wound and cause infection, such as the presence of urine or feces from incontinence, should be noted as well.

A doctor should be notified whenever a person:

- will be bedridden or immobilized for an extended time period

Pressure ulcer. *(Photograph by Michael English, M.D., Custom Medical Stock Photo. Reproduced by permission.)*

- is very weak or unable to move

- develops redness (inflammation) and warmth or peeling on any area of skin

Immediate medical attention is required whenever:

- skin turns black or becomes inflamed, tender, swollen, or warm to the touch

- the patient develops a fever during treatment

- a bedsore contains pus or has a foul-smelling discharge

Prompt medical attention can prevent surface pressure sores from deepening into more serious infections. The first step is always to reduce or eliminate the pressure that is causing bedsores. For minor bedsores, stages I and II, treatment involves relieving pressure, keeping the wound clean and moist, and keeping the area around the ulcer clean and dry. This is often accomplished with saline washes and the use of sterile medicated gauze dressings that both absorb the wound drainage and fight infection-causing bacteria. **Antiseptics**, harsh soaps, and other skin cleansers can damage new tissue and should be avoided. Only saline solution should be used to cleanse bedsores whenever fresh non-stick dressings are applied.

The patient's doctor may prescribe infection-fighting **antibiotics**, special dressings or drying agents, and/or lotions or ointments to be applied to the wound in a thin film three or four times a day. Warm whirlpool treatments are sometimes recommended for sores on the arm, hand, foot, or leg.

Typically, with the removal or reduction of pressure in conjunction with proper treatment and attention to the patient's general health, including good nutrition, bedsores should begin to heal two to four weeks after treatment begins.

Surgical options are often considered for non-healing wounds. When deep wounds are not responding well to standard medical procedures, consultation with a plastic surgeon may be needed to determine if reconstructive surgery is the best possible treatment. In a procedure called debriding, a scalpel may be used to remove dead tissue or other debris from Stage III and IV wounds. A surgical procedure called urinary (or fecal) diversion may also be used with incontinent patients to divert the flow of urinary or fecal material—this keeps the wound clean and encourages wound healing. Reconstruction involves the complete removal of the ulcerated area and surrounding damaged tissue (excision), debriding the bone, and reducing the amount of bacteria in the area with vigorous flushing (lavage) with saline solution. The surgical wound is then drained for a period of days until it is clear that no infection is present and that healing has begun. Plastic surgery may follow to close the wound with a flap (skin from another part of the body), providing a new tissue surface over the bone. For surgery to succeed, infection must not be present. Complications can occur after reconstructive surgery; these include bleeding under the skin (hematoma), wound infection, and the recurrence of pressure sores. Infection in deep wounds can progress to life-threatening systemic infection. **Amputation** may be required when a wound will not heal or when reconstructive surgery is not an option for a particular patient.

Alternatives

Zinc and vitamins A, C, E, and B complex provide necessary nutrients for the skin and help it to repair injuries and stay healthy. Large doses of vitamins or minerals should not be used without a doctor's approval.

A poultice made of equal parts of powdered slippery elm (*Ulmus fulva*), marsh mallow (*Althaea officinalis*), and echinacea blended with a small amount of hot water can relieve minor inflammation. An infection-fighting rinse of two drops of essential tea tree oil (Melaleuca) to every 8 oz (0.23 g) of water can also be administered. An herbal tea made from calendula (*Calendula officinalis*) is also an effective antiseptic and wound healing agent. Calendula cream can also be used.

Contrasting hot and cold compresses applied to the bedsore site can increase circulation to the area and help flush out waste products, speeding the healing process. The temperatures should be extreme (very hot and ice cold), yet tolerable to the skin. Hot compresses should be applied for three minutes, followed by 30 seconds of cold compress application, repeating the cycle three times. The cycle should always end with a cold compress.

Prevention

It is usually possible to prevent bedsores from developing or worsening. In 1989, the NPUAP set a goal that pressure sores be reduced by 50% by 2000. Because of the varying ways in which the number of cases were recorded during this timeframe, the NPUAP is finding it difficult to analyze accurate incident accounts. However even with the diversity of recording methods and the difficulties in comparing data, small group data indicates that progress has been made with the standardization of guidelines and care.

All patients recovering from illness or surgery or confined to a bed or wheelchair long-term should be inspected regularly; they should be bathed or should shower every day using warm water and mild soap; and patients should avoid cold or dry air. Bedridden patients who are either mentally unaware or physically unable to turn themselves, must be repositioned regularly by caregivers at least once every two hours while awake. People who use a wheelchair should be encouraged to shift their weight every 10 or 15 minutes, or be repositioned by caregivers at least once an hour. It is important to lift, rather than to drag, a person being repositioned. Bony parts of the body should not be massaged. Even slight friction can remove the weakened top layer of skin and damage blood vessels beneath it.

If the patient is bedridden, sensitive body parts can be protected by:

• sheepskin pads

• special cushions placed on top of a mattress

• a water-filled mattress

• a variable-pressure mattress with individually inflatable sections to redistribute pressure

Pillows or foam wedges can prevent a bedridden patient's ankles from irritating each other, and pillows placed under the legs from mid-calf to ankle can raise the heels off the bed. Raising the head of the bed slightly and briefly can provide relief, but raising the head of the bed more than 30 degrees can cause the patient to slide, thereby causing damage to skin and tiny blood vessels.

A person who uses a wheelchair should be encouraged to sit up as straight as possible. Pillows behind the head and between the legs can help prevent bedsores, as can a special cushion placed on the chair seat. Donut-shaped cushions should not be used because they restrict blood flow and cause tissues to swell.

Special support surfaces are manufactured and readily available for care in medical facilities or at home, including: air-filled mattresses and cushions, low-air loss beds, and air-fluidized beds. These devices give adequate support while reducing pressure on vulnerable skin. They have been shown to exert less pressure on the skin of compromised patients than do regular mattresses. Pa-

KEY TERMS

Anemia—Deficiency of overall blood, or reduced red cells and hemoglobin, the iron-bearing protein in the blood.

Debridement—Cutting away tissue from a wound.

Gangrene—Tissue death resulting from lack of nutrients and oxygen.

Granulocyte—A type of white cell.

Inflammation (inflamed)—Pain, heat, redness, swelling, and reduced function of tissue, often leading to infection.

Ischemia—Localized anemia, or lack of blood flow and oxygen delivery to a specific area, such as to the skin.

Soft tissue—Layers of cells that form the skin.

Ulceration—Death of tissue cells in a specific area, such as on skin.

tients using these devices and beds must still be repositioned every two hours.

Resources

ORGANIZATIONS

International Association of Enterstomal Therapy. 27241 La Paz Road, Suite 121, Laguna Niguel, CA 92656. (714) 476-0268.

National Pressure Ulcer Advisory Panel. 12100 Sunset Hills Road, Suite 130, Reston, VA 20190. (703) 464-4849. <http://www.npuap.org>.

OTHER

"Bed Sores." *American Health and Herbs Ministry.* March 15, 1998 [cited April 9, 2003]. <http://www.healthherbs. com>.

"Pressure Ulcers." *American Medical Association.* January 8, 2003 [cited April 9, 2003]. <http://www.nlm.nih.gov/ medlineplus>.

"Preventing Bedsores." *Mayo Clinic.* June 5, 2001 [cited February 20, 2003]. <http://www.mayoclinic.com>.

"Preventing Pressure Ulcers." *Atlanta Health Pages Library.* [cited April 9, 2003]. <http://www.healthpages.org/AHP/ LIBRARY/HLTHTOP/MISC/bedsore.htm>.

Maureen Haggerty
L. Lee Culvert

Betamethasone *see* **Corticosteroids**

Bicarbonate test *see* **Electrolyte tests**

Bile duct stone removal *see* **Endoscopic retrograde cholangiopancreatography**

Biliary stenting

Definition

A biliary stent is a plastic or metal tube that is inserted into a bile duct to relieve narrowing of the duct (also called bile duct stricture).

Purpose

Biliary stenting is used to treat obstructions that occur in the bile ducts. Bile is a substance that helps to digest fats and is produced by the liver, secreted through the bile ducts, and stored in the gallbladder. It is released into the small intestine after a fat-containing meal has been eaten. The release of bile is controlled by a muscle called the sphincter of Oddi found at the junction of the bile ducts and the small intestine.

There are a number of conditions, malignant or benign, that can cause strictures of the bile duct. Pancreatic cancer is the most common malignant cause, followed by cancers of the gallbladder, bile duct, liver, and large intestine. Noncancerous causes of bile duct stricture include:

- injury to the bile ducts during surgery for gallbladder removal (accounting for 80% of nonmalignant strictures)
- pancreatitis (inflammation of the pancreas)
- primary sclerosing cholangitis (an inflammation of the bile ducts that may cause pain, jaundice, itching, or other symptoms)
- gallstones

WHO PERFORMS THE PROCEDURE AND WHERE IS IT PERFORMED?

Biliary stenting is usually performed in the x-ray department of a hospital or outpatient facility in consultation with a general surgeon, a gastroenterologist (a medical doctor who specializes in the diagnosis and treatment of diseases of the digestive system), and/or an interventional radiologist (a medical doctor who specializes in the treatment of medical disorders using specialized imaging techniques).

- radiation therapy
- blunt trauma to the abdomen

Demographics

The overall incidence of bile duct stricture is not known. Approximately 0.2–0.5% of patients undergoing gallbladder surgery or other operations affecting the bile duct develop biliary stricture.

Description

A biliary stent is a thin, tube-like structure that is used to support a narrowed part of the bile duct and prevent the reformation of the stricture. Stents may be made of plastic or metal. The two most common methods that are used to place a biliary stent are **endoscopic retrograde cholangiopancreatography** (ERCP) and percutaneous transhepatic cholangiography (PTC).

ERCP

ERCP is an imaging technique used to diagnose diseases of the pancreas, liver, gallbladder, and bile ducts that also has the advantage of being used as a therapeutic device. The endoscope (a thin, lighted, hollow tube attached to a viewing screen) is inserted into a patient's mouth, down the esophagus, through the stomach, and into the upper part of the small intestine, until it reaches the spot where the bile ducts empty. At this point a small tube called a cannula is inserted through the endoscope and used to inject a contrast dye into the ducts; the term retrograde refers to the backward direction of the dye. A series of x rays are then taken as the dye moves through the ducts.

If the x rays show that a biliary stricture exists, a stent may be placed into a duct to relieve the obstruction.

In order to do this, special instruments are inserted into the endoscope and a sphincterotomy (a cut into the sphincter of Oddi) is performed to provide access to the bile ducts. In some cases, the biliary stricture may first be dilated (expanded) using a thin, flexible tube called a catheter, followed by a balloon-type device that is inflated. The stent is then inserted into the bile duct.

PTC

PTC is similar to ERCP in that the test is used to diagnose and treat obstructions affecting the flow of bile from the liver to the gastrointestinal tract. The procedure is generally reserved for patients who have undergone unsuccessful ERCP. A thin needle is used to inject a contrast dye through the skin and into the liver or gallbladder; x rays are taken while the dye moves through the bile ducts. If a biliary stricture becomes evident, a stent may then be placed. A hollow needle is introduced into the bile duct, and a thin guide wire inserted into the needle. The wire is guided to the area of obstruction; the stent is advanced over the wire and placed in the obstructed duct.

Diagnosis/Preparation

Prior to ERCP or PTC, the patient will be instructed to refrain from eating or drinking for at least six hours to ensure that the stomach and upper part of the intestine are free of food. The physician should be notified as to what medications the patient takes and if the patient has an allergy to iodine, which is found in the contrast dye. **Antibiotics** will be started prior to surgery and continued for several days afterward.

Aftercare

After the procedure, the patient is monitored for signs of complications. In the case of ERCP, the patient generally remains at the hospital or outpatient facility until the effects of the sedative wear off and to ensure no complications occur. After PTC, the patient is instructed to lie on his or her right side for at least six hours to reduce the risk of bleeding from the injection site. To ensure that the stent is functioning properly, the patient will be frequently assessed for symptoms that indicate the recurrence of biliary stricture. These symptoms include changes in stool or urine color, jaundice (yellowing of the skin), itching, and abnormal **liver function tests**.

Risks

Complications associated with ERCP include excessive bleeding, infection, pancreatitis, cholangitis (inflammation of the bile ducts), cholecystitis (inflammation of the gallbladder), and injury to the intestine. PTC may re-

KEY TERMS

Hepatic duct—A duct that carries bile from the liver.

Intestinal perforation—A hole in the intestinal wall.

Pancreas—An organ that secretes pancreatic juice into the upper part of the intestine; pancreatic juice is composed of specialized proteins that help to digest fats, proteins, and carbohydrates.

sult in bleeding, infection of the injection site, sepsis (spread of infection to the blood), or leakage of the dye into the abdomen. Complications specific to the stent include migration (movement of the stent out of the area in which it was placed), occlusion (blockage), and intestinal perforation.

Normal results

In more than 90% of patients, the placement of a biliary stent relieves the obstruction and allows the bile duct to drain properly.

Morbidity and mortality rates

The rate of serious complications with ERCP is approximately 11%, and 5–10% with PTC. Stent occlusion occurs in up to 25% of patients, and stent migration in up to 6%. Recurrence of biliary stricture occurs in 15–45% of patients after an average time of four to nine years.

Alternatives

The major alternative to biliary stenting is surgical repair of the stricture. The most common method is resection (removal) of the narrowed area followed by the creation of a connection between the bile duct and the middle portion of the small intestine (called a choledochojejunostomy) or the hepatic duct and the small intestine (called a hepaticojejunostomy). Surgical stricture repair results in a cure for 85–98% of patients and is associated with a low risk of complications.

Resources

BOOKS

Feldman, Mark, et al. *Sleisenger & Fordtran's Gastrointestinal and Liver Disease.* 7th ed. Philadelphia: Elsevier Science, 2002.

ORGANIZATIONS

American Gastroenterological Association. 7910 Woodmont Ave., 7th Floor, Bethesda, MD 20814. (301) 654–2055. <http://www.gastro.org>.

American Society for Gastrointestinal Endoscopy. 1520 Kensington Rd., Suite 202, Oak Brook, IL 60523. (630) 573–0600. <http://www.asge.org>.

Society of Interventional Radiology. 10201 Lee Highway, Suite 500, Fairfax, VA 22030. (800) 488–7284. <http://www.sirweb.org>.

OTHER

Pande, Hemant, Parviz Nikoomanesh, and Lawrence Cheskin. "Bile Duct Strictures." *eMedicine.* June 3, 2002 [cited May 1, 2003]. <http://www.emedicine.com/med/topic 3425.htm>.

Yakshe, Paul. "Biliary Disease." *eMedicine.* March 29, 2002 [cited April 7, 2003]. <http://www.emedicine.com/MED/topic225.htm>.

Stephanie Dionne Sherk

Bispectral index

Definition

The bispectral index (BIS) is one of several systems used in anesthesiology as of 2003 to measure the effects of specific anesthetic drugs on the brain and to track changes in the patient's level of sedation or hypnosis. In technical terms, the bispectral index itself is a complex mathematical algorithm that allows a computer inside an anesthesia monitor to analyze data from a patient's electroencephalogram (EEG) during surgery. BIS, which has been in use since 1997, is a type of automated direct measurement of the patient's condition, in comparison to the Glasgow Coma Scale and similar scoring systems, which are indirect assessments of sedation.

Purpose

Anesthetic depth

A brief discussion of anesthetic depth may be helpful in understanding people's interest in monitoring the brain's responses to anesthesia. Ever since the first modern anesthetics (ether, chloroform, and nitrous oxide) were used in the 1840s, doctors have been searching for a reliable method of measuring the depth of the patient's unconsciousness in order to guarantee the safety as well as the painlessness of surgery. Anesthetic drugs, whether inhaled or given intravenously, are toxic in high doses; too high a dose can stop the patient's breathing. On the other hand, too small a dose can result in the patient's coming to various degrees of awareness during surgery. Events of this type occur frequently enough to be publicized in general medical news sources as well as the professional literature. One Australian medical journal reports that postoperative recall of operations, including the patient's overhearing conversations among members of the **surgical team** as well as feeling helpless and experiencing physical pain, occurs in one of every 1,000 patients undergoing non-cardiac surgery and three of every 1,000 cardiac patients. An Israeli researcher gives the rate of accidental awareness during surgery as between 0.2% and 1.2% of patients. According to an American news account, "An estimated 40,000 to 200,000 mid-operative awakenings may occur each year in the United States alone." Research has indicated that patients' attitudes toward undergoing surgery are affected by the possibility of awakening during the procedure. A group of Australian researchers found that 56% of a group of 200 patients awaiting surgery had heard about awareness during operations, mostly from the mass media; 42.5% of the group expressed anxiety about it. Post-traumatic stress disorder (PTSD) is a common result of awareness episodes; a 2001 study done at Boston University reported that 56.3% of a group of patients who had awakened during surgery met the diagnostic criteria for PTSD—as late as 17 years after their operation.

There are several reasons for anesthesiologists' difficulty in evaluating dosages of anesthetic agents:

• The lack of a universally accepted definition of "consciousness." There are a number of scientific periodicals devoted solely to the study of human consciousness, as it concerns philosophers, psychologists, psychiatrists, and lawyers, as well as doctors involved in anesthesiology and critical care medicine. Some researchers emphasize the emotional or psychological dimensions of consciousness while others focus on physiological definitions—for example, the response of skin or muscle tissue to painful stimuli.

• The complex effects of anesthesia on the human organism. Scholarly debates about the nature of human consciousness are reflected in the variety of different goals that surgical anesthesia is expected to achieve. These goals are usually listed as blocking the nervous system's responses to pain (analgesia), inducing muscular relaxation and blocking reflexes (areflexia), keeping the patient asleep during the procedure (hypnosis), and preventing conscious recall of the procedure afterwards (amnesia). It is not always possible, however, to meet all four goals with the same degree of accuracy, since some

patients suffer from health conditions that require the anesthesiologist to keep them under lighter sedation in order to lower the risk of heart or circulation problems.

• The increased use of combinations of anesthetic agents rather than single drugs. At present, anesthesiologists rarely use inhaled anesthetics by themselves; most prefer what is known as balanced anesthesia, which combines inhaled and intravenous anesthetics. When different agents are used together, however, they are often synergistic, which means that they intensify each other's effects. This characteristic makes it more difficult for the anesthesiologist to predict how much of each drug will be needed during the operation.

• Changes in the patient's response to anesthesia over the course of the operation.

• Age- and sex-related differences in responsiveness to specific anesthetics. Anesthesiologists have become increasingly aware of the special needs of elderly patients, for example; they are more likely than younger patients to develop cardiovascular complications under anesthesia. With regard to sex, several studies have reported that women appear to emerge from anesthesia more rapidly than men after standardized anesthetic administration with the same agents.

• Large differences among individuals apart from age or sex groupings in regard to sensitivity to anesthesia.

Indirect measurements of consciousness

Indirect methods that allow an observer to assess a person's level of awareness have been used since the early 1970s. The earliest and most widely used instrument for evaluating impaired consciousness is the Glasgow Coma Scale (GCS), first published in the *Lancet* in 1974. The GCS evaluates the patient's responsiveness under three headings: eye response (four levels of responsiveness), verbal response (five levels), and motor (movement) response (six levels). A normally conscious individual would score 15, the maximum score. In practice, however, the total score on the GCS is usually broken down into three subscores for the three types of response measured; thus E2V2M3 would represent a total GCS score of 7. Total scores on the Glasgow Coma Scale are interpreted as follows: 13–14 indicates mild impairment of consciousness; 9–12 indicates moderate impairment; 8 or lower indicates coma.

There are about a dozen other scales that have been devised to measure consciousness in addition to the GCS; the two that are the most important in this context are the Ramsay Sedation Score, first published in 1974 as a measurement of sedation in patients receiving intravenous sedatives prior to surgery; and the Observer's Assessment of Alertness/Sedation Scale (OAA/SS), first used in 1990 for the same purpose as the Ramsay. These two instruments are significant because they are commonly used in research evaluations of the bispectral index and similar monitoring systems. The Ramsay Score is a six-point scale ranging from one ("patient agitated or restless") through six ("patient asleep; has no response to firm nailbed pressure or other noxious stimuli"). A score of 1 indicates inadequate sedation; 2–4, an acceptable level of sedation; and 5–6, oversedation.

The OAA/SS resembles the Glasgow Coma Scale in that it evaluates different categories of responsiveness, although the categories are different. The OAA/SS measures the patient's responsiveness to his or her name, quality of speech, degree of facial relaxation, and ability to focus the eyes.

Direct measurements of consciousness

A variety of different physiological responses have been used in attempts to measure the depth of a patient's unconsciousness under anesthesia. Most anesthesiologists use hemodynamic responses—the patient's blood pressure and heart rate—as basic guidelines for adjusting the amount of anesthetic delivered to the patient during surgery. Other direct measurements have been based on movements of the patient's body during surgery, hormonal responses, sweating, eye movement, and the reactivity of the eyes to light. One difficulty that has emerged from these attempts at direct measurement is that that they are not good predictors of the likelihood of awareness during surgery or recall of the procedure after surgery.

Another measurement that researchers have explored in their attempts to measure depth of anesthesia directly is the electroencephalogram, or EEG. The EEG is a complex recording of the electrical activity of the nerve cells in the brain. The first published paper on the EEG was written in 1929 by Dr. Hans Berger, an Austrian psychiatrist, on 73 recordings of brain waves using his son Klaus as the subject. Berger was the first to distinguish between alpha and beta brain waves, and to use the term EEG to describe the technique of **electroencephalography**. In 1931 Berger discovered that brain waves change in amplitude and frequency when a person is asleep or anesthetized; they slow down, shift to lower frequencies, and become more closely synchronized with one another. He also noted that such diseases as multiple sclerosis and Alzheimer disease affect a person's EEG.

Several attempts were made in the late 1980s and early 1990s to make use of what is known about changes in the EEG in order to monitor anesthetic depth. One attempt is known as spectral edge frequency, or SEF. SEF is the frequency just above 95% of the total power spectrum of electrical energy recorded on an EEG. It was thought that the spectral edge frequency would be useful in guiding adjustments of anesthetics administered during surgery. Unfortunately, SEF is difficult to use with balanced anesthesia; it is also difficult to correlate with such other measures of anesthetic depth as movement or memory of the procedure. Another method that has been tried is median frequency, which is based on the median frequency of the complex EEG electrical signal at any given moment. This method proved to have the same drawbacks as spectral edge frequency. The bispectral index can be understood historically as a slightly later and more sophisticated attempt to use EEG signals to monitor patients' responses to anesthesia.

Development of the bispectral index

The bispectral index was first developed in the early 1990s by applying bispectral analysis to EEG recordings. Bispectral analysis is a method of analyzing the mathematical relationships among the various components of an EEG signal (phase couplings) as well as measuring amplitudes and frequencies. To compile a database for the index, researchers recorded EEGs from several thousand patients and volunteers anesthetized with a range of commonly used anesthetics and anesthetic combinations. Each subject's depth of unconsciousness was evaluated on the basis of a modified version of the OAA/SS described earlier (in the volunteers) or the amount of drug concentration in blood serum (in the patients). Segments of the recorded EEGs were used to draw up a set of EEG features that were then tested for their ability to distinguish between different levels of sedation or unconsciousness. The index that resulted from this process was then tested on different EEG recordings from the researchers' larger database. It is scaled from 100 to 0 so that the BIS value decreases linearly with increasing doses of anesthesia.

It should be noted that the bispectral index is a work in progress. As new anesthetic agents are developed and used, the BIS algorithm is continually retested and refined. In addition, the algorithm is proprietary information, which means that it is kept secret by the company that developed it.

Description

When a patient is brought into the **operating room**, special BIS sensors are applied to his or her forehead. No additional gels or electrodes are required. The anesthesiologist can attach the sensors to the patient in less than 30 seconds, since preparing the patient's skin requires no more than an alcohol wipe to provide good electrical contact. The BIS system itself is integrated into patient monitoring devices produced by a number of different manufacturers that use enhanced EEG monitors. The BIS system displays both raw data from the EEG and a single number between 100 (indicating an awake patient) and 0 (indicating the absence of brain activity) that represents the patient's degree of sedation. The target number for most anesthetized patients is between 50 and 60.

Results

Current applications of BIS

BIS is presently used in intensive care units (ICUs) and some emergency departments as well as in operating rooms. According to company information, the bispectral index is used in about 26% of all hospital operating rooms in the United States as of late 2002. It is claimed that BIS reduces the risk of patient awareness during surgery as well as lowering hospital costs by speeding patient recovery and reducing the overuse of anesthetic agents.

Limitations of BIS

As of 2003, published studies of the bispectral index and other anesthetic monitoring systems presently available indicate that none of them can be considered a "gold standard" for preventing instances of patient awareness under anesthesia or for predicting the depth of anesthesia in a specific patient. Researchers have noted several specific limitations of the BIS system:

• BIS values are affected by the choice of anesthetic agent. This finding means that a patient with a BIS score of 60 anesthetized with one combination of agents may be more deeply sedated than another patient with the same score but anesthetized with a different combination of drugs. In addition, the BIS monitor appears unable to accurately track changes in consciousness produced by certain anesthetics, specifically ketamine and nitrous oxide.

• The changes in the BIS algorithm resulting from updating and refinement of the producer's database make it difficult to compare results obtained by different investigators using different versions of the BIS monitor. This fact also leaves hospital-based anesthesiologists uncertain as to whether findings based on earlier versions of the BIS system are still valid.

• BIS values are difficult to correlate with other measurements of anesthetic depth or altered consciousness. One group of Norwegian researchers found that BIS values had little relationship to serum blood concentrations of anesthetic agents. Other researchers in the United States have found that BIS scores showed wide variability when compared with Glasgow Coma Scores for emergency room patients.

• Standard BIS scores are not useful in monitoring special patient populations, particularly critically ill patients with unstable body temperatures and patients with dementia.

Alternatives

Other anesthesia monitoring systems that are in use as of 2003 include the Patient State Analyzer, or PSA 4000, which is also based on EEG data; and the A-Line (R) monitor, which processes signals derived from auditory stimuli. Current opinion among anesthesiologists appears to be that none of the present monitoring systems are sufficiently sensitive to guarantee that patients will not awaken during surgery while simultaneously preventing undesirable cardiovascular reactions, other stress responses, or overuse of anesthetic agents.

See also Anesthesiologist's role; Intensive care unit equipment; Sedation, conscious.

Resources

PERIODICALS

Baars, Bernard J. "The Brain Basis of a 'Consciousness Monitor.' A Breakthrough in Testing Unconsciousness During Anesthesia." *Science and Consciousness Review* 1 May 2002 [cited May 13, 2003]. <http://www.psych.pomona.edu/scr/news/articles/20020401.html>.

Blanchard, Amy R. "Sedation and Analgesia in Critical Care." *Postgraduate Medicine* 111 (February 2002): 59–60, 63–64, 67–70.

Drover, D. R., H. J. Lemmens, E. T. Pierce, et al. "Patient State Index: Titration of Delivery and Recovery from Propofol, Alfentanil, and Nitrous Oxide Anesthesia." *Anesthesiology* 97 (July 2002): 82–89.

Drummond, John C. "Monitoring Depth of Anesthesia: With Emphasis on the Application of the Bispectral Index and the Middle Latency Auditory Evoked Response to the Prevention of Recall." *Anesthesiology* 93 (September 2000): 876–882.

Frenzel, D., C. A. Greim, C. Sommer, et al. "Is the Bispectral Index Appropriate for Monitoring the Sedation Level of Mechanically Ventilated ICU Patients?" *Intensive Care Medicine* 28 (February 2002): 178–183.

Gill, M., S. M. Green, and B. Krauss. "Can the Bispectral Index Monitor Quantify Altered Level of Consciousness in Emergency Department Patients?" *Academic Emergency Medicine* 10 (February 2003): 175–179.

Hameroff, Stuart, MD. "Anesthesia: The 'Other Side' of Consciousness." *Consciousness and Cognition* 10 (June 2001): 217–229.

Hoymork, S. C., J. Raeder, B. Grimsmo, and P. A. Steen. "Bispectral Index, Predicted and Measured Drug Levels of Target-Controlled Infusions of Remifentanil and Propofol During Laparoscopic Cholecystectomy and Emergence." *Acta Anaesthesiological Scandinavica* 44 (October 2000): 1138–1144.

KEY TERMS

Algorithm—A procedure or formula for solving a problem. It is often used to refer to a sequence of steps used to program a computer to solve a specific problem.

Analgesia—Absence of the ability to feel pain. The term is also sometimes used to refer to pain relief without loss of consciousness. An analgesic is a drug that is given to relieve pain.

Anesthesia—Loss of the ability to feel pain, brought about by administration of a drug or such other medical interventions as hypnosis or acupuncture.

Anesthesiology—The branch of medicine that specializes in the study of anesthetic agents, their effects on patients, and their proper use and administration.

Areflexia—A condition in which the body's normal reflexes are absent. It is one of the objectives of general anesthesia.

Balanced anesthesia—The use of a combination of inhaled and intravenous drugs in anesthetizing patients.

Coma—A state of unconsciousness from which a person cannot be aroused, even by strong or painful stimuli.

Electroencephalogram (EEG)—A recording of the electrical activity of the nerve cells in the brain. The first such recording was made in 1929 by Hans Berger, an Austrian psychiatrist.

Hemodynamics—Measurement of the movements involved in the circulation of the blood; it usually includes blood pressure and heart rate.

Hypnosis—The term is used to refer to a specific verbal technique for refocusing a person's attention in order to change their perceptions, judgment, control of movements, and memory. A hypnotic medication is one that induces sleep.

Proprietary—Referring to a drug, device, or formula that is secret or sold only by the holder of the patent, trademark, or copyright. The algorithm used in BIS systems is proprietary information.

Sedation—A condition of calm or relaxation, brought about by the use of a drug or medication.

Sequela (plural, sequelae)—An abnormal condition or event resulting from a previous disease or disorder.

Synergistic—Enhancing the effects of another drug. Anesthetics given in combination are often synergistic.

Kalkman, Cor J., and John C. Drummond. "Monitors of Depth of Anesthesia, Quo Vadis?" *Anesthesiology* 96 (April 2002): 784–787.

Leslie, K., and P. S. Myles. "Awareness During General Anesthesia: Is It Worth Worrying About?" *Medical Journal of Australia* 174 (March 5, 2001): 212–213.

Leslie, K., L. Lee, P. S. Myles, et al. "Patients' Knowledge of and Attitudes Toward Awareness and Depth of Anesthesia Monitoring." *Anaesthesia and Intensive Care* 31 (February 2003): 63–68.

Muncaster, A. R., J. W. Sleigh, and M. Williams. "Changes in Consciousness, Conceptual Memory, and Quantitative Electroencephalographical Measures During Recovery from Sevoflurane- and Remifentanil-Based Anesthesia." *Anesthesia and Analgesia* 96 (March 2003): 720–725.

Osterman, J. E., J. Hopper, W. J. Heran, et al. "Awareness Under Anesthesia and the Development of Posttraumatic Stress Disorder." *General Hospital Psychiatry* 23 (July-August 2001): 198–204.

Renna, M., J. Handy, and A. Shah. "Low Baseline Bispectral Index of the Electroencephalogram in Patients with Dementia." *Anesthesia and Analgesia* 96 (May 2003): 1380–1385.

Riess, M. L., U. A. Graefe, C. Goeters, et al. "Sedation Assessment in Critically Ill Patients with Bispectral Index." *European Journal of Anaesthesiology* 19 (January 2002): 18–22.

Tassi, P., and A. Muzet. "Defining the States of Consciousness." *Neuroscience and Biobehavioral Reviews* 25 (March 2001): 175–191.

Welsby, Ian J., J. Mark Ryan, John V. Booth, et al. "The Bispectral Index in the Diagnosis of Perioperative Stroke: A Case Report and Discussion." *Anesthesia and Analgesia* 96 (February 2003): 435–437.

Wong, C. S. "What's the Matter of Depth of Anesthesia?" *Acta Anaesthesiologica Sinica* 39 (March 2001): 1–2.

ORGANIZATIONS

American Academy of Emergency Medicine (AAEM). 611 East Wells Street, Milwaukee, WI 53202. (800) 884-2236. <http://www.aaem.org>.

American Association of Nurse Anesthetists (AANA). 222 South Prospect Avenue, Park Ridge, IL 60068-4001. (847) 692-7050. <http://www.aana.com>.

American Society of Anesthesiologists (ASA). 520 N. Northwest Highway, Park Ridge, IL 60068-2573. (847) 825-5586. <http://www.asahq.org>.

American Society of Perianesthesia Nurses (ASPAN). 10 Melrose Avenue, Suite 110, Cherry Hill, NJ 08003. (877) 737-9696 or (856) 616-9600. <http://www.aspan.org>.

Center for Emergency Medicine. 230 McKee Place, Suite 500, Pittsburgh, PA 15213. (412) 647-5300. <http://www.centerem.com>.

Society for Technology in Anesthesia (STA). PMB 300, 223 North Guadalupe, Santa Fe, NM 87501. (505) 983-4923. <http://www.anestech.org>.

OTHER

Aspect Medical Systems White Paper. *Technology Overview: Bispectral Index*. Natick, MA: Aspect Medical Systems, 1997.

Greenwald, Scott D., Ph.D., Charles P. Smith, Jeffrey C. Sigl, Ph.D., et al. *Development of the EEG Bispectral Index (R) (BIS(R))*. Abstract presented at the first annual meeting of the Society for Technology in Anesthesia (STA). January 2000 [cited May 12, 2003]. <http://www.anestech.org/Publications/Annual_2000/Greenwald.html>.

Vuyk, Jaap, MD. *Does Bispectral Index Monitoring Optimize Intravenous Anaesthetic Drug Delivery?* Paper delivered on April 5, 2002 at the fifth annual meeting of the European Society for Intravenous Anaesthesia (Eurosiva) in Nice, France. <http://www.eurosiva.org/Archive/Nice/SpeakerAbstracts/Vuyk.htm>.

Rebecca Frey, Ph.D.

Bladder augmentation

Definition

Bladder augmentation, also known as augmentation cystoplasty, is reconstructive surgery to increase the reservoir capacity of the bladder. The procedure is very common and involves tissue grafts (anastomosis) from a section of the small intestine (ileum), stomach, or other substitutes that are attached to the urinary bladder by sewing or stapling. Whether due to chronic obstructive bladder damage, birth defects that resulted in small reservoir capacity, or dysfunction due to nerve innervation of the bladder muscle (sphincter), surgery is chosen only after a thorough medical work-up that involves assessment of the lower urinary tract, functional physiological evaluation, and anatomic assessment. Some laparoscopic methods (surgery with a fiber-optic instrument inserted through the abdomen) of bladder augmentation have been tried, but reports indicate that these are technically arduous and may not have the long-lasting effects of open surgery.

Purpose

Bladder dysfunction and incontinence may be due to problems with the reservoir capacity of the bladder or with the "gatekeeping" muscle (the sphincter), which, instructed

by the brain, allows urine to build up or to be released. Bladder augmentation is used to treat serious and irreversible forms of incontinence and to protect the upper urinary tract (kidney function) from reflexia (urine back up to the kidneys). Many candidates for the surgery are highly compromised individuals with other serious conditions like spinal cord injuries and multiple sclerosis, as well as patients likely to undergo **kidney transplantation**. Patients who undergo bladder augmentation must be free of bowel and urethral disease and be able to perform self-catheterization (able to place a urinary tube into their urethra).

Description

Standard augmentation involves segments of the bowel used to create a pouch or wider wall for the bladder in order to enhance its reservoir capacity. Often this reconstruction surgery is accompanied by procedures that tighten the neck of the bladder, as well. Milkulicz performed the first clinical augmentation cystoplasty using abdominal tissue in 1898. Couvelaire, in the 1950s, popularized bladder augmentation for the treatment of the contracted bladder due to tuberculosis. Until the 1970s it was thought that those with bladder dysfunction could be treated with bladder diversion, and that this procedure offered a simple and safe means of emptying the bladder. However, it was soon discovered that pressure from the bladder caused irreparable damage to the kidneys, with 50% of patients exhibiting such deterioration. The new diagnostic assessment of the bladder as well as the need for a new medical intervention for patients with severe bladder dysfunction opened the way for urinary tract reconstruction. Today, many techniques are available, along with new types of grafting substitutions.

The basic procedure involves open abdominal surgery with resection of a 10–20 in (25–30-cm) segment of ileum, cecum (first part of the large intestine), or the ileocecum (the junction of small and large intestines) cut down the middle (detubularized), and shaped into a U-configuration with a pouch at the bottom. This opening or pouch will be the "patch" for the bladder. During surgery, the bladder itself is also opened at the dome and cut at right angles to

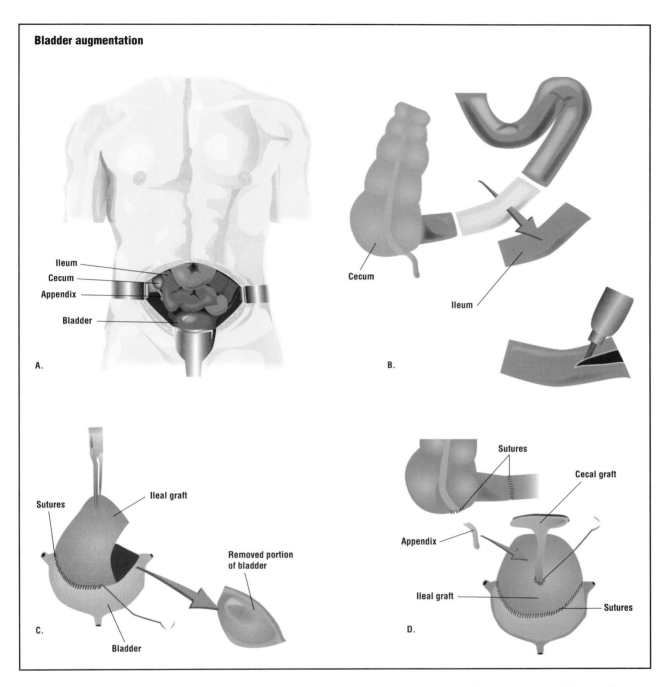

Bladder augmentation

A.

Ileum
Cecum
Appendix
Bladder

B.

Cecum
Ileum

C.

Sutures
Ileal graft
Removed portion
of bladder
Bladder

D.

Sutures
Cecal graft
Appendix
Ileal graft
Sutures

During a bladder augmentation procedure, an incision is made in the abdomen to expose the intestines and bladder (A). A section of ileum (small intestine) is removed and opened (B). After being sterilized, it is grafted onto the bladder to increase its capacity (C). The appendix and cecum (large intestine) may also be used (D). *(Illustration by GGS Inc.)*

create a clam-like shape. The open bowel "patch" is then attached to the bladder with sutures or stapling.

Diagnosis/Preparation

Patients selected for bladder augmentation are chosen after they undergo a thorough physical exam, x-ray tests, and bladder physiology tests, as well as a renal and bladder ultrasound for any dilation of the kidneys or ureters or kidney obstruction. A VCUG (holding and voiding urine) test is performed to assess the contour of the bladder and to assess for ureteral reflux (back up of urine to the kidneys). Finally, a CMG (cystometrogram) is performed in the physician's office to judge the pres-

QUESTIONS TO ASK THE DOCTOR

- How many bladder augmentation surgeries do you perform a year?
- What complications of this surgery do you think are the most likely and/or worrisome?
- Are there other patients with my underlying medical conditions who have had this surgery that I could contact?
- Is there a pre-op patient group with this hospital that could help me understand my rehabilitation and help with the compliance with the diet and self-catherization?

sure and volume levels at which the urine leakage occurs. Once the tests, as well as the history and physical exam are completed, treatment plans commence.

The patient should plan for up to two weeks in the hospital. The patient will have been on a low-residue diet for a few days before admission. Surgery will take place two to three days after hospital admittance. In the hospital, a general examination will be performed and blood taken. The bowel will need to be cleaned in preparation. Clear fluids will be given, as well as a strong laxative prior to surgery.

Aftercare

Early complications of surgery include cardiovascular, thrombo-embolic (blood clot), gastrointestinal, and respiratory complications associated with major abdominal surgery. Many patients require three months after surgery to allow their augmented bladder to establish itself. This involves a special diet for a few months as well as patient familiarity with the fact that the augmented bladder empties after the native bladder. Two weeks after surgery tests are performed to ensure that the patch is leak proof. Once a watertight reservoir is demonstrated, the catheters and drains that were introduced for surgery are removed.

Risks

Long term risks of the procedure include peptic ulceration of the bladder and perforation of the gastric segment. Spontaneous perforation is rare but it is life threatening and has a 25% mortality rate. Other risks include bacterial infections, metabolic changes, urinary tract infections, and urinary tract stones. Nocturnal incontinence is sometimes a problem after the surgery.

Normal results

Although some patients recover spontaneous voiding function, this does not occur with reliable predictability. Preoperatively, patients should be prepared for the likelihood that they will have to perform lifelong intermittent catherization and irrigation of the augmented bladder. Other effects are a special diet for up to three months and pain after surgery.

Morbidity and mortality rates

Reported surgical risks include 3–5.7% rate of adhesive small bowel obstruction requiring operative intervention, 5–6% incidence of wound infection, 0–3% reoperation rate for bleeding. Long term complications include a 50% unchanged bladder compliance and renal deterioration. No reduction in growth in children has been reported, but the procedure is not recommended for children who have not reached puberty, unless there is the threat of kidney damage.

Alternatives

Bladder augmentation is a medical treatment of last resort for those patients unable to avoid incontinence through medical alternatives. Other surgeries may be indicated if the individual is not a candidate for self-catherization or has other medical or psychological conditions that would rule out bladder augmentation.

Resources

BOOKS

Dewan, P., and M. E. Mitchell, eds. *Bladder Augmentation.* Oxford Press, 2000.

PERIODICALS

Abrams, P., S.K. Lowry, et al. "Assessment and Treatment of Urinary Incontinence." *Lancet* 355 (June 2000): 2153–58

Fantl, J. A., D. K. Newman, J. Colling, et al. "Urinary Incontinence in Adults: Acute and Chronic Management. Clinical Practice Guideline, Number 2, 1996." *Agency for Health Policy and Research Publications* (March 1996).

Greenwell, T. J., S. N. Venn, and A. R. Mundy. "Augmentation Cystoplasty." *British Journal of Urology International* 88, no. 6 (October 2001): 511–534.

Qucek, M. I., and D. A. Ginsberg. "Long-term Urodynamics Follow-up of Bladder Augmentation for Neurogenic Bladder." *Urology* 169 (January 2003): 195–198.

Rackley, R. R., and J. B. Abdelmalak. "Radical Prostatectomy: Laparoscopic Augmentation Cystoplasty." *Urological Clinics of America* 28 (August 2001).

ORGANIZATIONS

National Association for Continence. P.O. Box 8310 Spartanburg, SC 29305. (800) BLADDER, (252-3337). <http://www.nafc.org>.

KEY TERMS

Anamotosis—The surgical union of parts and especially hollow tubular parts.

Catherization—the use of or insertion of a catheter (as in or into the bladder, trachea, or heart).

Cystoplasty—Reconstructive surgery of the urinary bladder.

Neurogenic bladder—A urinary problem of neurological origin in which there is abnormal emptying of the bladder with subsequent retention or incontinence of urine.

Ureter—Either of the paired channels that carry urine from a kidney to the bladder.

National Kidney and Urologic Diseases Information Clearinghouse. 3 Information Way, Bethesda, MD 20892-3580. (301) 654-4415. <http://www.niddk.nih.gov>.

The Simon Foundation for Continence. P.O. Box 835 Wilmette, IL 60091. (800) 23SIMON (237-4666). <http://www.simon foundation.org>.

OTHER

"Bladder Augmentation." Dr. Rajhttp. [cited April 2003]. <http://www.drrajmd.com/treatments/treatments.htm>.

Carr, Michael, and M. E. Mitchell. "Bladder Augmentation." *Digital Urological Journal.* [cited April 2003]. <http://www.duj.com/Article/Carr/Carr.html>.

"Neurogenic Bladder." [cited April 2003]. <http://www.med.wayne.edu/urology/DISEASES/neurogenicbladder.html>.

Nancy McKenzie, Ph.D.

Bladder removal *see* **Cystectomy**

Bladder resection *see* **Transurethral bladder resection**

Bladder tumor antigen test *see* **Tumor marker tests**

Blepharoplasty

Definition

Blepharoplasty is a cosmetic surgical procedure that removes fat deposits, excess tissue, or muscle from the eyelids to improve the appearance of the eyes.

Purpose

The primary use of blepharoplasty is for improving the cosmetic appearance of the eyes. In some older persons, however, sagging and excess skin surrounding the eyes can be so extensive that it limits the range of vision. In those cases, blepharoplasty serves a more functional purpose.

Demographics

Approximately 100,000 blepharoplasty procedures are performed each year in the United States. The procedure is more common among women than men.

Description

Blepharoplasty can be performed on the upper or lower eyelid. It can involve the removal of excess skin and fat deposits and the tightening of selected muscles surrounding the eyelids. The goal is to provide a more youthful appearance and/or improve eyesight.

The surgeon will begin by deciding whether excess skin, fat deposits, or muscle looseness are at fault. While a person is sitting upright, the surgeon will mark where incisions will be made on the skin. Care will be taken to hide the incision lines in the natural skin folds above and below the eye. The surgeon will then inject a local anesthetic to numb the pain. Many surgeons also administer a sedative intravenously during the procedure.

After a small, crescent-shaped section of eyelid skin is removed, the surgeon will work to tease out small

WHO PERFORMS THE PROCEDURE AND WHERE IS IT PERFORMED?

Blepharoplasty procedures are performed by surgeons with specialized training in plastic and reconstructive surgery. They are most commonly performed in outpatient facilities or in private professional offices. The procedure may also be performed in a hospital.

In 2003, the average price of blepharoplasty for both upper lids was approximately $4,000. For both lower lids, the cost may be slightly higher. The cost for both upper and lower blepharoplasty was approximately $6,000. These prices usually include anesthesia and surgeon fees. Medications and lab work, as well as any revisionary work, are not included.

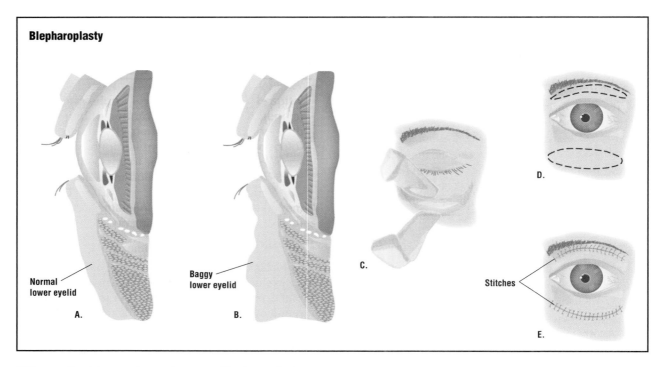

Blepharoplasty

Normal
lower eyelid

A.

Baggy
lower eyelid

B.

C.

D.

Stitches

E.

With age, the skin sags beneath the eye (B). To repair the area, the surgeon pinches the excess (C), then marks areas for removal (D). The incisions are closed with very fine stitches (E). *(Illustration by GGS Inc.)*

pockets of fat that have collected in the lids. If muscle looseness is also a problem, the surgeon may trim tissue or add a stitch to pull muscle tissue tighter. Then the incision is closed with stitches.

In some persons, fat deposits in the lower eyelid may be the only or primary problem. Such people may be good candidates for transconjunctival blepharoplasty. In this procedure the surgeon makes no incision on the surface of the eyelid, but instead enters from behind, through the inner surface of the lid, to tease out the fat deposits from a small incision. The advantage of this procedure is that there is no visible scar.

Diagnosis/Preparation

Before performing blepharoplasty, the surgeon will assess whether a person is a good candidate for the treatment. A thorough medical history is important. The surgeon will want to know about any history of thyroid disease, hypertension, or eye problems, which may increase the risk of complications.

Prior to surgery, surgeons and their candidates meet to discuss the procedure, clarify the results that can be achieved, and discuss potential problems that might occur. Having realistic expectations is important in any cosmetic procedure. People will learn, for example, that although blepharoplasty can improve the appearance of the eyelid, other procedures, such as a chemical peel,

will be necessary to reduce the appearance of wrinkles around the eye. Some surgeons prescribe vitamin C and vitamin K for 10 days prior to surgery in the belief that this helps the healing process. Candidates are also told to stop smoking in the weeks before and after the procedure, and to refrain from using alcohol or **aspirin**.

Aftercare

An antibiotic ointment is applied to the line of stitches each day for several days after surgery. Patients also take an antibiotic several times a day to prevent infection. Ice-cold compresses are applied to the eyes continuously for the first day following surgery, and several times a day for the next week or so, to reduce swelling. Some swelling and discoloration around the eyes is expected with the procedure. Persons should avoid aspirin or alcoholic beverages for one week and should limit their activities, including bending, straining, and lifting. The stitches are removed a few days after surgery. People can generally return to their usual activities within a week to 10 days.

Risks

As with any surgical procedure, blepharoplasty can lead to infection and scarring. Good care of the wound following surgery can minimize these risks. In cases where too much skin is removed from the eyelids, people may experience difficulty closing their eyes. Dry eye syndrome may develop, requiring the use of artificial tears to lubricate the eye. In a rare complication, called retrobulbar hematoma, a pocket of blood forms behind the eyeball.

Normal results

Most people can expect good results from blepharoplasty, with the removal of excess eyelid skin and fat producing a more youthful appearance. Some swelling and discoloration is expected immediately following the procedure, but this clears in time. Small scars will be left where the surgeon has made incisions; but these generally lighten in appearance over several months, and, if placed correctly, will not be readily noticeable.

Morbidity and mortality rates

If too much excess skin is removed from the upper eyelid, persons may be unable to close their eyes completely. Another surgery to correct the defect may be required. Similarly, too much skin can be removed from the lower eyelid, allowing too much of the white of the eye (the sclera) to show. In extreme cases, the lower lid may be pulled down too far, revealing the underlying tissue. This is called an ectropion and may require a second, corrective surgery. The eye's ability to make tears may also be compromised, leading to dry eye syndrome. Dry eye syndrome is potentially dangerous; in rare cases it leads to damage to the cornea of the eye and vision loss.

Alternatives

Some of the alternatives to blepharoplasty include losing some excess body fat, **exercise**, accepting one's body and appearance as it is, or using makeup to downplay or emphasize facial features.

See also Face lift; Liposuction.

Resources

BOOKS

Engler, Alan M. *BodySculpture: Plastic Surgery of the Body for Men and Women.* 2nd ed. Hudson Pub, 2000.

Irwin, Brandith, and Mark McPherson. *Your Best Face: Looking Your Best without Plastic Surgery.* Carlsbad, CA: Hay House, Inc, 2002.

Man, Daniel, and L. C. Faye. *New Art of Man: Faces of Plastic Surgery: Your Guide to the Latest Cosmetic Surgery Procedures.* 3rd ed. New York: BeautyArt Press, 2003.

Papel, I. D., and S. S. Park. *Facial Plastic and Reconstructive Surgery.* 2nd ed. New York: Thieme Medical Publishers, 2000.

PERIODICALS

Byrd, H. S., and J. D. Burt. "Achieving Aesthetic Balance in the Brow, Eyelids, and Midface." *Plastic and Reconstructive Surgery* 110 (2002): 926–939.

QUESTIONS TO ASK THE DOCTOR

- What will be the resulting appearance?
- Is the surgeon board certified in plastic and reconstructive surgery?
- How many blepharoplasty procedures has the surgeon performed?
- What is the surgeon's complication rate?

Cather, J. C., and A. Menter. "Update on Botulinum Toxin for Facial Aesthetics." *Dermatology Clinics of North America* 20 (2002): 749–761.

Oliva, M. S., A. J. Ahmadi, R. Mudumbai, J. L. Hargiss, and B. S. Sires. "Transient Impaired Vision, External Ophthalmoplegia, and Internal Ophthalmoplegia after Blepharoplasty under Local Anesthesia." *American Journal of Ophthalmology* 135 (2003): 410–412.

Yaremchuk, M. J. "Restoring Palpebral Fissure Shape after Previous Lower Blepharoplasty." *Plastic and Reconstructive Surgery* 111 (2003): 441–450.

ORGANIZATIONS

American Academy of Facial Plastic and Reconstructive Surgery. 310 S. Henry Street, Alexandria, VA 22314. Telephone: (703) 299-9291, Fax: (703) 299-8898. <http://www.facial-plastic-surgery.org>.

American Board of Plastic Surgery. Seven Penn Center, Suite 400, 1635 Market Street, Philadelphia, PA 19103-2204. (215) 587-9322. <http://www.abplsurg.org>.

American College of Plastic and Reconstructive Surgery. <http://www.breast-implant.org>.

American College of Surgeons. 633 North Saint Claire Street, Chicago, IL, 60611. (312) 202-5000. <http://www.facs.org>.

American Society for Aesthetic Plastic Surgery. 11081 Winners Circle, Los Alamitos, CA 90720. (800) 364-2147 or (562) 799-2356. <http://www.surgery.org>.

American Society for Dermatologic Surgery. 930 N. Meacham Road, P.O. Box 4014, Schaumburg, IL 60168-4014. (847) 330-9830. <http://www.asds-net.org>.

American Society of Plastic and Reconstructive Surgeons. 44 E. Algonquin Rd., Arlington Heights, IL 60005. (847) 228-9900. <http://www.plasticsurgery.org>.

American Society of Plastic Surgeons. 444 E. Algonquin Rd., Arlington Heights, IL 60005. (888) 475-2784. <http://www.plasticsurgery.org>.

OTHER

"Blepharoplasty." *American Society of Ophthalmic Plastic and Reconstructive Surgery.* [cited April 2003]. <http://www.asoprs.org/blepharoplasty.html>.

"Blepharoplasy." *Facial Plastic Surgery Network.* [cited March 2003]. <http://www.facialplasticsurgery.net/blepharoplasty.htm>.

"Eyelid Surgery (Blepharoplasty)." *Department of Otolaryngology/Head and Neck Surgery at Columbia University and New York Presbyterian Hospital.* 2002 [cited April 2003]. <http://www.entcolumbia.org/bleph.htm>.

Galli, Suzanne K. Doud, and Phillip J. Miller. "Blepharoplasty, Transconjunctival Approach." *emedicine.* September 11, 2001 [cited April 2003]. <http://www.emedicine.com/ent/topic95.htm>.

L. Fleming Fallon, Jr., MD, DrPH

Blood clot prevention *see* **Venous thrombosis prevention**

Blood count *see* **Complete blood count**

Blood crossmatching *see* **Type and screen**

Blood donation and registry

Definition

Blood donation, also called blood banking, refers to the process of collecting, testing, preparing, and storing whole blood and blood components intended primarily for **transfusion**. Blood donors are typically unpaid volunteers, but they may also be paid by commercial blood donation and processing enterprises, such as independent blood banks and donor centers. Blood registry refers to the collection and sharing of data about donated blood and donors. Donors who have been determined to be temporarily or permanently ineligible to donate blood are listed in a confidential national data base known as the Donor Deferral Register. The quality and safety of the U.S. blood supply is governed by physician-established guidelines for the practice of blood banking as found in the Standards of the American Association of Blood Banks (AABB) and through the organization's inspection and accreditation program. The Food and Drug Administration (FDA) controls federal licensure of blood banks. Hospital blood banks are also inspected by The College of American Pathologists (CAP) and the Joint Commission on Accreditation of Healthcare Organizations (JCAHC).

Purpose

Blood is collected, processed, stored, and distributed to maintain an adequate supply of whole blood and blood components for transfusion as needed. Blood replacement may be needed by people who have lost blood through accidents, burns, hemorrhage, or surgery. Blood or blood components are also used in the treatment of certain types of anemia, various disease conditions, and for medical research.

Healthy donors may be called upon to donate periodically to help maintain the overall blood supply or when their specific blood type is needed. People may sometimes donate blood to benefit a specific person. Directed donor blood is reserved for an intended recipient, such as a family member or friend; it is tested and processed as all other donated blood to ensure that it is appropriate for the recipient. People preparing for **elective surgery** may have their blood collected and held, and then returned to them if needed during their surgery. This process is known as **autologous blood donation**. Donors are advised to give blood only once in an eight-week period to maintain the iron stores in their blood. Autologous donors may donate more often if it is determined by their physician to be to their benefit.

The National Blood Data Resource Center reports that about 13.9 million units of whole blood (one unit of whole blood equals 450 ml, or about 1 pt) are donated annually in the United States, of which about 695,000 are autologous donations for elective surgery. The country's blood supply is donated by about eight million people, representing a broad cross section of the population, although fewer than 5% of those eligible donate. About half of the total amount needed is processed, stored, and delivered by the 36 regional blood centers of the American Red Cross; hospital blood banks, community blood centers, mobile blood drives, and independent blood banks collect, process, and distribute the other half.

Blood is donated as whole blood, collected in a plastic bag containing an anticoagulant that will keep the blood from clotting and allow it to be separated into multiple components. By dividing blood into components that each offer different clinical benefits, one unit of donated blood can meet the transfusion needs for more than one person. This practice is essential to meet the constant demand for blood; every year in the United States, more than four million people require blood transfusions. About 26 million transfusions are administered either as whole blood or components that have been prepared from whole blood. About 34,000 units per day, for example, are transfused as red cells.

Whole blood and blood components are used in various ways to meet the clinical needs of recipients. Whole blood is sometimes used to replace blood volume when a significant amount of blood has been lost through accidents or surgery. Red blood cells, which carry oxygen, are used to treat certain anemias and are often the preferred component when multiple transfusions are being administered to one person, as in open heart surgery or organ transplants. Platelets, part of the complex coagulation (clotting) system that helps control bleeding, are commonly used in the treatment of acute leukemia and some types of cancer. Fresh frozen plasma, which contains critical coagulation factors, is used to control bleeding in people who lack these factors. Cryoprecipitated (prepared from frozen plasma) antihemophilic factor (AHF) is transfused to provide a specific coagulation factor that is deficient in hemophilia and other diseases. Blood for transfusion is requested by physicians. Pretransfusion testing and issuance of blood and components to the recipients is performed by a transfusion service, which is commonly provided or supervised by a hospital blood bank.

Description

The actual process of donating whole blood takes about 20 minutes. The donor will either lie down or will sit in a special donor chair that elevates the lower body and legs. After selecting an appropriate vein, the phlebotomist (an individual trained in blood collection technique) will clean the arm well at the site of the needle puncture (venipuncture). With a tourniquet tightly in place on the donor's arm, a sterile needle is inserted into a vein. As the tourniquet is released, blood flows through plastic tubing into a plastic blood bag. The donor may be asked to open and close a fist to encourage blood to flow. Usually only one unit of blood is collected. Pressure is applied to the site of the venipuncture until the blood flow has been stopped. Donors are then escorted to an observation area, given light refreshments that include liquid, and allowed to rest. Positive identification of the donor and the blood bag from that donor are essential. The same unique identification number is assigned to the

Individual units of blood being stored in a blood bank.
(Custom Medical Stock Photo. Reproduced by permission.)

bag, all samples from the bag used for testing, and on all donor and testing records.

Plasma, the liquid portion of whole, anticoagulated blood in which blood cells, coagulation factors, and other blood constituents are suspended, is also collected. This is often done by commercial enterprises that sell it to companies manufacturing clotting factors and specific plasma protein products, or to companies and institutions engaged in medical research. Plasma is collected using a process known as apheresis, in which whole blood is collected, the desired blood component is removed, and the remainder is returned to the donor. Collecting plasma generally takes one to two hours. Apheresis may also be used to collect other blood components, such as platelets and granulocytes.

Different blood components vary in how long they can be stored. Red blood cells can be refrigerated for up to 42 days or coated with a protective agent and frozen at extremely low temperatures in liquid nitrogen, a process that preserves them for up to 10 years. Platelets must be used soon after they are prepared; they are stored at room temperature for no more than five days. Fresh frozen plasma and cryoprecipitated AHF can be kept for as long as one year.

To ensure the safety of the blood supply, a multi-tiered process of donor screening and deferral is employed. This involves donor education, taking a detailed **health history** of each prospective donor, and giving potential donors a simple **physical examination**, which includes measuring blood pressure and pulse rate, taking a few drops of blood to test for hemoglobin, the iron-bearing protein in blood, and also measuring blood cell volume. These tests will indicate general health and help ensure that donation will not contribute to anemia in the donor. At any point in the process, a potential donor may be "deferred," or determined to be ineligible to donate blood. This deferral may be temporary or permanent, depending on the reason. Potential donors are also encouraged to "self-defer," or voluntarily decline to donate, rather than put future blood recipients at risk.

In general, blood donors must be at least 17 years old (some states allow younger people to donate blood with their parents' consent), must weigh at least 110 lb (50 kg), and must be in good health. Donors with a history of heart, lung, or liver disease or who are pregnant are usually deferred. Donors can be disqualified if they are known to have engaged in behavior that put them at risk of infection (such as having had a tattoo, having had sex with people in high-risk groups, having used illegal intravenous drugs, having had certain diseases, or having been raped) or have spent time in specific parts of the world, such as areas where malaria may be prevalent.

Preparation

All donated blood is extensively tested before being distributed for use by transfusion services. The first step is determining the blood type, which is the primary indication of who can receive the blood. Blood is also screened for any irregular antibodies that could cause complications for the recipients. In addition, donor blood is screened for infectious diseases, such as hepatitis, AIDS, and syphilis, by testing for specific markers of these diseases that will appear in the blood of those infected. These include: Hepatitis B surface antigen (donors with this antigen are immune and can be accepted), hepatitis B core antigen, hepatitis C virus antibody, HIV-1 and HIV-2 antibodies, HIV p24 antigen, and HTLV-I and HTLV-II antibodies. Other tests may be performed if a recipient's doctor requests them.

In order to detect the greatest possible number of infections, when present at even the lowest levels in donor blood, these screening tests are extremely sensitive. For this reason, however, donors sometimes receive false positive test results. In these cases, more specific confirmatory tests are performed to help rule out false positive results. Blood found to be not suitable for transfusion is discarded, and all items coming into direct contact with donors are used only once and then discarded. Donors of infected blood are entered into the Donor Deferral Register to prevent subsequent donation of their blood at other blood donation facilities.

There are eight major blood types comprising four ABO groups (A, B, AB, and O), and the presence or absence of the Rh factor, designated as either type Rh positive (+) or type Rh negative (-). These types and their approximate distribution in the U.S. population are as follows: O+ (38%), O- (7%), A+ (34%), A- (6%), B+ (9%), B- (2%), AB+ (3%), AB- (1%). In an emergency, when there may be no time for compatibility testing, anyone can safely receive type O red blood cells, and people with this blood type are known as "universal donors." People with type AB blood, known as "universal recipients," can receive any type of red blood cells and can give plasma to all blood types. Receiving the wrong blood type can result in the destruction of red cells in the recipients body and even death. For this reason, the transfusion service must conduct more pre-transfusion testing to determine the compatibility of the donor blood with the blood of the recipient. This compatibility testing, known as type and cross match, begins with matching the major blood types. Additional testing will include antibody screening of the recipient and, if specific antibodies are found, testing of other blood groups (the MN group or Kell and Lewis groups, for example) will be done to find compatible donor blood.

Risks

Thanks to the use of a multi-tiered donor screening system and advances in the effectiveness of screening tests, the risk of transmitting infectious diseases to recipients via transfusion has been significantly diminished. Nonetheless, there is still a minuscule risk that blood recipients could contract human immunodeficiency virus (HIV), hepatitis, or other diseases via transfusion. Other diseases that are of particular concern to blood-collection agencies include: babesiosis, Chagas disease, human T-lymphotropic virus (HTLV-I and -II), cytomegalovirus (CMV), Lyme disease, malaria, Creutzfeldt-Jakob disease, and new variant Creutzfeldt-Jakob disease.

There are few risks to healthy donors when AABB standards for donation are followed. People who donate blood replace the fluid they lose within 24 hours and the red cells within two months. A person can safely donate blood once in eight weeks. Donors' blood will be tested prior to donation to determine their eligibility; those ineligible will be advised of the temporary or permanent reasons for being disqualified. Their names will be placed on the national deferral registry to prevent donation at other sites and to help protect the blood supply.

Medical professionals who draw the blood of eligible donors will advise donors of any necessary precautions following donation. Most blood donors suffer no significant after effects. Occasionally donors may feel faint or dizzy, nauseous, or have tenderness, redness, or a bruise where the needle was inserted to draw their blood. More serious complications, which rarely occur, may include fainting, muscle spasms, or nerve damage.

AABB standards are designed to protect donors and recipients and especially to help ensure that compatible blood is transfused to each recipient. The accurate labeling of blood, blood components, and donor records, and the recording of all data is essential from the time blood is collected, through testing and preparation, and through pre-transfusion testing and issuance of the blood or blood component. Autologous blood donors run a tiny risk of having the wrong blood returned to them due to clerical error. There is also a faint possibility of bacterial contamination of the autologous blood. These rare occurrences apply to all other transfusions as well.

Resources

BOOKS

McClatchey, Kenneth D., M.D., ed. "Section XI: Blood Transfusion Medicine." *Clinical Laboratory Medicine.* Baltimore: Williams & Wilkins, 1994.

Starr, Douglass. *Blood: An Epic History of Medicine and Commerce.* New York: Alfred A Knopf, 1998.

PERIODICALS

McKenna, C. "Blood Minded." *Nursing Times* (April 6, 2000): 27–28.

ORGANIZATIONS

American Association of Blood Banks. 8101 Glenbrook Road, Bethesda, MD 20814-2749. (301) 907-6977. <http://www.aabb.org>.

American Red Cross. 430 17th Street NW, Washington, D.C. 20006. <http://www.redcross.org>.

National Blood Data Resource Center. (301) 215-6506. <http://www.nbdrc.org>.

Peter Gregutt
L. Lee Culvert

Blood pressure measurement

Definition

Blood pressure measurement is the non-invasive measurement of the pressure exerted by the circulating blood on the walls of the body's arteries.

Purpose

The purpose of non-invasive blood pressure measurement is to detect any changes from normal values, which may indicate disease. Measurement is also performed to monitor the effectiveness of medication and other methods used to control elevated blood pressure.

Blood pressure should be routinely checked every one to two years and may be monitored more closely during illnesses that affect blood pressure or during medical treatments which may change blood pressure. Measurement can be taken as often as every few minutes.

Precautions

As there may be no prior knowledge of the patient's previous blood pressure for comparison, a wide range of normal values apply to patients of different ages. The inflated cuff can cause discomfort, and this should be taken into account when dealing with very ill patients. Patients with a history of sickle cell anemia should not have non-invasive blood pressure measurements made with a typical blood pressure cuff, because the sickling process can be initiated by the pressure on the arm. Blood pressure measurements should occur on a limb free of intravascular catheters and arterial venous fistulas (joined artery and vein) used for chronic dialysis.

Description

Blood pressure is usually recorded by measuring the force of the blood during the contraction of the ventricles

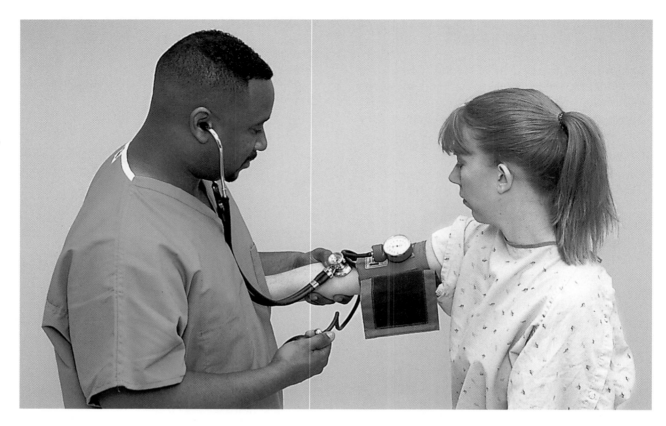

A health care provider takes the blood pressure of a patient with a stethoscope and inflatable cuff. *(From Fundamentals of Nursing, Standards & Practice, 1st edition by DELAUNE. (c) 1998. Reprinted with permission of Delmar Learning, a division of Thomson Learning: www.thomsonrights.com. Fax: 800-730-2215.)*

(lower chambers of the heart) as blood is pumped from the heart to the rest of the body (systolic pressure), and during the period when the heart is relaxed between beats and pressure is lowest (diastolic pressure).

The cardiac output, resistance, quality, and quantity of blood circulating through the heart, and the condition of the arterial walls are all factors that influence the blood pressure. Hypertension is an elevation in the blood pressure above normal values, with the diastolic pressure being the indicator most commonly used.

Hypotension is a reduction in the blood pressure below normal values. If a very high or very low pressure is taken, the blood pressure reading may be inaccurate and should be repeated immediately, prior to the initiation of medical treatment.

The non-invasive blood pressure is taken using a **sphygmomanometer**, a hand bulb pump, and a cuff.

The sphygmomanometer may be electronic or mercury-based. The mercury-based unit has a manually inflatable cuff attached by tubing to the unit that contains mercury and is calibrated in millimeters of mercury. The electronic unit is similar, but is mercury free and inflates

and deflates automatically with the reading displayed digitally. The electronic units are also calibrated to display the measurement in millimeters of mercury. Blood pressure can be measured with either unit, although electronic units are becoming more commonplace in both **home care** and clinical use.

Children and adults with smaller or larger than average-sized limbs require special sized cuffs appropriate for their needs. The blood pressure cuff is usually placed on the arm, but can also be used on the leg.

To record blood pressure, the patient may be seated or lying down. The cuff will be positioned so that it is level with the heart. With an electronic unit the cuff is placed in accordance with manufacturer instructions on the bare upper arm, on the bare wrist, or on the bare index finger.

If the blood pressure is monitored with a manual system, a cuff is placed level with the heart and wrapped firmly but not too tightly around the bare arm 1 in (2.5 cm) above the elbow, with any creases in the cuff smoothed out. Leg measurements, require the cuff to be positioned below the groin on the bare leg over the femoral artery.

176

Following the manufacturer's guidelines (electronic models), the cuff is inflated and then deflated automatically. The reading is displayed and recorded by the user. The results are charted with the systolic pressure first, then by the diastolic pressure in the following manner, xxx/xx (e.g., 120/70). A manual system requires a **stethoscope** be placed over the artery, the cuff is then inflated until the artery is occluded and no sound is heard through the stethoscope.

The cuff is then inflated a further 10 mm Hg above the last sound heard. The valve in the pump is slowly opened no faster than 5 mm Hg per second to deflate the pressure in the cuff to the point where a tapping sound is heard over the artery. This point is noted as the systolic pressure. The sounds continue as the pressure in the cuff is released and the artery is no longer occluded. At this point, the noises are no longer heard and this is noted as the diastolic pressure.

With children, the tapping noise changes to a soft muffled sound. That point is noted as the diastolic pressure, as commonly in children, sounds continue to be heard as the cuff deflates to zero.

Preparation

Medical staff should explain the procedure fully to the patient and reassure him or her that recording blood pressure is part of normal health checks and that it is necessary to ensure the patient's health is being correctly monitored. The appropriate-sized cuff should be used for the patient to give an accurate reading.

The test can be performed at any time, but is best performed when the patient has been resting for at least five minutes so that any exertion, such as climbing stairs prior to the test, will not unduly influence the outcome of the reading.

Devices should be checked and calibrated annually by a qualified technician to ensure accurate readings.

Aftercare

The patient should be made comfortable. The medical staff should be notified if the blood pressure measurement is above or below normal values so treatment can be initiated, continued, or adjusted. Repeated measurements are required for screening purposes and continuity of care.

Results

The normal values for blood pressure measurement is a systolic pressure of 120 mm Hg and a diastolic pressure of 70–80 mm Hg. Mild hypertension is a diastolic pressure above 90 mm Hg. The American Heart Association states that a systolic pressure above 130–139 mm Hg

---

KEY TERMS

Blood pressure—The pressure of the blood in the cardiovascular system measured in millimeters of mercury.

Diastolic—Minimum arterial blood pressure during ventricular rest.

Hypertension—High blood pressure.

Hypotension—Low blood pressure.

Systolic—Maximum arterial blood pressure during ventricular contraction.

---

needs to be watched carefully. Significant hypertension is a systolic pressure above 200 mm Hg. The blood pressure measurement is recorded and compared with normal ranges for the patient's age and medical condition. Based on the results, a decision is made as to whether any further action is required. Hypertension increases the risk of serious diseases such as heart attack and stroke.

Hypotension is demonstrated by with a systolic blood pressure under 80 mm Hg. Treatment options depend on the patient's current health and may include blood or saline administration. Drugs to improve heart rate and function may also be administered.

Resources

BOOKS

Nagel, Rob. "Measuring Blood Pressure." In *Body by Design: From the Digestive System to the Skeleton,* edited by Betz Des Chesnes. Farmington Hills, MI: UXL, 2000.

ORGANIZATIONS

Skeehan, Thomas, and Michael Jopling. "Monitoring the Cardiac Surgical Patient." In *The Practice of Cardiac Anesthesia,* 3rd edition. Edited by Frederick A. Hensley, Donald E. Martin, and Glenn P. Gravlee. Philadelphia: Lippincott Williams & Wilkins, 2003.

ORGANIZATIONS

American College of Nurse Practitioners. 503 Capitol Ct. NE #300, Washington, DC 20002. (202) 546-4825. acnp@nurse.org.

American Heart Association. AHA National Center, 7272 Greenville Avenue, Dallas, TX 752311. (800) AHA-USA1. <http://www.americanheart.org>.

OTHER

Cooper, Phyllis G. "Blood Pressure." *Clinical Reference Systems.* Annual 2000: 173.

National Library of Medicine. [cited April 2003]. <http://www.nlm.nih.gov>.

Margaret A Stockley, RGN
Allison J. Spiwak, MSBME

Blood pressure measurement device *see*
Sphygmomanometer

Blood removal *see* **Phlebotomy**

Blood salvage

Definition

Blood salvage is the recovery of a patient's own blood from the surgical site to be readministered to the patient.

Purpose

Pre-operative blood salvage can be performed prior to the surgical incision during the induction of anesthesia. This blood is collected to be administered post-operatively, because the clotting factors and platelets are protected from activation and destruction caused by the surgery. This procedure is most often used if cardiopulmonary bypass (use of a heart-lung machine) will be instituted. If the blood is not given to the patient, it will be discarded. Pre-operative blood donation or **autologous blood donation** is a coordinated donation process planned prior to a scheduled surgical procedure, but it is not considered blood salvage.

Blood salvage is performed during surgical procedures when the risk of significant blood loss is expected. The recovered blood is collected, processed, and readministered to the patient, decreasing or preventing the need for allogeneic (from a donor) blood product administration. If the blood is not given to the patient, it will be discarded.

Post-operative blood salvage is used to collect blood from the surgical cavity as the wound heals. The blood is collected, may or may not be processed, and returned to the patient. If the blood is not given to the patient, it will be discarded.

Administration of the patient's own blood eliminates the risk of transfusion-transmitted viral disease and **transfusion** reactions. Patients with multiple red blood cell antibodies or rare blood types benefit by blood salvage during the perioperative (during surgery) and post-operative period. Shortages of rare blood types can put the patient at risk for cardiovascular collapse caused if hemorrhage occurs during the surgical procedure.

Some Jehovah's Witnesses patients refuse allogeneic blood donation. Blood salvage provides an opportunity for autologous blood donation for these patients. Certain modifications in collection technique make autologous blood donation an acceptable treatment for members of this faith.

Neurological, vascular, cardiac, liver transplant, and orthopedic procedures make extensive use of blood salvage techniques. Patients having surgical procedures involving amniotic fluid, malignancies, bowel contamination, or microfibrillar collagen materials are not eligible for blood salvage. In the presence of amniotic fluid or bowel contamination, thorough rinsing of the surgical site may allow for blood salvage.

Description

Preoperative blood salvage

The patient will be provided with cardiac monitoring prior to the initiation of autologous blood collection. A venous access site will be gained with a catheter. The 500–1,000 ml of whole blood is collected into a transfusion container treated with anticoagulant. The container is properly labeled for the patient and clearly marked "AUTOLOGOUS DONOR." The blood can be stored for six hours if refrigerated, and will be destroyed if not used within that time.

Blood collected in this manner is not processed further, but stored for later administration. The whole blood product provides not only red blood cells, but more importantly, plasma proteins including clotting factors and platelets. This technique is most often associated with cardiopulmonary bypass, since the heart-lung machine can damage clotting factors and platelets. The pre-operative collection protects the blood components.

Perioperative blood salvage

During surgery, the surgeon uses suction in the surgical cavity to collect blood. Anticoagulant is mixed with the blood at the tip of the suction apparatus. The blood is filtered as it is collected into a container. From this collection container the blood may be placed into a transfusion container for direct administration to the patient. This blood will be anticoagulated and will contain all plasma proteins, including activated clotting factors and platelets. More commonly, the blood is processed by centrifugation. The blood is centrifuged to separate the red blood cells from the plasma. The plasma is removed as saline enters the centrifuge to wash the blood. Washing the blood removes anticoagulation, plasma-free hemoglobin, and plasma proteins, including activated clotting factors and platelets. This product is called washed packed red cells. After washing is complete, the blood is collected into a transfusion container free of anticoagulant since all clotting factors have been removed during washing. The container is properly labeled for the patient and clearly marked "AUTOLOGOUS DONOR." The blood can be stored for six hours if refrigerated, and will be destroyed if not used within that time.

KEY TERMS

Allogeneic—Blood and blood products collected from a blood donor for administration to a recipient.

Autologous—Blood and blood products collected from an individual for readministration to self.

Catheter—Patients experiencing open heart surgery will have at least one chest tube placed. This catheter is placed in the chest cavity and penetrates the chest wall to provide removal of blood from the chest cavity for collection and readministration. Used in joint surgery, it is a tube left in the joint cavity that penetrates the skin to provide connection to the blood collection apparatus.

Transfusion container—An administration bag made of polyvinyl chloride or other latex-free polymer for collection of blood products for administration to the patient. Use of the bag prevents air bubbles in the venous system, assuming there is no air trapped in the bag with the blood product.

Postoperative blood salvage

Postoperative blood salvage is used to remove shed blood from the surgical cavity that has been closed at the completion of the surgical procedure. At wound closure, a catheter is left in the cavity and penetrates the skin for connection to the collection reservoir. If the blood is collected from the chest cavity, no anticoagulation is required. If the blood is collected from a joint, it must receive anticoagulation during collection. The blood from the chest cavity is usually reinfused without additional processing, but may be washed. Blood collected from a joint must be washed prior to infusion. Washing involves centrifugation of the blood to separate the red blood cells from the plasma. In the plasma are the anticoagulant-free hemoglobin and plasma proteins, including activated clotting factors and platelets. Once the red blood cells and plasma are separated, saline is introduced to the centrifuge to displace the plasma with the end product collected into a transfusion container. The final product is called washed packed red blood cells. The container is properly labeled for the patient and clearly marked "AUTOLOGOUS DONOR." The blood can be stored for six hours if refrigerated, and will be destroyed if not used within that time.

Normal results

The patient will receive autologous blood donation when the red blood cell volume, as measured by hemo-globin or **hematocrit** values, falls below the desired level, commonly 18–21% or 6–7 g/dl, respectively. These values will be dictated by the physician in the orders for patient care.

If with the patient's condition is acceptable, autologous blood donation with preoperative blood collection occurs immediately following the termination of cardiopulmonary bypass. Treatment of low red cell volume is not best accomplished with this technique. Instead, this technique supports coagulation.

Blood collected postoperatively will be administered as need for maintenance of blood pressure or red cell volume.

The patient benefits from blood salvage by the elimination of the risk of blood-transmitted virus or blood transfusion reactions. Blood transfusion reactions are experienced by about 10% of recipients for each unit transfused.

Resources

BOOKS

Spiess, Bruce D., et al., eds. *Perioperative Transfusion Medicine*. Baltimore: Williams & Wilkins, 1998.

OTHER

"Guidance for Autologous Blood and Blood Components." *Autologous Blood and Blood Components*. Division of Blood and Blood Products, HFB-400, Bethesda, MD 20892. March 15, 1989 [cited April 3, 2003]. <http://www.fda.gov/cber/bldmem/031589.pdf>.

Allison Joan Spiwak, MSBME

Blood sugar test *see* **Glucose tests**

Blood thinners *see* **Anticoagulant and antiplatelet drugs**

Blood transfusion *see* **Transfusion**

Blood typing *see* **Type and screen**

Blood urea nitrogen test *see* **Kidney function tests**

Bloodless surgery

Definition

Bloodless surgery is an approach to health care that began in the 1960s as simple avoidance of the use of transfused blood. It has grown over the last four decades, however, to include changed attitudes toward blood conservation as well as new technologies that minimize the need for transfusions during surgery. The Center for Bloodless Medicine and Surgery at Hartford Hospital in Connecticut defines bloodless surgery as "...surgical and medical treatment without the administration of blood or blood-related products."

Purpose

The new interest in bloodless surgery has emerged from a variety of religious and social concerns as well as medical, legal, and economic issues.

Religious and ethical considerations

One of the earliest motivations for bloodless surgery was finding ways to treat Jehovah's Witnesses who needed **emergency surgery** without offending their beliefs about blood **transfusion**. Many of the larger bloodless surgery centers in the United States serve areas with a large population of Jehovah's Witnesses. The specific Biblical passages that Witnesses cite as the basis for their objections are Genesis 9: 4–5, in which God forbids eating animal "flesh with its blood"; and Acts 15:29, in which the Apostles ask their first converts to "abstain from blood" as well as from other forms of immorality. Mainstream commentators generally understand the first passage as referring to eating an animal that is still alive, and the second as referring to a controversy among early Christians between Jewish and Gentile converts. A group within the Jehovah's Witnesses community, the Associated Jehovah's Witnesses for Reform on Blood (AJWRB), is a good resource for readers interested in the range of views among contemporary Witnesses regarding blood transfusions and in the Witnesses' interpretation of the Bible.

Respect for the religious beliefs of a specific group, however, is related to a more general ethical concern for patients' rights. While a majority of bloodless surgical procedures are still requested by Jehovah's Witnesses, as of 2003 the proportion of other patients requesting bloodless surgery is rising and is expected to continue to increase. Whereas in 1998 only 10% of bloodless surgical procedures were performed on non-Witnesses, by the end of 2002 the proportion had risen to 30%. The number of medical centers in the United States that offer bloodless surgery has expanded from about 20 in 1996 to over 70 as of 2002. While the increased demand for bloodless procedures stems partly from concerns that will be discussed in the following sections, it also reflects changing attitudes on the part of patients. One nurse has described patients enrolling in bloodless surgery programs as "proactive" people who are aware that they have choices about health care and expect

medical professionals to respect their decisions. This attitude is a considerable change from the "doctor knows best" passive acceptance that characterized previous generations of patients. Hospitals with bloodless surgery centers emphasize the importance of patients' ethical rights to privacy and self-determination as well as their legal rights to refuse treatments that they find objectionable.

Patient safety

The most important non-religious reason that patients give for requesting bloodless surgery is concern about the safety of blood transfusions. These fears are related to the quality of the American blood supply as well as the process of blood transfusion itself.

• Bloodborne diseases. Many patients are afraid of contracting diseases such as AIDS and hepatitis from allogeneic (donated) blood. The risk of contracting these specific diseases has been vastly reduced over the past 40 years. According to Dr. Gregory Nuttall, chair of the Committee on Transfusion Medicine of the American Society of Anesthesiologists, the risk of contracting hepatitis from transfused blood has decreased from one chance in 10 in the 1960s to less than 1:100,000 by 2000. The risk of contracting HIV infection has been reduced by a factor of 10,000 since the virus was first identified in 1983. Unfortunately, these statistics do not reassure patients who are concerned about the possibility of being infected by disease agents that have not yet been identified as bloodborne. In addition, as of 2003 there is no way to screen potential blood donors for four diseases caused by parasites (malaria, babesiosis, Chagas' disease, and Lyme disease) and one disease caused by prions (Creutzfeldt-Jakob disease), even though the Centers for Disease Control (CDC) have recorded cases of transfusion-transmitted malaria, babesiosis, and Chagas' disease in the United States.

• Transfusion reactions related to **medical errors**. In contrast to the reduction of risk from infection, there has been little reduction of risk since 1960 of noninfectious serious hazards of transfusion, or NISHOT. NISHOT statistics include mistransfusion and ABO/Rh-incompatibility. Although transfusion errors are only a small percentage of all medical errors reported in North American hospitals, they are the most common cause of serious mortality and morbidity associated with blood transfusions. About 25 patients die each year in the United States from transfusion errors involving ABO-Rh incompatibility. These errors are due to misidentification of type-and-crossmatch samples, laboratory errors, or misidentification of the transfusion recipient. Even patients who donate their own blood (autologous donation) in preparation for **elective surgery** cannot be completely certain that their blood will be correctly labeled and used during their operation.

- Immune system reactions. Allogeneic blood has been shown to disrupt the immune system and reduce longevity in cancer patients. Other studies have shown that transfused donor blood suppresses the production of B-cells and T-cells in recipients.

- Availability of blood. Many healthcare professionals are concerned about the growing shortage of blood for surgical procedures in the United States. Some blood types are less common than others; in addition, there are often seasonal shortages of blood. In January 2003, the American Red Cross, American Association of Blood Banks, and the federal Department of Health and Human Services issued an urgent appeal for blood donations; many hospitals had less than a one-day supply when a seven-day supply is considered optimal. There is an increasing demand for blood; three million pints of blood are used in the United States every year just for elective surgery. In addition, many surgical procedures require large amounts of blood or blood products. According to the Center for Molecular and Cellular Therapy at the University of Minnesota, a liver transplant requires six to 10 units of red blood cells, 20 units of plasma, and 10 units of platelets, while a bone marrow transplant takes one to two units of red blood cells every other day for two to four weeks plus six to eight units of platelets daily for four to six weeks.

Economic issues

The cost of allogeneic blood transfusions is higher than most people realize. One hospital in New Jersey estimates that each blood transfusion costs the patient about $500. Another cost analysis published in the *American Journal of Surgery* concluded that even though the donated blood itself is free, the costs of preparing, storing, transporting, and unpackaging the blood come to $1,003 to $1,043 per patient receiving a transfusion—and this figure does not include treating the medical complications associated with allogeneic blood transfusion.

Demographics

A significant problem confronting blood banks in the United States is the growing proportion of older Americans in the general population. Their numbers are not matched by any corresponding increase in the donor population; it is estimated that only 5% of American adults give blood regularly. Although a wide cross-section of the public can be found at blood drives, several studies have shown that the statistically average donor is a college-educated married Caucasian male between the ages of 30 and 50 with an above-average income. As of 2003, the elderly comprise about 13% of the American population, but use about 25% of transfused blood. The aging of the so-called baby boomer generation, which represents a large segment of the population, is expected to lead to a critical shortage of blood by 2030. The rise in the number of complex orthopedic procedures associated with high-volume blood loss that are performed largely in elderly patients contributes to the likelihood of a severe blood shortage over the next two decades.

Another demographic change that affects the size of the population eligible to donate blood is the increased popularity of tourism and the rising number of people stationed in other countries by their employers or the military. People who have been exposed to or have a history of certain diseases from living abroad are either indefinitely or permanently deferred from giving blood. Detailed policies regarding donor deferral from the American Red Cross and the Department of Defense can be found in *All About Blood*, a booklet from the American Association of Blood Banks (AABB) that can be downloaded free of charge from the AABB web site.

Description

Bloodless surgery covers a wide variety of changes in medical practice as well as new equipment and technological innovations.

Preoperative assessment of patients

A patient seeking bloodless elective surgery is carefully evaluated for a history of unexpected bleeding or clotting problems after medical or dental procedures. He or she will also be asked about a family history of bleeding disorders.

The patient's blood will be tested to determine hemoglobin levels. In most cases, he or she will be given medications to build up hemoglobin levels prior to surgery. These are discussed in more detail below.

Care is taken to minimize the number and size of blood samples drawn for **presurgical testing**. The invention of microanalyzers allows hospital laboratories to run blood tests on samples of blood that are 30–60% smaller than those previously collected, and to use the same blood sample for multiple tests.

Reducing blood loss during surgery

NEW INSTRUMENTS AND SURGICAL TECHNIQUES. The invention of several types of new **surgical instruments** has allowed surgeons to perform a variety of procedures with minimal blood loss. Miniaturized endoscopes make it possible to perform surgery on the abdomen and spine through very small incisions, often shorter than 1 in (2.5 cm) in length. The invention of argon beam coagulators, electrocautery devices, and harmonic scalpels—which use a combination of ultrasound vibration and friction to clot blood at the same time as cutting—also help to make transfusions unnecessary. In addition, surgeons are being trained to use extra caution during surgery and to clamp or cauterize open blood vessels as quickly as possible.

PERFORMING DIFFICULT PROCEDURES IN STAGES. Blood transfusions can sometimes be avoided by scheduling lengthy surgical procedures in two stages. Although this approach requires additional exposure to general anesthesia, it can shorten the overall length of the patient's hospital stay. The patient can be discharged after the first operation relatively quickly and build up his or her hemoglobin levels before the second procedure. In addition, the second surgery can be completed without the need for allogeneic blood.

HYPOTENSION. Hypotension in surgery refers to the intentional lowering of the patient's arterial blood pressure during the procedure. Lowering blood pressure has been shown to reduce blood loss and the consequent need for transfusions. It also shortens the length of time spent in the **operating room**. The limitation of hypotension is that it cannot be used in surgical procedures requiring tissue grafting or in patients with coronary artery disease.

HEMODILUTION AND BLOOD SALVAGE TECHNIQUES. Hemodilution is a technique in which whole blood from the patient is withdrawn before surgery for temporary storage and replaced with crystalloid or colloid solutions that restore the normal fluid volume of the blood without adding new blood cells. The patient thus loses fewer red blood cells during surgery. At the close of the operation the patient's own blood is reinfused, thus minimizing the possibility of transfusion error or a transfusion reaction. Hemodilution has been approved and recommended by experts at the National Heart, Lung and Blood Institute (NHLBI) of the National Institutes of Health (NHI).

Blood salvage, which is also called autotransfusion, involves an automated recovery system that collects the patient's blood during surgery in a cell separation device. This device separates the red blood cells from other blood components, washes them, and concentrates them for reinfusion. As of 2003, however, autotransfusion cannot be used in patients with malignant tumors or active infections.

Reevaluation of postoperative anemia

Another change that has affected the frequency and number of blood transfusions is the reevaluation of anemia and its effects on the body. At one time patients were automatically given blood transfusions if their hemoglobin level fell below 10 g/dL. More recent studies have shown that patients can tolerate hemoglobin levels of 5 g/dL or even lower as long as the fluid volume of the blood is adequate. These findings have led medical professionals to question the wisdom of using blood as a "medication" for treating anemia. At present, the so-called transfusion trigger is a hemoglobin level of 7 g/dL, evaluated in the context of the patient's overall clinical condition.

Red cell substitutes

Researchers are presently investigating the possibility of manufacturing substitutes for red blood cells that would reduce the cost of transfusions while improving patient safety. As of 2002, the two approaches that have been explored are cell-free hemoglobin solutions and perfluorocarbon solutions. Neither approach has yielded satisfactory results so far; the hemoglobin solutions have a short half-life, and the perfluorocarbon solutions would be difficult to administer intravenously. Further research in this area is underway.

Diagnosis/Preparation
Administrative

Preparation for nonemergency bloodless surgery includes a registration process as well as medical preparation. In most American hospitals, a person who wants to register for bloodless surgery makes an appointment with the coordinator of the program. The coordinator, who is usually an RN, reviews the patient's request for bloodless care with him or her. The patient is then given an advance directive and enrollment form to sign. The documents are kept on file with the patient's preadmission chart. After the patient is admitted, he or she is given a red (or other distinctive color) wristband with the words "Do Not Administer Blood Products." Signs and stickers with the same warning are attached to the patient's bed and the front of the patient's chart. These identifiers are necessary because most hospitals with bloodless surgery programs do not operate special units; their patients are admitted to all **hospital services** together with other patients.

After the patient has signed the advance directive, he or she is given a copy that may be reproduced and given to friends or relatives in the event of an emergency. Some bloodless surgery centers give pre-enrolled patients wallet cards that can be attached to a driver's license, in the event that the patient needs emergency care and is unable to speak for him- or herself.

Medical

One of the basic components of bloodless surgery programs is presurgical treatment intended to boost the

KEY TERMS

Allogeneic blood—Blood that comes from a human donor other than the patient receiving the blood.

Autologous blood—The patient's own blood, drawn and set aside before surgery for use during surgery in case a transfusion is needed.

Autotransfusion—A technique for recovering blood during surgery, separating and concentrating the red blood cells, and reinfusing them in the patient. Autotransfusion is also known as blood salvage.

Electrocautery—A technique for sealing a blood vessel with a holder that contains a wire heated by electricity.

Erythropoetin—A hormone secreted chiefly by the kidney (in adults) that stimulates the production of red blood cells.

Harmonic scalpel—A scalpel that uses ultrasound technology to seal tissues while it is cutting.

Hemodilution—A technique in which the fluid content of the blood is increased without increasing the number of red blood cells.

Hemoglobin—The red pigment in red blood cells that carries oxygen.

Hypotension—In the context of bloodless surgery, the deliberate lowering of the patient's arterial blood pressure in order to decrease blood loss.

Plasma—The liquid portion of blood, as distinguished from blood cells. Plasma constitutes about 55% of blood volume.

Platelets—Disk-shaped structures found in blood that play an active role in blood clotting. Platelets are also known as thrombocytes.

oxygen-carrying capacity of the patient's blood. Patients are given erythropoetin, or EPO, several weeks before surgery. The usual dose is 600 units per kg of body weight once a week for three weeks. EPO is a hormone that stimulates the bone marrow to produce more red blood cells, as many as seven times the normal amount. The greater number of red cells increases the blood's ability to carry oxygen. In addition to the EPO, patients are given iron supplements, most commonly ferrous sulfate, iron dextran, or vitamin B.

Normal results

Patients who have been treated in bloodless surgery centers are generally satisfied with the care they receive. Hospitals have found that patients recover faster with fewer complications; several centers have reported that patients requiring inpatient procedures leave the hospital on average a full day earlier than patients who have had conventional transfusions.

See also Blood donation and registry; Transfusion.

Resources

BOOKS

Committee on Quality of Health Care in America, Institute of Medicine. *To Err Is Human: Building a Safer Health System.* Washington, DC: National Academy Press, 2000.

PERIODICALS

Cogliano, J., and D. Kisner. "Bloodless Medicine and Surgery in the OR and Beyond." *AORN Journal* 76 (November 2002): 830–837, 839, 841.

Dalton, John. "Bloodless Surgery Growing as Patients Demand Alternatives." *Health Industry Today*, December 1998.

Maness, C. P., S. M. Russell, P. Altonji, and P. Allmendinger. "Bloodless Medicine and Surgery." *AORN Journal* 67 (January 1998): 144–152.

Martyn, V., S. L. Farmer, M. N. Wren, et al. "The Theory and Practice of Bloodless Surgery." *Transfusion and Apheresis Science* 27 (August 2002): 29–43.

Nuttall, Gregory A., MD. "Keeping A Finger on the Pulse of Transfusion Practices." *American Society of Anesthesiologists Newsletter* 66 December 2002 [cited May 20, 2003]. <http://www.asahq.org/Newsletters/2002/12_02/nuttall.html>.

Ozawa, S., A. Shander, and T. D. Ochani. "A Practical Approach to Achieving Bloodless Surgery." *AORN Journal* 74 (July 2001): 34–40, 42–47, 50–54.

Yowler, Charles, MD. "Transfusion and Autotransfusion." *eMedicine* March 29, 2002 [cited May 21, 2003]. <http://www.emedicine.com/med/topic3215.htm>

ORGANIZATIONS

American Association of Blood Banks (AABB). 8101 Glenbrook Road, Bethesda, MD 20814-2749. (301) 907-6977. <http://www.aabb.org>.

American Red Cross (ARC) National Headquarters. 431 18th Street, NW. Washington, DC 20006. (202) 303-4498. <http://www.redcross.org>.

Associated Jehovah's Witnesses for Reform on Blood (AJWRB). P. O. Box 190089, Boise, ID 83719-0089. <http://www.ajwrb/org>.

Division of Blood Diseases and Resources. The National Heart, Lung and Blood Institute (NHLBI). Two Rockledge Center, Suite 10138, 6701 Rockledge Drive, MSC

7950, Bethesda, MD 20892-7950. <http://www.nhlbi.nih.gov/about/dbdr>.

National Blood Data Resource Center (NBDRC). 8101 Glenbrook Road, Bethesda, MD 20814-2749. (301) 215-6506. <http://www.nbdrc.org>.

Physicians and Nurses for Blood Conservation (PNBC). P. O. Box 217, 6-2400 Dundas Street West, Mississauga, ON L5K 2R8. (905) 608-1647. <http://www.pnbc.ca>.

Society for the Advancement of Blood Management (SABM). 350 Engle Street, Englewood, NJ 07631. (866) 894-3916. <http://www.sabm.org>.

OTHER

American Association of Blood Banks (AABB). *All About Blood*. Bethesda, MD: AABB, 2002.

Rebecca Frey, PhD

Bone grafting

Definition

Bone grafting is a surgical procedure that places new bone or a replacement material into spaces between or around broken bone (fractures) or in holes in bone (defects) to aid in healing.

Purpose

Bone grafting is used to repair bone fractures that are extremely complex, pose a significant risk to the patient, or fail to heal properly. Bone grafting is also used to help fusion between vertebrae, correct deformities, or provide structural support for fractures of the spine. In addition to **fracture repair**, bone grafting is used to repair defects in bone caused by congenital disorders, traumatic injury, or surgery for bone cancer. Bone grafts are also used for facial or cranial reconstruction.

Demographics

Degenerative diseases of the spine increase with age. People over age 50 are more likely to need a bone graft if their condition requires surgery. Traumatic injuries occur most often in people 18–44 years.

Description

Bone tissue is a matrix-like structure primarily composed of a protein called collagen. It is strengthened by hydroxyapatite, deposits of calcium and phosphate salts. Four types of bone cells are located within and around this matrix. Together, these four types of cells are responsible

for building the bone matrix, maintaining it, and remodeling the bone as needed. The four types of bone cells are:

• Osteoblasts, which produce the bone matrix.

• Osteocytes, mature osteoblasts that maintain the bone.

• Osteoclasts, which break down and remove bone tissue.

• Bone lining cells, which cover bone surfaces.

There are three ways that a bone graft can help repair a defect.

• Osteogenesis, the formation of new bone by the cells contained within the graft.

• Osteoinduction, a chemical process in which molecules contained within the graft (bone morphogenetic proteins, abbreviated as BMP) convert the patient's cells into cells capable of forming bone.

• Osteoconduction, a physical effect whereby the graft matrix configures a scaffold on which cells in the recipient form new bone.

Surgeons harvesting a sample of material for bone grafting. *(Custom Medical Stock Photo, Inc. Reproduced by permission.)*

The term "graft" commonly refers to an autograft or allograft. A graft made of bone from the patient's own body (e.g., hip bones or ribs) is an autograft. To obtain a piece of bone for an autograft, the patient undergoes surgery under general anesthesia. An incision is made over the crest of the hip bone, a piece of bone is removed, and the incision is stitched closed.

An allograft uses bone from a cadaver, which has been frozen and stored in a tissue bank. Allografts are used because of the inadequate amount of available autograft material, and the limited size and shape of a person's own bone. Bones for allografts are usually available from organ and tissues donated by healthy people who die unexpectedly. Occasionally, allograft bone may be provided by a living donor. Allograft bone is commonly used in reconstructive surgery of the hip, knee, and long bones, as well as cases of bone loss due to trauma or tumors. Using allograft tissue from another person eliminates the need for a second operation to remove autograft bone or tendon. It also reduces the risk of infection, and safeguards against temporary pain and loss of function at or near the secondary site.

To place an autograft or allograft, the surgeon makes an incision in the skin over the bone defect, and shapes the bone graft or replacement material to fit into it. After the graft is placed into the defect, it is held in place with pins, plates, or screws. The incision is stitched closed, and a splint or cast is often used to prevent movement of the bones while healing.

After the bone graft has been accepted by the body, the transplanted bone is slowly converted into new living bone or soft tissue, and incorporated into the body as a functional unit.

Bone grafts for spinal fusion

In surgery of the spine, especially **spinal fusion**, (also called arthrodesis), surgeons may decide to use bone grafts to assist in the healing and remodeling of the spine after surgery. Normally, small pieces of bone are placed into the space between the vertebrae to be fused, and sometimes larger solid pieces of bone provide immediate structural support. Spinal fusion involves the surgical treatment of abnormalities in the vertebrae, such as curvatures, scoliosis or kyphosis, or injuries (fractures). Bone grafts may be used in spinal fusion surgery involving the lower (lumbar) or upper (cervical) spine. Cervical spinal fusion joins selected bones in the neck.

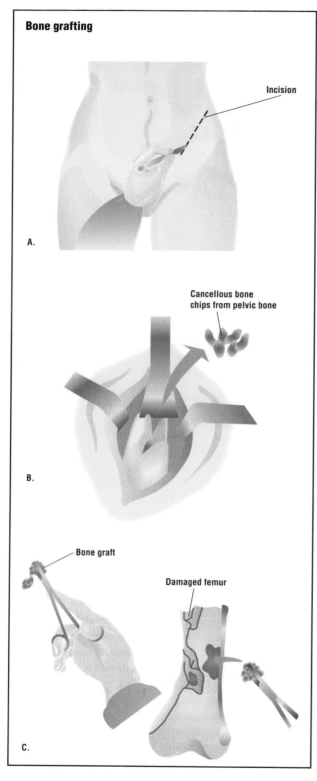

Bone grafting

A.

Incision

Cancellous bone
chips from pelvic bone

B.

Bone graft

Damaged femur

C.

For bone grafting, an incision is made in the donor's hip
(A). Pieces of bone are chipped off and removed (B). The
bone materials are then transferred to the recipient area, in
this case a femur that has been badly broken, to strengthen
the bone (C). *(Illustration by GGS Inc.)*

This surgery may also be performed by other means,
such as metal rods, which would not require bone grafts.

Diagnosis/Preparation

The surgeon does a clinical examination, and conducts tests to determine the necessity of a bone graft. Diagnostic tests determine the precise location of damage.
These tests include x rays, **magnetic resonance imaging**
(MRI), and computed tomography (CT) scan. They provide an image of the affected area, and indicate the exact
amount of damage that has occurred due to the fracture
or defect.

Orthopedic surgeries pose varying degrees of difficulty. The patient is instructed on what will take place
during the procedure, as well as risks involved. A consent form is obtained before surgery.

The following activities will help the patient prepare
for surgery.

• thorough physician consult before surgery

• banking some of his or her own blood in case a **transfusion** is needed

• eating well to achieve good nutritional status before
and after surgery

• following a recommended **exercise** program before and
after surgery.

• maintaining a positive attitude

• smoking cessation

Aftercare

Pain is normal for a few days following surgery, and
medication is given regularly to alleviate this problem.
The patient will likely have a urinary catheter.

The time required for convalescence after bone
grafts due to fractures or spinal fusion varies from one to
10 days. Vigorous exercise may be limited for up to three
months. Children heal faster than adults.

If a spinal fusion was performed, the patient may be
discharged from the hospital with a back brace or cast.
The family will be taught how to provide **home care** for
the patient. A splint or cast prevents injury or movement
while healing.

Risks

The risks for any surgical procedure requiring anesthesia include reactions to the medications and breathing
problems. Bleeding and infection are also risks of surgery.

There is little risk of graft rejection for autografts,
but there are drawbacks:

- additional surgical and anesthesia time (typically 30 minutes per procedure) to obtain or harvest the bone for grafting
- added costs for the additional surgery
- pain and infection at the site from which the graft is taken
- the relatively small amount of bone available for grafting
- surgical complications, such as infection and pain that sometimes last a longer period of time than the primary surgery (up to two years)

Allografts also have drawbacks:

- Bone variability because it is harvested from a variety of donors.
- Grafted bone may take longer to incorporate with the host bone (than in an autograft).
- Graft may be less effective than an autograft.
- Possibility of transferring diseases to the patient.
- Potential immune response complications (patient's immune system fighting against the grafted bone tissue). This problem is lessened through the use of anti-rejection drugs.

Normal results

Most bone grafts are successful in helping the bone defect to heal. The extent of recovery depends on the size of the defect and the condition of the bone surrounding the graft at the time of surgery. Severe defects take some time to heal, and may require further attention after the initial graft. Less severe bone defects should heal completely without serious complications. Repeat surgery is sometimes required if the condition recurs or complications develop.

If the bone graft is done on the face or head, the surgeries usually result in a more normal appearance.

Morbidity and mortality rates

Although bone harvested from the patient is ideal, postoperative morbidity is sometimes associated with hip bone or fibula (part of the knee) autografts. Morbidity of allografts is usually related to the graft incorporating more slowly, and less completely, into the body.

In one study of over 1,000 patients who received very large allografts after bone cancer surgery, researchers found that approximately 85% were able to return to work or normal physical activities without crutches. However, approximately 25% required a second operation because the first graft did not heal properly.

QUESTIONS TO ASK THE DOCTOR

- What should be done prepare for the graft?
- Who will provide education about the grafting process?
- How many attending surgeons are available to do this type of surgery?
- How long is hospitalization necessary?
- How long will recovery take?
- When will it be safe to resume normal activities?

Infections associated with bacterial contamination of allografts are rare. However, they can result in serious illness and death.

Alternatives

Despite the increase in the number of procedures requiring bone grafts, there is no ideal bone graft substitute. However, there are a variety of natural and synthetic replacement materials used instead of bone, including collagen (the protein substance of the white fibers of the skin, bone, and connective tissue); polymers, such as silicone and some acrylics; hydroxyapatite; calcium sulfate; and ceramics. Several new products are available or in development. They function as bone graft substitutes or extenders. Demineralized bone matrix (bone that has had its calcium removed) possesses some of the properties that the body uses to induce bone formation. Calcium hydroxyappetite products or coral have structures similar to bone, and act as scaffolding for new bone.

New BMP products are expected to be strong inducers of bone growth (osteoinductive). These new products will be relatively expensive, but will grow bone better than the patient's own bone, eliminating the need for bone graft harvesting. Bone morphogenetic proteins have been extracted from natural tissues and produced in the laboratory to stimulate bone production in animals and humans. Because they do not have the same drawbacks as grafts, surgeons are hopeful that they will soon be able to use BMP and laboratory produced BMP to aid in the generation and repair of bone.

The INFUSE Bone Graft (rhBMP-2) has received Food and Drug Administration approval, and has demonstrated better patient outcomes than hip autografts with regard to length of surgery, blood loss, hospital stay, re-

KEY TERMS

Allograft—Tissue for transplantation that is taken from another person.

Arthrodesis—Surgery that joins (or fuses) two bones so that the joint can no longer move; it may be done on joints such as the fingers, knees, ankles, or spine.

Autograft—Tissue for transplantation that is taken from the patient.

Bone morphogenetic proteins—A family of substances in human bones and blood that encourage the process of osteoinduction.

Computed tomography scan (CT)—A special type of x ray that can produce detailed pictures of structures inside the body.

Fusion—A union, joining together; e.g., bone fusion.

Hydroxyapatite—A calcium phosphate complex that is the primary mineral component of bone.

Magnetic resonance imaging (MRI)—A test that provides images of organs and structures inside the body using a magnetic field and pulses of radio wave energy. This form of imaging detects tumors, infection, and other types of tissue disease or damage, and helps diagnose conditions that affect

blood flow. The area of the body being studied is positioned inside a strong magnetic field.

Morbidity—A statistic that provides the rate at which an illness or abnormality occurs.

Mortality—The death rate, which reflects the number of deaths per unit of population in any specific region, age group, disease, or other classification, usually expressed as deaths per 1,000, 10,000, or 1,000,000.

Osteoblasts—Bone cells that build new bone tissue.

Osteoclasts—Bone cells that break down and remove bone tissue.

Osteoconduction—Provision of a scaffold for the growth of new bone.

Osteocytes—Bone cells that maintain bone tissue.

Osteogenesis—Growth of new bone.

Osteoinduction—Acceleration of new bone formation by chemical means. Also refers to the process of building, healing, and remodeling bone in humans.

Vertebra—The bones that make up the back bone (spine).

operation rate, median time to return to work, and fusion rates at six, 12, and 24 months following surgery.

Advances in tissue engineering have provided polymer based graft substitutes with degradable, porous, three-dimensional structure. New bone may be grown on these products; the grafts then slowly dissolve, leaving only the new bone behind.

See also Disk removal.

Resources

BOOKS

Beauchamp, Daniel R., M.D., Mark B. Evers, M.D., Kenneth L. Mattox, M.D., Courtney M. Townsend, and David C. Sabiston, eds. *Sabiston Textbook of Surgery: The Biological Basis of Modern Surgical Practice.* 16th edition. London: W B Saunders Co., 2001.

Branemark, Per-Ingvar, Philip Worthington, Kerstin Grondahl, and Christina Darle, eds. *Osseointegration and Autogenous Onlay Bone Grafts: Reconstruction of the Edentulous Atrophic Maxilla.* Chicago, IL: Quintessence Pub Co., 2001.

Laurencin, Cato T., ed. *Bone Graft Substitutes.* West Conshohocken, PA: American Society for Testing and Materials, 2003.

Lawrence, Peter F., Richard M. Bell, and Merril T. Dayton (Editors). *Essentials of General Surgery.* 2nd edition. Philadelphia, PA: Lippincott, Williams & Wilkins, 2000.

Lindholm, T. Sam, ed. *Advances in Skeletal Reconstruction Using Bone Morphogenetic Proteins.* River Edge, NJ: World Scientific Publishing Co., Inc., 2002.

PERIODICALS

Berg-Johnsen, J., and B. Magnaes. "Rib Bone Graft for Posterior Spinal Fusion in Children." *Acta Orthopaedica Scandinavic* 73, no.9 (December 2002): 260-7.

Cowan, N., J. Young, D. Murphy, and C. Bladen. "Double-blind, Randomized, Controlled Trial of Local Anesthetic Use for Iliac Crest Donor Site Pain." *Journal of Neuroscience Nursing* 34, no.4 (August, 2002): 205-10.

Kakibuchi, M., K. Fukuda, N. Yamada, K. Matsuda, K. Kawai, T. Kubo, et al. "A Simple Method of Harvesting a Thin Iliac Bone Graft for Reconstruction of the Orbital Wall." *Plastic Reconstruction Surgery* 111, no.2 (February 2003): 961-2.

Nelson C. L., J. H. Lonner, J. A. Rand, and P.A. Lotke. "Strategies of Stem Fixation and the Role of Supplemental Bone Graft in Revision Total Knee Arthroplasty." *Journal of Bone and Joint Surgery* American volume. 85-A Suppl 1 (2003): S52-7.

ORGANIZATIONS

American Association of Tissue Banks. 1350 Beverly Road, Suite 220-A, McLean, VA. 22101. (703) 827-9582, fax: (703) 356-2198. E-mail: aatb@aatb.org. <http://www.aatb.org/menu.htm>.

National Institutes of Health. 9000 Rockville Pike, Bethesda, MD. 20892. (301) 496-4000. Email: NIHInfo@OD.NIH.GOV. <http://www.nih.gov/>.

North American Spine Society. 22 Calendar Court, 2nd Floor, LaGrange, IL 60525. (877) Spine-Dr. E-mail: info@spine.org. <http://www.spine.org>.

OTHER

American Academy of Orthopaedic Surgeons (AAOS) and American Association of Tissue Banks (AATB). "What Can You Tell Me About Bone and Tissue Transplantation?" 2001. [cited March 19, 2003]. <http://orthoinfo.aaos.org/brochure/thr_report. cfm?Thread_ID=53&topcategory=About%20Ortho paedics&all=all>.

U.S. National Library of Medicine and the National Institutes of Health. *MEDLINE plus Health Information.* 2003 [cited March 13, 2003]. <http://www.nlm.nih.gov/medlineplus/html>.

Lisa Christenson, Ph.D.
Crystal H. Kaczkowski, M.Sc.

Bone lengthening/shortening *see* **Leg lengthening/shortening**

Bone marrow aspiration and biopsy

Definition

Bone marrow aspiration, also called bone marrow sampling, is the removal by suction of the soft, spongy semisolid tissue (marrow) that fills the inside of the long and flat bones. Bone marrow biopsy, or needle core biopsy, is the removal of a small piece (about 0.75 X 0.06 in, or 2 X 0.16 cm) of intact bone marrow. The bone marrow is where blood cells are made.

Purpose

Examination of the bone marrow may be the next step that follows an abnormal clinical finding, such as an abnormal **complete blood count** (CBC), and/or an abnormal peripheral blood smear. It may also be performed following an abnormal bone image such as the finding of a lesion on x rays.

A biopsy of bone marrow shows the intact tissue, so that the structure of the fat cells, lymphocytes, plasma cells, fibrous connective tissue cells, and other cells, and their relationships to each other, can be seen. A bone marrow biopsy is used to:

- diagnose and manage any form of leukemia or other myeloproliferative condition such as multiple myeloma
- rule out or confirm bone marrow infiltration by malignancies such as Hodgkin's disease, non-Hodgkin's lymphoma, and metastatic carcinoma
- monitor the effects of chemotherapy and the response or lack of response to treatment of blood disease
- evaluate the success of bone marrow transplantation
- diagnose certain genetic diseases (e.g., lipid storage disease)
- investigate pancytopenia (a decrease of all blood cells in peripheral blood), neutropenia (decreased phagocytic white blood cells), or thrombocytopenia (decreased platelets)
- diagnose an infection of unknown origin
- investigate rare anemias for which a cause cannot be found or which does not respond to treatment as anticipated
- obtain intact bone marrow for laboratory analysis
- diagnose some types of cancer or anemia and other blood disorders
- identify the source of an unexplained fever (e.g., granulomatous lesions)
- diagnose fibrosis of bone marrow and myeloma when bone marrow aspiration has failed to provide an appropriate specimen

The combination of aspiration and biopsy procedures are commonly used to ensure the availability of the best possible bone marrow specimen. The aspirate is collected at the same time as the bone core biopsy by attaching a syringe to the bone marrow needle and withdrawing the sample before the cutting blades are inserted and the bone core is removed. The aspirate is the sample of choice for studying and classifying the nucleated blood cells of the bone marrow (e.g., determining the ratio of immature white blood cells to red blood cells (M:E ratio). The biopsy is the only sample that shows the blood forming cells in relation to the structural and connective tissue elements (i.e., the microarchitecture) of the bone marrow. It provides the best sample for evaluating the cellularity of the bone marrow (the percentage of blood-forming tissue versus fat).

Description

Bone marrow aspiration and biopsy are performed by a pathologist, hematologist, or oncologist with special training in this procedure. The procedure may be performed on an outpatient basis. In adults, the specimen is usually taken from the posterior superior iliac crest (hip). The sternum (breastbone) may be used for aspiration, but is less desirable because it carries the risk of cardiac puncture. Other sites that are rarely used are the anterior superior iliac crest or a spinal column bone. When the patient is a child, the biopsy site is generally the anterior tibia, the larger of the two bones in the lower leg. A vertebra may also be used.

The skin covering the biopsy site is cleansed with an antiseptic, and the patient may be given a mild sedative. The patient is positioned, and a local anesthetic such as lidocaine is administered first under the skin with a fine needle and then around the bone at the intended puncture site with a somewhat larger gauge needle. When the area is numb, a small incision is made in the skin and the biopsy needle is inserted. Pressure is applied to force the needle through the outer bone, and a decrease in resistance signals entry into the marrow cavity. The needle most often used for bone marrow biopsy is a Jamshidi trephine needle or a Westerman-Jensen trephine needle. A syringe is placed on the top of the needle and 1–2 ml of the bone marrow is aspirated into the syringe. In some instances, the marrow cannot be aspirated because it is fibrosed or packed with neoplastic cells. The syringe is removed and the medical technologist uses this sample to prepare several smears containing small pieces of bone (spicules). Another syringe is fitted onto the needle hub and another sample of 3 ml is removed and transferred to a tube containing EDTA for analysis by flow cytometry, cytogenetic testing, or other special laboratory procedures. Following aspiration, the cutting blades are insert-

ed into the hollow of the needle until they protrude into the marrow. The needle is then forced over the tips of the cutting blades and the needle is rotated as it is withdrawn from the bone. This process captures the core sample inside the needle. A wire probe is inserted at the cutting end and the bone marrow sample is pushed through the hub of the needle onto sterile gauze. The specimen is used to make several preparations on glass slides or coverglasses and is transferred to a fixative solution.

In the laboratory, the aspirate slides are stained with Wright stain or Wright-Giemsa stain. The biopsy material is sectioned onto glass slides and stained with hematoxylin-eosin, Giemsa, and Prussian blue stains. Prussian blue stain is used to evaluate the amount of bone marrow iron, and the other stains are used to contrast cell structures under the microscope. In addition, special stains may be used that aid in the classification of malignant white blood cells.

Diagnosis/Preparation

The physician should be informed of any medication the patient is using and any heart surgery that the patient may have undergone.

Adults require no special preparation for this test. As for infants and children, they need physical and psychological preparation depending on the child's age, previous medical experiences, and level of trust.

Infant preparation

Before the test, parents should know that their child will most probably cry, and that restraints may be used. To provide comfort, and help their child through this procedure, parents are commonly asked to be present during the procedure. Crying is a normal infant response to an unfamiliar environment, strangers, restraints, and separation from the parent. Infants cry more for these reasons than because they hurt. An infant will be restrained by hand or with devices because they have not yet developed the physical control, coordination, and ability to follow commands as adults have. The restraints used thus aim to ensure the infant's safety.

Toddler preparation

Parents should prepare a toddler for bone marrow aspiration directly before the procedure, because toddlers have a very short attention span. Some general guidelines for parents include the following:

• Explain the procedure in a simple language, using concrete terms and avoiding abstract terminology.

• Make sure that the child understands where on his body the procedure will be performed and that it will be limited to that area.

- Allow the child to yell, cry, or express anything, especially pain, verbally.
- Describe how the test will feel.
- Stress the benefits of the procedure and anything that the child may find enjoyable afterwards, such as feeling better or going home.

Preschooler preparation

Parents should prepare a preschooler for bone marrow aspiration directly before the procedure, so that the child does not worry about it for days in advance. Explanations should be limited to 10 or 15 minutes, because preschoolers also have a limited attention span. Parents should also ensure that the child understands that the procedure is not a punishment. Some general guidelines for parents include the following:

- Explain the procedure in a simple language, using concrete terms and avoiding abstract terminology.
- Make sure that the child understands where on his or her body the procedure will be performed and that it will be limited to that area.
- Allow the child to yell, cry, or express anything, especially pain, verbally.
- Describe how the test will feel and be honest about any pain that may be felt.
- Allow the child to practice different positions or movements that will be required for the procedure.
- Stress the benefits of the procedure and anything that the child may find enjoyable afterwards, such as feeling better or going for a treat on the way home.
- Practice deep breathing and other relaxing exercises. Practice also to have the child hold your hand and tell him or her to squeeze it when he or she feels pain during the procedure.

School-age child preparation

Explanations should be limited to 20 minutes, and repeated if required. School-age children have a good concept of time, allowing for preparation in advance of the procedure. The older the child, the earlier a parent can start preparation. Guidelines for parents include the ones provided for preschoolers as well as the following:

- Suggest ways for maintaining control during the procedure. For example, counting, deep breathing, and relaxation (thinking of pleasant thoughts).
- Include the child in the decision-making process, for example, the time of day or the body site where the procedure will be performed. These of course depend on the scheduling constraints of your physician and the

---

QUESTIONS TO ASK THE DOCTOR

- What are the possible risks involved in this procedure?
- How many times will the procedure be required?
- How do I prepare for the procedure?
- Must I do anything special after the procedure?
- How long does it take to know the results?
- How many bone marrow aspirations/biopsies do you perform each year?

---

type of procedure being performed, but where possible, involve the child in the decisions.

- Encourage the child to participate in the procedure, for example by holding an instrument, if allowed by the attending hospital staff.
- Encourage the child to hold your hand or the hand of a nurse. Physical contact does help reduce pain and anxiety.

Adolescent preparation

An adolescent is best prepared by being provided with detailed information and reasons for the procedure. Adolescents should be encouraged to make as many decisions as possible. An adolescent may or may not wish a parent to be present during the procedure, and such wishes should be respected, since privacy is important during adolescence. Other guidelines include the following:

- Explain the procedure in correct medical terminology, and provide the reason for it. Ask the physician about the specific reason if you are not sure.
- To the best of your ability, describe the equipment that will be involved in concrete terms.
- Discuss potential risks because adolescents are usually quite concerned about any effects on appearance, mental function, and sexuality. These concerns should be addressed honestly and openly.

Aftercare

After the needle is removed, the biopsy site is covered with a clean, dry pressure bandage. The patient must remain lying down and is observed for bleeding for one hour. The patient's pulse, breathing, blood pressure, and temperature are monitored until they return to nor-

KEY TERMS

Antibodies—Proteins that are produced normally by specialized white blood cells after stimulation by a foreign substance (antigen) and that act specifically against the antigen in an immune response.

Aspiration—A procedure to withdraw fluid and cells from the body.

Connective tissue—Cells such as fibroblasts, and material such as collagen and reticulin, that unites one part of the body with another.

Fibrosis—A condition characterized by the presence of scar tissue, or reticulin and collagen proliferation in tissues to the extent that it replaces normal tissues.

Hematologist—A specialist who treats diseases and disorders of the blood and blood-forming organs.

Hematoma—Blood that collects under the skin, forms a blood clot, and causes swelling.

Hemorrhage—Heavy bleeding.

Immune system—Mechanism that protects the body from foreign substances, cells, and pathogens by producing the immune response, a concerted defense involving the thymus, spleen, lymph nodes, white blood cells including the B cells and T cells, and antibodies.

Lymphocytes—Type of white blood cells that are part of the immune system. The lymphocytes are composed of three main cell lines; B lymphocytes, T lymphocytes, and natural killer (NK) cells.

Myeloma (multiple myeloma)—A tumor of plasma cells that originates in bone marrow and usually spreads to more than one bone.

Needle biopsy—The procedure of using a large hollow needle to obtain a sample of intact tissue.

Pathologist—A medical doctor that specializes in identifying diseases by studying cells and tissues under a microscope.

Plasma cells—Cells in the blood and bone marrow that are formed from B lymphocytes, and that produce antibodies.

White blood cells (leukocytes)—Cells of the blood that are responsible for fighting infection.

---

mal. The biopsy site should be kept covered and dry for several hours.

The patient should be able to leave the clinic and resume most normal activities immediately. Patients who have received a sedative often feel sleepy for the rest of the day; so driving, cooking, and other activities that require clear thinking and quick reactions should be avoided. Walking or prescribed pain medications usually ease any discomfort felt at the biopsy site, and ice can be used to reduce swelling.

A doctor should be notified if the patient:

- feels severe pain for more than 24 hours after the procedure

- experiences persistent bleeding or notices more than a few drops of blood on the wound dressing

- has a temperature above 101°F (38.3°C)

- inflammation and pus at the biopsy site and other signs of infection

Risks

A small amount of bleeding and moderate discomfort often occur at the biopsy site. Rarely, reactions to anesthetic agents, infection, and hematoma (blood clot) or hemorrhage (excessive bleeding) may also develop. In rare instances, the heart or a major blood vessel is pierced when marrow is extracted from the sternum during bone marrow biopsy. This can lead to severe hemorrhage.

Normal results

Healthy adult bone marrow contains yellow fat cells, connective tissue, and red marrow that produces blood. Bone marrow is evaluated for cellularity, megakaryocyte production, M:E ratio, differential (classification of blood forming cells), iron content, lymphoid, bone, and connective tissue cells, and bone and blood vessel abnormalities. The bone marrow of a healthy infant is primarily red (75–100% cellularity), but the distribution of blood forming cells is very different than adult marrow. Consequently, age-related normal values must be used.

Microscopic examination of bone marrow can reveal leukemia, granulomas, myelofibrosis, myeloma, lymphoma, or metastatic cancers, bone marrow infection, and bone disease. Bone marrow evaluation is usually not needed to diagnose anemia, but may be useful in cases that cannot be classified by other means.

Resources

BOOKS

Montiel, Milka M. "Bone Marrow." In *Clinical Hematology and Fundamentals of Homeostasis.* 3rd ed., edited by Denise M. Harmening. Philadelphia: F. A. Davis Company, 1997.

Ryan, Daniel H. "Examination of the Marrow." In *Williams Hematology.* 6th ed., edited by Ernest Beutler, et al. New York, NY: McGraw-Hill, 2001.

PERIODICALS

Azar, D., C. Donaldson, and L. Dalla-Pozza. "Questioning the Need for Routine Bone Marrow Aspiration and Lumbar Puncture in Patients with Retinoblastoma." *Clinical and Experimental Ophthalmology* 31 (February 2003): 57–60.

Coop, J. "Bone Marrow Aspiration and Biopsy—2." *Nursing Times* 97 (August 2–8 2001): 45–46.

Coop, J. "Bone Marrow Aspiration and Biopsy—3." *Nursing Times* 97 (August 9–15, 2001): 43–44.

Cotelingam, James D. "Bone Marrow Interpretation: The Science and the Art." *Pathology Case Reviews* (September/ October 2000): 239–251.

Goldenberg, A. S., and J. J. Tiesinga. "Clinical Experience with a New Specimen Capturing Bone Marrow Biopsy Needle." *American Journal of Hematology* 68 (November 2001): 189–193.

Jubelirer, S. J., and R. Harpold. "The Role of the Bone Marrow Examination in the diagnosis of Immune Thrombocytopenic Purpura: Case Series and Literature Review." *Clinical and Applied Thrombosis/Homeostasis* 8 (January 2002): 73–76.

ORGANIZATIONS

The Leukemia & Lymphoma Society. 1311 Mamaroneck Avenue, White Plains, NY 10605. (914) 949-5213. <http://www.leukemia.org>.

National Cancer Institute Cancer Information Service. 31 Center Drive, Bethesda, MD 20892-2580. (800) 422-6237. <http://www.nci.nih.gov>.

National Marrow Donor Program. Suite 500, 3001 Broadway Street NE, Minneapolis, MN 55413-1753. (800) 627-7692. <http://www.marrow.org>.

OTHER

"Bone Marrow Biopsy." *Discoveryhealth.com.* June 2001 [cited April 2003]. <http://www.health.discovery.com/diseasesandcond/encyclopedia/1087.html>.

CanCareSA Bone Marrow Biopsy. July 1998 [cited April 2003]. <http://www.health.sa.gov.au/cancare/TREATS/TESTS/bmbiop.htm>.

"Diagnostic Tests: Bone Marrow Biopsy." *Harvard Family Health Guide.* [cited April 2003]. <http://www.health.harvard.edu/fhg/diagnostics/marrow/marrow.shtml>.

Mark A. Best
Monique Laberge, PhD

Bone marrow transplantation

Definition

The bone marrow—the sponge-like tissue found in the center of certain bones—contains stem cells that are the precursors of white blood cells, red blood cells, and platelets. These blood cells are vital for normal body functions, such as oxygen transport, defense against infection and disease, and clotting. Blood cells have a limited life span and are constantly being replaced; therefore, the production of healthy stem cells is vital.

In association with certain diseases, stem cells may produce too many, too few, or abnormal blood cells. Also, medical treatments may destroy stem cells or alter blood cell production. Blood cell abnormalities can be life-threatening.

Bone marrow transplantation involves extracting bone marrow containing normal stem cells or peripheral stem cells from a healthy donor, and transferring it to a recipient whose body cannot manufacture proper quantities of normal blood cells. The goal of the transplant is to rebuild the recipient's blood cells and immune system and hopefully cure the underlying disease.

Purpose

A person's red blood cells, white blood cells, and platelets may be destroyed or may be abnormal due to disease. Also, certain medical therapies, particularly chemotherapy or radiation therapy, may destroy a person's stem cells. The consequence to a person's health is severe. Under normal circumstances, red blood cells carry oxygen throughout the body and remove carbon dioxide from the body's tissues. White blood cells form the cornerstone of the body's immune system and defend it against infection. Platelets limit bleeding by enabling the blood to clot if a blood vessel is damaged.

A bone marrow transplant is used to rebuild the body's capacity to produce these blood cells and bring their numbers to normal levels. Illnesses that may be treated with a bone marrow transplant include both cancerous and noncancerous diseases.

Cancerous diseases may or may not specifically involve blood cells; but, cancer treatment can destroy the body's ability to manufacture new blood cells. Bone marrow transplantation may be used in conjunction with additional treatments, such as chemotherapy, for various types of leukemia, Hodgkin's disease, lymphoma, breast and ovarian cancer, renal cell carcinoma, myelodysplasia, myelofibrosis, germ cell cancer, and other cancers. Noncancerous diseases for which bone marrow trans-

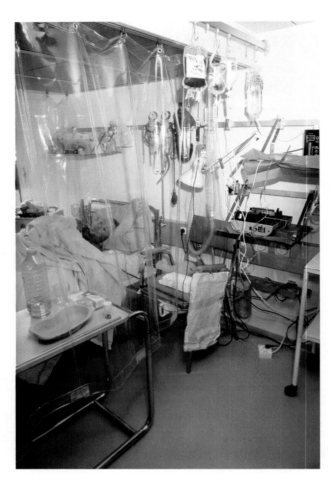

Patients who have undergone a bone marrow transplant are placed in sterile rooms to prevent infections. *(Custom Medical Stock Photo. Reproduced by permission.)*

plantation can be a treatment option include aplastic anemia, sickle cell disease, thalassemia, and severe immunodeficiency.

Demographics

The decision to prescribe a bone marrow transplant is based on the patient's age, general physical condition, diagnosis and stage of the disease. A person's age or state of health may prohibit use of a bone marrow transplant. The typical cut-off age for a transplant ranges from 40 to 55 years; however, a person's general health is usually the more important factor. Before undergoing a bone marrow transplant, the bone marrow transplant team will ensure that the patient understands the potential benefits and risks of the procedure.

The first successful bone marrow transplant took place in 1968 at the University of Minnesota. The recipient was a child with severe combined immunodeficiency disease and

the donor was a sibling. In 1973, the first unrelated bone marrow transplant was performed at Memorial Sloan-Kettering Cancer Center in New York City on a five-year-old patient with severe combined immunodeficiency disease. In 1984, Congress passed the National Organ Transplant Act which included language to evaluate unrelated marrow transplantation and determine if a national donor registry was feasible. The National Bone Marrow Donor Registry (NBMDR), now called the National Marrow Donor Program (NMDP), was established in 1986.

The NMDP Network has more than four million volunteer donors and has Donor Centers and Transplant Centers in 14 countries. About 40% of the transplants facilitated by the NMDP involve either a U.S. patient receiving bone marrow and/or stem cells from an international donor, or an international patient receiving bone marrow/stem cells from a U.S. donor.

The NMDP coordinates more than 130 stem cell transplants each month. Approximately 12,000 total bone marrow/stem cell transplants have been performed since the organization was founded.

Description

Types of bone marrow transplants

AUTOLOGOUS AND ALLOGENEIC TRANSPLANTS. Two important requirements for a bone marrow transplant are the donor and the recipient. Sometimes, the donor and the recipient may be the same person. This type of transplant is called an autologous transplant. It is typically used in cases in which a person's bone marrow is generally healthy but will be destroyed due to medical treatment for diseases such as breast cancer and Hodgkin's disease. Autologous transplants are also possible if the disease affecting the bone marrow is in remission. If a person's bone marrow is unsuitable for an autologous transplant, the bone marrow must be derived from another person in an allogeneic transplant.

An allogeneic bone marrow donor may be a family member or an unrelated donor. The donated bone marrow/peripheral stem cells must perfectly match the patient's bone marrow. The matching process is called HLA (human leukocyte antigens). Antigens are markers in cells that stimulate antibody production. HLA antigens are proteins on the surface of bone marrow cells. HLA testing is a series of blood tests that evaluate the closeness of tissue between the donor and recipient. If the donor and the recipient have very dissimilar antigens, the recipient's immune system regards the donor's bone marrow cells as invaders and launches a destructive attack against them. Such an attack negates any benefits offered by the transplant.

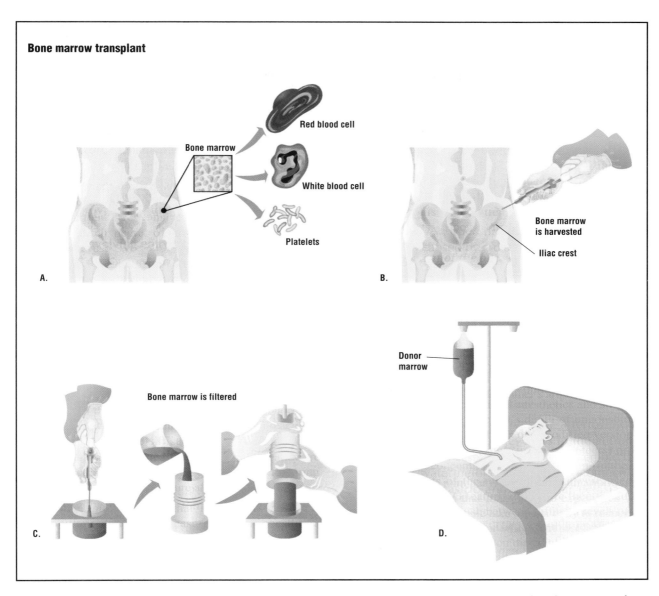

Bone marrow transplant

Bone marrow

Red blood cell

White blood cell

Platelets

A.

Bone marrow
is harvested

Iliac crest

B.

Bone marrow is filtered

C.

Donor
marrow

D.

Bone marrow consists of red blood cells, white blood cells, and platelets (A). In a bone marrow transplant, bone marrow is harvested from the donor's pelvic bone at the iliac crest (B). The marrow is filtered (C) before being introduced into a large vein in the recipient's chest via a catheter (D). *(Illustration by GGS Inc.)*

NON-MYEOBLATIVE ("MINI") ALLOGENEIC TRANS-PLANTS. A "mini" transplant involves receiving low-doses of chemotherapy and radiation therapy, followed by the infusion of a donor's bone marrow or peripheral stem cells. The goal is to suppress the patient's own bone marrow with low-dose chemotherapy and radiation therapy to allow the donor's cells to engraft. If there are cancer cells remaining in the patient's body, the donated cells are able to identify the cancer cells as foreign and trigger an immune response, killing the cancer cells. This is called the graft-versus-tumor effect. Mini transplants are still under investigation but are promising for the future.

PERIPHERAL BLOOD STEM CELL TRANSPLANTS. A relatively recent development in stem cell transplantation is the use of peripheral blood stem cells instead of cells from the bone marrow. Peripheral blood stem cells (PBSCs) are obtained from circulating blood rather than from bone marrow, but the amount of stem cells found in the peripheral blood is much smaller than the amount of stem cells found in the bone marrow. Peripheral blood stem cells can be used in either autologous or allogeneic transplants. The majority of PBSC transplants are autologous. However, clinical studies indicate that PBSCs are being used more frequently than bone marrow for allogeneic bone marrow transplantation.

WHO PERFORMS THE PROCEDURE AND WHERE IS IT PERFORMED?

Transplant physicians specially trained in bone marrow transplantation should perform this procedure. Bone marrow transplant physicians have extensive experience in hematology/oncology and bone marrow transplant.

Selecting a transplant center that has a multi-disciplinary team of specialists is important. The bone marrow transplant team should include transplant physicians, infectious disease specialists, pharmacologists, registered nurses and transplant coordinators. Other transplant team members may include registered dietitians, social workers, and financial counselors.

When selecting a transplant center, the patient should find out where the center is accredited. Some examples of accrediting organizations include The Foundation for the Accreditation of Cellular Therapy, the American Association of Blood Banking, the National Marrow Donor Program, and other state-level accreditation organizations.

Choosing a transplant center with experience is important. Here are some questions to consider when choosing a transplant center:

- How many bone marrow transplants are performed annually and what are the outcomes/survival rates of those transplants?

- Does the transplant center perform transplants for the patient's type of disease? How many has it performed to date?

- Does the transplant center have experience treating patients the same age as the patient considering transplant?

- What is the required patient and unrelated donor HLA matching level at this center?

- How much does a typical bone marrow transplant cost at this facility?

- Is financial help available?

- If the transplant center is far from the patient's home, will accommodations be provided for caregivers?

The advantages of PBSC transplants when compared to bone marrow transplants are: in allogeneic transplantation, haematopoietic and immune recovery are faster with PBSCs. In autologous transplantation, the use of PBSCs can result in faster blood count recovery. Also, some medical conditions exist in which the recipient cannot accept bone marrow transplants, but can accept PBSC transplants. Some possible disadvantages to PBSC transplant versus bone marrow transplantation are: so much more fluid volume is necessary to collect enough PBSCs that, at the time that the new stem cells are infused into the recipient, the fluid can collect in the lungs. Also, the time commitment for the donor for a PBSC transplant is considerable. When the PBSCs are being collected, several outpatient sessions are needed and each session lasts approximately two to four hours.

UMBILICAL CORD BLOOD TRANSPLANT. Umbilical cord blood transplant is a relatively new procedure in which umbilical cord blood from a newborn is used as the donor source. Umbilical cord blood is rich in stem cells, the cells that are needed for transplantation, and these cells are theoretically "immunologically naïve," reducing chances of rejection and making it a good source for donation. The matching criteria is the same as for bone marrow. Most programs to date use this procedure for a sibling or store cord blood for anonymous donation. Umbilical cord blood can be an excellent source for children. One potential problem with umbilical cord blood transplantation is the low volume of stem cells contained in the umbilical cord. In many instances, there is inadequate volume to safely use for a transplant in an adult recipient.

The transplant procedure

HLA MATCHING. There are only five major HLA classes or types—designated HLA-A, -B, -C, -D, and class III—but much variation within the groupings. For example, HLA-A from one individual may be similar to, but not the same as, HLA-A in another individual; such a situation can render a transplant from one to the other impossible.

HLA matching is more likely if the donor and recipient are related, particularly if they are siblings; however, an unrelated donor may be a potential match. Only in rare cases is matching HLA types between two people not an issue: if the recipient has an identical twin. Identical twins carry the same genes; therefore, the same antigens. A bone marrow transplant between identical twins is called a syngeneic transplant.

BONE MARROW TRANSPLANTATION. The bone marrow extraction, or harvest, is the same for autologous and allogeneic transplants. Harvesting is done under general anesthesia (i.e., the donor sleeps through the procedure), and discomfort is usually minimal afterwards. Bone marrow is drawn from the iliac crest (the part of the hip bone

QUESTIONS TO ASK THE DOCTOR

- What type of transplant is recommended for my condition?
- What are the potential benefits of bone marrow transplantation?
- Where does transplanted bone marrow come from?
- What types of tests are required to screen me for the bone marrow transplant?
- What is HLA/histocompatibility matching?
- What types of tests are used to screen potential bone marrow or peripheral stem donors?
- Are bone marrow or peripheral stem cell donors compensated?
- After my bone marrow transplant, can I contact an unrelated donor? How can I do this?
- Will my insurance provider cover the expenses of my bone marrow transplant?
- What types of questions should I ask my insurance provider to determine if the medical expenses of my bone marrow transplant will be covered?
- Whose insurance covers the medical expenses of the donor?
- How long does the insurance clearance process take?
- After bone marrow transplantation is approved as a treatment option for me, how long will I have to wait before I can receive the bone marrow transplant?
- What type of preparative regimen will I have before the bone marrow transplant?
- What are the side effects of the preparative regimen?

- What types of precautions must I follow before and after my bone marrow transplant?
- Will I have to have blood transfusions during the transplantation process?
- What are the risks and potential complications of bone marrow transplantation?
- What is Graft-versus-Host disease (GVHD) and can it be prevented?
- What are the signs of GVHD, rejection, and infection?
- How and when will I know if the bone marrow transplant was successful?
- How long will I have to stay in the hospital?
- What types of resources are available to me during my hospital stay and during my recovery at home?
- WHat types of medications will I have to take after my bone marrow transplant? How long will I have to take them?
- After I go home, how long will it take me to recover?
- When can I resume my normal activities?
- What type of follow-up care is recommended? How often will I need to go to follow-up appointments?
- Can I receive follow-up care from my primary physician, or do I need to go back to the center where I had my bone marrow transplant?
- If I live far away from my transplant center, do I have to stay near the transplant center during my recovery after I'm discharged? If yes, for how long? Will I receive help in making accommodations?

to either side of the lower back) with a special needle and a syringe. Several punctures are usually necessary to collect the needed amount of bone marrow, approximately 1–2 quarts. (This amount is only a small percentage of the total bone marrow and is typically replaced within four weeks.) The donor remains at the hospital for 24–48 hours and can resume normal activities within a few days.

If the bone marrow is meant for an autologous transplant, it is stored at -112– -320°F (-80– -196°C) until it is needed. If a patient's own bone marrow can be used for transplantation or if a donor is not found, peripheral stem cells may be harvested from the patient's circulat-

ing blood. Bone marrow for an allogeneic transplant is sometimes treated to remove the donor's T cells (a type of white blood cell) or to remove ABO (blood type) antigens; otherwise, it is transplanted without modification.

The bone marrow or peripheral stem cells are administered to the recipient via a catheter (a narrow, flexible tube) inserted into a large vein in the chest. The donor cells look like a bag of blood and are infused for about 20–30 minutes. During the infusion, the patient's blood pressure, pulse, and breathing are monitored. From the bloodstream, it migrates to the cavities within the bones where bone marrow is normally stored. If the

KEY TERMS

ABO antigen—Protein molecules located on the surfaces of red blood cells that determine a person's blood type: A, B, or O.

AML—Acute myelogenous leukemia, also called acute myelocytic leukemia. Malignant disorder where myeloid blast cells accumulate in the marrow and bloodstream.

Allogeneic—Referring to bone marrow transplants between two different, genetically dissimilar people.

Anemia—Decreased red cell production which results in deficiency in oxygen-carrying capacity of the blood.

Antigen—A molecule that is capable of provoking an immune response.

Aplastic anemia—A disorder in which the body produces inadequate amounts of red blood cells and hemoglobin due to underdeveloped or missing bone marrow.

Autologous—Referring to bone marrow transplants in which recipients serve as their own donors.

Blank—If an individual has inherited the same HLA antigen from both parents, the HLA typing is designated by the shared HLA antigen followed by a "blank"(-).

Blast cells—Blood cells in early stage of cellular development.

Blast crisis—Stage of chronic myelogenous leukemia where large quantities of immature cells are produced by the marrow and is not responsive to treatment.

Bone marrow—A spongy tissue located within flat bones, including the hip and breast bones and the skull. This tissue contains stem cells, the precursors of platelets, red blood cells, and white blood cells.

Bone marrow biopsy—A test involving the insertion of a thin needle into the breastbone or more commonly, the hip, in order to aspirate (remove) a sample of the marrow. A small piece of cortical bone may also be obtained for biopsy.

Bone marrow transplant—Healthy marrow is infused into people who have had high-dose chemotherapy for one of the many forms of leukemias, immunodeficiencies, lymphomas, anemias, metabolic disorders, and sometimes solid tumors.

Chemotherapy—Medical treatment of a disease, particularly cancer, with drugs or other chemicals.

Chest x ray—A diagnostic procedure in which a very small amount of radiation is used to produce an image of the structures of the chest (heart, lungs, and bones) on film.

transplant is successful, the bone marrow begins to produce normal blood cells once it is in place, or engrafted.

PERIPHERAL BLOOD STEM CELL TRANSPLANTATION. Before collection for a PBSC transplant, donors receive four injections daily of the drug G-CSF, or filgrastim. (Patients can give it to themselves at home if necessary.) These pretreatments stimulate the body to release stem cells into the blood. After these pretreatments, the donors' experience is similar to that of a whole blood donor's experience—PBSC donors' blood is collected at a clinic or hospital as an outpatient procedure. The differences are that several sessions will be needed over days or weeks and the blood is collected in a process called apheresis. The blood travels from one arm into a blood cell separator that removes only the stem cells, and the rest of the blood is returned back to the donor, in the other arm. The cells are then frozen for later use.

The PBSCs are administered to the recipient using the same methods as those used in bone marrow transplantation. As stated, the amount of fluid with PBSCs infused into the recipient's body can be an issue.

Costs

Bone marrow transplantation is an expensive procedure. (Bone marrow donors are volunteers and do not pay for any part of the procedure.) Insurance companies and health maintenance organizations (HMOs) may not cover the costs. Many insurance companies require pre-certification letters of medical necessity. As soon as bone marrow transplantation is discussed as a treatment option, it is important for the patient to contact his or her insurance provider to determine what costs will be covered.

Diagnosis/Preparation

Several tests are performed before the bone marrow transplant to identify any potential problems ahead of time. Tests include:

• tissue typing and a variety of blood tests

Chronic myelogenous leukemia (CML)—Also called chronic myelocytic leukemia, a malignant disorder that involves abnormal accumulation of white cells in the marrow and bloodstream.

Cytomegalovirus (CMV)—Virus that can cause pneumonia in post bone marrow transplant patients.

Computed tomography scan (CT or CAT scan)—Computed axial tomography, commonly known as a CAT scan, uses x rays and computers to produce an image of a cross-section of the body.

Conditioning—Process of preparing a patient to receive marrow donation, often through the use of chemotherapy and radiation therapy.

Confirmatory typing—Repeat tissue typing to confirm the compatibility of the donor and patient before transplant.

Donor—A healthy person who contributes bone marrow for transplantation.

Echocardiogram—An imaging procedure used to create a picture of the heart's movement, valves and chambers. The test uses high-frequency sound waves that come from a hand wand placed on your chest. Echocardiogram may be used in combination with Doppler ultrasound to evaluate the blood flow across the heart's valves. *Also see Transesophageal echocardiogram.*

Electrocardiogram (ECG, EKG)—A test that records the electrical activity of the heart using small electrode patches attached to the skin on the chest.

Graft versus host disease—A life-threatening complication of bone marrow transplants in which the donated marrow causes an immune reaction against the recipient's body.

Histocompatibility—The major histocompatibility determinants are the human leukocyte antigens (HLA) and characterize how well the patient and donor are matched.

HLA (human leukocyte antigen)—A group of protein molecules located on bone marrow cells that can provoke an immune response. A donor's and a recipient's HLA types should match as closely as possible to prevent the recipient's immune system from attacking the donor's marrow as a foreign material that does not belong in the body.

Hodgkin's disease—A type of cancer involving the lymph nodes and potentially affecting nonlymphatic organs in the later stage.

Immunodeficiency—A disorder in which the immune system is ineffective or disabled either due to acquired or inherited disease.

- chest x ray
- pulmonary function tests
- computed tomography scan (CT or CAT scan)
- heart function tests including an electrocardiogram and echocardiogram
- bone marrow biopsy
- skeletal survey

In addition, a complete dental exam is needed before the bone marrow transplant to reduce the risk of infection. Other precautions will be taken before the transplant to reduce the patient's risk of infection.

A triple lumen, central venous catheter (a slender, hollow flexible tube) is surgically inserted into a large vein in the chest during a simple outpatient procedure. The catheter is used to draw blood and infuse chemotherapy and other medications as well as donor cells, blood product, fluids, and sometimes nutritional solutions. The central venous catheter usually stays in place for about six months after the bone marrow transplant.

Hormone-like medications called colony stimulating factors may be given before the transplant to stimulate the patient's white blood cells. These medications stimulate the white blood cells to multiply, mature, and function. These medications also help the patient's white blood cells recover from chemotherapy and reduce the risk of infection.

A bone marrow transplant recipient can expect to spend three to four weeks in the hospital, depending on the rate of recovery. In preparation for receiving the transplant, the recipient undergoes "conditioning"—a preparative regimen (also called marrow ablation) in which the bone marrow and abnormal cells are destroyed. Conditioning rids the body of diseased cells and makes room for the marrow or peripheral stem cells to be transplanted. It typically involves chemotherapy and/or radiation treatment, depending on the disease being treated. Unfortunately, this treatment also destroys healthy cells and has many side effects such as extreme weakness, nausea, vomiting, and diarrhea. These side effects may continue for several weeks.

KEY TERMS (contd.)

Leukemia—A type of cancer that affects leukocytes, a particular type of white blood cell. A characteristic symptom is excessive production of immature or otherwise abnormal leukocytes.

Lymphoma—A type of cancer that affects lymph cells and tissues, including certain white blood cells (T cells and B cells), lymph nodes, bone marrow, and the spleen. Abnormal cells (lymphocyte/leukocyte) multiply uncontrollably.

Match—How similar the HLA typing, out of a possible six antigens, is between the donor and the recipient.

Mixed lymphocyte culture (MLC)—Test that measures level of reactivity between donor and recipient lymphocytes.

Myelodysplasia—Also called myelodysplastic syndrome. A condition in which the bone marrow does not function normally and can affect the various types of blood cells produced in the bone marrow. Often referred to as a preleukemia and may progress and become acute leukemia.

Myelofibrosis—An anemic condition in which bone marrow cells are abnormal or defective and become fibrotic.

Neuroblastoma—Solid tumor in children, may be treated by BMT.

Non-myeloblative allogeneic bone marrow transplant—Also called "mini" bone marrow transplants. This type of bone marrow transplant involves receiving low-doses of chemotherapy and radiation therapy, followed by the infusion of a donor's bone marrow or peripheral stem cells. The goal is to suppress the patient's own bone marrow with low-dose chemotherapy and radiation therapy to allow the donor's cells to engraft. If there are cancer cells remaining in the patient's body, the donated cells are able to identify the cancer cells as foreign and trigger an immune response, killing the cancer cells. This is called the graft-versus-tumor effect. Mini transplants are still under investigation but are promising for the future.

Peripheral stem cells—Stem cells that are taken directly from the circulating blood and used for transplantation. Stem cells are more concentrated in the bone marrow but they can also be extracted from the blood stream.

Peripheral stem cell transplant—The process of transplanting peripheral stem cells instead of using bone marrow. The stem cells in the circulating blood that are similar to those in the bone marrow are given to the patient after treatment to help the bone marrow recover and continue producing healthy blood cells. A peripheral stem cell transplant may also be used to supplement a bone marrow transplant.

Platelets—Fragments of a large precursor cell, a megakaryocyte found in the bone marrow. These fragments adhere to areas of blood vessel damage and release chemical signals that direct the formation of a blood clot.

Aftercare

A two- to four-week waiting period follows the marrow transplant before its success can begin to be judged. The marrow recipient is kept in isolation during this time to minimize potential infections. The recipient also receives intravenous antibiotic, antiviral, and antifungal medications, as well as blood and platelet transfusions to help fight off infection and prevent excessive bleeding. Blood tests are performed daily to monitor the patient's kidney and liver function, as well as nutritional status. Other tests are performed as necessary. Further side effects, such as nausea and vomiting, can be treated with other medications. Once blood counts are normal and the side effects of the transplant abate, the recipient is taken off **antibiotics** and usually no longer needs blood and platelet transfusions.

Following **discharge from the hospital**, the recipient is monitored through home visits by nurses or outpatient visits for up to a year. For the first several months out of the hospital, the recipient needs to be careful in avoiding potential infections. For example, contact with other people who may be ill should be avoided or kept to a minimum. Further blood transfusions and medications may be necessary, but barring complications, the recipient can return to normal activities about six to eight months after the transplant.

Risks

The procedure has a lower success rate the greater the recipient's age. Complications are exacerbated for people whose health is already seriously impaired, as in late-stage cancers.

Bone marrow transplants are accompanied by serious and life-threatening risks. Furthermore, they are not

Pulmonary function test—A test that measures the capacity and function of your lungs, as well as your blood's ability to carry oxygen. During the test, the patient breathes into a device called a spirometer.

Radiation therapy—The use of high-energy radiation from x rays, cobalt, radium, and other sources to kill cancer cells and shrink tumors. Radiation may come from a machine outside the body (external beam radiation therapy) or from materials called radioisotopes. Radioisotopes produce radiation and are placed in or near the tumor or in the area near the cancer cells. This type of radiation treatment is called internal radiation therapy, implant radiation, interstitial radiation, or brachytherapy. Systemic radiation therapy uses a radioactive substance, such as a radio labeled monoclonal antibody, that circulates throughout the body.

Recipient—The person who receives the donated blood marrow.

Red blood cells—Cells that carry hemoglobin (the molecule that transports oxygen) and help remove wastes from tissues throughout the body.

Remission—Disappearance of the signs and symptoms of cancer. When this happens, the disease is said to be "in remission." A remission can be temporary or permanent.

Sickle cell disease—An inherited disorder characterized by a genetic flaw in hemoglobin production. (Hemoglobin is the substance within red blood cells that enables them to transport oxygen.) The hemoglobin that is produced has a kink in its structure that forces the red blood cells to take on a sickle shape, inhibiting their circulation and causing pain. This disorder primarily affects people of African descent.

Stem cells—Unspecialized cells, or "immature" blood cells, that serve as the precursors of white blood cells, red blood cells, and platelets.

Syngeneic—Referring to a bone marrow transplant from one identical twin to the other.

Thalassemia—A group of inherited disorders that affects hemoglobin production. (Hemoglobin is the substance within red blood cells that enables them to transport oxygen.) Because hemoglobin production is impaired, a person with this disorder may suffer mild to severe anemia. Certain types of thalassemia can be fatal.

Umbilical cord blood transplant—A procedure in which the blood from a newborn's umbilical cord, which is rich in stem cells, is used as the donor source for bone marrow transplants. Currently, umbilical cord blood transplants are mainly used for sibling bone marrow transplants or to store blood for an anonymous donation. In most cases, umbilical cord blood does not contain enough stem cells to safely use for adult bone marrow transplants.

White blood cells—A group of several cell types that occur in the bloodstream and are essential for a properly functioning immune system.

---

always an absolute assurance of a cure for the underlying ailment; a disease may recur in the future.

Even in the absence of complications, the transplant and associated treatments are hard on the recipient. Bone marrow transplants are debilitating. A person's ability to withstand the rigors of the transplant is a key consideration in deciding to use this treatment.

In the short term, there is the danger of pneumonia or other infectious disease, excessive bleeding, or liver disorder caused by blocked blood vessels. The transplant may be rejected by the recipient's immune system, or the donor bone marrow may launch an immune-mediated attack against the recipient's tissues. This complication is called acute graft-versus-host disease, and it can be a life-threatening condition. Characteristic signs of the disease include fever, rash, diarrhea, liver problems, and a compromised immune system.

Approximately 25–50% of bone marrow transplant recipients develop long-term complications. Chronic graft-versus-host disease symptoms include skin changes such as dryness, altered pigmentation, and thickening; abnormal **liver function tests**; dry mouth and eyes; infections; and weight loss. Other long-term complications include cataracts (due to radiation treatment), abnormal lung function, hormonal abnormalities resulting in reduced growth or hypothyroidism, secondary cancers, and infertility.

Normal results

In a successful bone marrow transplant, the donor's marrow migrates to the cavities in the recipient's bones and produces normal numbers of healthy blood cells. Bone marrow transplants can extend a person's life, improve quality of life, and may aid in curing the underlying ailment.

Morbidity and mortality rates

Approximately 30% of people receiving allogeneic transplants do not survive. Autologous transplants have a much better survival rate—nearly 90%—but are not appropriate for all types of ailments requiring a bone marrow transplant. Furthermore, autologous transplants have a higher failure rate with certain diseases, specifically leukemia. At two years, the survival rate for patients with chronic myelogenous leukemia is 52% if they received a transplant in a chronic phase of their disease, 30% for patients in an accelerated phase and 15% for patients in the blast phase.

Alternatives

Complementary therapies are used along with standard cancer treatments. These treatments are aimed at bringing about some overall improvement in general health and well being. Complementary therapies can be helpful in managing symptoms and improving quality of life. They can be used to help alleviate pain; reduce nausea; strengthen muscles; and to decrease depression, anxiety, and stress. It is important to distinguish between alternative therapies (unproven methods promoted for use instead of mainstream treatment) and complementary therapies, which are used with standard treatment. Complementary therapies are noninvasive and soothing. However, before trying them, patients should check with their oncologist to make sure the complementary therapy will not interfere with standard cancer therapy or cause harm. Examples of complementary therapies are massage therapy, aromatherapy, meditation, yoga, biofeedback, music, art and dance therapies, group and individual therapy or counseling.

Hormone therapy is the treatment of cancer by removing, blocking, or adding hormones. Hormones are chemical substances produced by glands in the body that enter the bloodstream and cause effects in other tissues. Hormone therapies may be used to treat breast and prostate cancers. Hormone therapy may also be used in some situations for other cancers.

Immunotherapy, also called biological therapy, is a type of treatment that uses the body's immune system to fight cancer. The therapy mainly consists of stimulating the immune system with highly purified proteins that help it do its job more effectively.

Radiation therapy is the use of high-energy x rays, electron beams, or radioactive isotopes to attack cancer. Radiation therapy causes cancer cell death by ionization or by damaging the chromosomes in the cancer cells so they cannot multiply. Radiation therapy is a local treatment aimed directly at the cancer. Even though the radiation is aimed only at the cancer, it must often pass through skin and other organs to reach the tumor. Thus, some healthy cells may become damaged, too. The body however is able to repair the healthy cells that have been damaged and restore them to their proper function. Aside from its use as a single treatment, radiation therapy has been shown to enhance the effects of chemotherapy. It can be used in combination with chemotherapy to shrink a tumor. Successful radiation therapy depends on delivering the proper amount of radiation to the cancer in the best, and most effective way.

Resources

PERIODICALS

Dreger, P., and N. Schmitz. "Allogeneic Transplantation of Blood Stem Cells: Coming of Age?" *Annals of Hematology* 80, no. 3 (March 2001): 127–36.

Nuzhat, Iqbal, Donna Salzman, Audrey J. Lazenby, et al. "Diagnosis of Gastrointestinal Graft-Versus-Host Disease." *The American Journal of Gastroenterology* 95 (November 2000): 3034–3038.

ORGANIZATIONS

American Cancer Society. 1599 Clifton Road, NE, Atlanta, GA 30329. (800) 227-2345, (404) 320-3333. <http://www.cancer.org>.

American Society for Blood and Marrow Transplantation (ASBMT). 85 W. Algonquin Road, Suite 550 Arlington Heights, IL 60005. (847) 427-0224. mail@asbmt.org.

BMT Infonet (Blood and Marrow Transplant Information Network). 2900 Skokie Valley Road, Suite B, Highland Park, IL 60035. (847) 433-3313, (888) 597-7674. help@bmtinfonet.org. <http://www.bmtinfonet.org>.

Bone Marrow Transplant Branch, U.S. Department of Health and Human Services. <http://www.hrsa.gov/osp/dot/bone.htm>.

Bone Marrow Transplant Newsletter. 1985 Spruce Ave., Highland Park, IL, 60035. (847) 831-1913. <http://www.bmtnews.org>.

Cancercare. (800) 813-HOPE (4673). <http://www.cancercare.org>.

Health Resources and Services Administration. 5600 Fishers Lane, Rm. 14-45, Rockville, MD 20857. (301) 443-3376. comments@hrsa.gov. <http://www.hrsa.gov>.

International Bone Marrow Transplant Registry/Autologous Blood and Marrow Transplant Registry N. America. Health Policy Institute, Medical College of Wisconsin, 8701 Watertown Plank Road, P.O. Box 26509, Milwaukee, WI 53226. (414) 456-8325. ibmtr@mcw.edu.

Leukemia & Lymphoma Society, Inc. 1311 Mamaroneck Avenue White Plains, NY 10605. (914) 949-5213. <http://www.leukemia-lymphoma.org>.

Lymphoma Research Foundation of America. 8800 Venice Boulevard, Suite 207, Los Angeles, CA 90034. (800) 500-9976. (310) 204-7040. helpline@lymphoma.org. <http://www.lymphoma.org>.

National Bone Marrow Transplant Link. 20411 W. 12 Mile Road, Suite 108, Southfield, MI 48076. (800) LINK-BMT (800-546-5268). <http://comnet.org/nbmtlink/home2.html>.

National Foundation for Transplants. 1102 Brookfield, Suite 200, Memphis, TN, 38110. (800) 489-3863 or (901) 684-1697.<http://www.transplants.org>.

National Marrow Donor Program. Suite 500, 3001 Broadway Street Northeast, Minneapolis, MN 55413-1753. (800) MARROW-2. <http://www.marrow.org>.

National Organ and Tissue Donation Initiative. <http://www.organdonor.gov>.

Julia Barrett
Laura Ruth, PhD
Angela M. Costello

Bone repair *see* **Orthopedic surgery**

Bone x rays

Definition

Bone x rays are a diagnostic imaging test in which ionizing radiation passing through the bones enables an image to be produced on film.

Purpose

Bone x rays are ordered to detect bone disease or injury, such as in the case of broken bones, tumors, and other problems. They can determine bone density, texture, erosion, and changes in bone relationships. Bone x rays also evaluate the joints for such diseases as arthritis.

Description

X rays are a common diagnostic test in which a form of energy called x-ray radiation penetrates the patient's body. In bone x rays, electrical current passes through an x-ray tube and produces a beam of ionizing radiation that passes through the bone(s) being examined. This produces a picture of the inside of the body on film. The doctor reads the developed x ray on a wall-mounted light box or on a computer monitor.

Digital x rays are a new type of exam in which conventional equipment is used to take the x-ray picture, but the image is produced via computer. In a digital x ray, the image is created on a reusable plate. After being read by a laser reader, the information is sent in digital form to a storage unit that is connected to a computer network. The radiologist reads the x ray from there. An electronic report can then be sent to the patient's doctor. Electronic reports can also be generated with non-digital x-ray exams.

X rays can detect problems with bones that result from injury or disease caused by malfunction in the patient's bone chemistry. Bone injuries, especially broken bones (fractures), are common and can be accurately diagnosed by evaluation of bone x rays. X rays are especially helpful in diagnosing simple and incomplete fractures, which cannot be detected during a **physical examination**. X rays can also be used to check for bone position and alignment in a fracture. Some bone diseases can be definitively diagnosed with bone x rays, while others require additional, more sophisticated imaging tests.

Osteoporosis, a common bone disease, can be detected in bone x rays, but other tests, such as bone densitometry, may need to be ordered to determine the extent of the disease. In some cases, a bone biopsy (microscopic analysis of a small amount of tissue) is also done. For arthritis, a common ailment, x rays of the bone are occasionally used in conjunction with blood tests. In bone tumors, bone x rays can be helpful, but they may not be definitive when used alone.

Bone x rays are taken by a technologist or radiologist and interpreted by a radiologist. They are taken in a doctor's office, in a hospital, or in an outpatient clinic. Bone x rays generally take less than 10 minutes to complete. There is no pain or discomfort associated with the test, but some people find it difficult to remain still throughout the procedure.

During the test, the patient lies on a table. The technician taking the x ray checks the patient's position and places the x-ray machine over the part of the body being scanned. After asking the patient to remain still, the technician steps out of the area and presses a button to take the picture.

Preparation

The patient is asked to remove clothing, jewelry, and any other metal objects from the part of the body being x rayed. If appropriate, a lead shield is placed over another part of the body to minimize exposure to the radiation that is being used.

Aftercare

The patient can immediately resume normal activities once the technician has checked that the x-rays have processed well and that none need to be repeated. This takes just a few minutes.

Risks

The human body contains some natural radiation and is also exposed to radiation in the environment. There is a slight risk from exposure to radiation during bone x rays;

however, the amount of radiation is small and the risk of harm is very low. If reproductive organs are to be exposed to large amounts of radiation, genetic alterations could occur in the developing fetus. Excessive or repeated doses of radiation can cause changes in other types of body tissue. No radiation remains in the body after the x ray.

Normal results

Normal bones show no fractures, dislocations, or other abnormalities.

Results that indicate the presence of bone injury or disease differ in appearance, according to the nature of the injury or disease. For example, fractures show up as clear breaks in the bones, while osteoporotic bone has the same shape as normal bone on an x ray, but is less dense.

Resources

BOOKS

A Manual of Laboratory and Diagnostic Tests. 5th ed. Ed. Francis Fishback. Philadelphia: Lippincott, 1996.

"Tumors and Tumor-Like Lesions of the Bone." In *Current Medical Diagnosis and Treatment, 1996.* 35th ed. Ed. Stephen McPhee, et al. Stamford: Appleton & Lange, 1995.

Lori De Milto
Lee A. Shratter, MD

Bowel resection

Definition

Bowel resection is a surgical procedure in which a diseased part of the large intestine is removed. The pro-

cedure is also known as colectomy, colon removal, colon resection, or resection of part of the large intestine.

Purpose

The large bowel, also called the large intestine, is a part of the digestive system. It runs from the small bowel (small intestine) to the rectum, which receives waste material from the small bowel. Its major function is to store waste and to absorb water from waste material. It consists of the following sections, any of which may become diseased:

- Colon. The colon averages some 60 in (150 cm) in length. It is divided into four segments: the ascending colon, transverse colon, descending colon, and sigmoid colon. There are two bends (flexures) in the colon. The hepatic flexure is where the ascending colon joins the transverse colon. The splenic flexure is where the transverse colon merges into the descending colon.

- Cecum. This is the first portion of the large bowel that is joined to the small bowel. The appendix lies at the lowest portion of the cecum.

- Ascending colon. This segment is about 8 in (20 cm) in length, and it extends upwards from the cecum to the hepatic flexure near the liver.

- Transverse colon. This segment is usually more than 18 in (46 cm) in length and extends across the upper abdomen to the splenic flexure.

- Descending colon. This segment is usually less than 12 in (30 cm) long and extends from the splenic flexure downwards to the start of the pelvis.

- Sigmoid colon. An S-shaped segment that measures about 18 in (46 cm); it extends from the descending colon to the rectum.

The wall of the colon is composed of four layers:

- Mucosa. This single layer of cell lining is flat and regenerates itself every three to eight days. Small glands lie beneath the surface.

- Submucosa. The area between the mucosa and circular muscle layer that is separated from the mucosa by a thin layer of muscle, the muscularis mucosa.

- Muscularis propria. The inner circular and outer longitudinal muscle layers.

- Serosa. The outer, single-cell, thick covering of the bowel. It is similar to the peritoneum, the layer of cells that lines the abdomen.

The large intestine is also responsible for bacterial production and absorption of vitamins. Resection of a portion of the large intestine (or of the entire organ) may become necessary when it becomes diseased. The exact

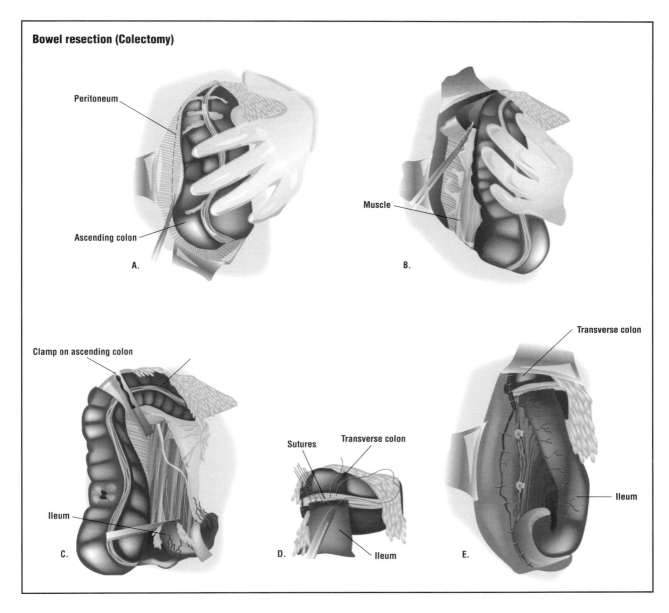

Bowel resection (Colectomy)

To remove a portion of the colon, or large intestine, and incision is made in the abdomen to expose the area (A). Tissues and muscles connecting the colon to surrounding organs are severed (B). The area to be removed is clamped and severed (C). The remaining portions of the bowel, the ileum (small intestine) and transverse colon, are connected with sutures (D). Muscles and tissues are repaired (E). *(Illustration by GGS Inc.)*

reasons for large bowel resection in any given patient may be complex and are always carefully evaluated by the treating physician or team. The procedure is usually performed to treat the following disorders or diseases of the large intestine:

• Cancer. Colon cancer is the second most common type of cancer diagnosed in the United States. Colon and rectum cancers, which are usually referred to as colorectal cancer, grow on the lining of the large intestine. Bowel resection may be indicated to remove the cancer.

• Diverticulitis. This condition is characterized by the inflammation of a diverticulum, especially of diverticula occurring in the colon, which may undergo perforation with abscess formation. The condition may be relieved by resecting the affected bowel section.

• Intestinal obstruction. This condition involves a partial or complete blockage of the bowel that results in the failure of the intestinal contents to pass through. It is usually treated by decompressing the intestine with suction, using a nasogastric tube inserted into the stomach or intestine. In cases where decompression does not relieve the symptoms, or if tissue death is suspected, bowel resection may be considered.

- Ulcerative colitis. This condition is characterized by chronic inflammation of the large intestine and rectum resulting in bloody diarrhea. Surgery may be indicated when medical therapy does not improve the condition. Removal of the colon is curative and also removes the risk of colon cancer. About 25–40% of ulcerative colitis patients must eventually have their colons removed because of massive bleeding, severe illness, rupture of the colon, or risk of cancer.

- Traumatic injuries. Accidents may result in bowel injuries that require resection.

- Pre-cancerous polyps. A colorectal polyp is a growth that projects from the lining of the colon. Polyps of the colon are usually benign and produce no symptoms, but they may cause rectal bleeding and develop into malignancies over time. When polyps have a high chance of becoming cancerous, bowel resection may be indicated.

- Familial adenomatous polyposis (FAP). This is a hereditary condition caused by a faulty gene. Most people discover that they have it at a young age. People with FAP grow many polyps in the bowel. These are mostly benign, but because there are so many, it is really only a question of time before one becomes cancerous. Since people with FAP have a very high risk of developing bowel cancer, bowel resection is thus often indicated.

- Hirschsprung's disease (HD). This condition usually occurs in children. It causes constipation, meaning that bowel movements are difficult. Some children with HD cannot have bowel movements at all; the stool creates a blockage in the intestine. If HD is not treated, stool can fill up the large intestine and cause serious problems such as infection, bursting of the colon, and even death.

Description

Bowel resection can be performed using an open surgical approach (colectomy) or laparoscopically.

Colectomy

Following adequate bowel preparation, the patient is placed under general anesthesia, which ensures that the patient is deep asleep and pain free during surgery. Because the effects of gravity to displace tissues and organs away from the site of operation are important, patients are carefully positioned, padded, and strapped to the operating table to prevent movement as the patient is tilted to an extreme degree. The surgeon starts the procedure by making a lower midline incision in the abdomen or, alternatively, he may prefer to perform a lateral lower transverse incision instead. He proceeds with the removal of the diseased portion of the large intestine, and then sutures or staples the two healthy ends back together before closing the incision. The amount of bowel removed can vary considerably, depending on the reasons for the operation. When possible, the procedure is performed to maintain the continuity of the bowel so as to preserve normal passage of stool. If the bowel has to be relieved of its normal digestive work while it heals, a temporary opening of the colon onto the skin of abdominal wall, called a **colostomy**, may be created. In this procedure, the end of the colon is passed through the abdominal wall and the edges are sutured to the skin. A removable bag is attached around the colostomy site so that stool may pass into the bag, which can be emptied several times during the day. Most colostomies are temporary and can be closed with another operation at a later date. However, if a large portion of the intestine is removed, or if the distal end of the colon is too diseased to reconnect to the proximal intestine, the colostomy is permanent.

Laparoscopic bowel resection

The benefits of laparoscopic bowel resection when compared to open colectomies include reduced postoperative pain, shorter hospitalization periods, and a faster return to normal activities. The procedure is also minimally invasive. When performing a laparoscopic procedure, the surgeon makes three to four small incisions in the abdomen or in the umbilicus (belly button). He inserts specialized **surgical instruments**, including a thin, telescope-like instrument called a laparoscope, in an incision. The abdomen is then filled with gas, usually carbon dioxide, to help the surgeon view the abdominal cavity. A camera is inserted through one of the tubes and displays images on a monitor located near the operating table to guide the surgeon as he works. Once an adequate view of the operative field is obtained, the actual dissection of the colon can start. Following the procedure, the small incisions are closed with sutures or surgical tape.

All colon surgery involves only three maneuvers that may vary in complexity depending on the region of the bowel and the nature of the disease. These three maneuvers are:

• retraction of the colon

• division of the attachments to the colon

• dissection of the mesentery

In a typical procedure, after retracting the colon, the surgeon proceeds to divide the attachments to the liver and the small bowel. Once the mesenteric vessels have been dissected and divided, the colon is divided with special stapling devices that close off the bowel while at the same time cutting between the staple lines. Alternatively, a laparoscopically assisted procedure may be selected, in which a small abdominal wall incision is made at this point to bring the bowel outside of the abdomen, allowing open bowel resection and reconnection using standard instruments. This technique is popular with many surgeons because an incision must be made to remove the bowel specimen from the abdomen, which allows the most time-consuming and risky parts of the procedure (from an infection point of view) to be done outside the body with better control of the colon.

Diagnosis/Preparation

Key elements of the **physical examination** before surgery focus on a thorough examination of the abdomen, groin, and rectum. Other common diagnostic tools used to evaluate medical conditions that may require bowel resection include imaging tests such as gastrointestinal barium series, **angiography**, computerized tomography (CT), **magnetic resonance imaging** (MRI), and endoscopy.

As with any surgery, the patient is required to sign a consent form. Details of the procedure are discussed with the patient, including goals, technique, and risks.

Blood and urine tests, along with various imaging tests and an electrocardiogram (EKG), may be ordered. To prepare for the procedure, the patient is asked to completely clean out the bowel. This is a crucial step if the bowel is to be opened safely within the peritoneal cavity, or even manipulated safely through small incisions. To empty and cleanse the bowel, the patient is usually placed on a low-residue diet for several days prior to surgery. A liquid diet may be ordered for at least the day before surgery, with nothing taken by mouth after midnight. A series of enemas and/or oral preparations (GoLytely or Colyte) may be ordered to empty the bowel of stool. Preoperative bowel preparation involving mechanical cleansing and administration of intravenous **antibiotics** immediately before surgery is the standard practice. The patient may also be given a prescription for oral antibiotics (neomycin, erythromycin, or kanamycin sulfate) the day before surgery to decrease bacteria in the intestine and to help prevent post-operative infection. A nasogastric tube is inserted through the nose into the stomach during surgery and may be left in place for 24–48 hours after surgery. This removes the gastric secretions and prevents nausea and vomiting. A urinary catheter (a thin tube inserted into the bladder) may be inserted to keep the bladder empty during surgery, giving more space in the surgical field and decreasing chances of accidental injury.

Aftercare

Postoperative care for the patient who has undergone a bowel resection, as with those who have had any major surgery, involves monitoring of blood pressure, pulse, respiration, and temperature. Breathing tends to be shallow because of the effect of anesthesia and the patient's reluctance to breathe deeply and experience pain that is caused by the abdominal incision. The patient is instructed how to support the operative site during deep breathing and coughing, and is given pain medication as necessary. Fluid intake and output is measured, and the operative site is observed for color and amount of wound drainage. The nasogastric tube will remain in place, attached to low intermittent suction until bowel activity resumes. Fluids and electrolytes are infused intravenously until the patient's diet can gradually be resumed, beginning with liquids and advancing to a regular diet as tolerated. The patient is generally out of bed approximately eight to 24 hours after surgery. Most patients will stay in the hospital for five to seven days, although laparoscopic surgery can reduce that stay to two to three days. Postoperative weight loss follows almost all bowel resections. Weight and strength are slowly regained over a period of months. Complete recovery from surgery may take two months. Laparoscopic surgery can reduce this time to one to two weeks.

The treating physician should be informed of any of the following problems after surgery:

• increased pain, swelling, redness, drainage, or bleeding in the surgical area

• headache, muscle aches, dizziness, or fever

• increased abdominal pain or swelling, constipation, nausea or vomiting, rectal bleeding, or black, tarry stools

Risks

Potential complications of bowel resection surgery include:

• excessive bleeding

• surgical wound infection

• incisional hernia (an organ projecting through the surrounding muscle wall, it occurs through the surgical scar)

• thrombophlebitis (inflammation and blood clot to veins in the legs)

• narrowing of the opening (stoma)

• pneumonia

• pulmonary embolism (blood clot or air bubble in the lung blood supply)

• reaction to medication

• breathing problems

• obstruction of the intestine from scar tissue

Normal results

Complete healing is expected without complications after bowel resection, but the period of time required for recovery from the surgery varies depending on the initial condition that required the procedure, the patient's overall health status prior to surgery, and the length of bowel removed.

Morbidity and mortality rates

Prognosis for bowel resection depends on the seriousness of the disease. For example, primary treatment for colorectal cancer consists of wide surgical resection of the colon cancer and lymphatic drainage after the bowel is prepared. The choice of operation for rectal cancer depends on the tumor's distance from the anus and gross extent; overall surgical cure is possible in 70% of these patients. In the case of ulcerative colitis patients, the colitis is cured by bowel resection and most people go on to live normal, active lives. As for Hirschsprung's disease patients, approximately 70–85% eventually achieve excellent results after surgery, with normal bowel habits and infrequent constipation.

Alternatives

Alternatives to bowel resection depend on the specific medical condition being treated. For most conditions where bowel resection is advised, the only alternative is medical treatment with drugs. In cases of cancer of the bowel, drug treatment alone will not cure the disease. Occasionally, it is possible to remove a rectal cancer from within the back passage without major surgery, but this only applies to very special cases. As for other conditions such as mild or moderate ulcerative colitis, drug therapy may represent an alternative to surgery; a combination of the drugs sulfonamide, sulfapyridine, and salicylate may help control inflammation. Similarly, most acute cases of diverticulitis are first treated with antibiotics and a liquid diet.

See also Laparoscopy; Small bowel resection.

Resources

BOOKS

Corman, M. L. *Colon and Rectal Surgery.* Philadelphia: Lippincott Williams & Wilkins, 1998.

Hampton, Beverly, and Ruth Bryant. *Ostomies and Continent Diversions.* St. Louis: Mosby Inc., 1992.

Michelassi, F., and J. W. Milsom, eds. *Operative Strategies in Inflammatory Bowel Disease.* New York: Springer Verlag, 1999.

Peppercorn, Mark, ed. *Therapy of Inflammatory Bowel Disease: New Medical and Surgical Approaches.* New York: Marcel Dekker, 1989.

PERIODICALS

Alves, A., Y. Panis, D. Trancart, J. Regimbeau, M. Pocard, and P. Valleur. "Factors Associated with Clinically Significant Anastomotic Leakage after Large Bowel Resection: Mul-

KEY TERMS

Anesthesia—A combination of drugs administered by a variety of techniques by trained professionals that provide sedation, amnesia, analgesia, and immobility adequate for the accomplishment of the surgical procedure with minimal discomfort, and without injury, to the patient.

Anus—The terminal orifice of the bowel.

Cancer—The uncontrolled growth of abnormal cells which have mutated from normal tissues.

Colectomy—The surgical removal of the colon or part of the colon.

Colon—Also called the large intestine, it is responsible for forming, storing and expelling waste matter.

Colostomy—The surgical construction of an artificial anus between the colon and the surface of the abdomen.

Diverticulum—A small, pouch-like structure that sometimes forms in the walls of the intestines and that can trap particles of food and become very inflamed and painful.

Enema—A liquid injected into the rectum.

Mesentery—The membranes, or one of the membranes (consisting of a fold of the peritoneum and enclosed tissues), that connect the intestines and their appendages with the dorsal wall of the abdominal cavity.

Ostomy—An operation to create an opening from an area inside the body to the outside.

Polyp—Growth, usually benign, protruding from a mucous membrane such as that lining the walls of the intestines.

Resection—Removal of a portion, or all, of an organ or other structure.

tivariate Analysis of 707 Patients." *World Journal of Surgery* 26 (April 2002): 499–502.

Miller, J., and A. Proietto. "The Place of Bowel Resection in Initial Debulking Surgery for Advanced Ovarian Cancer." *Australian and New Zealand Journal of Obstetrics and Gynaecology* 42 (November 2002): 535–537.

Sukhotnik, I., A. S. Gork, M. Chen, R. Drongowski, A. G. Coran, and C. M. Harmon. "Effect of Low Fat Diet on Lipid Absorption and Fatty-acid Transport following Bowel Resection." *Pediatric Surgery International* 17 (May 2001): 259–264.

Tabet, J., D. Hong, C. W. Kim, J. Wong, R. Goodacre, and M. Anvari. "Laparoscopic versus Open Bowel Resection for Crohn's Disease." *Canadian Journal of Gastroenterology* 15 (April 2001): 237–242.

Taylor, C., and C. Norton. "Information Booklets for Patients with Major Bowel Resection." *British Journal of Nursing* 19 (June–July 2000): 785–791.

ORGANIZATIONS

American Board of Colorectal Surgeons (ABCRS). 20600 Eureka Rd., Ste. 600, Taylor, MI 48180. (734) 282-9400. <http://www.abcrs.org>.

The American Society of Colorectal Surgeons (ASCRS). 85 West Algonquin, Suite 550, Arlington Heights, IL 60005. (847) 290 9184. <http://www.fascrs.org>.

United Ostomy Association, Inc. (UOA). 19772 MacArthur Blvd., Suite 200, Irvine, CA 92612-2405. (800) 826-0826. <http://www.uoa.org>.

OTHER

"Bowel Resection." *Patient & Family Education / NYU Medical Center.* <www.nmh.org/patient_ed_pdfs/pt_ed_bowel_resection_discharge.pdf.>.

"Bowel Resection with Colostomy." *Health Care Corporation of St. John's.* <www.hccsj.nf.ca/2002/Med_Services/Surgery/Procedures/bowel_resec_col.asp>.

"Colorectal Cancer." *ASCRS Homepage.* <www.fascrs.org>.

Kathleen D. Wright, RN
Monique Laberge, PhD

Bowel surgery with ostomy *see* **Colostomy**

Brain surgery *see* **Craniotomy**

Breast augmentation *see* **Breast implants**

Breast biopsy

Definition

A breast biopsy is the removal of breast tissue for examination by a pathologist. This can be accomplished surgically or by extracting, or withdrawing, tissue through a needle.

Purpose

A biopsy is recommended when a significant abnormality is found by **physical examination** or an imaging test. Examples of an abnormality can include a breast

Breast biopsy

Biopsy needle

Area of
calcification

Ribs

Breast tissue

A.

B.

Cavity within
region of
calcification

Sample

C.

During a needle biopsy on the breast, a local anesthetic is
used, and a needle with a looped end is inserted into the
potential tumor (A). A sample is taken (B), and the needle
withdrawn (C). The sample is sent to a laboratory for analysis. *(Illustration by GGS Inc.)*

lump felt during physical self-examination or tissue
changes noticed from a mammogram test. Before a biopsy
is performed, it is important to make sure that the threat of
cancer cannot be ruled out by a simpler, less invasive examination. A lump may be obviously harmless when examined by ultrasound. If less invasive tests are not conclusive, the presence of cancer or a variety of benign breast
conditions can be determined by using a biopsy.

Demographics

The American Cancer Society estimated that in
2003, 211,300 new cases of breast cancer would be diagnosed in the United States and 39,800 women would die
as a result of breast cancer. Approximately one in eight
women will develop breast cancer at some point in her
life. The risk of developing breast cancer increases with
age: women ages 30–40 have a one-in-252 chance,
women ages 40–50 a one-in-68 chance, women ages
50–60 a one-in-35 chance, and women ages 60–70 a
one-in-27 chance.

In the 1990s, the incidence of breast cancer was
higher among Caucasian women (113.1 cases per
100,000 women) than African American women (100.3
per 100,000). The death rate associated with breast cancer, however, was higher among African American
women (29.6 per 100,000) than Caucasian women (22.2
per 100,000). Death rates were lower among Hispanic
women (14.2 per 100,000), Native American women
(12.0), and Asian women (11.2 per 100,000).

Description

The type of biopsy recommended will depend on
whether the area can be felt, how well it can be seen on
mammogram or ultrasound, and how suspicious it feels
or appears. Specialized equipment is needed for different
types of biopsy and availability may vary.

Surgical biopsy

There are two major types of surgical breast biopsy:
excisional and incisional. An excisional biopsy is a surgical procedure where the entire area of concern and
some surrounding tissue is removed. It is usually done as
an outpatient procedure in a hospital or freestanding
surgery center. The patient may be awake and is sometimes given medication to make her drowsy. The area to
be operated on is numbed with local anesthetic. Infrequently, general anesthesia is used. An excisional biopsy
itself usually takes under one hour to perform. The total
amount of time spent at the facility depends on the type
of anesthesia used, whether a needle localization was
done, and the extent of the surgery.

If a mass is very large, an incisional biopsy may be performed. In this case, only a portion of the area is removed and sent for analysis. The procedure is the same as an excisional biopsy in other respects.

Needle biopsy

A needle biopsy removes part of the suspicious area for examination. There are two types: aspiration biopsy (using a fine needle) and large-core needle biopsy. Either of these may be called a percutaneous needle biopsy. Percutaneous refers to a procedure done through the skin.

A fine-needle aspiration biopsy uses a very thin needle to withdraw fluid and cells that can be studied. It can be done in a doctor's office, clinic, or hospital. Local anesthetic may be used, but is sometimes withheld, as its administration may be more painful than the biopsy needle. The area to place the needle may be located by touch without using specialized equipment. However, ultrasound guidance enables the physician to feel and see the lesion at the same time. The actual withdrawal of fluid and cells can be visualized as it occurs. This helps ensure that the specimen is taken from the right place.

A large-core needle biopsy uses a larger diameter needle to remove small pieces of tissue, usually about the size of a grain of rice. It can be done in a clinic or hospital that has the appropriate facilities. Local anesthetic is routinely used. Ultrasound or x ray is used for guidance of a large-core needle biopsy.

If the suspicious area is seen best with x ray, a stereotactic device is used. This means that x rays are taken from several angles. The information is fed into a computer that analyzes the data and guides the needle to the correct place. The patient may be sitting up, or she may be lying on her stomach, with her breast positioned through an opening in the table. The breast is held firmly but comfortably between a plastic paddle and a metal plate, similar to those used for mammograms. X rays may be taken before, during, and after the tissue is drawn into the needle to confirm that the correct spot is biopsied. This procedure may also be referred to as a stereotactic core biopsy, or a mammotomy.

Ultrasound is used to guide needle placement for some lesions. The patient lies on her back or side. After the area is numbed, sterile gel is applied. The physician places a transducer, an instrument about the size of an electric shaver, over the skin. This produces an image from the reflection of sound waves. A special needle, usually in a spring-loaded device, is used to obtain the tissue. The procedure is observed on a monitor as it is happening.

An abnormal pathology report indicates a cancer is present. If a fine-needle aspiration biopsy was performed,

WHO PERFORMS THE PROCEDURE AND WHERE IS IT PERFORMED?

The breast biopsy is usually performed by a surgeon or a radiologist, a medical doctor who specializes in the use of imaging techniques for diagnosis or treatment. The extracted tissue samples are analyzed by a pathologist, a medical doctor who has completed specialized training in the diagnosis of diseases from microscopic analysis of cells and tissues. Surgical biopsies are generally performed at a hospital or surgery center. Because needle biopsies are less invasive, they may be performed at a doctor's office, clinic, or hospital.

the pathologist has viewed individual cells under a microscope to see if they appear cancerous. Large-core needle biopsy and surgical biopsy will be able to give more information. This includes the type of cancer, whether or not it has invaded surrounding tissue, and how likely it is to spread quickly. There are some conditions that are not malignant but indicate high risk for future development of breast cancer. If these are identified, more frequent monitoring of the area may be recommended.

Diagnosis/Preparation

Sometimes an abnormality can be palpated during a self-examination or an examination by a health care professional. If an abnormality is not felt, there are other signs that indicate the need for medical attention. These include:

- severe breast pain
- changes in the size of a breast or nipple
- changes in the shape of both breast and nipple
- pitting, dumpling, or redness of the breast skin
- nipple redness, irritation, or inversion
- changes in the pattern of veins visible on the surface of the breast
- some types of nipple discharge

If the abnormality cannot be located easily, a wire localization may be done before the actual surgery. After local anesthetic is administered, a fine wire is placed in the area of concern. Either x ray or ultrasound guidance is used. The wire can then be followed to the area of concern. The patient is awake and usually sitting up.

A surgical breast biopsy may require the patient to have nothing to eat or drink for a period of time before the operation. This will typically be from midnight the night before, if general anesthesia is planned. No food restrictions are necessary for needle biopsy, although it is advisable to eat lightly before the procedure. This is especially important if the patient will be lying on her stomach for a stereotactic biopsy.

Aftercare

After a surgical biopsy, the incision will be closed with stitches and covered with a bandage. The bandage can usually be removed in one or two days. Stitches are taken out approximately one week afterward. Depending on the extent of the operation, normal activities can be resumed in approximately one to three days. Vigorous **exercise** may be limited for one to three weeks.

The skin opening for a needle biopsy is minimal. It may be closed with thin, clear tape (called a steri-strip) or covered with a small bandage. The patient can return to her usual routine immediately after the biopsy. Strenuous activity or heavy lifting is not recommended for 24 hours. Any bandages can be removed one or two days after the biopsy.

Risks

Infection is always a possibility when the skin is broken, although this rarely occurs. Redness, swelling, or severe pain at the biopsy site would indicate a possible infection. Another possible consequence of a breast biopsy is a hematoma. This is a collection of blood at the biopsy site; the body usually absorbs blood naturally. If the hematoma is very large and uncomfortable, it may need to be drained. A surgical breast biopsy may produce a visible scar on the breast, which may make future mammograms harder to interpret accurately.

A false negative pathology report is another risk. This means that no cancer was found when cancer was actually present. The incidence of this varies with the biopsy technique. In general, fine-needle aspiration biopsies have the highest rate of false negative results, but there may be variation in results between facilities.

Normal results

A normal pathology report indicates no malignancy is present. The tissue sample may be further classified as a benign breast condition, including tumor of the breast (fibroadenoma) and connective tissue that resembles fiber (fibrosis). Studies have demonstrated that approximately 80% of all breast biopsies result in a benign pathology report.

Morbidity and mortality rates

The reported rate of complications for image-guided percutaneous biopsy ranges is approximately 2%. Excessive bleeding occurs after approximately 0.5% of fine needle biopsies, 3% of small needle biopsies, and 5% to 10% of large needle biopsies. Infection occurs in approximately 1% of biopsy sites. Organ damage such as a collapsed lung (pneumothorax) occurs in approximately 0.5% of biopsies.

Alternatives

While a biopsy is the only way to determine definitively if a breast abnormality is cancerous, there are a number of procedures that may be used to rule out cancer so that a biopsy is not necessary. These include **mammography**, ultrasound imaging, and ductography (used for imaging the breast ducts and diagnosing the cause of abnormal nipple discharges).

Resources

PERIODICALS

Centers for Disease Control and Prevention. "Recent Trends in Mortality Rates for Four Major Cancers, by Sex and Race/Ethnicity." *Morbidity and Mortality Weekly Report,* 51, no. 3 (January 25, 2002): 49–53.

Marks, James S. and Nancy C. Lee. "Implementing Recommendations for the Early Detection of Breast and Cervical Cancer Among Low-income Women." *Morbidity and Mortality Weekly Report,* 49, no. RR02 (March 31, 2000): 35–55.

ORGANIZATIONS

American Cancer Society. 1599 Clifton Rd., NE, Atlanta, GA 30329-4251. (800) 227-2345. <http://www.cancer.org>.

National Cancer Institute. Building 31, Room 10A31, 31 Center Drive, MSC 2580, Bethesda, MD 20892-2580. (800) 422-6237. <http://www.nci.nih.gov>.

OTHER

Cardella, John F., et al. "Quality Improvement Guidelines for Image-Guided Percutaneous Biopsy in Adults." *Society of*

A silicone breast implant. *(Photograph by Peter A. Simon. Phototake. Reproduced by permission.)*

Cardiovascular and Interventional Radiology. November/December 1996 [cited March 11, 2003]. <http://www.scvir.org/clinical/T26.htm>.

"How is Breast Cancer Diagnosed?" *American Cancer Society.* 2003 [cited March 11, 2003]. <http://www.cancer.org/docroot/CRI/content/CRI_2_4_3X_How_is_breast_cancer_diagnosed_5.asp>.

"Lifetime Probability of Breast Cancer in American Women." *National Cancer Institute.* September 13, 2002 [cited March 11, 2003]. <http://cis.nci.nih.gov/fact/5_6.htm>.

Ellen S. Weber, MSN
Stephanie Dionne Sherk

Breast implants

Definition

Breast implantation is a surgical procedure for enlarging, or augmenting, the breast. Implants are breast-shaped pouches that are saccular in shape, made of a silicone outer shell, and filled with silicone gel or saline (salt water), are used.

Purpose

Breast implantation is usually performed to make normal breasts larger for cosmetic purposes. Sometimes a woman having a **breast reconstruction** after a mastectomy will need the opposite breast enlarged to make the breasts more symmetrical. Breasts that are very unequal in size due to trauma or congenital deformity may also be equalized with an enlargement procedure.

Male-to-female transsexuals may use breast implantation to achieve the physical appearance of a female.

Demographics

Breast enlargement is the second most common cosmetic surgical procedure practiced on women in the United States. It increased by 306% between 1992 and 1998. According to the American Society of Plastic and Reconstructive Surgeons, more than 125,000 breast augmentation procedures are performed each year.

Presently, more than two million, or approximately 8%, of women in the United States have breast implants. The majority of breast implant recipients are Caucasian women (95%), followed by African-American women (4%). The remaining women that have breast implants are Asian (0.5%) and other non-specified races (0.5%).

Description

Cosmetic breast enlargement or augmentation is usually performed as an outpatient procedure. It may be done under local or general anesthesia, depending on patient and physician preference. The incision is typically made through the armpit (axilla), along the fold line under the breast, or around the areola (the darkened area around the nipple); these techniques create the most inconspicuous scars. The implant is placed in one of two locations: between the breast tissue and underlying chest muscle, or under the chest muscle. The operation takes approximately one to two hours. The cost of a cosmetic procedure is rarely covered by insurance. However, if enlargement is part of breast reconstruction after a mastectomy, health plans may pay for some or all of it. The surgeon's fee ranges from $3,500 to $5,000, and up. The

Breast implants

A.

Sixteen injection sites
in the right breast

Sixteen injection sites
in the left breast

B.

Incision

C.

Fingers create pocket
under tissue with
blunt dissection

Pectoralis muscle

Pocket

Implant

Chest wall

D.

Injected saline

Implant inflated
to full size with
saline

E.

During a breast implant procedure, a local injection of anesthetic is administered at many points around the breast (A). An incision is made under the areola (B). The surgeon uses his fingers to create a pocket for the implant (C). The implant is placed under the pectoralis muscle of the chest (D), and is inflated to full size with saline injections (E). *(Illustration by GGS Inc.)*

procedure may also be called breast augmentation or augmentation mammoplasty.

Diagnosis/Preparation

The diagnosis for breast reconstruction is almost always visual. The underlying medical reasons include equalizing otherwise normal breasts that are markedly different in size, replacing all or part of breast tissue that has been removed during the course of cancer treatment, or replacing breast mass that has been lost due to injury. Underlying cosmetic reasons include personal preference for larger breasts among genetic females or the creation of breasts in male-to-female transsexuals.

Before any surgery is performed, the woman should have a clear understanding of what her new breasts will look like. She and her physician should agree about the desired final result. Many surgeons find it helpful to have the patient review before and after pictures of other patients, to clarify expectations. Computer modeling is often used to assess expected results.

A person in poor health or having a severe or chronic disease is not a good candidate for this procedure.

Aftercare

Many normal activities such as driving may be restricted for up to one week. Sutures are usually removed in seven to 10 days. Typically, a woman can resume all routines, including vigorous **exercise**, in about three weeks. The scars will be red for approximately one month, but will fade to their final appearance within one to two years.

Risks

Risks associated with this procedure are similar to those of any surgical procedure. These risks include bleeding, infection, reaction to anesthesia, or unexpected scarring. A breast enlargement may also result in decreased sensation in the breast or interference with breastfeeding. Implants can also make it more difficult to read and interpret mammograms, possibly delaying breast cancer detection. Also, the implant itself can rupture and leak, or become displaced. A thick scar that normally forms around the implant, called a capsule, can become very hard. This is called capsular contracture, and may result in pain and possible altered appearance of the breast. The chances that these problems will occur increase with the age of the implant.

There has been intermittent publicity about possible health risks associated with breast implants. Most concerns have focused on silicone gel-filled implants that

leaked or ruptured. In 1992, the Food and Drug Administration (FDA) restricted the use of this type of implant and ordered further studies. Today only saline-filled implants are used for cosmetic breast surgery. Recent studies have shown no evidence of long-term health risks from intact silicone implants. However, research on possible links between these implants and autoimmune or connective tissue diseases is continuing.

Normal results

Breasts of expected size and appearance are the normal results of this surgery. Normal scar formation should be expected. With any silicone prosthesis, a capsule usually forms around it. However, in some instances a mild form of capsular contraction ensues. Mild ridges that can be felt under the skin categorize this condition. The capsule contracts, which occurs occasionally, and can result in a hardening of the breast. There is no way to predict who will excessively scar.

Morbidity and mortality rates

In addition to scarring, other risks include infection, excessive bleeding, problems associated with anesthesia, rupturing of the implant, and leakage. There have been a total of 120,000 reports of ruptured silicone implants. Approximately 50,000 reports of breakage have been received for saline implants.

Deaths associated with breast augmentation are extremely rare. Most post surgical mortality has been attributed to anesthesia errors or overdoses of pain medications.

Alternatives

Alternatives to breast implant surgery include using external breast forms that fit into brassiere cups or are attached to the skin of the chest. Creams that allege to increase breast size usually produce no noticeable results. The use of creams containing hormones can lead to long-term hormonal imbalance. Reputable experts do not generally recommend these preparations for breast enlargement.

QUESTIONS TO ASK THE DOCTOR

- What will be the resulting appearance?
- Is the surgeon board certified in plastic and reconstructive surgery?
- How many procedures has the surgeon performed?
- What is the surgeon's complication rate?

Resources

BOOKS

Ball, Adrian S., and Peter M. Arnstein. *Handbook of Breast Surgery.* London: Edward Arnold, 1999.

Berger, Karen J., and John Bostwick. *A Woman's Decision: Breast Care, Treatment & Reconstruction,* 3rd edition. St. Louis: Quality Medical Publishers, 1998.

Bostwick, John. *Plastic and Reconstructive Breast Surgery.* 2nd edition. St. Louis: Quality Medical Publishers, 1999.

Engler, Alan M. *BodySculpture: Plastic Surgery of the Body for Men and Women,* 2nd edition. London: Hudson Pub., 2000.

PERIODICALS

Colville, R. J., N. R. McLean, C. A. Mallen, and L. McLean. "The Impact of Breast Augmentation on the Breast-screening Programme." *British Journal of Plastic Surgery,* 55, no. 7 (2002): 592–593.

Hudson, D. A. "Submuscle Saline Breast Augmentation: Are We Making Sense in the New Millennium?" *Aesthetic and Plastic Surgery* 26, no. 4 (2002): 287–290.

Jejurikar, S.S., J. M. Rovak, W. M. Kuzon Jr., K. C. Chung, S. V. Kotsis, and P. S. Cederna. "Evaluation of Plastic Surgery Information on the Internet." *Annals of Plastic Surgery* 49, no. 5 (2002): 460–465.

Smith, M., and K. Kent. "Breast Concerns and Lifestyles of Women." *Clinics in Obstetrics and Gynecology* 45, no. 4 (2002): 1129–1139.

ORGANIZATIONS

American Board of Plastic Surgery. Seven Penn Center, Suite 400, 1635 Market Street, Philadelphia, PA 19103-2204. (215) 587-9322. <http://www.abplsurg.org>.

American College of Plastic and Reconstructive Surgery. <http://www.breast-implant.org>.

American College of Surgeons. 633 North Saint Claire Street, Chicago, IL, 60611. (312) 202-5000. <http://www.facs.org>.

American Society for Aesthetic Plastic Surgery. 11081 Winners Circle, Los Alamitos, CA 90720. (800) 364-2147 or (562) 799-2356. <http://www.surgery.org/>.

American Society of Plastic Surgeons. 444 E. Algonquin Rd., Arlington Heights, IL 60005. (888) 475-2784. <http://www.plasticsurgery.org>.

KEY TERMS

Breast augmentation—Increase the size of breasts.

Contracture—Tissue change that is characterized by shortening of length, usually producing wrinkles or areas of thickening.

Transsexual—Person desiring to acquire the external appearance of a member of the opposite gender.

OTHER

American Society of Cosmetic Breast Surgery. *Information about Breast Surgery.* 2003 [cited February 24, 2003]. <http://www.breast-implant.org>.

National Library of Medicine. *Breast Implants.* 2003 [cited February 24, 2003]. <http://www.nlm.nih.gov/medlineplus/breastimplantsbreastreconstruction.htm>.

Public Broadcasting System. *Breast Implants on Trial.* 2003 [cited February 24, 2003]. <http://www.pbs.org/wgbh/pages/frontline/implants/cron.html>.

US Food and Drug Administration. *Breast Implants.* 2003 [cited February 24, 2003]. <http://www.fda.gov/cdrh/breast implants/labeling/mentor_patient_labeling_5900.htm>.

L. Fleming Fallon, Jr., MD, DrPH

Breast radiography *see* **Mammography**

Breast reconstruction

Definition

Breast reconstruction is a series of surgical procedures performed to recreate a breast. Reconstructions are commonly begun after portions of one or both breasts are removed as a treatment for breast cancer. A breast may need to be refashioned for other reasons such as trauma or to correct abnormalities that occur during breast development.

Purpose

Many experts consider reconstruction to be an integral component of the therapy for breast cancer. A naturally appearing breast offers a sense of wholeness and normalcy, which can aid in the psychological recovery from breast cancer. It eliminates the need for an external prosthesis (false breast), which many women find to be physically uncomfortable as well as inconvenient.

Woman with reconstructed breast (on left) following mastectomy. *(Biophoto Associates/Science Source. Reproduced by permission.)*

Demographics

Breast surgery, including reconstruction, is the second most commonly performed cosmetic surgical procedure practiced on women in the United States. It increased by 306% between 1992 and 1998. According to the American Society of Plastic and Reconstructive Surgeons, more than 125,000 breast augmentation or reconstruction procedures are performed each year.

Presently, more than two million, or approximately 8%, of women in the United States have **breast implants**. The majority of breast implant recipients are Caucasian women (95%), followed by African-American women (4%). The remaining women that have breast implants are Asian (0.5%) and other non-specified races (0.5%).

Description

Breast reconstruction is performed in two stages, with the ultimate goal of creating a breast that looks and feels as natural as possible. It is important to remember that while a good result may closely mimic a normal breast, there will inevitably be scars and some loss of sensation. The reconstructed breast cannot exactly match the original.

The first step is to create a structure called a breast mound. This can be accomplished using artificial materials called breast implants, or by using tissues from other parts of the woman's body. The second step involves creating a balance between the newly constructed breast and the breast on the opposite side. The nipple and areolar complex (darker area around the nipple) are recreated. This is usually done several months after the mound is created, to allow swelling to subside. Other procedures may be necessary, such as lifting the opposite breast (mastopexy) or making it larger or smaller to match the reconstructed breast.

Immediate or delayed reconstruction

While immediate reconstruction (IR) is not recommended for women with breast cancer who need to undergo other, more important treatments, breast reconstruction can be done almost anytime. It can be delayed, or it can be completed during the same procedure as the mastectomy. There are psychological benefits to IR. The ability to return to normal activities and routines is often enhanced when reconstruction follows immediately after mastectomy. A better final appearance may result from IR. There is less skin removal, often resulting in a short-

Breast reconstruction

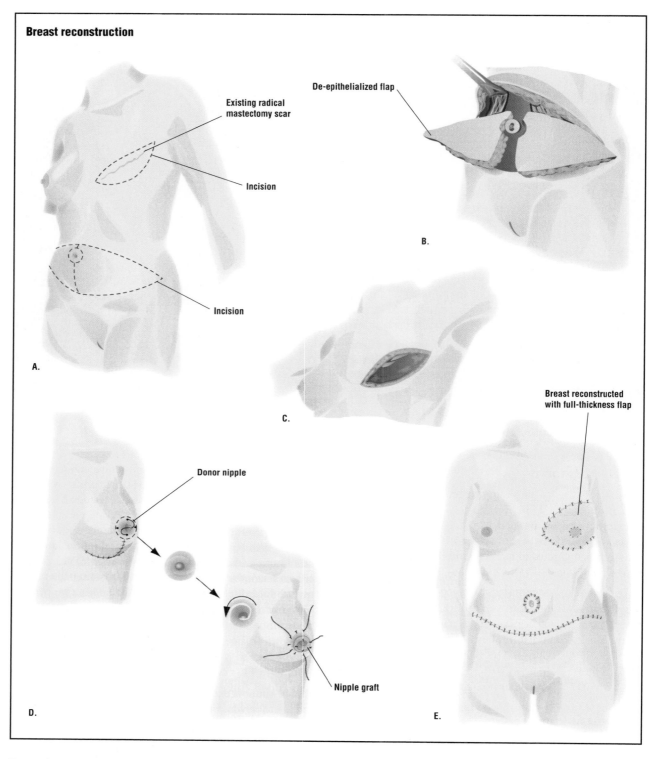

Existing radical
mastectomy scar

Incision

Incision

A.

De-epithelialized flap

B.

C.

Donor nipple

Nipple graft

D.

Breast reconstructed
with full-thickness flap

E.

Breast reconstruction is often performed after a mastectomy. In an autologous procedure, a section of tissue from the patient's abdomen (B) is used to create a natural-looking new breast. In a separate procedure, a layer of the patient's existing
nipple can be grafted onto the new breast (D). *(Illustration by GGS Inc.)*

er scar. The surgeon is better able to preserve the normal boundaries of the breast, so it is easier to more closely match the opposite breast.

The cost of IR is generally lower than the cost of delayed reconstruction (DR). There is one less operation and hospital stay. Surgeon's fees may be lower for a combined procedure than for two separate surgeries.

There are disadvantages of IR as well. The surgery itself is longer, resulting in more time under anesthesia. Postoperative pain and recovery time will be greater than for mastectomy alone.

Other authorities contend that delayed reconstruction (DR) offers different physical and psychological advantages. The initial mastectomy procedure alone takes less time, and has a shorter recovery period and less pain than mastectomy and IR. The woman has more time to adjust to her diagnosis and recover from additional therapy. She is better able to review and evaluate her options and to formulate realistic goals for reconstruction. Some reconstructive surgery requires blood transfusions. With DR, the patient can donate her own blood ahead of time (**autologous blood donation**), and/or arrange to have family and friends donate blood for her use (directed donation).

The psychological stress of living without a breast is a disadvantage of DR. The extra procedure needed to perform DR results in higher costs. Although initial recovery is faster, an additional recuperation period is required after the delayed operation.

Type of reconstruction

There are two basic choices for breast reconstruction. The breast tissue can be replaced with an implant, or the breast is created using some of the woman's own tissues (autologous reconstruction).

ARTIFICIAL IMPLANTS. In general, implant procedures take less time and are less expensive than autologous ones. Implants are breast-shaped pouches. They are made of silicone outer shells, which may be smooth or textured. The inside contains saline (salt water). Implants made prior to 1992 were filled with silicone gel. In 1992, the Food and Drug Association (FDA) discontinued the use of silicone as a filling material.

An implant may be a fixed-volume type, which cannot change its size. Implants that have the capacity to be filled after insertion are called tissue expanders. These may be temporary or permanent.

The initial procedure for any implant insertion uses the mastectomy incision to make a pocket of tissue, usually underneath the chest wall muscle. In DR, the mastectomy scar may be reopened and used for this purpose,

Breast reconstruction is normally performed by a surgeon with advanced training in plastic and reconstructive procedures. It is commonly, but not exclusively, performed as an outpatient procedure.

or a more cosmetic incision may be made. The implant is inserted into the pocket, the skin is stretched as needed, and sutured closed.

If there is inadequate tissue to achieve the desired size, or a naturally sagging breast is desired, a tissue expander is used. It resembles a partially deflated balloon, with an attached valve or port through which saline can be injected. After the initial surgical incision is healed, the woman returns to the doctor's office on a weekly or bi-weekly basis to have small amounts of saline injected. Injections can continue for about six to eight weeks, until the preferred size is obtained. In some cases, it may initially be overfilled and later partially deflated to allow for a more pliable, natural result. A temporary tissue expander is removed after several months and replaced with a permanent implant.

IR surgery using an implant takes approximately two to three hours, and usually requires up to a three-day hospital stay. Implant insertion surgery that is accomplished as part of DR takes one to two hours and can sometimes be done as an outpatient procedure. Alternatively, it may entail overnight hospitalization.

AUTOLOGOUS RECONSTRUCTION. Attached flap and free flap are two types of surgery where a woman's own tissue is used in reconstruction. An attached flap uses skin, muscle, and fat, leaving blood vessels attached to their original source of blood. The flap is maneuvered to the reconstruction site, keeping its original blood supply for nourishment; this is also known as a pedicle flap. The second kind of surgery is called a free flap, which also uses skin, muscle, and fat, but the surgeon severs the blood vessels and reattaches them to other vessels where the new breast is to be created. The surgeon uses a microscope to accomplish the delicate task of sewing blood vessels together (anastomosis). Sometimes, the term **microsurgery** is used to refer to free flap procedures. Either type of surgery may also be called a myocutaneous flap. This refers to the skin and muscle used.

The skin and muscle used in autologous reconstruction can come from one of several possible places on the body, including the abdomen (tummy tuck flap), the back (latissimus dorsi flap), or the buttocks (gluteus maximus free flap).

Finishing the reconstruction

Other procedures may be necessary to achieve the goal of symmetrical breasts. It may be necessary to make the opposite breast larger (augmentation), smaller (reduction), or higher (mastopexy). These, or any other refinements, should be completed before the creation of a nipple and areola. Tissue to form the new nipple may come from the reconstructed breast itself, the opposite breast, or a more distant donor site such as the inner thigh or behind the ear. The nipple and areolar construction is usually accomplished as an outpatient procedure. A final step, often done in the doctor's office, is tattooing the new nipple and areola to match the color of the opposite nipple and areola as closely as possible.

Insurance

Insurance coverage varies widely for breast reconstruction. Some policies will allow procedures on the affected breast, but refuse to pay for alterations to the opposite breast. Other plans may cover the cost of an external prosthesis or reconstructive surgery, but not both. The Women's Health and Cancer Rights Act of 1998 requires group health plans and health issuers to provide medical and surgical benefits with respect to mastectomy and to cover the cost of reconstructive breast surgery for women who have undergone a mastectomy.

Implants may pose additional insurance concerns. Some companies will withdraw coverage for women with implants, or add a disclaimer for future implant-related problems. Careful reading of insurance policies, including checking on the need for pre-approval and a **second opinion**, is strongly recommended.

Diagnosis/Preparation

The diagnosis for breast reconstruction is almost always made on a visual basis. The underlying medical reasons include replacing all or part of breast tissue that has been removed during the course of cancer treatment, replacing breast mass that has been lost due to injury, or equalizing otherwise normal breasts that are markedly different in size. Underlying cosmetic reasons include personal preference for larger breasts among genetic females or the creation of breasts in male-to-female transsexuals.

Routine preoperative preparations, such as having nothing to eat or drink the night before surgery, are needed for reconstructive procedures. Blood transfusions are often necessary for autologous reconstructive surgeries. The patient may donate her own blood and/or have family and friends donate blood for her use several weeks prior to the surgery.

Emotional preparation is also important. Breast reconstruction will not resolve a psychological problem the woman had before mastectomy, nor make an unstable relationship strong. An expectation of physical perfection is also unrealistic. A woman who cites any of these reasons for reconstruction shows that she has not been adequately informed or prepared. Complete understanding of the benefits and limitations of this surgery are necessary for a satisfactory result.

Not all women are good candidates for breast reconstruction. Overall poor physical health, or specific problems such as cigarette smoking, obesity, high blood pressure, or diabetes, will increase the chance of complications. Also, a difficult or prolonged recovery period or failure of the reconstruction may be a result. A woman's physical ability to cope with major surgery and recuperation should also be considered.

Aftercare

The length of the hospital stay, recovery period, and frequency of visits to the doctor after surgery vary considerably with the different types of reconstruction. In general, autologous procedures require longer hospitalization and recovery times than implant procedures. For all surgical procedures, bandages and drainage tubes remain in place for at least a day. Microsurgical or free flap procedures are most closely monitored in the first day or two after surgery. The circulation to the breast may be checked as often as every hour. Complete breast reconstruction requires at least one additional surgery to create a nipple and areola. Scars may remain red and raised for a month or longer. They will fade to their final appearance within one to two years. The true, final appearance of the breasts usually will not be visible for at least one year.

Risks

Some women have reported various types of autoimmune-related connective tissue disorders, which they attribute to their implants—usually involving silicone gel implants. Lawsuits have been filed against the manufacturers of these implants. Food and Drug Administration (FDA) guidelines, issued in 1992, now greatly restrict their use, primarily to women who need to replace an existing silicone gel-filled implant. In addition, recipients must sign a consent form that details the potential risks of silicone gel-filled implants and become enrolled in a long-range study. Saline is now the filling of choice for breast implants. Saline-filled implants are permitted for all uses, although manufacturers must continue to collect data on possible risks.

The FDA issued a status report on Breast Implant Safety in 1995, and revised it in March 1997. It noted that studies to date have not shown a serious increase in the risk of recognized autoimmune diseases in women with silicone gel-filled breast implants. It also addressed concerns about other complications and emphasized the need for further study of this issue.

There are a number of risks common to any surgical procedure, such as bleeding, infection, anesthesia reaction, or unexpected scarring. Hematoma (accumulation of blood at the surgical site), or seroma (collection of fluid at the surgical site) can delay healing if they are not drained. Any breast reconstruction also poses a risk of asymmetry and the possible need for an unplanned surgical revision. Persistent pain is another potential complication of all types of breast reconstruction.

Implants have some unique problems that may develop. A thick scar, called a capsule, forms around the implant as part of the body's normal reaction to a foreign substance. Capsular contracture occurs when the scar becomes firm or hardened. This may cause pain accompanied by changes in the texture or appearance of the breast. Implants can rupture and leak, deflate, or become displaced. The chances of capsular contracture or rupture increase with the age of the implant. These complications can usually be remedied with **outpatient surgery** to loosen the capsule and remove or replace the implant as needed. There is some evidence that using implants with textured surfaces may decrease the incidence of these problems. An implant tends to remain firm indefinitely. It will not grow larger or smaller as a woman's weight changes. Asymmetry can develop if a woman gains or loses a large amount of weight.

The autologous procedures all carry a risk of flap failure, which is a loss of blood supply to the tissue forming the new breast. If a large portion of the flap develops inadequate blood supply, another reconstructive technique may be necessary. Tummy tuck flap procedures can result in decreased muscle tone and weakness in the abdomen, or lead to an abdominal hernia. Arm weakness may occur after latissimus dorsi flap surgery.

Normal results

A normal result of breast reconstruction depends on the woman's goals and expectations. It will not be the same as the breast it replaces. In general, the reconstructed breast should be similar in size and shape to the opposite breast, but will have less sensation and be less mobile than a natural breast. A reconstruction using an implant will usually be firmer and rounder than the other breast. It may feel cooler to the touch, depending on the amount of tissue over it. Scars are unavoidable, but should be as inconspicuous as possible.

Morbidity and mortality rates

Normal scar formation should be expected. With any silicone prosthesis, a capsule usually forms around it. However, in some instances a mild form of capsular contraction may develop. Mild ridges that can be felt under the skin categorize this condition. If the capsule contracts, as occasionally occurs, it results in a hardening of the breast. There is no way to predict who will excessively scar. Other risks include infection, excessive bleeding, problems associated with anesthesia, rupturing of the implant, and leakage. There have been a total of 120,000 reports of ruptured silicone implants. Approximately 50,000 reports of breakage have been received for saline implants.

Deaths associated with breast reconstruction are extremely rare. Most post-surgical mortality has been attributed to anesthesia errors or overdoses of pain medications.

Alternatives

Alternatives to breast reconstruction surgery include using external breast forms that fit into brassiere cups or are attached to the skin of the chest. Creams that allege to increase breast size usually produce no noticeable results. The use of creams containing hormones can lead to long-term hormonal imbalances. Reputable experts do not generally recommend these preparations for breast enlargement.

Resources

BOOKS

Ball, Adrian S., and Peter M. Arnstein. *Handbook of Breast Surgery.* London: Edward Arnold, 1999.

Berger, Karen J., and John Bostwick. *A Woman's Decision: Breast Care, Treatment & Reconstruction,* 3rd edition. St. Louis: Quality Medical Publshers, 1998.

Bostwick, John. *Plastic and Reconstructive Breast Surgery,* 2nd edition. St. Louis: Quality Medical Publishers, 1999.

Engler, Alan M. *BodySculpture: Plastic Surgery of the Body for Men and Women,* 2nd edition. London: Hudson Pub., 2000.

KEY TERMS

Autologous—From the same person; an autologous breast reconstruction uses the woman's own tissues, while an autologous blood transfusion is blood removed then transfused back to the same person at a later time.

Capsular contracture—Thick scar tissue around a breast implant, which may tighten and cause discomfort and/or firmness.

Flap—A section of tissue moved from one area of the body to another.

Free flap—A section of tissue is detached from its blood supply, moved to another part of the body, and reattached by microsurgery to a new blood supply.

Mastectomy—Removal of all or a portion of breast tissue.

Mastopexy—Surgical procedure to lift up a breast; may be used on opposite breast to achieve symmetrical appearance with a reconstructed breast.

Pedicle flap—Also called an attached flap; a section of tissue, with its blood supply intact, which is maneuvered to another part of the body.

PERIODICALS

Colville, R. J., N. R. McLean, C. A. Mallen, and L. McLean. "The Impact of Breast Augmentation on the Breast-screening Programme." *British Journal of Plastic Surgery,* 55, no. 7 (2002): 592–593.

Hudson, D. A. "Submuscle Saline Breast Augmentation: Are We Making Sense in the New Millenium?" *Aesthetic and Plastic Surgery* 26, no. 4 (2002): 287–290.

Jejurikar, S. S., J. M. Rovak, W. M. Kuzon Jr, K. C. Chung, S. V. Kotsis, and P. S. Cederna. "Evaluation of Plastic Surgery Information on the Internet." *Annals of Plastic Surgery* 49, no. 5 (2002): 460–465.

Smith, M., and K. Kent. "Breast Concerns and Lifestyles of Women." *Clinics in Obstetrics and Gynecology* 45, no. 4 (2002): 1129–1139.

ORGANIZATIONS

American Board of Plastic Surgery. Seven Penn Center, Suite 400, 1635 Market Street, Philadelphia, PA 19103-2204. (215) 587-9322. <http://www.abplsurg.org/>.

American College of Plastic and Reconstructive Surgery. <http://www.breast-implant.org>.

American College of Surgeons. 633 North Saint Claire Street, Chicago, IL 60611. (312) 202-5000. <http://www.facs.org/>.

American Society for Aesthetic Plastic Surgery. 11081 Winners Circle, Los Alamitos, CA 90720. (800) 364-2147 or (562) 799-2356. <http://www.surgery.org/>.

American Society of Plastic Surgeons. 444 E. Algonquin Rd., Arlington Heights, IL 60005. (888) 475-2784. <http://www.plasticsurgery.org/>.

OTHER

American Society of Cosmetic Breast Surgery. *Information about Breast Surgery.* [cited February 24, 2003] <http://www.breast-implant.org>.

National Library of Medicine. *Breast Implants.* [cited February 24, 2003] <http://www.nlm.nih.gov/medlineplus/breast implantsbreastreconstruction.htm>.

Public Broadcasting System *Breast Implants on Trial.* [cited February 24, 2003] <http://www.pbs.org/wgbh/pages/frontline/implants/cron.html>.

U.S. Food and Drug Administration. *Breast Implants.* [cited February 24, 2003] <http://www.fda.gov/cdrh/breast implants/labeling/mentor_patient_labeling_5900.htm>.

L. Fleming Fallon, Jr., MD, DrPH

Breast reduction

Definition

Breast reduction is a surgical procedure performed to decrease the size of the breasts.

Purpose

Women with very large breasts (macromastia, or mammary hyperplasia) seek breast reduction for relief of back, shoulder, and neck pain. They may also feel uncomfortable about their breast size and have difficulty finding clothing that will fit properly. Additionally, breast reduction may be needed after reconstructive surgery following the surgical removal of cancerous breast tissue (mastectomy), to make the breasts more symmetric.

Men who have enlarged breasts (gynecomastia) may also be candidates for breast reduction surgery. However, excessive alcohol intake, marijuana use, or using anabolic steroids may cause gynecomastia. Surgery is not recommended for men who continue to use these products.

Demographics

According to the American Society of Plastic Surgeons, more than 70,000 women underwent breast reduction surgery in 1999, while fewer than 40,000 women had the procedure performed in 1992. Breast reduction

Breast reduction

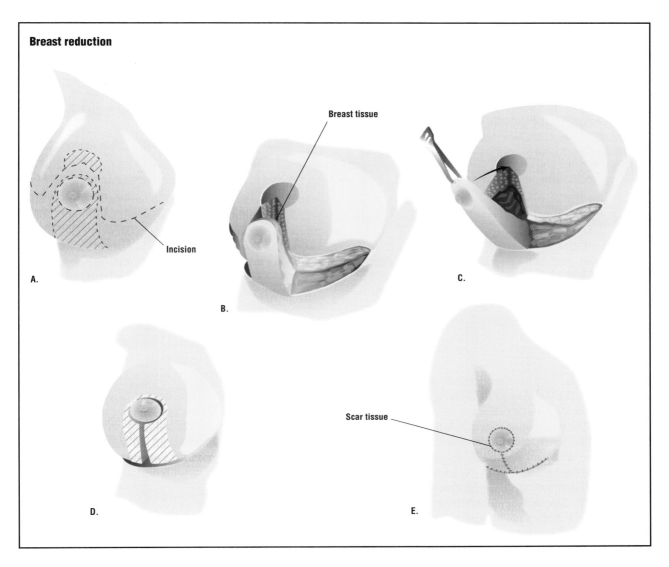

Breast tissue

Incision

A.

B.

C.

Scar tissue

D.

E.

In a breast reduction surgery, the breast tissue is cut along predetermined lines and (A) excess tissue is removed (B). The nipple is placed higher on the breast (C), and the two sides of the incision are brought together (D), removing any excess skin (E). *(Illustration by GGS Inc.)*

surgery is becoming more common each year. Women most likely to undergo breast reduction range in age from 19 to 50.

Description

Breast reduction is also called reduction mammoplasty. It is most often performed in a hospital, under general anesthetic. However, studies have suggested that an outpatient procedure, using local anesthetic and mild sedation, may be appropriate for some persons. The operation requires approximately two to four hours. The most commonly made incision encircles the areola (darkened area around the nipple) and extends down-

ward and around the underside of the breast. This produces the least conspicuous scar. Excess tissue, fat, and skin are removed, and the nipple and areola are repositioned. In certain cases, **liposuction** (fat suctioning) is used to remove extra fat from the armpit area. A hospital stay of up to three days may be needed for recovery.

Breast reduction surgery for males with gynecomastia is similar to that described for females.

If deemed medically necessary, breast reduction is covered by some insurance plans. However, a specified amount of breast tissue may need to be removed in order to qualify for coverage. Surgeon's fees range from $5,000 to $6,500, or more.

Diagnosis/Preparation

Consultation between surgeon and patient is important to ensure that there is understanding and agreement with the expected final results of the procedure. Measurements and photographs may be taken. Many doctors also recommend a mammogram before the operation to ensure that there is no cancer.

Aftercare

After the surgery, an elastic bandage or special supportive bra is placed over gauze bandages and drainage tubes. The bandages and tubes are removed in a day or two. The bra is worn around the clock for several weeks. Stitches are removed one to three weeks after the operation. Normal activities, including sexual relations, may be restricted for several weeks. Scars will typically remain red and perhaps raised for up to several months, but will gradually fade and become less noticeable. It may take up to a year before the breasts achieve their final position and size.

Risks

Breast reduction surgery is not recommended for women whose breasts are not fully developed or who plan to breastfeed.

Risks common to any operation include bleeding, infection, anesthesia reactions, or unexpected scarring. Breast reduction may result in decreased feeling in the breasts or nipples and/or impaired ability to breastfeed. When healing is complete, the breasts may be slightly uneven, or the nipples may be asymmetric. However, this is consistent with normal breast tissue.

Normal results

Smaller breast size should be achieved and, with that, the accompanying pain and discomfort should be alleviated. Self-esteem should be improved for both females and males having breast reduction surgery.

Morbidity and mortality rates

Deaths associated with breast reduction surgery are extremely rare. Most post-surgical mortality has been attributed to anesthesia errors, overdoses of pain medications, or postoperative infections.

In very rare cases, the skin of the breast or nipple does not heal properly and additional surgery is necessary to graft skin. Approximately 10% of women experience some loss of sensation in their nipples.

Permanent scars are left after breast reduction surgery. At first, the scars usually appear red and raised but will become less obvious over time. Women who smoke often experience more prominent scars. This is because smoking interferes with the healing process.

Alternatives

There are no alternatives to surgery as a way to reduce breast tissue, although significant weight loss can decrease the size of the breast.

Resources

BOOKS

Ball, Adrian S., and Peter M. Arnstein. *Handbook of Breast Surgery.* London: Edward Arnold, 1999.

Berger, Karen J., and John Bostwick. *A Woman's Decision: Breast Care, Treatment & Reconstruction,* 3rd edition. St. Louis: Quality Medical Publshers, 1998.

Bostwick, John. *Plastic and Reconstructive Breast Surgery,* 2nd edition. St. Louis: Quality Medical Publishers, 1999.

Engler, Alan M. *BodySculpture: Plastic Surgery of the Body for Men and Women,* 2nd edition. London: Hudson Pub., 2000.

PERIODICALS

Chao, J. D., H. C. Memmel, J. F. Redding, L. Egan, L. C. Odom, and L. A. Casas. "Reduction Mammaplasty Is a Functional Operation, Improving Quality of Life in Symptomatic Women: A Prospective, Single-center Breast

Reduction Outcome Study." *Plastic and Reconstructive Surgery* 110, no. 7 (2002): 1644–1654.

Jejurikar, S. S., J. M. Rovak, W. M. Kuzon Jr, K. C. Chung, S. V. Kotsis, and P. S. Cederna. "Evaluation of Plastic Surgery Information on the Internet." *Annals of Plastic Surgery* 49, no. 5 (2002): 460–465.

Johansson, A. S., H. Wennborg, L. Blomqvist, D. Isacson, and E. Kylberg. "Breastfeeding after Reduction Mammoplasty and Augmentation Mammoplasty." *Epidemiology* 14, no. 1 (2003): 127–129.

Qiao, Q., J. Sun, C. Liu, Z. Liu, and R. Zhao. "Reduction Mammaplasty and Correction of Ptosis: Dermal Bra Technique." *Plastic and Reconstructive Surgery* 111, no. 3 (2003): 1122–1130.

Smith, M., and K. Kent. "Breast Concerns and Lifestyles of Women." *Clinics in Obstetrics and Gynecology* 45, no. 4 (2002): 1129–1139.

Spear, S. L., C. V. Pelletiere, A. J. Wolfe, T. N. Tsangaris, and M. F. Pennanen. "Experience with Reduction Mammaplasty Combined with Breast Conservation Therapy in the Treatment of Breast Cancer." *Plastic and Reconstructive Surgery* 111, no. 3 (2003): 1102–1109.

ORGANIZATIONS

American Board of Plastic Surgery. Seven Penn Center, Suite 400, 1635 Market Street, Philadelphia, PA 19103-2204. (215) 587-9322. <http://www.abplsurg.org/>.

American College of Plastic and Reconstructive Surgery. <http://www.breast-implant.org>.

American College of Surgeons. 633 North Saint Claire Street, Chicago, IL 60611. (312) 202-5000. <http://www.facs.org/>.

American Society for Aesthetic Plastic Surgery. 11081 Winners Circle, Los Alamitos, CA 90720. (800) 364-2147 or (562) 799-2356. <http://www.surgery.org/>.

American Society of Plastic Surgeons. 444 E. Algonquin Rd., Arlington Heights, IL 60005. (888) 475-2784. <http://www.plasticsurgery.org/>.

OTHER

"Breast Implants." *U.S. Food and Drug Administration.* [cited February 24, 2003] <http://www.fda.gov/cdrh/breast implants/labeling/mentor_patient_labeling_5900.htm>.

"Breast Implants and Breast Reconstruction." *National Library of Medicine.* [cited March 20, 2003]. <http://www.nlm.nih.gov/medlineplus/breastimplantsbreastreconstruction.htm>.

"Implants on Trial." *Public Broadcasting Systems.* [cited March 20, 2003] <http://www.pbs.org/wgbh/pages/frontline/implants/cron.html>.

"Information about Breast Surgery." *American Society of Cosmetic Breast Surgery.* [cited March 20, 2003] <http://www.breast-implant.org>.

L. Fleming Fallon, Jr., MD, DrPH

Breast x ray *see* **Mammography**

Bronchoscopy

Definition

Bronchoscopy is a procedure in which a hollow, flexible tube called a bronchoscope is inserted into the airways through the nose or mouth to provide a view of the tracheobronchial tree. It can also be used to collect bronchial and/or lung secretions and to perform tissue biopsy.

Purpose

During a bronchoscopy, the physician can visually examine the lower airways, including the larynx, trachea, bronchi, and bronchioles. The procedure is used to examine the mucosal surface of the airways for abnormalities that might be associated with a variety of lung diseases. Its use may be diagnostic or therapeutic.

Bronchoscopy may be used to examine and help diagnose:

• diseases of the lung, such as cancer or tuberculosis

Instruments used in bronchoscopy procedures. *(Custom Medical Stock Photo. Reproduced by permission.)*

• congenital deformity of the lungs

• suspected tumor, obstruction, secretion, bleeding, or foreign body in the airways

• airway abnormalities, such as tracheal stenoses

• persistent cough, or hemoptysis, that includes blood in the sputum

Bronchoscopy may also be used for the following therapeutic purposes:

• to remove a foreign body in the lungs

• to remove excessive secretions

Bronchoscopy can also be used to collect the following biopsy specimens:

• sputum

• tissue samples from the bronchi or bronchioles

• cells collected from washing the lining of the bronchi or bronchioles

If the purpose of the bronchoscopy is to take tissue samples or biopsy, a forceps or bronchial brush are used to obtain cells. Alternatively, if the purpose is to identify an infectious agent, a bronchoalveolar lavage can be performed to gather fluid for culture purposes. If any foreign matter is found in the airways, it can be removed as well.

The instrument used in bronchoscopy, a bronchoscope, is a slender, flexible tube less than 0.5 in (2.5 cm) wide and approximately 2 ft (0.3 m) long that uses fiberoptic technology (very fine filaments that can bend and carry light). There are two types of bronchoscopes, a standard tube that is more rigid and a fiberoptic tube that is more flexible. The rigid instrument does not bend, does not see as far down into the lungs as the flexible one, and may carry a greater risk of causing injury to nearby structures. Because it can cause more discomfort than the flexible bronchoscope, it usually requires general anesthesia. However, it is useful for taking large samples of tissue and for removing foreign bodies from the airways. During the procedure, the airway is never blocked since oxygen can be supplied through the bronchoscope.

Demographics

In 2000, the National Hospital Discharge Survey and the National Survey of Ambulatory Surgery Reports outlined the following rates for bronchoscopy with or without biopsy at short-stay hospitals in the United States:

• Both sexes: 8.9 per 10,000 population

• Males: 10.6 per 10,000 population

• Females: 7.3 per 10,000 population

According to the National Cancer Institute, cancer of the lung and bronchi is the second most common cancer among both men and women and is the leading cause of cancer death in both sexes in the United States. Among men, lung cancer incidence rates per 100,000 people range from a low of approximately 14 among American Indians to a high of 117 among African Americans. Between these two extremes, rates fall into two groups ranging from 42 to 53 for Hispanics, Japanese, Chinese, Filipinos, and Koreans and from 71 to 89 for Vietnamese, Caucasians, Alaska natives, and Hawaiians. The range among women is much narrower, from a rate of about 15 among Japanese to nearly 51 among Alaska Natives, only a three-fold difference. Rates for the remaining female populations fall roughly into two groups with low rates of 16–25 for Korean, Filipino, Hispanic, and Chinese women, and rates of 31–44 among Vietnamese, Caucasian, Hawaiian, and African American women. The rates among men are about two to three times greater than the rates among women in each of the racial/ethnic groups.

Description

Bronchoscopy is usually performed in an endoscopy room, but may also be performed at the bedside. The patient is placed on his back or sits upright. A pulmonologist, a specialist trained to perform the procedure, sprays an anesthetic into the patient's mouth or throat. When anesthesia has taken effect and the area is numb, the bronchoscope is inserted into the patient's mouth and passed into the throat. If the bronchoscope is passed through the nose, an anesthetic jelly is inserted into one nostril. While the bronchoscope is moving down the throat, additional anesthetic is put into the bronchoscope to anesthetize the lower airways. The physician observes the trachea, bronchi, and the mucosal lining of these passageways looking for any abnormalities that may be present. If samples are needed, a bronchial lavage may be performed, meaning that a saline solution is introduced to flush the area prior to collecting cells for laboratory

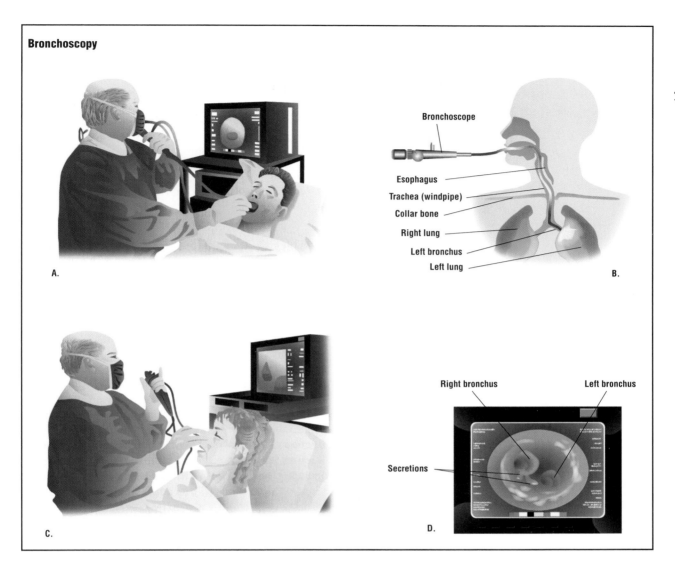

Bronchoscopy (label top-left of figure)

- Bronchoscope
- Esophagus
- Trachea (windpipe)
- Collar bone
- Right lung
- Left bronchus
- Left lung

A.   B.

- Right bronchus
- Left bronchus
- Secretions

C.   D.

Bronchoscopy can be performed via the patient's mouth (A) or through the nose (C). During the procedure, the scope is fed down the trachea and into the bronchus leading to the lungs (B), providing the physician with a view of internal structures (D). *(Illustration by GGS Inc.)*

analysis. Very small brushes, needles, or forceps may also be introduced through the bronchoscope to collect tissue samples from the lungs.

Preparation

The patient should fast for six to 12 hours prior to the procedure and refrain from drinking any liquids the day of the procedure. Smoking should be avoided for 24 hours prior to the procedure and patients should also avoid taking any **aspirin** or ibuprofen-type medications. The bronchoscopy itself takes about 45–60 minutes. Prior to the bronchoscopy, several tests are usually done, including a **chest x ray** and blood work. Sometimes a bronchoscopy is done under general anesthesia, in which case the patient

will have an intravenous (IV) line in the arm. More commonly, the procedure is performed under local anesthesia, which is sprayed into the nose or mouth. This is necessary to inhibit the gag reflex. A sedative also may be given. A signed consent form is necessary for this procedure.

Aftercare

After the bronchoscopy, the **vital signs** (heart rate, blood pressure, and breathing) are monitored. Sometimes patients have an abnormal reaction to anesthesia. Any sputum should be collected in an emesis basin so that it can be examined for the presence of blood. If a biopsy was taken, the patient should not cough or clear the throat as this might dislodge any blood clot that has

QUESTIONS TO ASK THE DOCTOR

- What will happen during the procedure?
- Will it hurt?
- How long will the test last?
- How many bronchoscopies do you perform each year?
- Are there any risks associated with the procedure?

formed and cause bleeding. No food or drink should be consumed for about two hours after the procedure or until the anesthesia wears off. There is a significant risk for choking if anything (including water) is ingested before the anesthetic wears off, and the gag reflex has returned. To test if the gag reflex has returned, a spoon is placed on the back of the tongue for a few seconds with light pressure. If there is no gagging, the process is repeated after 15 minutes. The gag reflex should return in one to two hours. Ice chips or clear liquids should be taken before the patient attempts to eat solid food.

Patients are informed that after the anesthetic wears off the throat may be irritated for several days.

Patients should notify their health care provider if they develop any of these symptoms:

- hemoptysis (coughing up blood)
- shortness of breath, wheezing, or any trouble breathing
- chest pain
- fever, with or without breathing problems

Risks

Use of the bronchoscope mildly irritates the lining of the airways, resulting in some swelling and inflammation, as well as hoarseness caused from abrading the vocal cords. If this abrasion is more serious, it can lead to respiratory difficulty or bleeding of the lining of the airways.

The bronchoscopy procedure is also associated with a small risk of disordered heart rhythm (arrhythmia), heart attacks, low blood oxygen (hypoxemia), and pneumothorax (a puncture of the lungs that allows air to escape into the space between the lung and the chest wall). These risks are greater with the use of a rigid bronchoscope than with a fiberoptic bronchoscope. If a rigid tube is used, there is also a risk of chipped teeth. The risk of transmitting infectious disease from one patient to another by the bronchoscope is also present. There is also a risk of infec-

tion from endoscopes inadequately reprocessed by the automated endoscope reprocessing (AER) system. The Centers for Disease Control (CDC) reported cases of patient-to-patient transmission of infections following bronchoscopic procedures using bronchoscopes that were inadequately reprocessed by AERs. Investigation of the incidents revealed inconsistencies between the reprocessing instructions provided by the manufacturer of the bronchoscope and the manufacturer of the AER; or that the bronchoscopes were inadequately reprocessed.

Normal results

If the results of the bronchoscopy are normal, the windpipe (trachea) appears as smooth muscle with C-shaped rings of cartilage at regular intervals. There are no abnormalities either in the trachea or in the bronchi of the lungs.

Bronchoscopy results may also confirm a suspected diagnosis. This may include swelling, ulceration, or deformity in the bronchial wall, such as inflammation, stenosis, or compression of the trachea, neoplasm, and foreign bodies. The bronchoscopy may also reveal the presence of atypical substances in the trachea and bronchi. If samples are taken, the results could indicate cancer, disease-causing agents, or other lung diseases. Other findings may include constriction or narrowing (stenosis), compression, dilation of vessels, or abnormal branching of the bronchi. Abnormal substances that might be found in the airways include blood, secretions, or mucous plugs.

Morbidity and mortality rates

Bronchoscopy belongs to the group of procedures associated with highest inpatient mortality with a 12.7% mortality rate.

Alternatives

Depending upon the purpose of the bronchoscopy, alternatives may include a chest x ray or a computed tomography (CT) scan. If the purpose is to obtain biopsy specimens, one option is to perform surgery, which carries greater risks. Another option is percutaneous biopsy guided by CT.

Resources

BOOKS

Bolliger, C. T., and P. N. Mathur, eds. *Interventional Bronchoscopy.* (Progress in Respiratory Research, Vol. 30). Basel: S. Karger Publishing, 1999.

Koppen, W., J. F. Turner, and A. C. Mehta, eds. *Flexible Bronchoscopy.* 2nd ed. Oxford: Blackwell Publishers, 2004.

Loeb, S., ed. *Illustrated Guide to Diagnostic Tests.* Springhouse, PA: Springhouse Corporation, 1994.

KEY TERMS

Anesthetic—A drug that causes loss of sensation. It is used to lessen the pain of surgery and medical procedures.

Biopsy—Procedure that involves obtaining a tissue specimen for microscopic analysis to establish a precise diagnosis.

Bronchi—The network of tubular passages that carry air to the lungs and allow air to be expelled from the lungs.

Bronchioles—Small airways extending from the bronchi into the lobes of the lungs.

Bronchoalveolar lavage—Washing cells from the air sacs at the end of the bronchioles.

Computed tomography (CT)—A special radiographic imaging technique that uses a computer to acquire multiple x rays into a two-dimensional sectional image.

Emesis basin—A basin used to collect a patient's sputum or vomit.

Endoscope—A highly flexible viewing instrument.

Endoscopy—The visual inspection of any cavity of the body using an endoscope.

Hemoptysis—The The expectoration of blood or of blood containing sputum.

Larynx—The voice box.

Lavage—Washing out.

Neoplasm—A new growth or tumor.

Sputum—Matter ejected from the lungs, bronchi, and trachea through the mouth.

Stenosis—Narrowing of a duct or canal.

Trachea—The windpipe.

Tracheobronchial—Pertaining both to the tracheal and bronchial tubes or to their junction.

Pagana, Kathleen D., and Timothy J. Pagana. *Diagnostic Testing and Nursing Implications.* 5th ed. St. Louis: Mosby, 1999.

PERIODICALS

Diette, G. B., N. Lechtzin, E. Haponik, A. Devrotes, and H. R. Rubin. "Distraction Therapy with Nature Sights and Sounds Reduces Pain during Flexible Bronchoscopy: A Complementary Approach to Routine Analgesia." *Chest* 123 (March 2003): 941–948.

Nakamura, C. T., J. F. Ripka, K. McVeigh, N. Kapoor, and T. G. Keens. "Bronchoscopic Instillation of Surfactant in Acute Respiratory Distress Syndrome." *Pediatric Pulmonology* 31, no. 4 (April 2001): 317–320.

Starobin, D., G. Fink, D. Shitrit, G. Izbicki, D. Bendayan, I. Bakal, and M. R. Kramer. "The Role of Fiberoptic Bronchoscopy Evaluating Transplant Recipients with Suspected Pulmonary Infections: Analysis of 168 Cases in a Multi-organ Transplantation Center." *Transplantation Proceedings* 35 (March 2003): 659–660.

Wu, K. H., T. T. Man, K. L. Wong, C. F. Lin, C. C. Chen, and C. R. Cheng. "Bronchoscopy and Anesthesia for Preschool-aged Patients: A Review of 228 Cases." *Internal Surgery* 87 (October-December 2002): 252–255.

Yang, C. C., and K. S. Lee. "Comparison of Direct Vision and Video Imaging during Bronchoscopy for Pediatric Airway Foreign Bodies." *Ear, Nose, and Throat Journal* 82 (February 2003): 129–133.

ORGANIZATIONS

American College of Chest Physicians. 3300 Dundee Road, Northbrook, IL 60062. (800) 343-2227.

The Association of Perioperative Registered Nurses, Inc. (AORN). 2170 South Parker Rd, Suite 300, Denver, CO 80231-5711. (800) 755-2676. <http://www.aorn.org/>.

OTHER

"Bronchoscopy." *Medline Plus.* [cited April 2003]. <http://www.nlm.nih.gov/medlineplus/ency/article/003857.htm>.

Public Health Advisory: Infections from Endoscopes Inadequately Reprocessed by an Automated Endoscope Reprocessing System. U. S. Food and Drug Administration, Center for Devices and Radiological Health. September 1999 [cited April 2003]. <http://www.fda.gov/cdrh/safety/endoreprocess.html>.

Maggie Boleyn, RN, BSN
Monique Laberge, Ph D

BUN test *see* **Kidney function tests**

Bunionectomy

Definition

A bunionectomy is a surgical procedure to excise, or remove, a bunion. A bunion is an enlargement of the joint at the base of the big toe and is comprised of bone and soft tissue. It is usually a result of inflammation and irritation from poorly fitting (narrow and tight) shoes in

Bunionectomy

A. *Incision*

B. *Bursa / Bony overgrowth*

C. *Phalanx*

D. *Gauze pad / Sutures*

A bunion results in a bony overgrowth in the foot, causing the big toe to curve outward. To repair this, an incision is made in the top of the foot (A). The overgrowth and fluid-filled sac called a bursa are removed (B). The phalanx bone of the big toe is shortened to straighten it (C). The foot is realigned, and the incision is closed (D). *(Illustration by GGS Inc.)*

conjunction with an overly mobile first metatarsal joint and over-pronation of the foot. Over time, a painful lump appears at the side of the joint, while the big toe appears to buckle and move sideway towards the second toe. New bone growth can occur in response to the inflammatory process, and a bone spur may develop. Therefore, the development of a bunion may involve soft tissue as well as a hard bone spur. The intense pain makes walking and other activities extremely difficult. Since

the involved joint is a significant structure in providing weight-bearing stability, walking on the foot while trying to avoid putting pressure on the painful area can create an unstable gait.

Purpose

A bunionectomy is performed when conservative means of addressing the problem, including properly fitting, wide-toed shoes, a padded cushion against the joint, orthotics, and anti-inflammatory medication, are unsuccessful. As the big toe moves sideways, it can push the second toe sideways as well. This can result in extreme deformity of the foot, and the patient may complain not only of significant pain, but of an inability to find shoes that fit.

Demographics

Bunion formation can be hereditary, which means that if the individual's mother or father had the condition, he or she is at an increased risk of developing one as well. Bunions can also be a result of a congenital deformity, which means that the individual was born with an anatomical condition that made the development of a bunion more likely. Women are nine to 10 times more likely to develop bunions than men. The American Orthopaedic Foot & Ankle Society reports a study estimating that about 88% of women wear shoes that are too small and that 55% have developed bunions. The condition may begin to form in adolescence. Other conditions that contribute to bunion formation include flat-footedness, a tight Achilles tendon, and rheumatoid arthritis. The earlier the diagnosis, the better the chance that significant deformity will be avoided.

Description

Bunions become more common later in life. One reason is that with age the foot spreads and proper alignment is not maintained. In addition, the constant friction of poorly fitting shoes against the big toe joint creates a greater problem over time. Ignoring the problem in its early stages leads to a shifting gait that further aggravates the situation.

Once surgery has been decided on, the extent of the procedure will depend on the degree of deformity that has taken place. There are several different surgical techniques, mostly named after the surgeons who developed them, such as McBride, Chevron, and Keller. The degree and angle of deformity as well as the patient's age and physical condition play a significant role in the surgeon's choice of technique, which will determine how much tissue is removed and whether or not bone repositioning will occur. If bone repositioning is done, that part of the surgery is referred to as an osteotomy (*osteo* means bone). The type of anesthesia, whether ankle block (the most common, in which the foot is numb but the patient is awake), general, or spinal, will depend on the patient's condition and the anticipated extent of the surgery. For surgery done on an ambulatory basis, the patient will usually be asked to arrive one to two hours before the surgery and stay for about two to three hours after the procedure. The procedure itself may take about an hour.

The surgeon will make an incision over the swollen area at the first joint of the big toe. The enlarged lump will be removed. The surgeon may need to reposition the alignment of the bones of the big toe. This may require more than one incision. The bone itself may need to be cut. If the joint surfaces have been damaged, the surgeon may hold the bones together with screws, wires, or metal plates. In severe cases, the entire joint may need to be removed and a joint replacement inserted. If pins were used to hold the bones in place during recovery, they will be removed a few weeks later. In some mild cases, it may be sufficient to repair the tendons and ligaments that are pulling the big toe out of alignment. When finished, the surgeon will close the incision with sutures and may apply steri-strips as an added reinforcement. A compression dressing will be wrapped around the surgical wound. This helps to keep the foot in alignment as well as help reduce postoperative swelling.

Diagnosis/Preparation

Intense pain at the first joint of the big toe is what most commonly brings the patient to the doctor. Loss of toe mobility may also have occurred. Severe deformity of the foot may also make it almost impossible for the patient to fit the affected foot into a shoe. The condition may be in either foot or in both. In addition, there may be a crackling sound in the joint when it moves. Diagnosis of a bunion is based on a **physical examination**, a detailed history of the patient's symptoms and their development over time, and x rays to determine the degree of deformity. Other foot disorders such as gout must be ruled out. The patient history should include factors that increase the pain, the patient's level of physical activity, occupation, amount of time spent on his or her feet, the type of shoe most frequently worn, other health conditions such as diabetes that can affect the body's ability to heal, a thorough medication history, including home remedies, and any allergies to food, medications, or environmental aspects. The physical exam should include an assessment while standing and walking to judge the degree to which stability and gait have been affected, as well as an assessment while seated or lying down to measure range of motion and anatomical integrity. An examination of the foot itself will check for the presence of unusual calluses, which indicate abnormal patterns of friction. Circulation in the affected foot will be noted by checking the skin color and temperature. A neurological assessment will also be conducted.

Conservative measures are usually the first line of treatment and target dealing with the acute phase of the condition, as well as attempting to stop the progression of the condition to a more serious form. Measures may include:

- rest and elevation of the affected foot
- eliminating any additional pressure on the tender area, perhaps by using soft slippers instead of shoes
- soaking the foot in warm water to improve blood flow
- use of anti-inflammatory oral medication
- an injection of a steroidal medication into the area surrounding the joint
- systematic use of an orthotic, either an over-the-counter product or one specifically molded to the foot
- the use of a cushioned padding against the joint when wearing a shoe

If these measures prove unsuccessful, or if the condition has worsened to significant foot deformity and altered gait, then a bunionectomy is considered. The doctor may use the term *hallux valgus* when referring to the bunion. *Hallux* means big toe and *valgus* means bent outward. In discussing the surgical option, it is important for the patient to clearly understand the degree of improvement that is realistic following surgery.

X rays to determine the exact angle of displacement of the big toe and potential involvement of the second toe will be taken. The angles of the two toes in relation to each other will be noted to determine the severity of the condition. Studies in both a standing as well as a seated or lying down position will be considered. These will guide the surgeon at the time of the surgery as well. In addition, blood tests, an EKG, and a chest x-ray will most likely be ordered to be sure that no other medical condition has gone undiagnosed that could affect the success of the surgery and the patient's recovery.

Aftercare

Recovery from a bunionectomy takes place both at the surgical center as well as in the patient's home. Immediate post-surgical care is provided in the surgical recovery area. The patient's foot will be monitored for bleeding and excessive swelling; some swelling is considered normal. The patient will need to stay for a few hours in the recovery area before being discharged. This allows time for the anesthesia to wear off. The patient will be monitored for nausea and vomiting, potential aftereffects of the anesthesia, and will be given something light to eat, such as crackers and juice or ginger ale, to see how the food is tolerated. Hospital policy usually requires that the patient have someone drive them home, as there is a safety concern after having undergone anesthesia. In addition, the patient will most likely be on pain medication that could cause drowsiness and impaired thinking.

It is important to contact the surgeon if any of the following occur after discharge from the surgical center:

- fever
- chills
- constant or increased pain at the surgical site
- redness and a warmth to the touch in the area around the dressing
- swelling in the calf above the operated foot
- the dressing has become wet and falls off
- the dressing is bloody

While the patient can expect to return to normal activities within six to eight weeks after the surgery, the foot is at increased risk for swelling for several months.

When the patient can expect to bear weight on the operated foot will depend on the extent of the surgery. The milder the deformity, the less tissue is removed and the sooner the return to normal activity level. During the six-to-eight-week recovery period, a special shoe, boot, or cast may be worn to accommodate the surgical bandage and to help provide stability to the foot.

Risks

All surgical procedures involve some degree of risk. The most likely problems to occur in a bunionectomy are infection, pain, nerve damage to the operated foot, and the possibility that the bunion will recur. Sharing all pertinent past and present medical history with the **surgical team** helps to lower the chance of a complication. In addition to the risk of the surgery itself, anesthesia also has risks. It is important to share with the anesthesia team the list of all the vitamins, herbs, and supplements, over-the-counter medications, and prescription medications that the patient is taking.

Normal results

The expected result will depend on the degree of deformity that has occurred prior to surgery, the patient's medical condition and age, and the adherence to the recovery regimen prescribed. Some degree of swelling in the foot is normal for up to six months after the surgery. Once wound healing has taken place, the surgeon may recommend exercises or physical therapy to improve foot strength and range of motion. It is important to be realistic about the possible results before consenting to the surgery. Since over-pronation of the foot is not corrected with the surgery, orthotics to help keep the foot/feet in alignment are usually prescribed.

Morbidity and mortality rates

According to the American Orthopaedic Foot & Ankle Society, less than 10% of patients undergoing bunionectomy experience complications, and 85–90% of patients feel the surgery was successful.

Alternatives

It may be possible to avoid surgery by preventing bunion growth from worsening. Wearing shoes that are the right size and shape is a key factor. Try on new shoes in the afternoon when the foot is more tired and perhaps has some fluid buildup. Rather than going by size alone, make sure the shoe fits well, and that there is proper arch support. Additionally, there should be enough space in the toe box for the toes to wiggle around.

KEY TERMS

Excision—The surgical removal of a damaged or diseased part of the body.

Incision—A surgical incision is a cut into the body or an organ of the body to create an opening such as to remove a lump.

Metatarsal joint—Having to do with the bones of the foot.

Orthotic—A device designed to be inserted into a shoe to help keep the foot in proper alignment, stabilize the heel, support the arch, and distribute body weight more evenly over the foot.

Pronation—The foot leans toward the inside of the foot, towards the center of the body.

If diagnosed early, an injection of a steroidal anti-inflammatory medication around the joint may be enough to decrease the irritation in the area and allow the joint to recuperate. This, along with proper shoes, may halt progression of the condition. If there is no pain accompanying the bunion, surgery is not necessary. Some people find that a cream containing the same ingredient as found in chili peppers, capsaicin, applied locally to the joint can decrease the pain. However, once deformity and its accompanying severe pain has occurred, it is unlikely that surgery can be avoided.

Resources

BOOKS

Barker, L. Randol, John R. Burton, and Phillip D. Zieve, eds. *Principles of Ambulatory Medicine.* 5th edition. Baltimore: William & Wilkins, 1999.
Skinner, Harry B. *Current Diagnosis & Treatment in Orthopedics.* Appleton & Lange, 2000.

ORGANIZATIONS

American Orthopaedic Foot & Ankle Society. 2517 Eastlake Avenue East, Seattle, WA 98102. <http://www.aofas.org>.
American Podiatric Medical Association. <http://www.apma.com>.

Esther Csapo Rastegari, RN, BSN, EdM

Burch procedure *see* **Retropubic suspension**

Bypass surgery *see* **Coronary artery bypass graft surgery**

C-reactive protein tests *see* **Cardiac marker tests**

C-section *see* **Cesarean section**

CABG surgery *see* **Coronary artery bypass graft surgery**

Cancer surgery *see* **Surgical oncology**

Carcinoembryonic antigen test *see* **Tumor marker tests**

Cardiac blood pool scan *see* **Multiple-gated acquisition (MUGA) scan**

Cardiac catheterization

Definition

Cardiac catheterization (also called heart catheterization) is a diagnostic and occasionally therapeutic procedure that allows a comprehensive examination of the heart and surrounding blood vessels. It enables the physician to take angiograms, record blood flow, calculate cardiac output and vascular resistance, perform an endomyocardial biopsy, and evaluate the heart's electrical activity. Cardiac catheterization is performed by inserting one or more catheters (thin flexible tubes) through a peripheral blood vessel in the arm (antecubital artery or vein) or leg (femoral artery or vein) under x-ray guidance.

Purpose

Cardiac catheterization is most commonly performed to examine the coronary arteries, because heart attacks, angina, sudden death, and heart failure most often originate from disease in these arteries. Cardiac catheterization may reveal the presence of other conditions, including enlargement of the left ventricle; ventric-

ular aneurysms (abnormal dilation of a blood vessel); narrowing of the aortic valve; insufficiency of the aortic or mitral valve; and septal defects that allow an abnormal flow of blood from one side of the heart to the other.

Symptoms and diagnoses that may be associated with the above conditions and may lead to cardiac catheterization include:

- chest pain characterized by prolonged heavy pressure or a squeezing pain
- abnormal results from a treadmill stress test
- myocardial infarction (heart attack)
- congenital heart defects
- valvular disease

Cardiac catheterization with coronary **angiography** is recommended in patients with angina (especially unstable angina); suspected coronary artery disease; suspected silent ischemia and a family history of heart attack; congestive heart failure; congenital heart disease; and pericardial (lining outside the heart) disease. Catheterization is also recommended for patients with suspected valvular disease, including aortic stenosis (narrowing) or regurgitation, and mitral stenosis or regurgitation.

Patients with congenital cardiac defects are also evaluated with cardiac catheterization to visualize the abnormal direction of blood flow associated with these diseases. In addition, the procedure may be performed after acute myocardial infarction (heart attack); before major noncardiac surgery in patients at high risk for cardiac problems; before cardiac surgery in patients at risk for coronary artery disease; and before such interventional technologies and procedures as stents and percutaneous transluminal coronary **angioplasty** (PTCA) or closure of small openings between the atria (upper chambers), called atrial septal defects.

Left- and right-side catheterization

Cardiac catheterization can be performed on either side of the heart to evaluate different functions. Testing the right side of the heart allows the physician to evaluate tricuspid and pulmonary valve function, in addition to measuring blood pressures and collecting blood samples from the right atrium, right ventricle (lower chamber), and pulmonary artery. Catheterization of the left side of the heart is performed to test the blood flow in the coronary arteries, as well as the level of function of the mitral and aortic valves and left ventricle.

Coronary angiography

Coronary angiography, which is also known as coronary arteriography, is an imaging technique that involves injecting a dye into the vascular system to outline the heart and coronary vessels. Angiography allows the visualization of any blockages, narrowing, or abnormalities in the coronary arteries. If these signs are visible, the cardiologist may assess the patient's readiness for coronary bypass surgery, or a less invasive approach such as dilation of a narrowed blood vessel by surgery or the use of a balloon (angioplasty). Because some interventions may be performed during cardiac catheterization, the procedure is considered therapeutic as well as diagnostic.

Outpatient catheterization

Cardiac catheterization is usually performed in a specially designed cardiac catheterization suite in a hospital, so that any procedural complications may be handled rapidly and effectively. Cardiac catheterization may also be performed on patients presenting to the emergency department with chest pain or chest injuries. The procedure may be performed on an outpatient basis, depending on the patient's pre- and post-catheterization condition. As of 2000, however, the American Heart Association (AHA) and the American College of Cardiology (ACC) issued a joint statement denying approval of the use of separate cardiac catheterization laboratories that are not part of a hospital, on the grounds that a small number of patients having the procedure on an outpatient basis will have unexpected reactions or complications.

Demographics

Coronary artery disease is the first-ranked cause of death for both men and women in the United States. More than 1.5 million cardiac catheterizations are performed every year in the United States, primarily to diagnose or monitor heart disease. There is an expected growth to more than three million procedures by 2010.

Description

Cardiac anatomy

The heart consists of four chambers separated by valves. The right side of the heart, which consists of the right atrium (upper chamber; sometimes called the right auricle) and the right ventricle (lower chamber), pumps blood to the lungs. The left side of the heart, which consists of the left atrium and the left ventricle, simultaneously pumps blood to the rest of the body. The right and left coronary arteries, which are the first vessels to branch off from the aorta, supply blood to the heart. The left anterior descending coronary artery supplies the front of the heart; the left circumflex coronary artery wraps around and supplies the left side and the back of the heart; and the right coronary artery supplies the back of the heart. There is, however, a considerable amount of variation in the anatomy of the coronary arteries.

Catheterization procedure

The patient lies face up on a table during the catheterization procedure, and is connected to a **cardiac monitor**. The insertion site is numbed with a local anesthetic, and access to the vein or artery is obtained using a needle. A sheath, a rigid plastic tube that facilitates insertion of catheters and infusion of drugs, is placed in the puncture site. Under fluoroscopic guidance, a guidewire (a thin wire that guides the catheter insertion) is threaded through a brachial or femoral artery to the heart. The catheter, a flexible or preshaped tube approximately 32–43 in (80–110 cm) long, is then inserted over the wire and threaded to the arterial side of the heart. The patient may experience pressure as the catheter is threaded into the heart. The contrast agent, or dye, used for imaging is then injected so that the physician can view the heart and surrounding vessels. The patient may experience a hot, flushed feeling or slight nausea following injection of the contrast medium. Depending on the type of catheterization (left or right heart) and the area being imaged, different catheters with various shapes and ends are used.

The radiographic/fluoroscopic system has an x-ray subsystem and video system with viewing monitors that allow the physician to observe the procedure in real time using fluoroscopy as well as taking still x rays for documentation purposes. Most newer systems use a digital angiography system that allows images to be recorded, manipulated, and stored digitally on a computer.

The procedure usually lasts about two or three hours. If further intervention is necessary, an angioplasty, stent implantation, or other procedure can be performed. At the end of the catheterization, the catheter and sheath are removed, and the puncture site is closed using a sealing device or manual compression to stop the bleeding. One commonly used sealing device is called Perclose, which allows the doctor to sew up the hole in the groin. Other devices use collagen seals to close the hole in the femoral artery.

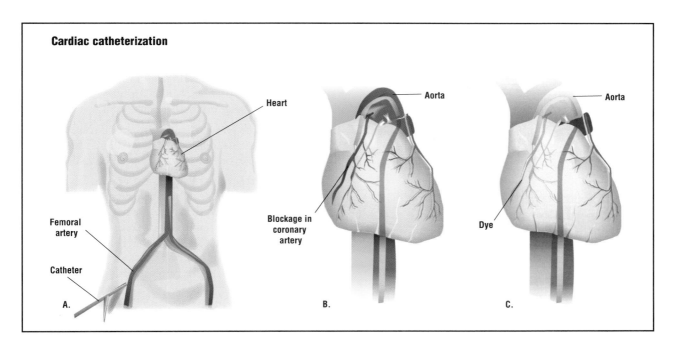

Cardiac catheterization

During cardiac catherization, a catheter is fed into the femoral artery of the upper leg (A). The catheter is fed up to coronary arteries to an area of blockage (B). A dye is released, allowing visualization of the blockage (C). *(Illustration by GGS Inc.)*

Diagnosis/Preparation

Before undergoing cardiac catheterization, the patient may have had other noninvasive diagnostic tests, including an electrocardiogram (ECG), **echocardiography**, computed tomography (CT), **magnetic resonance imaging** (MRI), laboratory studies (e.g., blood work), and/or nuclear medicine cardiac imaging. The results of these noninvasive tests may have indicated a need for cardiac catheterization to confirm a suspected cardiac condition, further define the severity of a previously diagnosed condition, or establish the need for an interventional procedure (e.g., cardiac surgery).

Patients should give the physician or nurse a complete list of their regular medications, including **aspirin** and **nonsteroidal anti-inflammatory drugs** (NSAIDs), because they can affect blood clotting. Diabetics who are taking either metformin or insulin to control their diabetes should inform the physician, as these drugs may need to have their dosages changed before the procedure. Patients should also notify staff members of any allergies to shellfish containing iodine, iodine itself, or the dyes commonly used as contrast agents before cardiac catheterization.

Because cardiac catheterization is considered surgery, the patient will be instructed to fast for at least six hours prior to the procedure. A mild sedative may be administered about an hour before the procedure to help the patient relax. If the catheter is to be inserted through the groin, the area around the patient's groin will be shaved and cleansed with an antiseptic solution.

Aftercare

While cardiac catheterization may be performed on an outpatient basis, the patient requires close monitoring following the procedure; the patient may have to remain in the hospital for up to 24 hours. The patient will be instructed to rest in bed for at least eight hours immediately after the test. If the catheter was inserted into a vein or artery in the leg or groin area, the leg will be kept extended for four to six hours. If a vein or artery in the arm was used to insert the catheter, the arm will need to remain extended for a minimum of three hours.

Most doctors advise patients to avoid heavy lifting or vigorous **exercise** for several days after cardiac catheterization. Those whose occupation involves a high level of physical activity should ask the doctor when they could safely return to work. In most cases, a hard ridge will form over the incision site that diminishes as the site heals. A bluish discoloration under the skin often occurs at the point of insertion but usually fades within two weeks. The incision site may bleed during the first 24 hours following surgery. The patient may apply pressure to the site with a clean tissue or cloth for 10–15 minutes to stop the bleeding.

The patient should be instructed to call the doctor at once if tenderness, fever, shaking, or chills develop, which may indicate an infection. Other symptoms requiring medical attention include severe pain or discoloration in the leg, which may indicate that a blood vessel was damaged.

Risks

Cardiac catheterization is categorized as an invasive procedure that involves the heart, its valves, and coronary arteries, in addition to a large artery in the arm or leg. Cardiac catheterization is contraindicated (not advised) for patients with the following conditions:

- A bleeding disorder, or anticoagulation treatment with Coumadin (sodium warfarin); these may adversely affect bleeding and clotting during the catheterization procedure.
- Renal insufficiency or poor kidney functioning (especially in diabetic patients), which may worsen following angiography.
- Severe uncontrolled hypertension.
- Severe peripheral vascular disease that limits access to the arteries.
- Untreated active infections, severe anemia, electrolyte imbalances, or coexisting illnesses that may affect recovery or survival.
- Endocarditis (an inflammatory infection of the heart's lining that often affects the valves).

Radiation hazards

Cardiac catheterization involves radiation exposure for staff members as well as the patient. The patient's dose of radiation is minimized by using lead shielding in the form of blankets or pads over certain body parts and by choosing the appropriate dose during fluoroscopy. To monitor staff members' exposure to radiation, they wear radiation badges that detect exposure and lead aprons that shield the body. The radiographic/fluoroscopic system may be equipped with movable lead shields that do not interfere with access to the patient and are placed between staff members and the source of radiation during the procedure.

Morbidity and mortality rates

As with all invasive procedures, cardiac catheterization involves some risks. The most serious complications include stroke and myocardial infarction. Other complications include cardiac arrhythmias, pericardial tamponade, vessel injury, and renal failure. One study demonstrated a total risk of major complications under 2% for all patients. The risk of death from cardiac catheterization has been demonstrated at 0.11%. The most common complications resulting from cardiac catheterization are

vascular related, including external bleeding at the arterial puncture site, hematomas, and pseudoaneurysms.

The patient may be given anticoagulant medications to lower the risk of developing an arterial blood clot (thrombosis) or of blood clots forming and traveling through the body (embolization).

The risk of complications from cardiac catheterization is higher in patients over the age of 60; those who have severe heart failure; or those with advanced valvular disease.

Allergic reactions related to the contrast agent (dye) and anesthetics may occur in some patients during cardiac catheterization. Allergic reactions may range from minor hives and swelling to severe shock. Patients with allergies to seafood or penicillin are at a higher risk of allergic reaction; giving antihistamines prior to the procedure may reduce the occurrence of allergic reactions to contrast agents.

Normal results

Normal findings from a cardiac catheterization will indicate no abnormalities in the size or configuration of the heart chamber, the motion or thickness of its walls, the direction of blood flow, or motion of the valves. Smooth and regular outlines indicate normal structure of the coronary arteries.

The measurement of intracardiac pressures, or the pressure in the heart's chambers and vessels, is an essential part of the catheterization procedure. Pressure readings that are higher than normal are significant for a patient's overall diagnosis. Pressure readings that are lower, other than those resulting from shock, are usually not significant.

The ejection fraction is also determined by performing a cardiac catheterization. The ejection fraction is a comparison of the quantity of blood ejected from the heart's left ventricle during its contraction phase with the quantity of blood remaining at the end of the left ventricle's relaxation phase. The cardiologist will look for a normal ejection fraction reading of 60–70%.

Abnormal results are obtained by viewing the still and live motion x rays during cardiac catheterization for evidence of coronary artery disease, poor heart function, disease of the heart valves, and septal defects.

The most prominent sign of coronary artery disease is narrowing or blockage (stenosis) in the coronary arteries, with narrowing greater than 50% considered significant. A clear indication for intervention by angioplasty or surgery is a finding of significant narrowing of the left main coronary artery and/or blockage or severe narrowing in the high left anterior descending coronary artery.

A finding of impaired wall motion is an additional indicator of coronary artery disease, an aneurysm, an enlarged heart, or a congenital heart problem. Using an

KEY TERMS

Aneurysm—An abnormal dilatation of a blood vessel, usually an artery. It may be caused by a congenital defect or weakness in the vessel's wall.

Angiography—A procedure that allows x-ray examination of the heart and coronary arteries following injection of a radiopaque substance (often referred to as a dye or contrast agent).

Angioplasty—A procedure in which a balloon catheter is used to mechanically dilate the affected area of a diseased artery and enlarge the constricted or narrowed segment; it is an alternative to vascular surgery.

Aortic valve—The valve between the heart's left ventricle and ascending aorta that prevents regurgitation of blood back into the left ventricle.

Arrhythmia—A variation in the normal rhythm of the heartbeat.

Catheter—A flexible or pre-shaped curved tube, usually made of plastic, used to evacuate fluids from or inject fluids into the body.

Computed tomography (CT)—A diagnostic imaging procedure that uses x rays to produce cross-sectional images of the anatomy.

Coronary bypass surgery—A surgical procedure that places a shunt to allow blood to travel from the aorta to a branch of the coronary artery at a point below an obstruction.

Echocardiography—An ultrasound examination of the heart.

Fluoroscopy—A diagnostic imaging procedure that uses x rays and contrast agents to visualize anatomy and motion in real time.

Hematoma—An accumulation of clotted blood that may occur in the tissue around a catheter insertion site.

Ischemia—A localized deficiency in the blood supply, usually caused either by vasoconstriction or by obstacles to the arterial blood flow.

Magnetic resonance imaging (MRI)—A diagnostic imaging procedure that uses a magnetic field to produce anatomical images.

Mitral valve—The bicuspid valve that lies between the left atrium and left ventricle of the heart.

Percutaneous transluminal coronary angioplasty (PTCA)—A cardiac intervention in which an artery blocked by plaque is dilated, using a balloon catheter to flatten the plaque and open the vessel; it is also called balloon angioplasty.

Pericardial tamponade—The collection of blood in the sac surrounding the heart that causes compression.

Pseudoaneurysm—A dilation of a blood vessel that resembles an aneurysm.

Pulmonary valve—The heart valve that separates the right ventricle and the opening into the pulmonary artery.

Septum—The muscular wall that separates the two sides of the heart; an opening in the septum that allows blood to flow from one side to the other is called a septal defect.

Shunt—A passageway (or an artificially created passageway) that diverts blood flow from one main route to another.

Stent—A small tube-like device made of stainless steel or other material, used to hold open a blocked artery.

Tricuspid valve—The right atrioventricular valve of the heart; it has three flaps, whereas the mitral valve has only two.

---

ejection fraction test that measures wall motion, cardiologists regard an ejection fraction reading under 35% as increasing the risk of complications while also decreasing the possibility of a successful long- or short-term outcome from surgery.

Detecting the difference in pressure above and below the heart valve can verify the presence of valvular disease. The greater the narrowing, the higher the difference in pressure.

To confirm the presence of septal defects, measurements are taken of the oxygen content on both the left and right sides of the heart. The right heart pumps unoxygenated blood to the lungs, and the left heart pumps blood containing oxygen from the lungs to the rest of the body. Elevated oxygen levels on the right side indicate the presence of a left-to-right atrial or **ventricular shunt**. Low oxygen levels on the left side indicate the presence of a right-to-left shunt.

Alternatives

Other methods of visualization are available that limit radiation exposure, by using ultrasound imaging to observe the coronary arteries. Imaging of general cardiac architecture and valvular function can be visualized by noninvasive cardiac ultrasound. Cardiac ultrasound and Doppler ultrasound can be used together to observe valvular insufficiency and stenosis. Areas of poor myocardial function can also be evaluated by ultrasound.

Nuclear medicine scans of the heart can show the perfusion of blood to a region of the myocardium. If blockages of the coronary artery exist, blood flow will be reduced. By adding a radioactive marker to the blood, images are generated to show areas of poor perfusion. Combined with exercise, these tests can accurately demonstrate cardiovascular disease. However, the imaging process can take several hours, and the patient is still internally exposed to high levels of radiation.

Resources

BOOKS

Bennett, J. Claude, and Fred Plum, eds. "Cardiac Catheterization and Angiography." In *Cecil Textbook of Medicine*. 20th ed. Vol. 1. Philadelphia: W. B. Saunders Company, 1996.
"Diagnostic Cardiovascular Procedures: Invasive Procedures." In *The Merck Manual of Diagnosis and Therapy*, 17th ed, Ed. Mark H. Beers, and Robert Berkow. Whitehouse Station, NJ: Merck Research Laboratories, 1999.
Segen, Joseph C., and Joseph Stauffer. "Cardiac Catheterization." In *The Patient's Guide To Medical Tests: Everything You Need To Know About The Tests Your Doctor Prescribes*. New York: Facts On File, Inc., 1998.

PERIODICALS

Norris, Teresa G. "Principles of Cardiac Catheterization." *Radiologic Technology* 72, no. 2 (November-December 2000): 109–136.
Scanlon, Patrick J, et al. *ACC/AHA Guidelines for Coronary Angiography* 33, no. 6 (May 1999): 1756–1824.
Segal, A. Z., et al. "Stroke as a Complication of Cardiac Catheterization: Risk Factors and Clinical Features." *Neurology* 56 (April 2001): 975–977.

ORGANIZATIONS

American College of Cardiology. Heart House, 9111 Old Georgetown Road, Bethesda, MD 20814-1699. (800) 253-4636. <http://www.acc.org>.
American Heart Association National Center. 7272 Greenville Avenue, Dallas, TX 75231. (800) AHA-USA1. <http://www.americanheart.org>.

OTHER

Cardiology Channel. *Cardiac Catheterization.* <http://www.cardiologychannel.com/cardiaccath/>.

Jennifer E. Sisk, MA
Allison J. Spiwak, MSBME

Cardiac exercise stress testing *see* **Stress test**

Cardiac mapping *see* **Electrophysiology study of the heart**

Cardiac marker tests

Definition

Cardiac marker tests identify blood chemicals associated with myocardial infarction (MI), commonly known as a heart attack. The myocardium is the middle layer of the heart wall composed of heart muscle. Infarction is tissue death caused by an interruption in the blood supply to an area.

Purpose

Cardiac markers help physicians to assess acute coronary syndromes and to identify and manage high-risk patients. Creatine kinase-MB (CK-MB), myoglobin, homocysteine, C-reactive protein (CRP), troponin T (cTnT), and troponin I (cTnI) are all used for assessment of the suspected acute myocardial infarction. CK-MB, cTnT, and cTnI may also be used to identify and manage high-risk patients.

Precautions

C-reactive protein results may be affected by the use of oral contraceptives, NSAIDs, steroids, salicylates, and intrauterine devices (IUDs). Homocysteine levels may be affected by smoking, diabetes, and coffee.

Description

Creatine kinase (CK)

Creatine kinase is an enzyme responsible for transferring a phosphate group from ATP to creatine. It is composed of M and/or B subunits that form CK-MM, CK-MB, and CK-BB isoenzymes. Total CK (the activity of the MM, MB, and BB isoenzymes) is not myocardial-specific. However, the MB isoenzyme (also called CK-2) comprises about 40% of the CK activity in cardiac muscle and 2% or less of the activity in most muscle groups and other tissues. In the proper clinical setting, MB is both a sensitive and specific marker for myocardial infarction. MB usually becomes abnormal three to four hours after an MI, peaks in 10–24 hours, and returns to normal within 72 hours. However, an elevated serum MB may occur in people with severe skeletal muscle damage (such as in muscular dystrophy or a crush injury) and renal failure. In such cases, the CK index (MB divided by total CK) is very helpful. If the index is under 4%, a nonmyocardial cause of a high MB should be suspected. CK-MB is considered the benchmark for cardiac markers of myocardial injury. Measurement of CK-MB may be performed via electrophoresis or immunoassays; the latter demonstrates better analytical sensitivity and better precision.

CK-MB forms can be used to determine whether **thrombolytic therapy** (such as treatment with tissue plasminogen activator to dissolve a blood clot in the coronary artery) has succeeded. MB forms are different molecular forms of MB found in the circulation. When MB is released into the blood, part of the M subunit is removed by an enzyme in the plasma. This results in a molecule called CK-2_1. This is the prevalent form of MB in the blood. CK-2_2 is the unmodified cardiac form of MB. After successful thrombolytic therapy, the unmodified form of MB is rapidly flushed into the blood, causing it to become the dominant form.

Myoblobin

Myoglobin is a protein found in both skeletal and myocardial muscle. It is released rapidly after tissue injury and may be elevated as early as one hour after myocardial injury, though it may also be elevated due to skeletal muscle trauma. However, if myoglobin values do not rise within three to four hours after a person shows acute symptoms, it is highly unlikely that he or she had an MI. There are several measurement methods available.

Troponin T and troponin I

Troponin C, I, and T are proteins that form the thin filaments of muscle fibers and regulate the movement of contractile proteins in muscle tissue. Skeletal and cardiac forms are structurally distinct, and antibodies can be produced that react only with the cardiac forms of troponin I and troponin T.

Cardiac troponin T (cTnT) and cardiac troponin I (cTnI) are the newest additions to the list of cardiac markers. Cardiac troponins are specific to heart muscle. They have enabled the development of assays (tests) that can detect heart muscle injury with great sensitivity and specificity. While these markers have been used mainly to aid in the diagnosis of chest-pain patients with nondiagnostic electrocardiograms, they are also used as prognostic indicators of a MI. According to the American Heart Association, "Several studies have identified a measurable relationship between cardiac troponin levels and long-term outcome after an episode of chest discomfort. They suggest that these tests may be particularly useful to evaluate levels of risk. In other words, it's possible that the results of a troponin test could be used to identify people at either low risk or high risk for later, serious heart problems."

Several commercially available quantitative (measures amounts) immunoassays are available for the measurement of cTnI and cTnT. There is also a qualitative (positive or negative) cTnI test, targeted at bedside testing.

C-reactive protein (CRP)

CRP is a protein found in serum or plasma at elevated levels during a inflammatory processes. The protein can be measured via a variety of methods for the quantitative or semiquantitative determination of C-reactive protein in human serum.

CRP binds to part of the capsule of *Streptococcus pneumoniae*. It is a sensitive marker of acute and chronic inflammation and infection, and in such cases is increased several hundred-fold. Several recent studies have demonstrated that CRP levels are useful in predicting the risk for a thrombotic event (such as a blood clot causing MI). These studies suggest that a high-sensitivity assay for CRP be used that is capable of measuring the very low level normally found in serum (0.1–2.5 mg/L). Heart patients who have persistent CRP levels between 4 and 10 mg/L, with clinical evidence of low-grade inflammation, should be considered to be at increased risk for thrombosis. People can be stratified into four groups of increased risk based upon the quartile in which their CRP levels fall.

Homocysteine

Homocysteine is an amino acid. According to the American Heart Association, studies have shown that too much homocysteine in the blood is related to a higher risk of coronary heart disease, stroke, and peripheral vascular disease; and that it may also have an effect on atherosclerosis. High levels of homocysteine are the result of a lack of certain B vitamins, inheritance, or dietary excess and have been implicated in vascular-wall injury. It is believed that laboratory testing for plasma homocysteine levels can improve the assessment of risk, particularly in patients with a personal or family history of cardiovascular disease, but in whom the well-established risk factors (smoking, high blood cholesterol, high blood pressure, physical inactivity, obesity, and diabetes) do not exist.

Preparation

These assays require a sample of blood, which is typically obtained via a standard vein puncture procedure. Homocysteine tests require the patient to fast.

Aftercare

Discomfort or bruising may occur at the puncture site, or the person may feel dizzy or faint. Applying pressure to the puncture site until the bleeding stops reduces bruising. Warm packs to the puncture site relieve discomfort.

Risks

There are no complications associated with these tests.

Results

Normal results vary, based on the laboratory and method used. Unless otherwise specified, the following information is from the American College of Cardiology and the American Heart Association.

- Total CK: Reference value is 38–174 units/L for men and 96–140 units/L for women. The values begin to rise within four to six hours and peak at 24 hours. Values return to normal within three to four days.

- CK-MB: Reference value is 10–13 units/L. The values begin to rise within three to four hours and peak at 10–24 hours. Values return to normal within two to four days.

- Troponin T: Reference value is less than 0.1 ng/mL. The values begin to rise within two to four hours and peak at 10–24 hours. Values return to normal within five to 14 days.

- Troponin I: Reference value is less than 1.5 ng/mL. The values begin to rise within two to four hours and peak at 10–24 hours. Values return to normal within five to 10 days.

- CK-MB forms: Reference value is a ratio of 1.5 or greater. The values begin to rise within two to four hours and peak at six to 12 hours. Values return to normal within 12–24 hours.

- Myoglobin: Reference value is less than 110 ng/mL. The values begin to rise within one to two hours and peak at four to eight hours. Values return to normal within 12–24 hours.

- Homocysteine: The normal fasting level for plasma is 5–15 micromol/L. Moderate, intermediate, and severe hyperhomocysteinemia refer to concentrations between 16 and 30, between 31 and 100, and less than 100 micromol/L, respectively.

- C-reactive protein: According to the U.S. Food and Drug Administration, in healthy people, reference values are below 5 mg/dL; in various diseases, this threshold is often exceeded within four to eight hours after an acute inflammatory event, with CRP values reaching approximately 20–500 mg/dL.

Resources

BOOKS

Henry, J. B. *Clinical Diagnosis and Management by Laboratory Methods.* 20th ed. Philadelphia: W. B. Saunders, 2001.

Wallach, Jacques. *Interpretation of Diagnostic Tests.* 7th ed. Philadelphia: Lippincott Williams & Wilkins, 2000.

KEY TERMS

Cardiac marker—A substance in the blood that rises following a myocardial infarction.

Diagnostic window—A cardiac marker's timeline for rising, peaking, and returning to normal after a heart attack.

Isoenzymes—Structurally related forms of an enzyme.

Myocardial infarction (MI)—Commonly known as a heart attack, a myocardial infarction is an episode in which some of the heart's blood supply is severely cut off or restricted, causing the heart muscle to suffer and die from lack of oxygen.

Myoglobin—A protein that holds oxygen in heart and skeletal muscle. It rises after damage to either of these muscle types.

Wu, A., ed. *Cardiac Markers.* Washington, DC: American Association of Clinical Chemistry (AACC) Press, 1998.

PERIODICALS

Ogedegbe, Henry O. "Biochemical Markers in Risk Stratification and Diagnosis of Acute Coronary Syndromes." *Laboratory Medicine* (January 2002): 42–53.

OTHER

"ACC/AHA Guidelines for the Management of Patients with Acute Myocardial Infarction," American College of Cardiology and the American Heart Association, 1999.

American Heart Association [cited June 30, 2003]. <http://www.americanheart.org/>.

Victoria E. DeMoranville
Mark A. Best

Cardiac monitor

Definition

The cardiac monitor is a device that shows the electrical and pressure waveforms of the cardiovascular system for measurement and treatment. Parameters specific to respiratory function can also be measured. Because electrical connections are made between the cardiac monitor and the patient, it is kept at the patient's bedside.

Purpose

The cardiac monitor continuously displays the cardiac electrocardiogram (EKG) tracing. Additional monitoring components allow cardiovascular pressures and cardiac output to be monitored and displayed as required for patient diagnosis and treatment. Oxygen saturation of the arterial blood can also be monitored continuously. Most commonly used in emergency rooms and critical care areas, bedside monitors can be interconnected to allow for continual observation of several patients from a central display. Continuous cardiovascular and pulmonary monitoring allows for prompt identification and initiation of treatment.

Description

The monitor provides a visual display of many patient parameters. It can be set to sound an alarm if any parameter changes outside of an expected range determined by the physician. Parameters to be monitored may include, but are not limited to, electrocardiogram, noninvasive blood pressure, intravascular pressures, cardiac output, arterial blood oxygen saturation, and blood temperature.

Equipment required for continuous cardiac monitoring includes the cardiac monitor, cables, and disposable supplies such as electrode patches, pressure transducers, a pulmonary artery catheter (Swan-Ganz catheter), and an arterial blood saturation probe.

Preparation

As the cardiac monitor is most commonly used to monitor electrical activity of the heart, the patient can expect the following preparations. The sites selected for electrode placement on the skin will be shaved and cleaned causing surface abrasion for better contact between the skin and electrode. The electrode will have a layer of gel protected by a film, which is removed prior to placing the electrode to the skin. Electrode patches will be placed near or on the right arm, right leg, left arm, left leg, and the center left side of the chest. The cable will be connected to the electrode patches for the measurement of a five-lead electrocardiogram. Additional configurations are referred to as three-lead and 12-lead electrocardiograms. If noninvasive blood pressure is being measured, a blood pressure cuff will be placed around the patient's arm or leg. The blood pressure cuff will be set to inflate manually or automatically. If manual inflation is chosen, the cuff will only inflate at the prompting of the health care provider, after which a blood pressure will be displayed. During automatic operation, the blood pressure cuff will inflate at timed intervals and the display will update at the end of each measurement.

Disposable pressure transducers require a reference to atmosphere, called zeroing, which is completed before monitoring patient pressures. This measurement will

Cardiac monitors display such vital signs as heart rate, pulse, and blood pressure for patients in the intensive care unit. *(Photograph by Hank Morgan. Science Source/Photo Researchers. Reproduced by permission.)*

occur once the patient is comfortably positioned since the transducer must be level with the measurement point. The pressure transducer will then be connected to the indwelling catheter. It may be necessary for as many as four or five pressure transducers to be connected to the patient.

The arterial blood saturation probe will be placed on the finger, toe, ear, or nasal septum of the patient, providing as little discomfort as possible, while achieving a satisfactory measurement.

Aftercare

After connecting all equipment, the health care provider will observe the monitor and evaluate the quality of the tracings, while making size and position adjustments as needed. The provider will confirm that the monitor is detecting each heartbeat by taking an apical pulse and comparing the pulse to the digital display. The upper and lower alarm limits should be set according to physician orders, and the alarm activated. A printout may be recorded for the medical record, and labeled with patient name, room number, date, time, and interpretation of the strip.

Maintenance and replacement of the disposable components may be necessary as frequently as every eight hours, or as required to maintain proper operation. The arterial saturation probe can be repositioned to suit patient comfort and to obtain a tracing. All connections will be treated in a gentle manner to avoid disruption of the signal and to avoid injury to the patient.

Normal results

The monitor will provide waveforms and/or numeric values associated with the patient status. These may include, but are not limited to, heart rate, arterial blood

KEY TERMS

Artifact—Extra electrical activity typically caused by interference.

Cardiomyopathies—Diseases of the heart muscle; usually refers to a disease of obscure etiology.

Electrodes—Adhesive pads that are placed on the skin and attached to the leads.

Lead—Color-coded wires that connect the electrode to the monitor cable.

QRST complex—The combined waves of an electrocardiogram for monitoring the heart.

pressure, central venous pressure, pulmonary artery pressure, pulmonary capillary wedge pressure, left atrial pressure, cardiac output, arterial blood saturation, and blood temperature. Furthermore, these values can be used to calculate other values, or parameters, or used to diagnose and treat the patient's condition.

Patient movement may cause measurement errors; the patient will be requested to remain motionless. Depending on the mobility of the patient, assistance should be provided by the health care provider prior to changing from a laying down position to sitting or standing.

As the patient's condition improves, the amount of monitoring equipment may be decreased. However, the electrocardiogram and arterial blood saturation probe should be expect to remain attached until discharge is imminent.

Resources

BOOKS

Cahill, Matthew. "Providing Cardiovascular Care." In *Nursing Photobook.* Springhouse, PA: Springhouse Corporation, 1996.

Marriott, Henry J. L. *Pearls and Pitfalls in Electrocardiography: Pithy, Practical Pointers,* 2nd ed. Baltimore: Williams and Wilkins, 1998.

Milford, Cheryl, and Gladys Purvis. "Cardiovascular Care" In *Nursing Procedures,* 3rd ed. Springhouse, PA: Springhouse Corporation, 2000.

Skeehan, Thomas, and Michael Jopling. "Monitoring the Cardiac Surgical Patient." In *A Practical Approach to Cardiac Anesthesia,* 3rd edition, edited by Frederick A. Hensley, Donald E. Martin, and Glenn P. Gravlee. Philadelphia, PA: Lippincott Williams & Wilkins, 2003.

Woods, Susan, and Erika Sivarajan. *Cardiac Nursing,* 4th ed. Philadelphia: Lippincott, 2000.

PERIODICALS

Perry, A., et al. "Measuring the Costs and Benefits of Heart Disease Monitoring." *Heart* 83 (June 2000): 651–656.

ORGANIZATIONS

American Association of Critical-Care Nurses. 101 Columbia, Aliso Viejo, CA 92656-4109. (800) 899-2226. <http://www.aacn.org/>.

The American College of Cardiology. Heart House, 9111 Old Georgetown Road, Bethesda, MD 20814-1699. (800) 253-4636. <http://www.acc.org>.

American Heart Association. 7272 Greenville Ave., Dallas, TX 75231-4596. (800) 242-1793. <http://www.amhrt.org>.

Applied Biometrics. P.O. Box 3170, Burnsville, MN 55337. (952) 890-1123.

OTHER

Advanced Cardiac Monitoring: Ventricular Ectopy vs. Aberrancy. Videotape. RamEx, Inc.

Maggie Boleyn, RN, BSN
Allison Spiwak, MS

Cardiopulmonary bypass machine *see*
Heart-lung machines

Cardiopulmonary resuscitation

Definition

Cardiopulmonary resuscitation, commonly called CPR, combines rescue breathing (one person breathing into another person) and chest compression in a lifesaving procedure performed when a person has stopped breathing or a person's heart has stopped beating.

Purpose

When performed quickly enough, CPR can save lives in such emergencies as loss of consciousness, heart attacks or heart "arrests," electric shock, drowning, excessive bleeding, drug overdose, and other conditions in which there is no breathing or no pulse. The purpose of CPR is to bring oxygen to the victim's lungs and to keep blood circulating so oxygen gets to every part of the body. When a person is deprived of oxygen, permanent brain damage can begin in as little as four minutes and death can follow only minutes later.

Description

There are three physical symptoms that indicate a need for CPR to be performed immediately and for emergency medical support to be called: unconsciousness, not breathing, and no pulse detected.

Figure A

Figure D

Figure B

Figure C

Figure E

Figure F

CPR in basic life support. Figure A: The victim should be flat on his back and his mouth should be checked for debris. Figure B: If the victim is unconscious, open airway, lift neck, and tilt head back. Figure C: If victim is not breathing, begin artificial breathing with four quick full breaths. Figure D: Check for carotid pulse. Figure E: If pulse is absent, begin artificial circulation by depressing sternum. Figure F: Mouth-to-mouth resuscitation of an infant. *(Illustration by Electronic Illustrators Group.)*

Unconsciousness

Unconsciousness is when the victim seems to be asleep but has lost all awareness and is not able to respond to questions or to touch or gentle shaking. A sleeping person will usually respond to a loud noise, shouting, or gentle shaking. An unconscious person will not respond to noise or shaking. When unconscious, a person can not cough or clear the throat, which can block the windpipe and cause suffocation and death. People with a major illness or injury or who have had recent surgery are at risk for losing consciousness. If the person has fainted, which is brief unconsciousness, the cause may be dehydration (lack of body fluids), low blood pressure, or low blood sugar. This is a temporary condition. If the victim is known to have diabetes, a bit of fruit juice may revive the person once they have regained consciousness.

Just before a person loses consciousness, symptoms may include:

• lack of response to voice or touch

• disorientation or stupor

• light-headedness

• headache

• sleepiness

Not breathing

Not breathing, which is also called apnea, is the lack of spontaneous breathing. It requires immediate medical attention. The victim may become limp and lifeless, have a seizure, or turn blue. Prolonged apnea is called respiratory arrest. In children, this can lead quickly to cardiac arrest in which the heart stops beating. In adults, cardiac arrest usually happens first and then respiratory arrest. The common causes of apnea in adults are obstructive sleep apnea (something blocks the airway during sleep), choking, drug overdose, near-drowning, head injury, heart irregularities (arrhythmia, fibrillation) or cardiac arrest, nervous system disorders, or metabolic disorders. In children the causes may be different, such as prematurity, bronchial disturbances or pneumonia, airway blockage or choking on a foreign object, holding the breath, seizures, meningitis, regurgitating food, or asthma attacks.

No pulse detected

If the rescuer is unable to detect a pulse or has difficulty in feeling a pulse it can be an indication of the use of improper technique by the rescuer, or shock or cardiac arrest in the victim. If a sudden, severe decrease occurs in pulse quality (such as pulse weakness) or pulse rate (how many beats in a minute) when other symptoms are also present, life-threatening shock is suspected. The res-cuer may need to explain to a doctor or medical professional where on the victim's body the pulse was measured, if the pulse is weak or absent altogether, and what other symptoms are present.

Medical help and CPR are needed immediately if any of these symptoms is found. Time is critical. A local emergency number should be called immediately. If more than one person is available to help, one can call 911 or a local emergency medical service, while the other person begins CPR. Ideally, someone CPR certified performs the procedure. Local medical personnel, a hospital, or the American Heart Association teaches special accredited CPR courses. If a critically ill patient or post-operative patient is being cared for at home, it is a good idea for a family member to take a CPR course to be better prepared to help in case of an emergency.

The steps usually followed in CPR are as follows:

• If the victim appears to be unconscious with either no breathing or no pulse, the person should be shaken or tapped gently to check for any movement. The victim is spoken to loudly, asking if he or she is OK. If there is no response, emergency help must be called and CPR begun immediately.

• The victim is placed on his or her back on a level surface such as the ground or the floor. The victim's back should be in a straight line with the head and neck supported slightly by a rolled up cloth, small towel, or piece of clothing under the neck. A pillow should not be used to support the head. The victim's clothing should be loosened to expose the chest.

• The rescuer kneels next to the victim, tilts the victim's head back, lifts the jaw forward, and moves the tongue forward or to the side, making sure it does not block the opening to the windpipe. The victim's mouth must be kept open at all times, reopening as necessary.

• The rescuer listens close to the victim's mouth for any sign of breathing, and watches the chest for movement. If the victim is found to be breathing, and has perhaps fainted, he or she can be placed in the recovery position until medical assistance arrives. This is done by straightening the victim's legs and pulling the closest arm out away from the body with the elbow at a right angle or 3 o'clock position, and the other arm across the chest. The far leg should be pulled up over the victim's body with the hip and knee bent. This allows the victim's body to be rolled onto its side. The head should be tilted back slightly to keep the windpipe open. The head should not be propped up.

• If the victim is not breathing, rescue breathing begins, closing the victim's nostrils between a thumb and index finger, and covering the victim's mouth with the rescuer's mouth. Two slow breaths, about two seconds each, are breathed into the victim's mouth with a pause in between. This is repeated until the chest begins to rise. The victim's head should be repositioned as often as necessary during the procedure. The mouth must remain open and the tongue kept away from the windpipe.

- When the chest begins to rise, or the victim begins to breathe on his or her own, the rescuer looks for signs of circulation, such as coughing or movement. If a healthcare professional has arrived by this time, the pulse will be checked before resuming resuscitation.

- If chest compressions are needed to restart breathing, the rescuer will place the heel of a hand above the lowest part of the victim's ribcage where it meets the middle-abdomen. The other hand will be placed over the heel of the first hand, with fingers interlocked. Keeping the elbows straight, the rescuer will lean his or her shoulders over the hands and press down firmly about 15 times. It is best to develop an up-and-down rhythm, keeping the hands firmly on the victim's chest.

- After the compressions, the rescuer will give the victim two long breaths. The sequence of 15 compressions and two breaths will be repeated until there are signs of spontaneous breathing and circulation or until professional medical help arrives.

Precautions

There are certain important precautions for rescuers to remember in order to protect the victim and get the best result from CPR. These include:

- Do not leave the victim alone.

- Do not give chest compressions if the victim has a pulse. Chest compression when there is normal circulation could cause the heart to stop beating.

- Do not give the victim anything to eat or drink.

- Avoid moving the victim's head or neck if spinal injury is a possibility. The person should be left as found if breathing freely. To check for breathing when spinal injury is suspected, the rescuer should only listen for breath by the victim's mouth and watch the chest for movement.

- Do not slap the victim's face, or throw water on the face, to try and revive the person.

- Do not place a pillow under the victim's head.

The description above is not a substitute for CPR training and is not intended to be followed as a procedure.

Normal results

Successful CPR will restore breathing and circulation in the victim. Medical attention is required immedi-

---

KEY TERMS

Apnea—A period of no breathing, sometimes sudden, sometimes prolonged.

Arrest—A sudden stopping of the function of a body organ, such as no breathing (respiratory arrest) or no beating of the heart (cardiac arrest).

Cardiopulmonary—Involving both heart and lungs.

Circulation—The passage of blood and delivery of oxygen through the veins and arteries of the body.

Respiratory—Referring to breathing in and breathing out and the function of the lungs.

Resuscitation—Reviving an unconscious person or restoring breathing.

Shock—A sudden reducing of function in major body systems such as circulation and respiration.

---

ately even if successful CPR has been performed and the victim is breathing freely.

Prevention

Loss of consciousness is an emergency that is potentially life threatening. To avoid loss of consciousness and protect themselves from emergency situations, people at risk can follow these general guidelines:

- People with known conditions or diseases, such as diabetes or epilepsy, should wear a medical alert tag or bracelet.

- People with diabetes should avoid situations that will lower their blood sugar level.

- People who feel weak, become dizzy or light-headed, or have ever fainted, should avoid standing in one place too long without moving.

- People who feel faint, can lie down or sit with their head lowered between their knees.

- Risk factors that contribute to heart disease should be reduced or eliminated. People can reduce risks if they stop smoking, lower blood pressure and cholesterol, lose weight, and reduce stress.

- Illegal recreational drugs should be avoided.

- Seeing a doctor regularly and being aware of any disease conditions or risk factors can help prevent or complicate illness, as can seeking and following the doctor's advice about diet and exercise.

- Using seat belts and driving carefully can help avoid accidental injury.

• People with poor eyesight or those who have difficulty walking because of disability, injury, or recovery from illness, can use a cane or other assistance device to help them avoid falls and injury.

Resources

ORGANIZATIONS

American CPR Training. <http://www.cpr-training-classes.com>.

American Heart Association, National Center. 7272 Greenville Avenue, Dallas, TX 75231. <http://www.americanheart.org>.

OTHER

Emergency Cardiovascular Care. [cited April 2003]. <http://www.cpr-ecc.org>.

Severson, Todd. "Cardiopulmonary Resuscitation." *Medline Plus.* April 2003 [cited April 2003]. <http://www.nlm.nih.gov/medlineplus>.

L. Lee Culvert

Cardioversion

Definition

Cardioversion refers to the process of restoring the heart's normal rhythm by applying a controlled electric shock to the exterior of the chest. Abnormal heart rhythms are called arrhythmias or dysrhythmias.

Purpose

When the heart beats too fast, blood no longer circulates effectively in the body. Cardioversion is used to stop this abnormal beating so that the heart can begin its normal rhythm and pump more efficiently.

Demographics

Cardioversion is used to treat many types of fast and/or irregular heart rhythms. Most often, cardioversion is used to treat atrial fibrillation or atrial flutter. Life-saving cardioversion can be used to treat ventricular tachycardia and ventricular fibrillation.

Abnormal heart rhythms are slightly more common in men than in women and the prevalence of abnormal heart rhythms, especially atrial fibrillation, increases with age. Atrial fibrillation is relatively uncommon in people under age 20.

Description

Elective cardioversion is usually scheduled ahead of time. After arriving at the hospital, an intravenous (IV)

catheter will be placed in the arm to deliver medications and fluids. Oxygen may be given through a face mask.

In some people, a test called a transesophageal echocardiogram (TEE) may need to be performed before the cardioversion to make sure there are no blood clots in the heart.

A short-acting general anesthetic will be given through the IV to put the patient to sleep. During the five or 10 minutes of anesthesia, an electric shock is delivered through paddles or patches placed on the exterior of the chest and sometimes on the back. It may be necessary for the doctor to administer the shock two or three times to stop the abnormal heartbeat and allow the heart to resume a normal rhythm. During the procedure, the patient's breathing, blood pressure, and heart rhythm are continuously monitored.

Diagnosis/Preparation

Diagnosis of abnormal heart rhythms

A doctor may be able to detect an irregular heart beat during a physical exam by taking the patient's pulse. In addition, the diagnosis may be based upon the presence of certain symptoms, including:

• palpitations (feeling of skipped heart beats or fluttering in the chest)
• pounding in the chest
• shortness of breath
• chest discomfort
• fainting
• dizziness or feeling light-headed
• weakness, fatigue, or feeling tired

Not everyone with abnormal heart rhythms will experience symptoms, so the condition may be discovered upon examination for another medical condition.

DIAGNOSTIC TESTS. Tests used to diagnose an abnormal heart rhythm or determine its cause include:

- blood tests

- chest x rays

- electrocardiogram

- ambulatory monitors such as the Holter monitor, loop recorder and transtelephonic transmitter

- stress test

- echocardiogram

- cardiac catheterization

- electrophysiology study (EPS)

- head-upright tilt table test

- nuclear medicine test, such as a **MUGA scan** (multiple-gated acquisition scanning)

Preparation for cardioversion

MEDICATION GUIDELINES.

- Medication to thin the blood (blood thinner or anticoagulant) is usually given for at least three weeks before elective cardioversion.

- The patient should take all usual medications as prescribed, unless other instructions have been given.

- Patients who take diabetes medications or anticoagulants should ask their doctor for specific instructions.

EATING AND DRINKING GUIDELINES. The patient should not eat or drink anything for six to eight hours before the procedure.

OTHER GUIDELINES. It is advisable to arrange for transportation home, because drowsiness may last several hours and driving is not permitted after the procedure.

Do not apply any lotion or ointments to your chest or back before the procedure.

Aftercare

The patient generally wakes quickly after the procedure. Medical personnel will monitor the patient's heart rhythm for a few hours, after which the patient is usually sent home. The patient should not drive home; driving is not permitted for 24 hours after the procedure.

Medications

The doctor may prescribe anti-arrhythmic medications (such as beta-blockers, digitalis, or calcium chan-

QUESTIONS TO ASK THE DOCTOR

- Why is this procedure being performed?

- What are the potential benefits of the procedure?

- What are the risks of the procedure?

- Can I take my medications the day of the procedure?

- Can I eat or drink the day of the procedure? If not, how long before the procedure should I stop eating or drinking?

- When can I drive after the procedure?

- What should I wear the day of the procedure?

- Will I be awake during the procedure?

- What kinds of monitors are used during the procedure to evaluate my condition?

- Will I have to stay in the hospital after the procedure?

- When can I resume my normal activities?

- When will I find out the results?

- What if the procedure was not successful?

- If I've had the cardioversion procedure once, can I have it again to correct an abnormal heart rhythm, if necessary?

- Will I have any pain or discomfort after the procedure? If so, how can I relieve this pain or discomfort?

- Are there any medications, foods or activities I should avoid to prevent my symptoms from recurring?

nel blockers) to prevent the abnormal heart rhythm from returning.

Some patients may be prescribed anticoagulant medication, such as warfarin and **aspirin**, to reduce the risk of blood clots.

The medications prescribed may be adjusted over time to determine the best dosage and type of medication so the abnormal heart rhythm is adequately controlled.

Discomfort

Some chest wall discomfort may be present for a few days after the procedure. The doctor may recommend that the patient take an over-the-counter pain re-

KEY TERMS

Ablation—The removal or destruction of tissue.

Ablation therapy—A procedure used to treat arrhythmias, especially atrial fibrillation. During the procedure, a catheter (small, flexible tube) is inserted in a vein and threaded to the heart. High-frequency electrical energy is delivered through the catheter to disconnect the pathway causing the abnormal heart rhythm in the heart.

Ambulatory monitors—Small portable electrocardiograph machines that record the heart's rhythm. Ambulatory monitors include the Holter monitor, loop recorder, and transtelephonic transmitter. Each type of monitor has specific features related to the length of recording time and the ability to send the recordings over the phone.

Antiarrhythmic—Medication used to treat abnormal heart rhythms.

Anticoagulant—A medication, also called a "blood thinner," that prevents blood from clotting. This type of medication is used for people at risk of stroke or blood clots.

Arrhythmia—An irregular heart rhythm.

Atria—The right and left upper chambers of the heart.

Atrial fibrillation—A condition in which the upper chamber of the heart quivers instead of pumping in an organized way.

Atrial flutter—A rapid pulsation of the upper chambers of the heart (atrium) that interferes with normal heart function. Atrial flutter is usually more organized and regular than atrial fibrillation, although it often converts to atrial fibrillation. Atrial

flutter occurs most often in people with heart disease and in the first week after heart surgery.

Cardiac catheterization—An invasive procedure used to create x rays of the coronary arteries, heart chambers and valves. During the procedure, a catheter is inserted into an artery in the groin or arm and is guided to the heart. Contrast material (dye) is injected into the catheter to produce the x ray images.

Echocardiogram—An imaging procedure used to create a picture of the heart's movement, valves and chambers. The test uses high-frequency sound waves that come from a hand wand placed on your chest. Echocardiogram may be used in combination with Doppler ultrasound to evaluate the blood flow across the heart's valves. *Also see Transesophageal echocardiogram.*

Electrocardiogram (ECG, EKG)—A test that records the electrical activity of the heart using small electrode patches attached to the skin on the chest.

Electrophysiology study (EPS)—A test that evaluates the electrical activity within the heart. The test is used to help the doctor determine the cause of the abnormal heart rhythm and find the best treatment. During the test, the doctor may safely reproduce the abnormal heart rhythm and give the patient medications to determine which medication works best to control the abnormal heart rhythm.

Head-upright tilt table test—A test used to determine the cause of fainting spells. During the test, the patient is tilted at different angles on special

liever such as ibuprofen to relieve discomfort. Skin irritation may also be present after the procedure. Skin lotion or ointment can be used to relieve irritation.

Risks

Cardioverters have been in use for many years and the risks are few. The unlikely risks that remain include those instances when the device delivers greater or lesser power than expected or when the power setting and control knobs are not set correctly. Unfortunately, in about 50% of cases, the heart prefers its abnormal rhythm and reverts to it within one year, despite cardioversion. Cardioversion can be repeated for some patients whose abnormal heart rhythm returns.

Normal results

About 90% of cardioversions are successful and, at least for a time, restore the normal heart rhythm safely and prevent further symptoms.

Morbidity and mortality rates

The 2002 Rate Control vs. Electrical Cardioversion for Persistent Atrial Fibrillation (RACE) study, published in *The New England Journal of Medicine* indicated that controlling a patient's heart rate is as important as controlling the patient's heart rhythm to prevent death and complications from cardiovascular causes. The study also concluded that anticoagulant therapy is important to table for a period time. During the test, the patient's heart rhythm, blood pressure and other measurements are evaluated with changes in position.

Implantable cardioverter-defibrillator (ICD)—An electronic device that is surgically placed to constantly monitor the patient's heart rate and rhythm. If a very fast, abnormal heart rate is detected, the device delivers electrical energy to the heart to beat in a normal rhythm again.

Maze procedure—A surgical procedure used to treat atrial fibrillation. During the procedure, precise incisions are made in the right and left atria to interrupt the conduction of abnormal impulses. When the heart heals, scar tissue forms and the abnormal electrical impulses are blocked from traveling through the heart.

Nuclear imaging—Method of producing images by detecting radiation from different parts of the body after a radioactive tracer material is administered.

Pacemaker—A small electronic device implanted under the skin. This device sends electrical impulses to the heart to maintain a suitable heart rate and prevent slow heart rates.

Pulmonary vein isolation—A surgical procedure used to treat atrial fibrillation. During the procedure, a radio frequency probe, microwave probe or cryoprobe is inserted and under direct vision, used to create lesion lines in the heart to interrupt the conduction of abnormal impulses.

Stress test—A test used to determine how the heart responds to stress. It usually involves walking on a treadmill or riding a stationary bike at increasing

levels of difficulty, while the electrocardiogram, heart rate and blood pressure are monitored. If the patient is unable to walk on a treadmill or ride a stationary bike, medications may be used to produce similar results.

Transesophageal echocardiogram (TEE)—An invasive imaging procedure used to create a picture of the heart's movement, valves and chambers. The test uses high-frequency sound waves that come from a small transducer passed down the patient's throat. TEE may be used in combination with Doppler ultrasound to evaluate the blood flow across the heart's valves.

Ventricles—The lower, pumping chambers of the heart. The heart has two ventricles: the right and the left ventricle.

Ventricular fibrillation—An erratic, disorganized firing of impulses from the ventricles, the lower chambers of the heart. The ventricles quiver instead of pumping in an organized way, preventing blood from pumping through the body. Ventricular fibrillation is a medical emergency that must be treated with cardiopulmonary resuscitation (CPR) and defibrillation as soon as possible.

Ventricular tachycardia—A rapid heart beat, usually over 100 beats per minute. Ventricular tachycardia originates from the lower chambers of the heart (ventricles). The rapid rate prevents the heart from filling adequately with blood, so less blood is able to pump through the body. Ventricular tachycardia can be a serious type of arrhythmia and may be associated with more symptoms.

reduce the risk of stroke and is appropriate therapy for patients who have recurring, persistent atrial fibrillation even after they were treated with cardioversion. In patients who did not receive anticoagulant therapy after cardioversion, there was a 2.4% increase of embolic events (such as stroke or blood clots), even though there were no signs of these events prior to the procedure.

Alternatives

Atrial fibrillation and atrial flutter often revert to normal rhythms without the need for cardioversion. Healthcare providers usually try to correct the heart rhythm with medication or recommend lifestyle changes before recommending cardioversion.

Lifestyle changes often recommended to treat abnormal heart rhythms include:

• quitting smoking

• avoiding activities that prompt the symptoms of abnormal heart rhythms

• limiting alcohol intake

• limiting or not using caffeine (Caffeine products may produce more symptoms in some people with abnormal heart rhythms.)

• avoiding medications containing stimulants, such as some cough and cold remedies (These medications contain ingredients that may cause abnormal heart rhythms. Read all medication labels and ask a doctor or pharmacist for specific recommendations.)

If cardioversion is not successful in restoring the normal heart rhythm, other treatments for abnormal heart rhythms include:

• permanent pacemakers

• implantable cardioverter-defibrillator

• ablation therapy

• heart surgery, including the Maze procedure and the pulmonary vein isolation procedure

Resources

BOOKS

McGoon, Michael D., ed., and Bernard J. Gersh, MD. *Mayo Clinic Heart Book: The Ultimate Guide to Heart Health, Second Edition.* New York: William Morrow and Co., Inc., 2000.

Topol, Eric J., MD. *Cleveland Clinic Heart Book: The Definitive Guide for the Entire Family from the Nation's Leading Heart Center.* New York: Hyperion, 2000.

Trout, Darrell, and Ellen Welch. *Surviving with Heart: Taking Charge of Your Heart Care.* Colorado: Fulcrum Publishing, 2002.

PERIODICALS

The New England Journal of Medicine 347, no. 23 (December 5, 2002): 1834–1840.

ORGANIZATIONS

American College of Cardiology. Heart House. 9111 Old Georgetown Rd., Bethesda, MD 20814-1699. (800) 253-4636 ext. 694 or (301) 897-5400. <http://www.acc.org>.

American Heart Association. 7272 Greenville Ave. Dallas, TX 75231. (800) 242-8721 or (214) 373-6300. <http://www.americanheart.org>.

The Cleveland Clinic Heart Center, The Cleveland Clinic Foundation. 9500 Euclid Avenue, F25, Cleveland, Ohio, 44195. (800) 223-2273 ext. 46697 or (216) 444-6697. <http://www.clevelandclinic.org/heartcenter>.

Heart Information Network. <http://www.heartinfo.org> .

HeartCenterOnline. <http://www.heartcenteronline.com> .

National Heart, Lung and Blood Institute. National Institutes of Health. Building 1. 1 Center Dr., Bethesda, MD 20892. E-mail: NHLBIinfo@rover.nhlbi. <http://www.nhlbi.nih.gov>.

North American Society of Pacing and Electrophysiology. 6 Strathmore Rd., Natick, MA 01760-2499. (508) 647-0100. <http://www.naspe.org> .

Dorothy Elinor Stonely
Angela M. Costello

Carotid artery stenting *see* **Endovascular stent surgery**

Carotid endarterectomy

Definition

Carotid endarterectomy (CEA) is a surgical procedure that is performed to remove deposits of fat, called plaque, from the carotid arteries in the neck. These two main arteries, one on each side of the neck, deliver blood and oxygen to the brain. Plaque builds up in large- and medium-sized arteries as people get older, more in some people than others depending on lifestyle and hereditary factors. This build up is a vascular disease called atherosclerosis, or hardening of the arteries. When this happens in either one or both of the carotid arteries, they can become narrowed, a condition called stenosis. During a carotid endarterectomy, a surgeon removes the fatty deposits to correct the narrowing and to allow blood and oxygen to flow freely to the brain.

Purpose

Carotid endarterectomy is a protective procedure intended to reduce the risk of stroke, a vascular condition also known as a cardiovascular accident (CVA). In studies conducted by the National Institute of Neurological Disorders and Stroke (NINDS), endarterectomy has proven to be especially protective for people who have already had a stroke, and for people who are at high risk for stroke or who have already been diagnosed with significant stenosis (between 50% and 70% blockage).

Demographics

The National Stroke Association reports that two-thirds of stroke victims are over age 65. Risk is shown to double with each 10 years over age 55. Men are more at risk than women, although most stroke survivors over age 65 are women, which may be partly because there are more women than men in this age group. African Americans have been shown to be at greater risk for stroke than other racial groups in the United States. Risk is also higher in people who have a family history of stroke as well as people with diabetes, because of the circulatory problems associated with diabetes. People with high blood pressure, also called hypertension, have four to six times the risk of stroke.

Nearly 700,000 strokes occur in the United States each year, with about 150,000 deaths, making stroke the third leading cause of death behind heart disease and cancer. Stroke is also responsible for the high number of disabled adults in the United States; two million stroke survivors have some permanent disability. The annual cost to the country for treating stroke and disabilities caused by stroke is about $40 billion.

Carotid endarterectomy

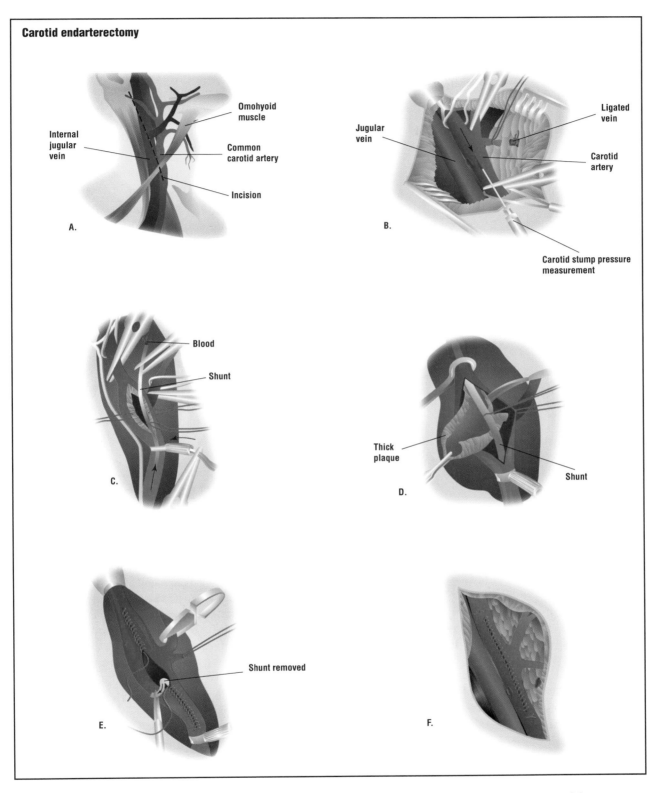

A.
Internal jugular vein
Omohyoid muscle
Common carotid artery
Incision

B.
Jugular vein
Ligated vein
Carotid artery
Carotid stump pressure measurement

C.
Blood
Shunt

D.
Thick plaque
Shunt

E.
Shunt removed

F.

In a carotid endarterectomy, the carotid artery is access through an incision in the neck (A). A measurement of the pressure inside the vessel is taken to assess the degree of blockage (B). The carotid is clamped above and below the incision, and a shunt is inserted to maintain blood flow (C). Plaque lining the artery is removed (D). The shunt is taken out (E), and the incisions are repaired (F). *(Illustration by GGS Inc.)*

Description

The presence of fatty deposits in the carotid arteries of the neck is the most significant risk factor for ischemic stroke, which represents 80% of all strokes. A stroke can be either ischemic, which is an interruption of blood flow in a narrowed carotid artery, or hemorrhagic, which involves bleeding in the brain. Carotid endarterectomy is performed as prevention of ischemic strokes.

Some people at high risk for ischemic stroke have disturbing symptoms that can occur periodically and last from minutes to up to 24 hours, and then disappear. These episodes are called transient ischemic attacks (TIA). The symptoms are the same as actual stroke symptoms. The symptoms of TIA and ischemic stroke may include:

• Numbness, muscle weakness, or paralysis of the face, arm, or leg, usually on one side of the body, and usually occurring suddenly.

• speech or vision difficulties

• sudden loss of understanding, confusion

• lightheadedness or fainting spells

• loss of balance with difficulty walking and moving; poor coordination

• severe headache with no obvious cause, either sudden or persistent

About 35% of people who have TIAs will have a stroke within five years. The risk of stroke goes up with age and is greatest in people whose blood pressure is higher than normal. High blood pressure stresses the walls of blood vessels, particularly when the vessels are blocked with plaque and so space for blood to pass is reduced.

Carotid endarterectomy has been performed since the 1950s as a stroke-prevention method. During the 1990s, about 130,000 carotid endarterectomies were performed each year in the United States. Because the surgery itself presents a high risk of complications, surgeons will look at the possible benefits and risks for each patient and compare them with such medical treatment as drug therapy to reduce plaque, cholesterol, and blood pressure. Carotid endarterectomy is typically performed on those who will benefit most from the surgery and who have the lowest risk for postoperative complications. Good candidates include:

• People who have already had one or more TIA episodes in a six-month period, with 70% narrowing of the carotid arteries supplying the part of the brain affected by the TIA.

• People who have had a mild stroke in the past six months but who are not significantly disabled and whose carotid arteries are at least 70% narrowed.

• People who have not had a stroke or TIA, but their carotid arteries are narrowed 60% or more and they have low risk of complication from having the surgery.

Carotid endarterectomy is not recommended for:

• People whose risk of complications from the surgery is greater than the intended benefits. The presence of other problems such as heart disease may increase risk.

• People who have had a TIA but their carotid arteries are less than 50% narrowed.

• People who have had a stroke or TIA because arteries other than the carotid arteries are blocked.

• People whose carotid arteries are blocked above a point on the neck where they can be reached easily during surgery.

The endarterectomy procedure takes about an hour to perform. General anesthesia is usually administered. A vascular surgeon or neurosurgeon will usually perform the surgery. During the procedure, a small incision is made in the neck below the jaw to expose the carotid artery. Blood that normally flows through the artery must be diverted in order to perform the surgery. This is accomplished by rerouting the blood through a tube (shunt) connecting the vessels below and above the surgical site. The carotid artery is opened and the waxy fat deposit is removed, sometimes in one piece. If the carotid artery is observed to be too narrow or too damaged to perform the critical job of delivering blood to the brain, a graft using a vein from the patient's leg may be created and stitched (grafted) onto the artery to enlarge or repair it. The shunt is then removed, and incisions in the blood vessels, the carotid artery, and the skin are closed.

Diagnosis/Preparation

Diagnosis

The presence and degree of stenosis in the carotid artery must be determined before a doctor decides that carotid endarterectomy is necessary. Carotid stenosis can sometimes be detected in a routine checkup, especially when a detailed history reveals to the doctor that the patient has experienced symptoms of TIA or stroke. The doctor will use a **stethoscope** to listen to blood flow in the carotid artery and may hear an abnormal rushing sound called a "bruit" (pronounced "brew-ee") that will indicate narrowing in the artery. The absence of sound, however, does not mean there is no risk. More extensive testing will most likely have to be done to determine the degree of stenosis and the potential of risk for the patient. These tests may include:

• Ultrasound imaging with Doppler—a painless, noninvasive imaging test that measures sound waves directed into the body and returned to the ultrasound machine as echoes. Usually these echoes are visualized as an image on a screen; Doppler captures the sound as the echoes bounce off of moving blood in the carotid artery, giving some indication of the amount of blockage as the ultrasound probe moves up and down the arteries on each side of the neck.

• Computed tomography (CT) or computer-assisted tomography (CAT scan)—a series of cross-sectional x rays of the head and brain that can rule out other causes for the symptoms but cannot detect carotid artery stenosis.

• Oculoplethysmography (OPG)—a procedure that measures the pulsing of arteries behind the eye, which can show carotid artery blockage.

• Arteriography and digital subtraction **angiography** (DSA)—special x-ray procedures using dye in the patient's vascular system. These tests are invasive and can actually cause a stroke, but they do indicate more exactly what degree of stenosis is present. The doctor will have to weigh the extent of risk and how much the patient will benefit from the tests.

• Magnetic resonance angiography (MRA)—an imaging test that does not use dyes or x rays and relies on special computer software and powerful magnetic fields to create a highly detailed image of the inside of the brain's arteries.

Preparation

If carotid ultrasonography or arteriography procedures were not performed earlier to diagnose carotid stenosis, these tests will be performed before surgery to evaluate the amount of plaque and the extent and location of narrowing in the patient's carotid arteries. Other blood vessels in the body are also evaluated. If other arteries show significant signs of artherosclerosis or damage, the patient's risk for surgery may be too great, and the procedure will not be performed. **Aspirin** therapy or other clot-prevention medication may be prescribed before surgery. Any underlying medical condition such as high blood pressure or heart disease will be treated prior

QUESTIONS TO ASK THE DOCTOR

• Why do I need this surgery?

• How will the surgery improve my condition?

• What kind of anesthesia will I be given?

• What are the risks of having this surgery?

• Is there anything I can do, myself, to get in shape for the surgery and to improve my chances of successful surgery?

• How many of these procedures have you performed? How many of the surgery patients had complications after surgery?

• How can I expect to feel after surgery? How long will it take me to recover?

• What are my chances of developing this problem again after the surgery?

• If the surgery is not successful, what will my options be?

to carotid endarterectomy to help achieve the best result from the surgery. Upon **admission to the hospital**, routine blood and urine tests will be performed.

Aftercare

A person who has had carotid endarterectomy will be monitored in a hospital **recovery room** immediately after the surgery and will then go to an **intensive care unit** at least overnight to be observed for any sign of complications. The total hospital stay may be two to three days. When the patient returns home, activities can be resumed gradually, as long as they are not strenuous. During recuperation, the patient's neck may ache slightly. The doctor may recommend against turning the head often or too quickly during recovery. The most important thing people can do after endarterectomy is to follow their doctor's guidelines for stroke prevention, which will reduce the progression of artherosclerosis and avoid repeat narrowing of the carotid artery. Repeat stenosis (restenosis) has been shown to occur frequently in people who do not make the necessary changes in lifestyle such as in diet, **exercise**, and quitting smoking or excessive use of alcohol. The benefits of the surgery may only be temporary if underlying disease such as artherosclerosis high blood pressure, or diabetes, is not also treated.

Risks

Serious risks are associated with carotid endarterectomy. They involve complications that can arise during or following the surgery, as well as underlying conditions that led to blockage of the patient's arteries in the first place. Stroke is the most serious postoperative risk. If it occurs within 12 to 24 hours after surgery, the cause is usually an embolism, which is a clot or tissue from the endarterectomy site. Other major complications that can occur are:

• heart attack or other heart problems

• death

• breathing difficulties

• high blood pressure

• nerve injury, which can cause problems with vocal cords, saliva management, and tongue movement

• bleeding within the brain

• restenosis, the continuing buildup of plaque, which can occur from five months to 13 years after surgery

The risks of carotid endarterectomy surgery depend upon age, overall health, and the skill and experience levels of the surgeons treating the patient. The likelihood of complications is lower when the surgeon performing the procedure has acknowledged skills and experience. According to the Stroke Council of the American Heart Association, surgery is best performed by a surgeon who has only had complications occur in less than 3% of patients. Hospitals, too, should be able to show that fewer than 3% of their patients undergoing endarterectomy have had complications. These recommendations are based not only on skill levels, but also on the ability to accurately weigh the stroke risks for each patient against the potential risk of complication because of age, hereditary factors, and the presence of underlying conditions or diseases.

Normal results

The desired outcome of carotid endarterectomy is improved blood flow to the brain and a reduced risk of stroke. The National Stroke Association has reported that successful carotid endarterectomy surgery reduces risk of stroke by as much as 80% in people who have had either transient ischemic attacks or symptoms of stroke, or who have been diagnosed with 70% or more arterial blockage. Studies of people who have no symptoms but have been found to have stenosis from 60% to 99%, show that endarterectomy surgery also reduces the risk of stroke by more than 50%. These groups of people at higher risk for stroke will benefit most from having carotid endarterectomy. The benefit for people who have lesser degrees of blockage is shown to be much lower than that of high-risk stroke candidates. Surgery is not indicated for people with artery narrowing less than 50%.

Morbidity and mortality rates

Death and disabling stroke occur more often in symptomatic and asymptomatic patients at high risk for stroke who have not been treated with carotid endarterectomy surgery. A well-respected study, the North American Symptomatic Carotid Endarterectomy Trial (NASCET), along with a corresponding European study (ECST), showed that death or disabling stroke are reduced by 48% among those with severe stenosis (greater than 70%) when they undergo carotid endarterectomy surgery. In patients with less severe stenosis (50–69%), endarterectomy was shown to reduce risk by 27%. Patients with less than 50% stenosis were actually harmed by surgery, increasing the risk of death or disability by 20%. The conclusion of the study was that death and disability could be reduced overall if carotid endarterectomy was performed only on patients with the more severe stenosis who are also surgically fit, and that that the procedure should be performed only by surgeons whose complication rates are less than 6%.

Alternatives

The carotid endarterectomy removes plaque directly from blocked arteries and there is no alternative way to mechanically remove plaque. However, there are alternative ways to prevent the buildup of plaque and thus help to prevent stroke or heart attack. Certain vitamin deficiencies in older people are known to promote high levels of homocysteine, an amino acid that contributes to atherosclerosis, putting people at greater risk for stroke or heart attack. Certain nutritional supplements have been shown to reduce homocysteine levels.

Nutritional supplements and alternative therapies that are sometimes recommended to help reduce risks and promote good vascular health include:

• Folic acid, which helps lower homocysteine levels and increases the oxygen-carrying capacity of red blood cells.

• Vitamins B_6 and B_{12}, which help lower homocycteine levels; B6 is also a mild diuretic and helps to balance fluids in the body.

• Antioxidant vitamins C and E, which work together to promote healthy blood vessels and improve circulation.

• Angelica, an herb that contains coumadin, a recognized anticoagulant, which may help to prevent clot formation in the blood (blood thinner).

• Essential fatty acids, which help reduce blood pressure and cholesterol, and maintain elasticity of blood vessels.

• Chelation therapy, which can be used to break up plaque and improve circulation.

Resources

BOOKS

Caplan, L. R. *American Heart Association Family Guide to Stroke Treatment, Recovery, and Prevention.* New York: Times Books, 1994.

Moore, R. D. *The High Blood Pressure Solution: A Scientifically Proven Program for Preventing Strokes and Heart Disease,* 2nd Edition. Portland, OR: Inner Traditions, 2001.

PERIODICALS

Harrar, S. "Brain Attack." *Prevention Magazine* 20 September 2002.

ORGANIZATIONS

National Institute of Neurological Disorders and Stroke (NINDS). National Institutes of Health, Bethesda, MD 20892. <http://www.ninds.nih.gov>.

National Stroke Association. 9707 E. Easter Lane, Englewood, CO 80112. (800) Strokes or (303) 649-9299. <http://www.stroke.org>.

OTHER

Carotid Endarterectomy: Questions and Answers. Harvard Medical School and Aetna. <www.intelihealth.com>.

Carotid Endarterectomy: What to Think About. Healthwise, Inc., Boise, ID. <www.laurushealth.com/newsearch>.

Uncontrollable Stroke Risk Factors and Controllable Stroke Risk Factors. National Stroke Association, Stroke Prevention Guidelines. <www.stroke.org>.

L. Lee Culvert

Carpal tunnel release

Definition

A carpal tunnel release is a surgical procedure performed to relieve pressure on the nerve located inside the carpal tunnel, an area in the wrist that supplies nerve function to the fingers. The condition for which the release is performed is called carpal tunnel syndrome.

Purpose

Carpal tunnel syndrome is a relatively common problem affecting the wrist and hand. Individuals afflicted with carpal tunnel syndrome complain of numbness, tingling, and pain in the hand, with pain radiating up into the arm, shoulder, and even the neck. Some patients may experience an aching or burning sensation in the affected hand. The fingers may feel swollen, although they are no larger in size. If the condition is left unattended, symptoms may begin to awaken the individuals during sleep. If left unattended medically, muscle weakness can develop, leading to an inability to grasp objects or engage in any action requiring the opposition of the thumb and the other fingers in the affected hand. It is known as a repetitive stress injury, as it most commonly occurs in individuals who engage in motions that require the hands to repeat the same movements over and over again, especially with strong, forceful hand movements or ones that involve vibrating tools. Many individuals develop carpal tunnel syndrome in both hands. For some the condition is worse in the dominant hand.

Demographics

Individuals who perform repetitive wrist movements, either at work or play, are at risk of developing carpal tunnel syndrome. Repetitive movements include computer work, typing, computer games, sports such as tennis, scanning items at the supermarket checkout, playing musical instruments for extended periods of time on a daily basis, assembly-line work, especially that requiring heavy gripping or the use of vibrating machinery, and the use of power tools such as for lawn care. It is more common in women, perhaps as much as three to seven times more than in men, especially during pregnancy, and also in individuals who are obese, or have diabetes or rheumatoid arthritis. It is also more common with advancing age. Carpal tunnel release is one of the most common hand surgeries performed in the United States.

Description

The carpal tunnel is a channel inside the hand, on the palm side, that surrounds and protects the main nerve

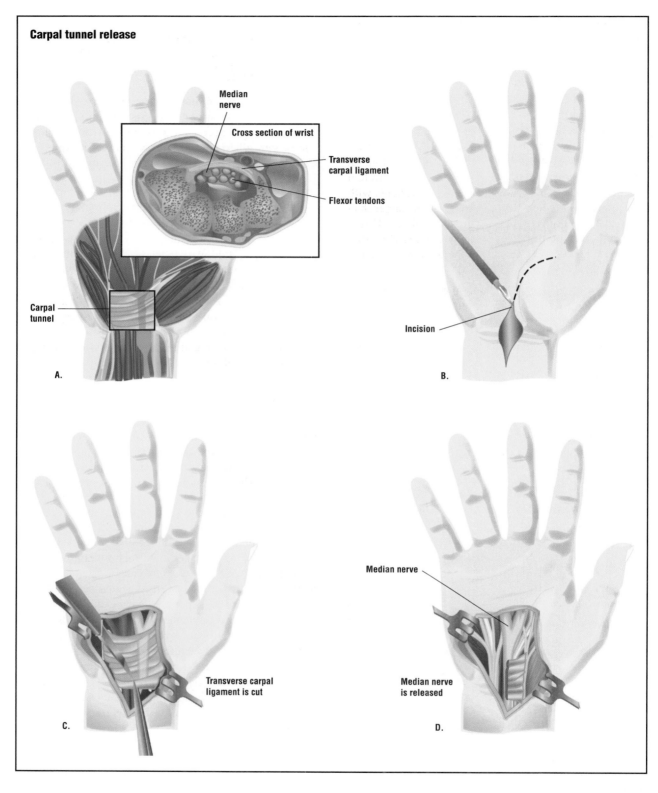

Carpal tunnel release

Median
nerve

Cross section of wrist

Transverse
carpal ligament

Flexor tendons

Carpal
tunnel

A.

Incision

B.

Transverse carpal
ligament is cut

C.

Median nerve

Median nerve
is released

D.

To perform a carpal tunnel release, the surgeon makes an incision in the palm of the hand, above the area of the carpal tunnel (B). The carpal ligament going across the hand is severed (C), releasing pressure on the median nerve (D). *(Illustration by GGS Inc.)*

and the tendons that help bend the fingers. This nerve is called the median nerve. The symptoms start gradually and continue to increase if the problem is not addressed. Numbness and tingling in the fingers are usually the first signs of the condition. It may come on while driving, sleeping, holding a telephone, or reading a book. It may also occur after a long bicycle ride, which involves gripping the handlebars. The pain or tingling might begin to travel up the arm to the shoulder. The individual may appear clumsy, drop objects, or have difficulty holding on to a glass. There may be a decrease in the ability to feel sensations in the hand. Once the problem interferes with daily activity, including sleep, or persists for longer than two weeks, it is important to seek medical advice. This is because the symptoms, even if they are not terribly disabling, can become permanent, as the damage to the tissues themselves becomes permanent.

Because of the nerve innervation routes, the one finger that is not involved in carpal tunnel syndrome is the pinkie.

Conditions associated with carpal tunnel syndrome, or that appear to put the individual at higher risk for developing the condition include:

- obesity
- pregnancy
- certain thyroid conditions
- arthritis, especially rheumatoid
- diabetes
- menopause
- taking oral contraceptives
- conditions involving hormonal changes
- gout
- cigarette smoking

Conditions such as carpal tunnel syndrome are sometimes referred to as cumulative trauma disorders. In these disorders, the injury is not related to one major incident that causes damage, such as a fall that results in a fractured limb, but is the build up of small microtraumas, in which the affected area is repeatedly damaged. Each small injury causes the area to become irritated or inflamed, and there is not enough time in between injuries for complete healing to occur. Treatment focuses on relieving the compression of the nerve and decreasing or eliminating the irritation and inflammation of the area. A term often associated with microtraumas or repetitive stress injuries is ergonomics, which means the way in which the body is set up to perform a certain function. If the function is typing, an ergonomic assessment would include looking at the height of the desk, the height of the chair in which one is sitting to work at the desk, the

height of the hands in relation to the work area, such as the keyboard, and the angle of the wrist, elbow, hips, and knees. An ergonomically designed work station would have all components at the right height and angle for work so that there is no strain put on any joint as it performs its necessary function, and therefore no injury can take place. For those who use vibrating tools at work, special gloves exist that are padded and designed to decrease the effect of the vibration.

Diagnosis/Preparation

The diagnosis of carpal tunnel syndrome most commonly occurs because the individual seeks medical advice for numbness and tingling in the hand, especially while holding a telephone, newspaper, or holding onto the steering wheel, or has experienced dropping objects. A thorough medical and medication history and a **physical examination**, especially for checking the nerve pathway functioning in the arms and hands, are essential components of a full diagnostic workup for carpal tunnel syndrome. It is important to be able to rule out other medical conditions such as a pinched nerve in the neck, which may present with similar symptoms. A complete account of symptoms, including which fingers are involved, is important because the median nerve, the nerve involved in carpal tunnel syndrome, does not innervate the little finger. The timing of the symptoms is also important, because it indicates what activities set off the symptoms, such as while reading a book or having the hands placed on the steering wheel. Symptoms often occur at night because the hand gets set in a certain position for extended periods of time. Many people find that their hand is numb when they wake up in the morning, or that they wake up during the night with pain in the affected hand. To get relief, the individual may hang the hand off the bed, rub the hand, or shake it until the tingling goes away. Since, for many sufferers, the symptoms are worse at night than during the day, it may take time to associate the symptoms with the problem causing

QUESTIONS TO ASK THE DOCTOR

- Can I expect a full recovery?
- Will I be able to return to my regular work?
- Can both wrists be done at the same time?
- Is this a work-related condition?
- How soon will I be able to drive?
- When can I return to playing sports?
- How many of these surgeries have you performed?
- What complications have you seen in the surgeries you performed?
- What other complications might I encounter?

them. For some people, the symptoms come on, especially at first, only at work, because that is where the hand has to exert more than usual force in an awkward position. For others, the symptoms may come on when engaging in a hobby such as painting, gardening, knitting, woodworking, lifting weights, or playing a musical instrument. What begins as periodic symptoms may progress to constant symptoms, and mundane tasks such as unscrewing a bottle top or turning a key in a lock become extremely painful, or even impossible to perform. The doctor will want to try to elicit the symptoms by placing the hands in the same position as when the symptoms come on naturally.

Carpal tunnel syndrome is sometimes referred to as entrapment neuropathy, which means that a nerve, in this case the median nerve, is entrapped or compressed. In carpal tunnel syndrome, the median nerve is compressed, usually by swelling and inflammation, as it passes from the forearm into the hand through the carpal tunnel. The compression puts pressure on the nerve, which is what elicits the tingling and numbness felt by the patient. Compression can arise from a condition that causes the carpal tunnel to become smaller or narrower, or by something such as fluid retention, which would increase the volume inside the tunnel. In addition to trying to assess what nerve is involved in the problem, the doctor will want to see if strength in the hand has been affected. As part of the neurological exam, the doctor may tap at the base of the crease of the wrist. If this tapping brings on tingling in all the fingers except the pinkie, it is said that the Tinel's sign was positive. A positive Phalen test occurs when the two hands are placed back-to-back and held in that position for 60 seconds, bringing on symp-

toms. By extending the hands out of that position, symptoms are relieved. If these tests are positive, the doctor may want to order nerve conduction studies, although it is possible for conduction tests to be normal when the individual suffers from carpal tunnel syndrome.

Treatment

Once diagnosed, the first line of treatment for carpal tunnel syndrome is usually conservative in nature. This means that surgery is reserved as a last resort. Initial treatment may include taking frequent rest breaks from aggravating activity (if the activity cannot be completely avoided), anti-inflammatory medication, physical therapy, and using a splint or brace to keep the wrist in a neutral position; the splint is usually worn at night. Activities that bring on the symptoms are eliminated, avoided, or altered in some way to change the stress on the nerve. Tests to rule out conditions such as hypothyroidism may be conducted. If the problem is work-related, an assessment of the work environment from an ergonomic standpoint will be important. Work positions and tools used may need to be modified or changed completely.

If symptoms persist after conservative treatment, the injection of a corticosteroidal medication may be the next line of treatment suggested. This is an anti-inflammatory medication, but because it is injected directly into the area affected, it has a greater impact than medication that is taken orally. If injections are being considered, it is important that the doctor have considerable skill and experience in administering these injections, with a thorough understanding of the anatomy of the wrist and hand. After the injection, a restriction on any wrist movement will be imposed for several days, usually followed by the wearing of a wrist splint for about one month. Finally, hand and wrist exercises to stretch the tendons as well as increase hand strength may be recommended. While the injection tends to give good short-term results, long-term results are less promising. When symptoms are not relieved by these more conservative measures, then surgery may be the next step. It is estimated that about one third of patients will not respond to conservative treatment and will require surgery.

Surgery may be performed in the more tradition fashion, or endoscopically. In traditional surgical treatment, an incision is made in the palm of the hand to openly expose the underlying structures. In endoscopic surgery, a smaller incision is made in the palm or wrist into which endoscopic instruments are inserted. In both techniques, entry into the carpal tunnel is made and the tissue called the transverse carpal ligament is cut, which stops the compression on the median nerve from continuing. Extreme caution is taken to avoid cutting additional anatomical structures or damaging the surrounding nerves. Early reports on endoscopic surgeries showed an earlier return to work and routine activities, but with a higher incidence of nerve and tendon injuries. However, in 2002, several studies were reported showing endoscopic surgery to be comparable or superior to open excision surgery, without a higher rate of complications.

Aftercare

Initial **postoperative care** while the individual is still in the surgical center involves making sure that circulation in the hands and fingers has not been compromised. There should be a strong radial (wrist) pulse, and the fingers should be their normal skin color and warm to the touch. The individual should be able to move all fingers equally, and there should be no edema.

Once discharged, it will be important for the patient to be aware of signs of complications. Contact the surgeon with symptoms such as:

• fever

• pale or bluish color to the operated hand

• if the operated hand feels significantly colder than the non-operated hand

• inability or difficulty moving the fingers in the operated hand

• numbness in the operated hand

• bleeding from the bandaged hand

• swelling of the operated arm

A splint may be worn for about a month to help keep the wrist in a neutral position. This may be followed by exercises to both stretch and strengthen the hand, fingers, and wrist. Any accommodations in the work or home environment will need to be made to prevent further problems.

Risks

All surgical procedures involve some risk of infection through the operated site. Sharing all pertinent past and present medical history with the **surgical team** helps to lower the chance of a complication. In addition to the risk of the surgery itself, there are the risks associated with anesthesia. In carpal tunnel release surgery, anesthesia is more localized, which lowers the chance of complications. Nonetheless, it is important to share with the anesthesia team the list of all the vitamins, herbs, and supplements, over-the-counter medications, and prescription medications that the patient is taking. Drug interactions can be significant, especially if the anesthesia team does not have all the necessary information to make the best anesthesia choices for a particular patient. Complications such as nerve damage are linked with poor surgical technique.

KEY TERMS

Dominant hand—The hand that the individual prefers to use for most activities, especially writing.

Edema—The abnormal accumulation of fluid in the body tissues.

Endoscopic—Surgery done making a few small incisions and inserting specialized instruments, one of which is a camera, that function as extended hands of the surgeon.

Innervate—Means to carry nerve impulses to a particular body part.

Neurosurgeon—A surgeon who specializes in dealing with nerve-related conditions.

Normal results

Whether or not a full recovery is achieved depends on several factors. The most important factor is if there has been permanent damage to the nerve or tissue fibers. If muscle atrophy occurred because the condition went untreated for a significant period of time, full recovery is unlikely. If no permanent damage resulted, then full recovery would be expected. Recovery is expected to take about six to eight weeks. Occupational rehabilitation may take an additional month. Those for whom the condition was work-related will need to address the causative factors before returning to work.

Morbidity and mortality rates

The research literature does not indicate a significant mortality risk with carpal tunnel release. Morbidity complications are small, and it is a safe enough procedure to be done during pregnancy. Nerve block anesthesia decreases morbidity and offers pain relief from the wrist to the fingertips. A 2001 Swedish study showed a 91% patient satisfaction rate with the release surgery several years after the surgery was done. According to a 2002 study, recurrent scar formation was the most common complication. Individuals considering surgery should investigate the complication rates with the surgeon, as well as the surgeon's and the facility's record.

Alternatives

Conservative treatment is the main alternative to surgery. A "wait and see" method is not a realistic form of treatment, as symptoms worsen over time, and the risk of permanent damage exists. Some acupuncturists treat carpal tunnel syndrome with success, though research studies have not been done in this area. A 2002 British study looked at the use of the homeopathic medicine, Arnica, for postoperative pain following carpal tunnel release. In the 37 patients tested, researchers found a significant decrease in pain reported by those taking the Arnica. A July 1998 study reported that about 70% of patients who undertook a specific **exercise** program for their carpal tunnel condition reported good results, and they were able to avoid surgery.

Resources

BOOKS

Barker, L. Randol, John R. Burton, and Phillip D. Zieve, eds. *Principles of Ambulatory Medicine,* 5th edition. Baltimore, MD: William & Wilkins, 1999.

Fihn, Stephan D. and Dawn E. DeWitt. *Outpatient Medicine.* Philadelphia: W. B. Saunders Company, 1998.

PERIODICALS

Braun, R. M., M. Rechnic, and E. Fowler. "Complications Related to Carpal Tunnel Release." *Hand Clinics* 18, no. 2 (May 2002): 347–57.

Filippi, R., R. Reisch, D. El-Shki, and P. Grunert. "Uniportal Endoscopic Surgery of Carpal Tunnel Syndrome: Technique and Clinical Results." *Minimally Invasive Neurosurgy* 45, no. 2 (June 2002): 78–83.

Jeffrey, S. L. and H. J. Belcher. "Use of Arnica to Relieve Pain after Carpal-tunnel Release Surgery." *Alternative Therapies in Health and Medicine* 8, no. 2 (March/April 2002): 66–68.

ORGANIZATIONS

Mayo Clinic. 200 First St. S.W., Rochester, MN 55905. (507) 284-2511. <http://www.mayoclinic.com>.

Esther Csapo Rastegari, RN, BSN, EdM

Castration *see* **Orchiectomy**

CAT scan *see* **CT scans**

Cataract cryotherapy *see* **Cryotherapy for cataracts**

Catheterization, cardiac *see* **Cardiac catheterization**

Catheterization, female

Definition

Urinary catheterization is the insertion of a catheter through the urethra into the urinary bladder for withdrawal of urine. Straight catheters are used for intermittent withdrawals, while indwelling (Foley) catheters are inserted and retained in the bladder for continuous drainage of urine into a closed system.

Purpose

Intermittent catheterization is used for the following reasons:

- Obtaining a sterile urine specimen for diagnostic evaluation.
- Emptying bladder contents when an individual is unable to void (urinate) due to urinary retention, bladder distention, or obstruction.
- Measuring residual urine after urinating.
- Instilling medication for a localized therapeutic effect in the bladder.
- Instilling contrast material (dye) into the bladder for cystourethralgraphy (x-ray study of the bladder and urethra).
- Emptying the bladder for increased space in the pelvic cavity to protect the bladder during labor and delivery or during pelvic and abdominal surgery.
- Monitoring accurately the urinary output and fluid balance of critically ill patients.

Indwelling catheterization is used for the following reasons:

- Providing palliative care for incontinent persons who are terminally ill or severely impaired, for whom bed and clothing changes are uncomfortable.
- Managing skin ulceration caused or exacerbated by incontinence.
- Maintaining a continuous outflow of urine for persons undergoing surgical procedures that cause a delay in bladder sensation, or for individuals with chronic neurological disorders that cause paralysis or loss of sensation in the perineal area.
- Keeping with standard preoperative preparation for **urologic surgery** and procedures for bladder outlet obstruction.
- Providing relief for persons with an initial episode of acute urinary retention, allowing the bladder to regain its normal muscle tone.

Demographics

As of 2002, experts estimated that approximately 96 million urinary catheters are sold annually throughout the world. Women are more likely than men to use them.

Description

The female urethral orifice is a vertical, slit-like, or irregularly ovoid (egg-shaped) opening, 0.16–0.2 in (4–5 mm) in diameter, located between the clitoris and the vagina. The urinary meatus (opening) is concealed between the labia minora, which are the small folds of tissue that need to be separated to view the opening and insert a catheter. With proper positioning, good lighting, and gloved hands, these anatomical landmarks can be identified. Perineal care or cleansing may be required to ensure a clean procedural environment.

Catheterization of the female patient is traditionally performed without the use of local anesthetic gel to facilitate catheter insertion. But since there are no lubricating glands in the female urethra (as are found in the male urethra), the risk of trauma from a simple catheter insertion is increased. Therefore, an ample supply of an anesthetic or antibacterial lubricant should be used.

Once the catheter is inserted, it is secured as appropriate for the catheter type. A straight catheter is typically secured with adhesive tape. An indwelling catheter is secured by inflating a bulb-like device inside of the bladder.

Diagnosis/Preparation

Health-care practitioners performing the catheterization should have a good understanding of the anatomy and physiology of the urinary system, be trained in antiseptic techniques, and have proficiency in catheter insertion and catheter care.

After determining the primary purpose for the catheterization, practitioners should give the woman to be catheterized and her caregiver a detailed explanation. Women requiring self-catheterization should be instructed and trained in the technique by a qualified health professional.

Sterile disposable catheterization sets are available in clinical settings and for home use. These sets contain most of the items needed for the procedure, such as antiseptic agent, perineal drapes, gloves, lubricant, specimen container, label, and tape. Anesthetic or antibacterial lubricant, catheter, and a drainage system may need to be added.

Catheter choices

TYPES. Silastic catheters have been recommended for short-term catheterization after surgery because they are known to decrease incidence of urethritis (inflammation of the urethra). However, due to lower cost and acceptable outcomes, latex is the catheter of choice for long-term catheterization. Silastic catheters should be reserved for individuals who are allergic to latex products.

There are additional types of catheters:

• PTFE (plastic)-coated latex indwelling (Foley) catheters

• hydrogel-coated latex indwelling catheters

• pure silicone indwelling catheters

• silicone-coated latex indwelling catheters

SIZE. The diameter of a catheter is measured in millimeters. Authorities recommend using the narrowest and softest tube that will serve the purpose. Rarely is a catheter larger than size 18 F(rench) required, and sizes 14 or 16 F are used more often. Catheters greater than size 16 F have been associated with patient discomfort and urine bypassing. A size 12 catheter has been successfully used in children and in female patients with urinary restriction.

DRAINAGE SYSTEM. The health-care provider should discuss the design, capacity, and emptying mechanism of several urine drainage bags with the patient. For women with normal bladder sensation, a catheter valve for intermittent drainage may be an acceptable option.

PROCEDURE. When inserting a urinary catheter, the health-care provider will first wash the hands and put on gloves and clean the skin of the area around the urethra. An anesthetic lubricating gel may be used. The catheter is threaded up the urethra and into the bladder until the urine starts to flow. The catheter is taped to the upper thigh and attached to a drainage system.

Aftercare

Women using intermittent catheterization to manage incontinence may require a period of adjustment as they try to establish a catheterization schedule that is adequate for their normal fluid intake.

Antibiotics should not be prescribed as a preventative measure for women at risk for urinary tract infection (UTI). Prophylactic use of antibacterial agents may lead to the development of drug-resistant bacteria. Women who practice intermittent self-catheterization can reduce their risk for UTI by using antiseptic techniques for insertion and catheter care.

The extended portion of the catheter should be washed with a mild soap and warm water to keep it free of accumulated debris.

Risks

Complications that may occur include:

• Trauma or introduction of bacteria into the urinary system, leading to infection and, rarely, septicemia.

• Trauma to the urethra or bladder from incorrect insertion or attempting to remove the catheter with the balloon inflated. Repeated trauma may cause scarring or stricture (narrowing) of the urethra.

• Passage of urine around the catheter. Inserting a different catheter size can minimize this problem.

Sexual activity and menopause can also compromise the sterility of the urinary tract. Irritation of the urethra during intercourse promotes the migration of perineal bacteria into the urethra and bladder, causing UTIs. Postmenopausal women may experience more UTIs than younger women. The presence of residual urine in the bladder due to incomplete voiding provides an ideal environment for bacterial growth.

Urinary catheterization should be avoided whenever possible. Clean intermittent catheterization, when practical, is preferable to long-term catheterization.

Catheters should not be routinely changed. Each woman should be monitored for indication of obstruction, infection, or complications before the catheter is changed. Some women require weekly catheter changes, while others may need one change in several weeks. Fewer catheter changes will reduce trauma to the urethra and reduce the incidence of UTI.

Because the urinary tract is normally a sterile system, catheterization presents the risk of causing a UTI. The catheterization procedure must be sterile, and the catheter must be free from bacteria.

Frequent intermittent catheterization and long-term use of indwelling catheterization predisposes a woman to UTI. Care should be taken to avoid trauma to the urinary meatus or urothelium (urinary lining) with catheters that are too large or inserted with insufficient use of lubricant. Women with an indwelling catheter must be reassessed periodically to determine if alternative treatment will be more effective in treating the problem.

Normal results

A catheterization program that includes correctly inserted catheters and is appropriately maintained will usually control urinary incontinence.

The woman and her caregiver should be taught to use **aseptic technique** for catheter care. Nursing interventions and patient education can make a difference in the incidence of urinary tract infections in hospitals, **nursing homes**, and **home care** settings.

The sexuality of a woman with an indwelling catheter for continuous urinary drainage is seldom considered. If the patient is sexually active, the practitioner must explain that intercourse can take place with the catheter in place. The woman or her partner can be taught to remove the catheter before intercourse and replace it with a new one afterwards.

Morbidity and mortality rates

Injuries resulting from catheterization are infrequent. Deaths are extremely rare. Both complications are usually due to infections that result from improper catheter care.

Alternatives

An alternative to catheterization is to use a pad to absorb voided urine.

See also Catheterization, male.

Resources

BOOKS

Altman, M. *Urinary Care/Catheterization.* Albany, NY: Delmar, 2003.

Gearhart, John P. *Pediatric Urology.* Totawa, NJ: Humana Press, 2003.

Hanna, P. M., S. B. Malkowicz, and A. J. Wein. *Clinical Manual of Urology, 3rd edition.* New York: McGraw Hill, 2001.

Laycock, J., and J. Haslam. *Therapeutic Management of Incontinence and Pelvic Pain.* New York: Sringer-Verlag, 2001.

Newman, Diane K. *Managing and Treating Urinary Incontinence.* Baltimore, MD: Health Professions Press, 2002.

PERIODICALS

Wilde, M. H. and B. L. Cameron. "Meanings and Practical Knowledge of People with Long-term Urinary Catheters."

KEY TERMS

Catheter—A tube for evacuating or injecting fluid.

Contaminate—To make an item unsterile or unclean by direct contact.

Foley catheter—A double-channel retention catheter; one channel provides for the inflow and outflow of bladder fluid, the second (smaller) channel is used to fill a balloon that holds the catheter in the bladder.

Incontinence—The inability to retain urine or control one's urine flow.

Intermittent catheterization—Periodic catheterization to facilitate urine flow.

Perineal area—The genital area between the vulva and anus in a woman.

Urethra—The tube that allows passage of urine out of the urinary bladder.

Urethritis—Inflammation of the urinary bladder.

Urinary retention—The inability to void (urinate) or discharge urine.

Septicemia—An infection in the blood.

Journal of Wound Ostomy Continence Nursing 30(1) (2003): 33–43.

Johnson, J. R. "Safety of urinary catheters." *Journal of the American Medical Association,* 289(3) (2003): 300–301.

Munasinghe, R. L., V. Nagappan, and M. Siddique. "Urinary Catheters: A One-point Restraint?" *Annals of Internal Medicine* 138(3) (2003): 238–239.

Winder, A. "Intermittent Self-catheterisation." *Nursing Times* 98(48) (2002): 50.

ORGANIZATIONS

American Board of Urology. 2216 Ivy Road, Suite 210, Chaarlottesviille, VA 22903. (434) 979-0059. <http://www.abu.org/>.

American Foundation for Urologic Disease. 1128 North Charles Street, Baltimore, MD 21201. (800) 242-2383. <http://www.afud.org/>.

American Urological Association. 1120 North Charles Street, Baltimore, MD 21201. (410) 727-1100. <http://www.auanet.org/>.

National Health Service of Great Britain. <http://www.nhsdirect.nhs.uk/nhsdoheso/display.asp?sTopic=Urinaryc>.

National Kidney and Urologic Diseases Information Clearinghouse. 3 Information Way, Bethesda, MD 20892. (800) 891-5390. <http://www.niddk.nih.gov/health/kidney/nkudic.htm/>.

OTHER

AdvancePCS. [cited February 28, 2003] <http://www.buildingbetterhealth.com/topic/topic100587629>.

Harvard Pilgrim Health Care. [cited February 28, 2003] <http://www.intelihealth.com/IH/ihtIH/WSHPO000/25792/31681.html>.

Mount Clemens General Hospital, Mt. Clemens, MI. [cited February 28, 2003] <http://www.mcgh.org/Health_Information/Articles/URINARYCATHETERIZATION.htm>.

Wayne State University. [cited February 28, 2003] <http://www.dmc.org/health_info/topics/urin5266.html>.

L. Fleming Fallon, Jr, MD, DrPH

Catheterization, male

Definition

Urinary catheterization is the insertion of a catheter through the urethra into the urinary bladder for withdrawal of urine. Straight catheters are used for intermittent withdrawals, while indwelling (Foley) catheters are inserted and retained in the bladder for continuous drainage of urine into a closed system.

Purpose

Intermittent catheterization is used for the following reasons:

- Obtaining a sterile urine specimen for diagnostic evaluation.
- Emptying bladder contents when an individual is unable to void (urinate) due to urinary retention, bladder distention, or obstruction.
- Measuring residual urine after urinating.
- Instilling medication for a localized therapeutic effect in the bladder.
- Instilling contrast material (dye) into the bladder for cystourethralgraphy (x-ray study of the bladder and urethra).
- Emptying the bladder for increased space in the pelvic cavity to protect the bladder during labor and delivery or during pelvic and abdominal surgery.
- Monitoring accurately the urinary output and fluid balance of critically ill patients.

Indwelling catheterization is used for the following reasons:

- Providing palliative care for incontinent persons who are terminally ill or severely impaired, for whom bed and clothing changes are uncomfortable.
- Managing skin ulceration caused or exacerbated by incontinence.

- Maintaining a continuous outflow of urine for persons undergoing surgical procedures that cause a delay in bladder sensation, or for individuals with chronic neurological disorders that cause paralysis or loss of sensation in the perineal area.

- Included in standard preoperative preparation for **urologic surgery** and procedures for bladder outlet obstruction.

- Providing relief for persons with an initial episode of acute urinary retention, allowing their bladder to regain its normal muscle tone.

Demographics

As of 2002, experts estimate that approximately 96 million urinary catheters are sold annually throughout the world. Men are less likely than women to use them.

Description

The male urethral orifice (urinary meatus) is a vertical, slit-like opening, 0.15–0.2 in (4–5 mm) long, located at the tip of the penis. The foreskin of the penis may conceal the opening. This must be retracted to view the opening to be able to insert a catheter. With proper positioning, good lighting, and gloved hands, these anatomical landmarks can be identified. Perineal care or cleansing may be required to ensure a clean procedural environment.

The male urethra is longer than the female urethra and has two curves in it as it passes through the penis to the bladder. Catheterization of the male patient is traditionally performed without the use of local anesthetic gel to facilitate catheter insertion. Glands along the urethra provide some natural lubrication. Older men may require lubrication. In such an instance, an anesthetic or antibacterial lubricant should be used.

Once the catheter is inserted, it is secured as appropriate for the catheter type. A straight catheter is typically secured with adhesive tape. An indwelling catheter is secured by inflating a bulb-like device inside of the bladder.

Diagnosis/Preparation

Health-care practitioners performing the catheterization should have a good understanding of the anatomy and physiology of the urinary system, be trained in antiseptic techniques, and have proficiency in catheter insertion and catheter care.

After determining the primary purpose for the catheterization, practitioners should give the male patient and his caregiver a detailed explanation. Men requiring self-catheterization should be instructed and trained in the technique by a qualified health professional.

Sterile disposable catheterization sets are available in clinical settings and for home use. These sets contain most of the items needed for the procedure, such as antiseptic agent, gloves, lubricant, specimen container, label, and tape. Anesthetic or antibacterial lubricant, catheter, and a drainage system may need to be added.

Catheter choices

TYPES. Silastic catheters have been recommended for short-term catheterization after surgery because they are known to decrease incidence of urethritis (inflammation of the urethra). However, due to lower cost and acceptable outcomes, latex is the catheter of choice for long-term catheterization. Silastic catheters should be reserved for individuals who are allergic to latex products.

There are additional types of catheters:

- PTFE (plastic)-coated latex indwelling (Foley) catheters
- hydrogel-coated latex indwelling catheters
- pure silicone indwelling catheters
- silicone-coated latex indwelling catheters

SIZE. The diameter of a catheter is measured in millimeters. Authorities recommend using the narrowest and softest tube that will serve the purpose. Rarely is a catheter larger than size 18 F(rench) required, and sizes 14 or 16 F are used more often. Catheters greater than size 16 F have been associated with patient discomfort and urine bypassing. A size 12 F catheter has been successfully used in children and in male patients with urinary restriction.

DRAINAGE SYSTEM. The health-care provider should discuss the design, capacity, and emptying mechanism of several urine drainage bags with the patient. For men with normal bladder sensation, a catheter valve for intermittent drainage may be an acceptable option.

PROCEDURE. When inserting a urinary catheter, the health care provider will first wash the hands and put on gloves and clean the tip of the penis. An anesthetic lubricating gel may be used. The catheter is threaded up the urethra and into the bladder until the urine starts to flow. The catheter is taped to the upper thigh and attached to a drainage system.

Aftercare

Men using intermittent catheterization to manage incontinence may require a period of adjustment as they try to establish a catheterization schedule that is adequate for their normal fluid intake.

Antibiotics should not be prescribed as a preventative measure for men at risk for urinary tract infection (UTI). Prophylactic use of antibacterial agents may lead to the development of drug-resistant bacteria. Men who practice intermittent self-catheterization can reduce their risk for UTI by using antiseptic techniques for insertion and catheter care.

The extended portion of the catheter should be washed with a mild soap and warm water to keep it free of accumulated debris.

Risks

Phimosis is constriction of the prepuce (foreskin) so that it cannot be drawn back over the glans penis. This may make it difficult to identify the external urethral meatus. Care should be taken when catheterizing men with phimosis to avoid trauma from forced retraction of the prepuce or by incorrect positioning of the catheter.

Complications that may occur from a catheterization procedure include:

• Trauma or introduction of bacteria into the urinary system, leading to infection and, rarely, septicemia.

• Trauma to the urethra or bladder from incorrect insertion or attempting to remove the catheter with the balloon inflated. Repeated trauma may cause scarring or stricture (narrowing) of the urethra.

• Passage of urine around the catheter. Inserting a different catheter size can minimize this problem.

The presence of residual urine in the bladder due to incomplete voiding provides an ideal environment for bacterial growth.

Urinary catheterization should be avoided whenever possible. Clean intermittent catheterization, when practical, is preferable to long-term catheterization.

Catheters should not be routinely changed. Each man should be monitored for indication of obstruction, infection, or complications before the catheter is changed. Some men require daily or weekly catheter changes, while others may need one change in several weeks. Fewer catheter changes will reduce trauma to the urethra and reduce the incidence of UTI.

QUESTIONS TO ASK THE DOCTOR

• Will the catheterization be intermittent or indwelling?

• If intermittent, who will change the catheter and how long will it remain in place?

• If indwelling, how often will the catheter be changed and who will change it?

• Who will teach me or my caregiver how to insert and remove the catheter, monitor it, and perform routine care?

Because the urinary tract is normally a sterile system, catheterization presents the risk of causing a UTI. The catheterization procedure must be sterile and the catheter must be free from bacteria.

Frequent intermittent catheterization and long-term use of indwelling catheterization predisposes a man to UTI. Care should be taken to avoid trauma to the urinary meatus or urothelium (urinary lining) with catheters that are too large or inserted with insufficient use of lubricant. Men with an indwelling catheter must be reassessed periodically to determine if alternative treatment will be more effective in treating the problem.

Normal results

A catheterization program that includes correctly inserted catheters and is appropriately maintained will usually control urinary incontinence.

The man and his caregiver should be taught to use **aseptic technique** for catheter care. Nursing interventions and patient education can make a difference in the incidence of urinary tract infections in hospitals, **nursing homes**, and **home care** settings.

The sexuality of a man with an indwelling catheter for continuous urinary drainage is seldom considered. If the patient is sexually active, the man or his partner can be taught to remove the catheter before intercourse and replace it with a new one afterwards.

Morbidity and mortality rates

Injuries resulting from catheterization are infrequent. Deaths are extremely rare. Both complications are usually due to infections that result from improper catheter care.

KEY TERMS

Catheter—A tube for evacuating or injecting fluid.

Contaminate—To make an item unsterile or unclean by direct contact.

Foley catheter—A double-channel retention catheter. One channel provides for the inflow and outflow of bladder fluid, the second (smaller) channel is used to fill a balloon that holds the catheter in the bladder.

Incontinence—The inability to retain urine or control one's urine flow.

Intermittent catheterization—Periodic catheterization to facilitate urine flow. The catheter is removed when the bladder is sufficiently empty.

Urethra—The tube that allows passage of urine out of the urinary bladder.

Urethritis—Inflammation of the urinary bladder.

Urinary retention—The inability to void (urinate) or discharge urine.

Septicemia—An infection in the blood.

Alternatives

An alternative to catheterization is to use a pad to absorb voided urine.

See also Catheterization, female.

Resources

BOOKS

Altman, M. *Urinary Care/Catheterization*. Albany, NY: Delmar, 2003.

Gearhart, John P. *Pediatric Urology*. Totawa, NJ: Humana Press, 2003.

Hanna, P. M., S. B. Malkowicz, and A. J. Wein. *Clinical Manual of Urology, 3rd edition*. New York: McGraw Hill, 2001.

Laycock, J. and J. Haslam. *Therapeutic Management of Incontinence and Pelvic Pain*. New York: Sringer-Verlag, 2001.

Newman, Diane K. *Managing and Treating Urinary Incontinence*. Baltimore, MD: Health Professions Press, 2002.

PERIODICALS

Johnson, J. R. "Safety of Urinary Catheters." *Journal of the American Medical Association* 289(3) (2003): 300–301.

Munasinghe, R. L., V. Nagappan V, and M. Siddique. "Urinary Catheters: A One-point Restraint?" *Annals of Internal Medicine* 138(3) (2003): 238–239.

Wilde, M. H. and B. L. Cameron. "Meanings and Practical Knowledge of People with Long-term Urinary Catheters." *Journal of Wound Ostomy Continence Nursing* 30(1) (2003): 33–43.

Winder, A. "Intermittent Self-catheterisation." *Nursing Times* 98(48) (2002): 50.

ORGANIZATIONS

American Board of Urology. 2216 Ivy Road, Suite 210, Chaarlottesviille, VA 22903. (434) 979-0059. <http://www.abu.org/>.

American Foundation for Urologic Disease. 1128 North Charles Street, Baltimore, MD 21201. (800) 242-2383. <http://www.afud.org/>.

American Urological Association. 1120 North Charles Street, Baltimore, MD 21201. (410) 727-1100. <http://www.auanet.org/>.

National Health Service of Great Britain. <http://www.nhsdirect.nhs.uk/nhsdoheso/display.asp?sTopic=Urinaryc>.

National Kidney and Urologic Diseases Information Clearinghouse. 3 Information Way, Bethesda, MD 20892. (800) 891-5390. <http://www.niddk.nih.gov/health/kidney/nkudic.htm/>.

OTHER

AdvancePCS. [cited February 28, 2003] <http://www.buildingbetterhealth.com/topic/topic100587629>.

Harvard Pilgrim Health Care. [cited February 28, 2003] <http://www.intelihealth.com/IH/ihtIH/WSHPO000/25792/31681.html>.

Mount Clemens General Hospital, Mt. Clemens, MI. [cited February 28, 2003] <http://www.mcgh.org/Health_Information/Articles/URINARYCATHETERIZATION.htm>.

Wayne State University. [cited February 28, 2003] <http://www.dmc.org/health_info/topics/urin5266.html>.

L. Fleming Fallon, Jr, MD, DrPH

CBC *see* **Complete blood count**

Cephalosporins

Definition

Cephalosporins are a type of antibiotic, or medicines that kill bacteria or prevent their growth.

Purpose

Cephalosporins are used to treat infections in different parts of the body—the ears, nose, throat, lungs, sinuses, and skin, for example. Physicians may prescribe these drugs to treat pneumonia, strep throat, staph infections, tonsillitis, bronchitis, and gonorrhea. These drugs will *not* work for colds, flu, and other infections caused by viruses.

Cephalosporins are also commonly used for surgical prophylaxis—prevention of bacterial infection during or immediately after surgery. For this purpose, a single injection may be given during the surgical procedure. In some cases, the cephalosporin may be continued for 24 to 48 hours after surgery. If, in spite of all precautions, an infection develops, the **antibiotics** may be continued until the infection has resolved.

Description

Examples of cephalosporins are cefaclor (Ceclor), cefadroxil (Duricef), cefazolin (Ancef, Kefzol, Zolicef), cefixime, (Suprax), cefoxitin (Mefoxin), cefprozil (Cefzil), ceftazidime (Ceptaz, Fortaz, Tazicef, Tazideme), cefuroxime (Ceftin) and cephalexin (Keflex). These medicines are available only with a physician's prescription. They are sold in tablet, capsule, liquid, and injectable forms.

Cephalosporins are sometimes referred to as first, second, and third generation. Each "generation" is effective against more types of bacteria than the one before it. In addition, each subsequent generation is better at getting into the central nervous system (the brain and spinal cord).

Cephalosporins are chemically similar to penicillins, and to other types of antibiotics called cephamycins.

Recommended dosage

The recommended dosage depends on the type of cephalosporin. The physician who prescribed the drug or the pharmacist who filled the prescription should be consulted for the correct dosage.

The following recommendations do not apply when cephalosporins are given as a single intravenous dose prior to or during surgery. The recommendations should be considered if the drugs are used afterwards to treat a surgical infection, particularly if the cephalosporins are given by mouth.

Cephalosporins should be taken exactly as directed by the physician. The patient should never take larger, smaller, more frequent, or less frequent doses than prescribed. The drug should be taken for exactly as long as directed. No doses of the drug should be saved to take for future infections, because the medicine may not be right for other kinds of infections, even if the symptoms are the same. In addition, all of the medicine should be taken to treat the infection for which it was prescribed. The infection may not clear up completely if too little medicine is taken. Taking this medicine for too long, on the other hand, may open the door to new infections that do not respond to the drug.

Some cephalosporins work best when taken on an empty stomach. Others should be taken after meals. The physician who prescribed the medicine or the pharmacist who filled the prescription should give instructions as to how to take the medicine.

When given for surgical prophylaxis, it used to be common practice to give a dose of a cephalosporin as soon as the patient has been called to the **operating room**. More recently, the practice has been to give a single dose during the surgical procedure. This works just as well as the "on call" dose, and lowers the amount of antibiotic that the patient must take.

Precautions

The following recommendations do not apply when cephalosporins are given as a single intravenous dose prior to or during surgery. They should be considered if the drugs are used afterwards to treat a surgical infection, particularly if the cephalosporins are given by mouth.

Certain cephalosporins should not be combined with alcohol or with medicines that contain alcohol. Abdominal or stomach cramps, nausea, vomiting, facial flushing, and other symptoms may result within 15–30 minutes and may last for several hours. Alcoholic beverages as well as other medicines that contain alcohol should be avoided while being treated with cephalosporins and for several days after treatment ends.

Special conditions

People with certain medical conditions or who are taking certain other medicines can have problems if they take cephalosporins. Before taking these drugs, be sure to let the physician know about any of these conditions:

ALLERGIES. Severe allergic reactions to this medicine may occur. Anyone who is allergic to cephalosporins of any kind should not take other cephalosporins. Anyone who is allergic to penicillin should check with a physician before taking any cephalosporin. The physician should also be told about any allergies to foods, dyes, preservatives, or other substances. The type of allergic reaction should be discussed in detail, since some people have reactions to a drug that are not truly allergies. These people may be able to take cephalosporins safely.

DIABETES. Some cephalosporins may cause false positive results on urine sugar tests for diabetes. People with diabetes should check with their physicians to see if they need to adjust their medication or their diets.

PHENYLKETONURIA. Oral suspensions of cefprozil contain phenylalanine. People with phenylketonuria (PKU) should consult a physician before taking this medicine.

PREGNANCY. Women who are pregnant or who may become pregnant should check with their physicians before using cephalosporins.

KEY TERMS

Bronchitis—Inflammation of the air passages of the lungs.

Colitis—Inflammation of the colon (large bowel).

Gonorrhea—A sexually transmitted disease (STD) that causes infection in the genital organs and may cause disease in other parts of the body.

Inflammation—Pain, redness, swelling, and heat that usually develop in response to injury or illness.

Phenylketonuria—(PKU) A genetic disorder in which the body lacks an important enzyme. If untreated, the disorder can lead to brain damage and mental retardation.

Pneumonia—A disease in which the lungs become inflamed. Pneumonia may be caused by bacteria, viruses, or other organisms, or by physical or chemical irritants.

Sexually transmitted disease—A disease that is passed from one person to another through sexual intercourse or other intimate sexual contact. Also called STD.

Staph infection—Infection with *Staphylococcus* bacteria. These bacteria can infect any part of the body.

Strep throat—A sore throat caused by infection with *Streptococcus* bacteria. Symptoms include sore throat, chills, fever, and swollen lymph nodes in the neck.

Tonsillitis—Inflammation of a tonsil, a small mass of tissue in the throat.

BREASTFEEDING. Cephalosporins may pass into breast milk and may affect nursing babies. Women who are breast-feeding and who need to take this medicine should check with their physicians. They may need to stop breast-feeding until treatment is finished.

OTHER MEDICAL CONDITIONS. Before using cephalosporins, people with any of these medical problems should make sure their physicians are aware of their conditions:

• History of stomach or intestinal problems, especially colitis. Cephalosporins may cause colitis in some people.

• Kidney problems. The dose of cephalosporin may need to be lower.

• Bleeding problems. Cephalosporins may increase the chance of bleeding in people with a history of bleeding problems.

• Liver disease. The dose of cephalosporin may need to be lower.

USE OF CERTAIN MEDICINES. Taking cephalosporins with certain other drugs may affect the way the drugs work or may increase the chance of side effects.

Side effects

The patient should get medical attention immediately if any of these symptoms develop while taking cephalosporins:

• shortness of breath

• pounding heartbeat

• skin rash or hives

• severe cramps or pain in the stomach or abdomen

• fever

• severe watery or bloody diarrhea (may occur up to several weeks after stopping the drug)

• unusual bleeding or bruising

Other rare side effects may occur. Anyone who has unusual symptoms during or after treatment with cephalosporins should contact his or her physician.

Interactions

Some cephalosporins cause diarrhea. Certain diarrhea medicines, such as diphenoxylate-atropine (Lomotil), may make the problem worse. Check with a physician before taking any medicine for diarrhea caused by taking cephalosporins.

Birth control pills may not work properly when taken at the same time as cephalosporins. To prevent pregnancy, other methods of birth control in addition to the pills are advised while taking cephalosporins.

Taking cephalosporins with certain other drugs may increase the risk of excess bleeding. Among the drugs that may have this effect when taken with cephalosporins are:

• blood-thinning drugs (anticoagulants) such as warfarin (Coumadin)

• blood viscosity-reducing medicines such as pentoxifylline (Trental)

• the antiseizure medicines divalproex (Depakote) and valproic acid (Depakene)

Cephalosporins may also interact with other medicines. When this happens, the effects of one or both of the drugs may change or the risk of side effects may be greater. Anyone who takes cephalosporins should let the physician know all other medicines he or she is taking.

Resources

BOOKS

AHFS: Drug Information. Washington, DC: American Society of Healthsystems Pharmaceuticals, 2003.

Reynolds, J. E. F. (ed). *Martindale The Extra Pharmacopoeia* 31st Edition. London: The Pharmaceutical Press, 1993.

Schwartz, S., G. T. Shires, and others (editors). *Principles of Surgery.* New York: McGraw Hill, 1999.

PERIODICALS

Barie, P. S. "Modern surgical antibiotic prophylaxis and therapy—less is more." *Surgical Infections* 1, no. 1 (2000): 23–29.

Cosgrove, S. E., K. S. Kaye, G. M. Eliopoulous, and Y. Carmeli. "Health and economic outcomes of the emergence of third-generation cephalosporin resistance in Enterobacter species." *Archives of Internal Medicine.* 162, no. 2 (January 28, 2002): 185–190.

OTHER

Blondel-Hill, Edith, Susan Fryters, and others. "Recommended Drug Regimes for Surgical Prophylaxis," in *Bugs and Drugs Antimicrobial Pocket Reference 2001.* Capital Health, 2000. [cited June 30, 2003]. <http://www.dobugsneeddrugs.org/healthcare/antimicrobial/RecommendedDrugRegi mensfor-SurgicalProphylaxis.pdf>.

Nancy Ross-Flanigan
Sam Uretsky

Cerclage, cervical *see* **Cervical cerclage**

Cerebral aneurysm repair

Definition

Cerebral aneurysm repair involves corrective treatment of an abnormal blood-filled sac formed by localized expansion of an artery or vein within the brain. These sacs tend to form at the juncture between a primary vessel and a branch. If the vessel involved is an artery, the lesion is also known as a berry aneurysm because of its round, berry-like appearance.

Purpose

The purpose of the surgical treatment of cerebral aneurysms is to isolate the weakened vessel area from the blood supply. This is commonly done through the strategic placement of small, surgical clips to the neck of the lesion. Thus, the aneurysm becomes isolated from the normal circulation without damaging adjacent ves-

sels or their branches and shrinks in size to become undetectable, a process known as aneurysm obliteration.

Demographics

Cerebral, or brain, aneurysms occur in about 2% of the American population. An estimated 15–33% of these patients have more than one aneurysm present. Occurrence of certain other medical conditions appears to increase the chances of developing aneurysms. These conditions include polycystic kidneys, systemic lupus erythematosus (SLE or lupus), and Ehlers-Danlos syndrome (EDS), a genetic disease that affects collagen, which is a primary component of connective tissue. Aneurysms in children are very rare, strongly suggesting that the condition develops, enlarges, and becomes symptomatic over a person's lifetime.

Other less frequent causes of aneurysms are infectious material from the heart, trauma, brain tumor, and brain arteriovenous malformation (AVM), a defect of the brain's circulatory system that results in the abnormal direct movement of blood from the arteries to the veins of the brain. The average age of cerebral aneurysm rupture is in the fifth decade of life and occurs more often in women than men by a slight margin. Environmental factors known to increase the chances of aneurysm development and rupture are cigarette smoking, excess alcohol consumption, and atherosclerotic heart disease. Some families have a definite genetic predisposition; in such families, aneurysms may run as high as 10%.

Diagnosis/Preparation

Cerebral aneurysms become apparent in two general ways: from rupture followed by bleeding within the brain, or from enlargement and compression on surrounding critical brain structures, which leads to symptoms. The most life-threatening presentation is bleeding and is often described clinically as subarachnoid hemorrhage (SAH), a term derived from the anatomic area of the brain that becomes contaminated with blood when an aneurysm ruptures. The surface of the brain is covered by three thin membranous layers, or meninges, called the dura mater, the pia mater, and the arachnoid. The dura mater adheres to the skull, while the pia mater adheres to the brain. The arachnoid lies between the other two meninges. The space between the pia mater and the arachnoid is known as the subarachnoid space and is normally filled with cerebrospinal fluid. SAH occurs when blood leaks into this space, contaminating the cerebrospinal fluid. About half of all SAH result from a ruptured cerebral aneurysm.

Clinically, the rupture causes the sudden explosive onset of a very severe headache that patients describe as the worst headache of their life. Other symptoms can in-

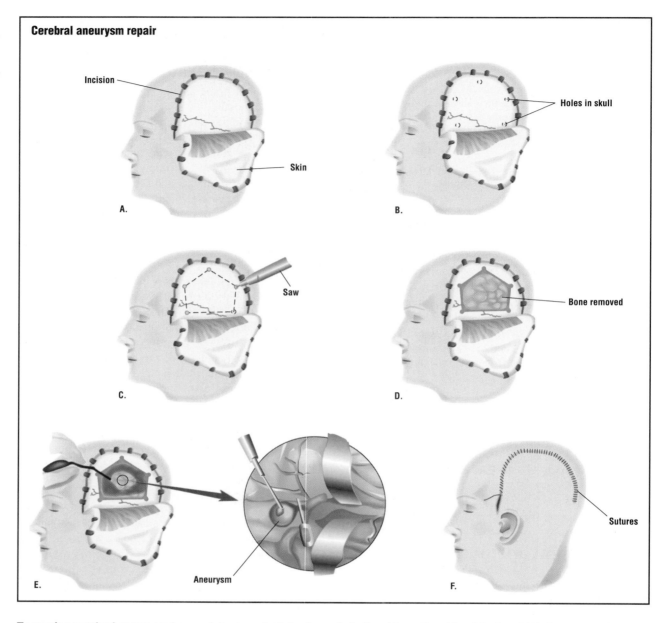

Cerebral aneurysm repair

To repair a cerebral aneurysm by craniotomy, an incision is made in the skin on the side of the head (A). Small holes are drilled in the skull (B), and a special saw is used to cut the bone between the holes (C). The bone is removed (D), and the aneurysm is treated (E). The bone is replaced, and the skin is sutured closed (F). *(Illustration by GGS Inc.)*

clude short-term loss of consciousness, neck stiffness, back pain, nausea or vomiting, and an inability to tolerate bright light. Sometimes a seizure can occur. About 40% of patients have symptoms and signs prior to the actual rupture, including minor headaches or dizziness, which are thought to result from swelling of the aneurysm or minor bleeding that occurs prior to the full rupture. Unfortunately, many of these events go undetected.

Rupture of a cerebral aneurysm is an emergency situation. About 10% of people with SAH die within the first day, and without treatment, 25% succumb within the next three months. More than half of those who survive have significant neurological damage. Partial paralysis, weakness, or numbness may linger or be permanent, as may vision and speech problems.

When SAH is suspected, a computerized tomography (CT) scan is performed to confirm the diagnosis by visualizing the bleeding. The aneurysm itself is only rarely seen using this test. CT scanning is positive (detects the bleeding) in more than 90% of patients within the first 24 hours after the event, and for more than 50% within the first week. As time goes on, however, the bleeding becomes harder and harder to detect using this imaging method. If no bleeding is detected, a second test that could be performed is a lumbar puncture (LP), which involves drawing cerebrospinal fluid through a needle from the lower back of the patient. If SAH has occurred, the collected cerebrospinal fluid will contain blood and could be discolored yellow, caused by the presence of breakdown products of the blood cells. Other more sophisticated tests can also be performed to confirm the presence of blood and its breakdown products in the sample.

The definitive test for a cerebral aneurysm is a fluoroscopic angiogram, as it can often directly document the aneurysm, particularly its location and size. This procedure involves the placement of fluorescent material into the vein or artery of concern that increases the contrast between vessels and surrounding tissue so that their path can be clearly seen. The vessel is accessed through the insertion of a catheter in the femoral (leg) artery and threading it through the heart and into the blood vessels of the brain. A microcatheter is threaded through the larger one and used to deliver the contrast material to the precise location of the suspected aneurysm. Digital subtraction removes the bony structures from the image and leaves only the vessels. Generally, when SAH is suspected, a full cerebral angiogram that studies all four of the major cerebral arteries is performed. Modern angiograms are able to identify 85% of all cerebral aneurysms, with another 10% visible upon a second test seven to 10 days later. If this test is negative, magnetic resonance imagining (MRI), which is in some ways a more sensitive test, is often recommended.

If an aneurysm presents without rupture, some symptoms include seizures, double vision, progressive blindness in one eye, numbness on one side of the face, difficulty speaking, or, occasionally, hydrocephalus (accumulation of cerebrospinal fluid in the brain). Because of the sensitivity of available scanning techniques (particularly MRI), many aneurysms are discovered even before symptoms develop. This raises the issue of whether non-ruptured, asymptomatic aneurysms should be surgically treated.

Many health professionals view an unruptured aneurysm as a potential time bomb. In general, there is a 3% per year cumulative risk of rupture once an aneurysm is identified, or stated another way, about 0.5–0.75% of all aneurysms rupture each year. Each rupture brings with it the very high probability of serious neurological damage or even death. Furthermore, there are certain aneurysms that rupture more commonly than others, and environmental factors such as smoking and high blood pressure con-

tribute to these events. However, all other things being equal, research indicates that by 10 years after diagnosis, there is an approximately 30% chance the aneurysm will rupture. Yet, the surgery itself carries significant risk. Whether or not to treat an unruptured aneurysm is a difficult decision and should be made only after careful consideration of the many influencing factors.

After diagnosis with a cerebral aneurysm, a patient will be put on strict bed rest and receive medication to avoid complications, keep blood pressure under control, and for pain relief.

Description

The exact timing for surgical treatment of cerebral aneurysms is historically a controversial subject in **neurosurgery** and is dependent on many factors including patient age, aneurysm size, aneurysm location, density of SAH, and whether the patient is comatose. Research indicates that early treatment, within the first 48 hours after hemorrhage, is generally associated with better outcomes, particularly because of the reduction of two serious complications of rupture: re-bleeding and vasospasm.

Re-bleeding is the most important cause of death if a patient survives the initial bleed and will happen in approximately 50% of all patients with a ruptured aneurysm who do not undergo surgical treatment. The peak occurrence of re-bleeding is within the first few days after rupture. About 60% of patients who re-bleed die.

The second major cause of death after rupture is vasospasm, a condition where the arteries at the base of the brain become irritated and constrict so tightly that blood cannot flow to critical brain regions. This spasm may result in further brain damage or induce re-bleeding, and much of the medical treatment after the aneurysm ruptures and prior to surgical treatment is designed to prevent this complication.

The procedure itself begins with general anesthesia of the patient and shaving of the area of the skull where the **craniotomy**, or opening of the skull bone, will occur.

QUESTIONS TO ASK THE DOCTOR

- What are the risks of treatment of my aneurysm?
- What are the chances of recovery using this surgical treatment method?
- What are the risks if the aneurysm is left to heal on its own?
- What are the specific characteristics of my aneurysm and how does this affect the decision to treat the problem?
- Is inventional radiology a possible means of treating my aneurysm?

The exact position of the opening depends on the approach that the neurosurgeon will use to reach the aneurysm. The approach varies with the exact location of the aneurysm within the brain's cardiovascular system.

Once the bone flap is removed, the various layers of tissue are cut away to expose the brain. Blocking brain tissue is gently retracted back to expose the area containing the abnormal vessel formation. Surgical techniques performed through a microscope are then utilized to dissect the aneurysm away from the feeding vessels and expose the neck to receive the clip. Clips are manufactured in various types, sizes, shapes, and lengths to accommodate the needs for the various positions, shapes, and sizes of aneurysms. Clips are made of different kinds of materials, with titanium being popular because the material will not interfere with later **magnetic resonance imaging** (MRI) testing.

The clip is placed on the neck of the aneurysm in order to isolate it from the normal circulation. Careful clip placement will stop the flow of blood into the aneurysm, causing it to deflate or obliterate. Proper placement causes aneurysm obliteration and avoids damage to the adjacent vessels or their branches. Once the clip is in place, the brain tissue is carefully lowered back into place, the various layers sutured closed, and the bone flap is reseated for healing. The skin and other outer layers are also sutured closed. Bandages protect the area during healing.

Aftercare

Many times a postoperative angiogram is performed to confirm good clip placement, total obliteration of the aneurysm, and continued blood flow through the neighboring vessels. Because of the unpredictable nature of

vessel behavior and the individual structure of each aneurysm, unexpected findings are seen in approximately 19% of postoperative angiograms. Patients stay in the hospital an average of 9.3 days after this procedure.

Risks

A major risk during surgery is a second rupture of the aneurysm during the procedure. Intraoperative rupture is very serious and associated with an approximately 30–35% morbidity and mortality of the patient. It is particularly dangerous if it occurs during the administration of the anesthesia or the opening of the dura mater because there will be a delay before the surgeon can control the bleeding.

Although much rarer than without surgical treatment, re-bleeding can occur even after surgery, particularly with improper placement of the clip. If too close to the parent vessel, the clip can block blood flow and promote brain damage in that area. If it is too far away from the parent vessel, a condition known as an aneurysmal rest can develop that will swell and rupture later. This re-bleeding can also be described as a stroke, and occurs in between 1% and 10% of surgical patients.

Again rarer than without treatment, patients having their aneurysm clipped can also develop vasospasm after the procedure. The presence of vasospasm increases the occurrence of re-bleeding as well, making it a particularly dangerous complication. Treatments for vasospasm include giving medications that relax the smooth muscles in vessel walls, administering intravenous fluids to increase blood volume, or using drugs to increase blood pressure. In some cases, it may be necessary to open the vessel with a balloon catheter, a procedure called **angioplasty**. Angioplasty carries with it its own significant risks, including the formation of blood clots and rupture of the artery, and is effective only in some cases.

Other risks of the surgical treatment of cerebral aneurysms include neurological damage over and above what had occurred with the rupture. Special surgical procedures such as the use of temporary clips on the parent vessel, reduction of the patient's blood pressure, and administration of drugs that increase the brain tissue's ability to survive without oxygen are some techniques that minimize the amount of damage. Hypothermia (reduction of the patient's temperature during surgery) is sometimes also utilized to reduce the chance of this risk.

As this surgery involves opening of the cranium (skull), the procedure carries an increased risk of infection of brain and spinal tissues. This surgery also has all the risks of any other invasive procedure, such as infection at the incision site, and risks associated with anesthesia.

Normal results

If the postoperative angiogram indicates the clip has been properly placed, the aneurysm has been totally obliterated, and vasospasm is avoided, most patients do extremely well. However, the results of the surgery are always limited by the amount of neurological damage that occurred with the rupture itself, as much of the damage is nonreversible with current treatment methods. This issue is not a consideration with elective repair of a pre-rupture aneurysm.

Morbidity and mortality rates

Despite advances in **microsurgery**, anesthetic techniques, and critical care, the morbidity and mortality rates of SAH remains high at 25–35% and 40–50%, respectively. Age and neurologic status on hospital admission continue to be the best predictors of outcome.

In contrast, the operative mortality rate for elective clipping is close to 0, with morbidity ranging between 0% and 10%, especially if the surgeon is experienced in the procedure and utilizes the latest microsurgical techniques. In this situation, morbidity is most closely related to aneurysm size and location. Generally, elective clipping of an unruptured aneurysm is associated with better outcomes than ruptured aneurysms because the brain has not been damaged by the SAH prior to the procedure.

Alternatives

A promising new alternative to open surgery is the use of inventional neuroradiology to treat aneurysms. The greatest advantages to this technique are that it is less invasive and requires less recovery time in most patients. This technique is also more effective than craniotomy for certain positions of aneurysms or for patients that have complicating conditions that would make them unable to tolerate the stress of the more traditional surgery. The decision of whether an aneurysm should be treated surgically with a clip or through inventional neuroradiological techniques should be made as a team by the neurosurgeon and the endovascular radiologist.

Inventional neuroradiology, also known as endovascular neuroradiology, utilizes fluoroscopic **angiography**, described as a diagnostic imaging technique. Besides delivering the contrast material, the catheter can be used to place small coils, known as Gugliemlimi detachable coils, within the neck of the aneurysm using a delivery wire. Once the coil has been maneuvered into place, an electrical charge is sent through the delivery wire. This charge disintegrates the stainless steel of the coil, separating it from the delivery wire, which is removed from the body, leaving the coil. Anywhere from one to 30 coils may be

necessary to block the neck of the aneurysm from the normal circulation and obliterate it, as occurs with the clip procedure. Although more research is needed to compare the two procedures, recent results indicate that intervention surgery for ruptured aneurysms may be safer than the traditionally more invasive procedure and may increase the chances of survival without disability after SAH.

> ## KEY TERMS
>
> **Computerized tomography (CT)**—A method of visualizing bleeding that has occurred in the brain.
>
> **Fluoroscopic angiogram**—A method of precisely visualizing the brain cardiovascular system and its defects, including aneurysms.
>
> **Gugliemlimi detachable coils**—A new method of treating aneurysms that is minimally invasive.
>
> **Magnetic resonance imaging (MRI)**—A method of visualizing the vessels in the brain that is particularly effective at locating unruptured aneurysms.
>
> **Subarachnoid hemorrhage**—Bleeding from a ruptured blood vessel in the brain that contaminates the cerebrospinal fluid.
>
> **Stroke**—A brain attack that can be caused by bleeding in the brain.
>
> **Vasospasm**—A deadly side effect of aneurysm rupture where the vessels in the brain spontaneously constrict; can cause brain damage or death.

Resources

BOOKS

Aldrich, E. Francois, et al. "Neurosurgery." In *Textbook of Surgery,* edited by Courtney m. Townsend. Philadelphia: W.B. Saunders Company, 2001.

Hoff, Julian T. and Michael F. Boland. "Neurosurgery." In *Principles of Surgery, Vol. 2,* edited by Seymour I. Schwartz. New York: McGraw-Hill, 1999.

PERIODICALS

"International Subarachnoid Aneurysm Trial (ISAT) of Neurosurgical Clipping versus Endovascular Coiling in 2143 Patients with Ruptured Intracranial Aneurysms: A Randomised Trial." *The Lancet* 360, no. 9342 (October 2002): 1267.

Pope, Wendi L. "Cerebral Vessel Repair with Coils & Glue." *Nursing* (July 2002): 47–49.

ORGANIZATIONS

American Association of Neurological Surgeons. <http://www.aans.org>.

American Society of Interventional and Therapeutic Neuroradiology. <http://www.asitn.org>.

OTHER

Greenberg, Mark S. *Handbook of Neurosurgery,* 1997 [cited March 1, 2003]. <http://www.grgraphics.com/site/HBNS/chapters/SAH/SAH_001.html>.

Michelle Johnson, MS, JD

Cerebrospinal fluid (CSF) analysis

Definition

Cerebrospinal fluid (CSF) analysis is a set of laboratory tests that examine a sample of the fluid surrounding the brain and spinal cord. This fluid is an ultrafiltrate of plasma. It is clear and colorless. It contains glucose, electrolytes, amino acids, and other small molecules found in plasma, but has very little protein and few cells. CSF protects the central nervous system from injury, cushions it from the surrounding bone structure, provides it with nutrients, and removes waste products by returning them to the blood. CSF is withdrawn from the subarachnoid space through a needle by a procedure called a lumbar puncture or spinal tap. CSF analysis includes tests in clinical chemistry, hematology, immunology, and microbiology. Usually three or four tubes are collected. The first tube is used for chemical and/or serological analysis and the last two tubes are used for hematology and microbiology tests. This reduces the chances of a falsely elevated white cell count caused by a traumatic tap (bleeding into the subarachnoid space at the puncture site), and contamination of the bacterial culture by skin germs or flora.

Purpose

The purpose of a CSF analysis is to diagnose medical disorders that affect the central nervous system. Some of these conditions are:

- meningitis and encephalitis, which may be viral, bacterial, fungal, or parasitic infections

- metastatic tumors (e.g., leukemia) and central nervous system tumors that shed cells into the CSF

- syphilis, a sexually transmitted bacterial disease

- bleeding (hemorrhaging) in the brain and spinal cord

- multiple sclerosis, a degenerative nerve disease that results in the loss of the myelin coating of the nerve fibers of the brain and spinal cord

- Guillain-Barré syndrome, a demyelinating disease involving peripheral sensory and motor nerves

Routine examination of CSF includes visual observation of color and clarity and tests for glucose, protein, lactate, lactate dehydrogenase, red blood cell count, white blood cell count with differential, syphilis serology (testing for antibodies indicative of syphilis), Gram stain, and bacterial culture. Further tests may need to be performed depending upon the results of initial tests and the presumptive diagnosis. For example, an abnormally high total protein seen in a patient suspected of having a demyelinating disease such as multiple sclerosis dictates CSF protein electrophoresis and measurement of immunoglobulin levels and myelin basic protein.

GROSS EXAMINATION. Color and clarity are important diagnostic characteristics of CSF. Straw, pink, yellow, or amber pigments (xanthochromia) are abnormal and indicate the presence of bilirubin, hemoglobin, red blood cells, or increased protein. Turbidity (suspended particles) indicates an increased number of cells. Gross examination is an important aid to differentiating a subarachnoid hemorrhage from a traumatic tap. The latter is often associated with sequential clearing of CSF as it is collected; streaks of blood in an otherwise clear fluid; or a sample that clots.

GLUCOSE. CSF glucose is normally approximately two-thirds of the fasting plasma glucose. A glucose level below 40 mg/dL is significant and occurs in bacterial and fungal meningitis and in malignancy.

PROTEIN. Total protein levels in CSF are normally very low, and albumin makes up approximately two-thirds of the total. High levels are seen in many conditions including bacterial and fungal meningitis, multiple sclerosis, tumors, subarachnoid hemorrhage, and traumatic tap.

LACTATE. The CSF lactate is used mainly to help differentiate bacterial and fungal meningitis, which cause increased lactate, from viral meningitis, which does not.

LACTATE DEHYDROGENASE. This enzyme is elevated in bacterial and fungal meningitis, malignancy, and subarachnoid hemorrhage.

WHITE BLOOD CELL (WBC) COUNT. The number of white blood cells in CSF is very low, usually necessitating a manual WBC count. An increase in WBCs may occur in many conditions including infection (viral, bacterial, fungal, and parasitic), allergy, leukemia, multiple sclerosis, hemorrhage, traumatic tap, encephalitis, and Guillain-Barré syndrome. The WBC differential helps to distinguish many of these causes. For example, viral infection is usually associated with an increase in lymphocytes, while bacterial and fungal infections are associated with an increase in polymorphonuclear leukocytes (neutrophils). The differential may also reveal eosinophils associated with allergy and ventricular shunts; macrophages with ingested bacteria (indicating meningitis), RBCs (indicating hemorrhage), or lipids (indicating possible cerebral infarction); blasts (immature cells) that indicate leukemia; and malignant cells characteristic of the tissue of origin. About 50% of metastatic cancers that infiltrate the central nervous system and about 10% of central nervous system tumors will shed cells into the CSF.

RED BLOOD CELL (RBC) COUNT. While not normally found in CSF, RBCs will appear whenever bleeding has occurred. Red cells in CSF signal subarachnoid hemorrhage, stroke, or traumatic tap. Since white cells may enter the CSF in response to local infection, inflammation, or bleeding, the RBC count is used to correct the WBC count so that it reflects conditions other than hemorrhage or a traumatic tap. This is accomplished by counting RBCs and WBCs in both blood and CSF. The ratio of RBCs in CSF to blood is multiplied by the blood WBC count. This value is subtracted from the CSF WBC count to eliminate WBCs derived from hemorrhage or traumatic tap.

GRAM STAIN. The Gram stain is performed on a sediment of the CSF and is positive in at least 60% of cases of bacterial meningitis. Culture is performed for both aerobic and anaerobic bacteria. In addition, other stains (e.g. the acid-fast stain for *Mycobacterium tuberculosis*, fungal culture, and rapid identification tests [tests for bacterial and fungal antigens]) may be performed routinely.

SYPHILIS SEROLOGY. This involves testing for antibodies that indicate neurosyphilis. The fluorescent treponemal antibody-absorption (FTA-ABS) test is often used and is positive in persons with active and treated syphilis. The test is used in conjunction with the VDRL test for nontreponemal antibodies, which is positive in most persons with active syphilis, but negative in treated cases.

Precautions

In some circumstances, a lumbar puncture to withdraw a small amount of CSF for analysis may lead to serious complications. Lumbar punctures should be performed only with extreme caution, and only if the benefits are thought to outweigh the risks. In people who have bleeding disorders, lumbar puncture can cause hemorrhage that can compress the spinal cord. If there is increased spinal column pressure, as may occur with a brain tumor and other conditions, removal of CSF can cause the brain to herniate, compressing the brain stem and other vital structures and leading to irreversible brain damage or death. Bacteria introduced during the puncture may cause meningitis. For this reason, **aseptic technique**

must be followed strictly, and a lumbar puncture should never be performed at the site of a localized skin lesion.

Specimens should be handled with caution to avoid contamination with skin flora. They should be refrigerated if analysis cannot be performed immediately.

Description

Lumbar puncture is performed by inserting the needle between the fourth and fifth lumbar vertabrae (L4-L5). This location is used because the spinal cord stops near L2, and a needle introduced below this level will miss the cord. In rare instances, such as a spinal fluid blockage in the middle of the back, a physician may perform a spinal tap in the cervical spine.

Aftercare

After the procedure, the site of the puncture is covered with a sterile bandage. The patient should remain lying down for four to six hours after the lumbar puncture. **Vital signs** should be monitored every 15 minutes for four hours, then every 30 minutes for another four hours. The puncture site should be observed for signs of weeping or swelling for 24 hours. The neurological status of the patient should also be evaluated for such symptoms as numbness and/or tingling in the lower extremities.

Risks

The most common side effect after the removal of CSF is a headache. This occurs in 10–30% of adult patients and in up to 40% of children. It is caused by a decreased CSF pressure related to a small leak of CSF through the puncture site. These headaches usually are a dull pain, although some people report a throbbing sensation. A stiff neck and nausea may accompany the headache. Lumbar puncture headaches typically begin within two days after the procedure and persist from a few days to several weeks or months.

Normal results

- Gross appearance: Normal CSF is clear and colorless.

- CSF opening pressure: 50–175 mm H_2O.

- Specific gravity: 1.006–1.009.

- Glucose: 40–80 mg/dL.

- Total protein: 15–45 mg/dL.

- LD: 1/10 of serum level.

- Lactate: less than 35 mg/dL.

- Leukocytes (white blood cells): 0–5/microL (adults and children); up to 30/microL (newborns).

KEY TERMS

Encephalitis—An inflammation or infection of the brain and spinal cord caused by a virus or as a complication of another infection.

Demyelination—The loss of myelin with preservation of the axons or fiber tracts. Central demyelination occurs within the central nervous system, and peripheral demyelination affects the peripheral nervous system as with Guillain-Barré syndrome.

Guillain-Barré syndrome—A demyelinating disease involving nerves that affect the extremities and causing weakness and motor and sensory dysfunction.

Meningitis—An infection of the membranes that cover the brain and spinal cord.

Multiple sclerosis—A disease that destroys the covering (myelin sheath) of nerve fibers of the brain and spinal cord.

Spinal canal—The cavity or hollow space within the spine that contains the spinal cord and the cerebrospinal fluid.

Subarachnoid—The space underneath the anachnoid membrane, a thin membrane enclosing the brain and spinal cord.

Treponeme—A term used to refer to any member of the genus *Treponema,* which is an anaerobic bacteria consisting of cells, 3–8 μm in length, with acute, regular, or irregular spirals and no obvious protoplasmic structure.

Vertebrae—The bones of the spinal column. There are 33 along the spine, with five (called L1-L5) making up the lower lumbar region.

- Differential: 60–80% lymphocytes; up to 30% monocytes and macrophages; other cells 2% or less. Monocytes and macrophages are somewhat higher in neonates.
- Gram stain: negative.
- Culture: sterile.
- Syphilis serology: negative.
- Red blood cell count: Normally, there are no red blood cells in the CSF unless the needle passes through a blood vessel on route to the CSF.

Resources

BOOKS

Braunwald, Eugene, et al., eds., "Approach to the Patient with Neurologic Disease." In *Harrison's Principles of Internal Medicine.* 15th ed. New York: McGraw-Hill, 2001.

Henry, J. B. *Clinical Diagnosis and Management by Laboratory Methods.* 20th ed. Philadelphia, PA: W. B. Saunders, 2001.

Kee, Joyce LeFever. *Handbook of Laboratory and Diagnostic Tests.* 4th ed. Upper Saddle River, NJ: Prentice Hall, 2001.

Smith, Gregory P., and Carl R. Kieldsberg. *Cerebrospinal, Synovial, and Serous Body Fluids.* Philadelphia, PA: W. B. Saunders, 2001.

Wallach, Jacques. *Interpretation of Diagnostic Tests.* 7th ed. Philadelphia, PA: Lippincott Williams & Wilkins, 2000.

OTHER

National Institutes of Health. March 14, 2003 [cited April 5, 2003]. <http://www.nlm.nih.gov/medlineplus/encyclopedia.html>.

Victoria E. DeMoranville
Mark A. Best

Cerebrospinal fluid shunt *see* **Ventricular shunt**

Cervical biopsy *see* **Cone biopsy**

Cervical cerclage

Definition

A cervical cerclage is a minor surgical procedure in which the opening to the uterus (the cervix) is stitched closed in order to prevent a miscarriage or premature birth.

Purpose

Approximately 10% of pregnancies end in preterm delivery, defined as a delivery that occurs before week 37 of pregnancy (the average pregnancy lasts 40 weeks). Premature birth is a major cause of serious health problems in neonates (newborn babies), including respiratory distress, difficulty regulating body temperature, and infection. More than 85% of long-term disabilities in otherwise healthy babies and 75% of deaths among newborns occur as a result of preterm delivery.

A woman with an incompetent cervix is 3.3 times more likely to deliver prematurely. The cervix is the neck-shaped opening at the lower part of the uterus and is normally closed tight during pregnancy until the baby is ready to be delivered, at which point it expands (dilates) to roughly 4 in (10 cm) in diameter. An incompetent cervix is prone to dilating and/or effacing (shortening) prematurely during the second trimester. The growing fetus subsequently places too great a strain on the cervix, leading to miscarriage (loss before week 20 of pregnancy) or premature delivery (loss after week 20). Approximately 1% of women will be diagnosed with an incompetent cervix (one in 500–2,000 pregnancies). It is the cause of 25% of losses during the second trimester.

A doctor might recommend a cerclage be performed if a woman has one or more of the following risk factors:

• a previous preterm delivery

• previous trauma or surgery to the cervix

• early rupture of membranes ("breaking water")

• hormonal influences

• abnormalities of the uterus or cervix

• exposure as a fetus to diethylstilbestrol (DES), a synthetic hormone that was used in the mid-twentieth century to treat recurrent miscarriages

Demographics

Racial and socioeconomic factors influence a woman's risk of delivering prematurely: African-American women are at more risk (16–18%) than white women (7–9%); women under 18 and over 35 are also at greater risk. Less educated women are more likely to deliver prematurely. Smoking during pregnancy is associated with a 20–30% greater risk of delivering prematurely. Male fetuses are more likely to be born prematurely and have a higher rate of fetal death than female fetuses (a difference of 2.8–9.8%).

Description

Elective cervical cerclage is a minor surgical procedure that is generally performed between 12 and 14 weeks of pregnancy (at the beginning of the second trimester) before symptoms of premature labor begin. Emergent cerclages are those placed later in pregnancy when cervical changes have already begun.

The patient will usually receive regional (epidural or spinal) anesthesia during the procedure, although general anesthesia is sometimes used. Spinal anesthesia involves inserting a needle into a region between the vertebrae of the lower back and injecting numbing medications. An epidural is similar to a spinal except that a catheter is inserted so that numbing medications may be administered as needed. Some women experience a drop in blood pressure when a regional anesthetic is administered; this effect can be countered with fluids and/or medications.

While there are numerous techniques for performing cerclage, the McDonald and Shirodkar techniques are the most common. The McDonald cerclage involves stitching the cervix with a 0.2 in (5 mm) band of suture. The cer-

clage is placed high on the cervix when the lower part has already started to efface. The stitch is usually removed around week 37 of pregnancy. The classic Shirodkar procedure involves a permanent "purse-string" stitch around the cervix; because it will not be removed, a **cesarean section** will be necessary to deliver the baby. Most Shirodkar cerclages are now performed with a modified technique that allows the sutures to be later removed.

Some less common methods of cerclage include:

• Hefner (or Wurm) cerclage (usually reserved for later in pregnancy when there is little cervix to work with)

• abdominal cerclage (a permanent stitch performed through an abdominal incision instead of the vagina; reserved for when a vaginal cerclage has failed or is not possible)

• Lash cerclage (a permanent stitch performed before pregnancy because of trauma to the cervix or an anatomical abnormality)

Diagnosis/Preparation

Diagnosis of an incompetent cervix is usually done by medical history and/or by examination (manually during a pelvic exam or using ultrasound technology). Some symptoms of an incompetent cervix used to decide if a cerclage is necessary are:

• cervical dilation

• shortening of the cervix

• funneling of 25% or more (when the internal opening of the cervix has begun to dilate but the external opening remains closed)

Women who are more than 1.5 in (4 cm) dilated, who have already experienced rupture of membranes, or whose fetus has died are ineligible for cerclage.

Before the procedure may be performed, there are a number of preparatory steps that must be taken. A complete medical history will be taken. A cervical exam will

QUESTIONS TO ASK THE DOCTOR

- How many cerclages do you perform each year?
- What is your rate of complications?
- Why is cerclage recommended for my particular condition?
- What are my options for anesthesia?
- After the cerclage is placed, do I have to alter my day-to-day routine?
- What alternatives to cerclage are available to me?

be necessary to assess the state of the cervix; usually a transvaginal (through the vagina) ultrasound will be performed. No food or drink will be allowed after midnight before the day of surgery to avoid nausea and vomiting during and after the procedure. The patient will also be instructed to avoid sexual intercourse, tampons, and douches for 24 hours before the procedure. Before the procedure is performed, an intravenous (IV) catheter will be placed in order to administrate fluids and medications.

Aftercare

After the cerclage has been placed, the patient will be observed for at least several hours (sometimes overnight) to ensure that she does not go into premature labor. The patient will then be allowed to return home, but will be instructed to remain in bed or avoid physical activity for two to three days. Follow-up appointments will usually take place so that her doctor can monitor the cervix and stitch and watch for signs of premature labor.

Risks

While cerclage is generally a safe procedure, there are a number of potential complications that may arise during or after surgery. These include:

- risks associated with regional or general anesthesia
- premature labor
- premature rupture of membranes
- infection of the cervix
- infection of the amniotic sac (chorioamnionitis)
- cervical rupture (may occur if the stitch is not removed before onset of labor)
- injury to the cervix or bladder
- bleeding

Normal results

The success rate for cervical cerclage is approximately 80–90% for elective cerclages, and 40–60% for emergent cerclages. A cerclage is considered successful if labor and delivery is delayed to at least 37 weeks (full term).

Morbidity and mortality rates

Approximately 1–9% of women will experience premature labor after cerclage. The risk of chorioamnionitis is 1–7%, but increases to 30% if the cervix is dilated greater than 1.2 in (3 cm). The risks associated with premature delivery, however, are far greater. Babies born between 22 and 25 weeks of pregnancy are at significant risk of moderate to severe disabilities (46–56%) or death (approximately 10–30% survive at 22 weeks, increasing to 50% at 24 weeks, and 95% by 26 weeks).

Alternatives

Depending on her specific condition, a woman may have some alternative therapies available to her to avoid or delay premature labor. These include:

- Bed rest. At least 20% of pregnant women in the United States have at least one week of bed rest prescribed to them at some point of their pregnancy. The idea of bed rest is to avoid putting unnecessary pressure on the cervix.
- Tocolytics. These are drugs that are designed to stop or delay labor. Ritrodrine, terbutaline, and magnesium sulfate are some common tocolytics.
- **Antibiotics.** Some infections are associated with a high risk of preterm labor (e.g., upper genital tract infection). Antibiotics may be successful in preventing preterm labor from occurring by treating the infection.

Resources

BOOKS

Enkin, Murray, et al. *A Guide to Effective Care in Pregnancy and Childbirth,* 3rd ed. Oxford: Oxford University Press, 2000.

PERIODICALS

Goldenberg, Robert L. "The Management of Preterm Labor." *Obstetrics & Gynecology* 100, no. 5 (November 2002): 1020–37.

MacDonald, Hugh. "Perinatal Care at the Threshold of Viability." *American Academy of Pediatrics* 110, no. 5 (November 2002): 1024–7.

Matijevic, Ratko, Branka Olujic, Jasua Tumbri, and Asim Kurjak. "Cervical Incompetence: The Use of Selective and Emergency Cerclage." *Journal of Perinatal Medicine* 29 (2001): 31–5.

Weismiller, David G. "Preterm Labor." *American Family Physician* February 1, 1999: 593–604.

ORGANIZATIONS

American Academy of Family Physicians. 8880 Ward Parkway, Kansas City, MO 64114. (816) 333-9700. <http://www.aafp.org>.

American Board of Obstetrics and Gynecology. 2915 Vine Street, Dallas, TX 75204. (214) 871-1619. <http://www.abog.org>.

American College of Obstetricians and Gynecologists. 409 12th St., SW, PO Box 96920, Washington, DC 20090-6920. <http://www.acog.org>.

OTHER

Bernstein, Peter S. "Controversies in Obstetrics: Cervical Cerclage." *Third World Congress on Controversies in Obstetrics, Gynecology, and Infertility.* 2002 [cited March 1, 2003]. <http://www.medscape.com/viewprogram/1964>.

Pincock, Stephen. "Cervical Cerclage Associated with Good Pregnancy Outcome." *Reuters Health.* February 13, 2003 [cited March 1, 2003]. <http://www.medscape.com/viewarticle/449414>.

"Shortened Cervix in Second Trimester Possible Warning Sign for Premature Birth." *National Institute of Child Health and Development.* September 18, 2001 [cited March 1, 2003]. <http://www.nichd.nih.gov/new/releases/cervix.cfm>.

Starzyk, Kathryn A. and Carolyn M. Salafia. "A Perinatal Pathology View of Preterm Labor." *Medscape Women's Health eJournal.* 2000 [cited March 1, 2003]. <http://www.medscape.com/viewarticle/408936_1>.

Weiss, Robin Elise. "The Incompetent Cervix." [cited March 1, 2003.] <http://pregnancy.about.com/library/weekly/aa011298.htm>.

Stephanie Dionne Sherk

Cervical cryotherapy

Definition

Cervical **cryotherapy** is a procedure which involves freezing an area of abnormal tissue on the cervix. This tissue gradually disappears and the cervix heals. One cervical cryotherapy is usually sufficient to destroy the abnormal tissue.

Purpose

Cervical cryotherapy is a standard method used to treat cervical dysplasia, meaning the removal of abnormal cell tissue on the cervix.

Description

Cervical cryotherapy, or freezing, usually lasts about five minutes and causes a slight amount of discomfort. The procedure is usually performed in an outpatient setting.

Cervical cryotherapy is done by placing a small freeze-probe (cryoprobe) against the cervix that cools the cervix to sub-zero temperatures. The cells destroyed by freezing are shed afterwards in a heavy watery discharge. The main advantage of cryotherapy is that it is a simple procedure that requires inexpensive equipment.

The cryogenic device consists of a gas tank containing a refrigerant and non-explosive, non-toxic gas (usually nitrous oxide). The gas is delivered using flexible tubing through a gun-type attachment to the cryoprobe.

Diagnosis/Preparation

Women who undergo cervical cryotherapy typically have had an abnormal Pap smear which has led to a diag-

WHO PERFORMS THE PROCEDURE AND WHERE IS IT PERFORMED?

Cervical cryotherapy can be done in the treating physician's office. The physician is usually a gynecologist.

QUESTIONS TO ASK
THE DOCTOR

- How is cervical cryotherapy performed?
- Why is cryotherapy required?
- What are the risks of cryotherapy?
- Is cryotherapy painful?
- What is the purpose of my cryotherapy?
- How long will it take to recover from the surgery?
- What are the after-effects of cryotherapy?
- How much cervical cryotherapy do you perform each year?

nosis of cervical squamous dysplasia and usually confirmed by biopsy after an adequate colposcopic exam.

Preparation for cervical cryotherapy involves scheduling the procedure when the patient is not experiencing heavy menstrual flow. Ibuprofen, ketoprofen, or naproxen sodium may be given before cryotherapy to decrease cramping. If there is any doubt about the pregnancy status, a pregnancy test is performed.

Aftercare

Cervical cryotherapy is often followed by a heavy and often odorous discharge during the first month after the procedure. The discharge is due to the dead tissue cells leaving the treatment site, and Aminocerv cream may be prescribed. The patient should abstain from sexual intercourse and not use tampons for a period of three weeks after the procedure. Excessive **exercise** should also be avoided to lessen the occurrence of post-therapy bleeding.

Risks

The following risks have been associated with cervical cryotherapy:

- Uterine cramping. Often occurs during the cryotherapy but rapidly subsides after treatment.

- Bleeding and infection. Rare, but incidences have been reported.

- More difficult Pap smears. Future Pap smears and **colposcopy** may be more difficult after cryotherapy.

Normal results

A normal result is no recurrence of the abnormal cervix cells. The first follow-up Pap smear is done with-

in three to six months. If normal, Pap smears are repeated every six months for two years. If any, recurrences usually occur within two years of treatment. Another option is to replace the initial and each yearly Pap smear with a colposcopic examination.

If a follow-up Pap smear is abnormal, a colposcopy with biopsy is usually performed. Other treatment methods, usually the loop electrocautery excision procedure (LEEP) are then used if persistent disease is discovered.

Following the procedure, it is considered normal to experience the following:

- slight cramping for two to three days
- watery discharge requiring several pad changes daily
- bloody discharge, especially 12–16 days after the procedure

Alternatives

Alternatives to cryotherapy include:

- Laser treatment. A carbon dioxide laser focuses a beam of light to vaporize the abnormal cells. This technique can be used in the physician's office with very little discomfort.

- Loop electrocautery excision procedure (LEEP). This procedure uses a fine wire loop with an electric current flowing through it to remove the desired area of the cervix. Loop excision is usually done under local anesthesia and causes very little discomfort.

See also Colposcopy; Cone biopsy; Cryotherapy.

Resources

BOOKS

Handley, J. *What Your Doctor May Not Tell You about HPV and Abnormal Pap Smears.* New York: Warner Books, 2002.

Platzer, W., et al. *Vaginal Operations: Surgical Anatomy and Technique.* Philadelphia: Lippincott, Williams and Wilikins, 1996.

Rushing, L., and N. Joste. *Abnormal Pap Smears: What Every Woman Needs to Know.* Amherst, NY: Prometheus Books, 2001.

PERIODICALS

Sparks, R. A., D. Scheid, V. Loemker, E. Stader, K. Reilly, R. Hamm, and L. McCarthy. "Association of Cervical Cryotherapy with Inadequate Follow-up Colposcopy." *Journal of Family Practice* 51 (June 2002): 526–529.

Tate, D. R. and R. J. Anderson. "Recrudescence of Cervical Dysplasia among Women Who are Infected with the Human Immunodeficiency Virus: A Case-control Analysis." *American Journal of Obstetrics and Gynecology* 186 (May 2002): 880–882.

ORGANIZATIONS

American Society for Colposcopy and Cervical Pathology. 20 West Washington St., Suite 1, Hagerstown, MD 21740. (301) 733-3640. <http://www.asccp.org/index.html>

KEY TERMS

Biopsy—Procedure that involves obtaining a tissue specimen for microscopic analysis to establish a precise diagnosis.

Cervix—Opening of the uterus (womb) that leads into the vagina.

Colposcopy—Examination of the cervix through a magnifying device to detect abnormal cells.

Cryotherapy—The therapeutic use of cold to reduce discomfort, or remove abnormal tissue.

Dysplasia—Abnormality of development, or change in size, shape, and organization of adult cells.

Electrocautery—The cauterization of tissue using an electric current that generates heat.

Loop electrocautery excision procedure (LEEP)—Electrocautery performed to excise abnormal cervical tissue.

Pap smear—A test performed using a special stain applied on a smear taken from the cervix.

Squamous cells—Scaly or plate-like cells.

National Association for Women's Health. 300 W. Adams Street, Suite 328, Chicago, IL 60606-5101. (312) 786-1468. <http://www.nawh.org>

OTHER

"Cervical Cancer Prevention." *JHPIEG*. September 2002 [cited April 2003]. <http://www.jhpiego.jhu.edu/cecap>.

"Cytopathology." *The Internet Pathology Laboratory for Medical Education* [cited April 2003]. <http//www-medlib.med.utah.edu/WebPath/TUTORIAL/CYTOPATH/CYTOPATH.html>.

Mayeaux Jr., E. J., M.D. "Cervical Cryotherapy Atlas." *LSUHSC-S Family Medicine Server* [cited April 2003]. <http://lib-sh.lsumc.edu/fammed/atlases/cryo.html>.

National Women's Health Information Center [cited April 2003]. <http://www.4woman.org>.

"What is cervical dysplasia?" *AMA Medical Library* [cited April 2003]. <http://www.medem.com>.

Monique Laberge, Ph. D.

Cesarean section

Definition

A cesarean section is a surgical procedure in which incisions are made through a woman's abdomen and uterus to deliver her baby.

Purpose

Cesarean sections, also called c-sections or cesarean deliveries, are performed whenever abnormal conditions complicate labor and vaginal delivery, threatening the life or health of the mother or the baby. Dystocia, or difficult labor, is the other common cause of c-sections. The procedure is performed in the United States on nearly one of every four babies delivered—more than 900,000 babies each year. The procedure is often used in cases where the mother has had a previous c-section.

The most common reason that a cesarean section is performed (in 35% of all cases, according to the United States Public Health Service) is the woman has had a previous c-section. The "once a cesarean, always a cesarean" rule originated when the uterine incision was made vertically (termed a "classical incision"); the resulting scar was weak and had a risk of rupturing in subsequent deliveries. Today, the incision is almost always made horizontally across the lower end of the uterus (called a low transverse incision), resulting in reduced blood loss and a decreased chance of rupture. This kind of incision allows many women to have a vaginal birth after a cesarean (VBAC).

The second most common reason that a c-section is performed (in 30% of all cases) is difficult childbirth due to non-progressive labor (dystocia). Difficult labor is commonly caused by one of the three following conditions: abnormalities in the mother's birth canal; abnormalities in the position of the fetus; or abnormalities in the labor, including weak or infrequent contractions. The mother's pelvic structure may not allow adequate passage for birth. When the baby's head is too large to fit through the pelvis, the condition is called cephalopelvic disproportion (CPD).

Another 12% of c-sections are performed to deliver a baby in a breech presentation (buttocks or feet first). Breech presentation is found in about 3% of all births.

In 9% of all cases, c-sections are performed in response to fetal distress, which refers to any situation that threatens the baby such as the umbilical cord wrapped around the baby's neck. This may appear on the fetal heart monitor as an abnormal heart rate or rhythm. Fetal brain damage can result from oxygen deprivation. Fetal distress is often related to abnormalities in the position of the fetus or abnormalities in the birth canal, causing reduced blood flow through the placenta.

The remaining 14% of c-sections are indicated by other serious factors. One is prolapse of the umbilical cord: the cord is pushed into the vagina ahead of the baby and becomes compressed, cutting off blood flow to the baby. Another is "placental abruption," whereby the placenta separates from the uterine wall before the baby is

Baby emerging from the mother's abdomen during a cesarean section. *(Photograph by John Smith. Custom Medical Stock Photo. Reproduced by permission.)*

born, cutting off blood flow to the baby. The risk of this is especially high in multiple births (twins, triplets, or more). A third factor is "placenta previa," in which the placenta covers the cervix partially or completely, making vaginal delivery impossible. In some cases requiring c-section, the baby is in a transverse position, lying horizontally across the pelvis, perhaps with a shoulder in the birth canal.

The mother's health may make delivery by c-section the safer choice, especially in cases of maternal diabetes, hypertension, genital herpes, malignancies of the genital tract, and preeclampsia (high blood pressure related to pregnancy).

Choosing cesarean section

A 1997 survey of female obstetricians found that 31% would choose to have a c-section without trial of labor if they had an uncomplicated pregnancy. This finding mirrors a growing movement to allow women the right to choose c-section over vaginal delivery, even when no indications for c-section exist.

There are a number of reasons why a woman might choose a c-section in the absence of the usual indications. These include:

- Convenience. A scheduled c-section would allow a woman to choose the time and date of delivery to avoid conflicting with work or family obligations.

- Fear of childbirth. A woman might fear the pain of labor and delivery and feel that a scheduled c-section would allow her to circumvent it.

- Avoiding risks of vaginal delivery. Certain risks inherent to vaginal delivery (urinary or rectal incontinence, sexual dysfunction, dystocia) are avoided in a c-section.

Demographics

Women of higher socioeconomic status are more likely to have a c-section, 22.9%, compared to 13.2% of women who live in low-income families. C-section rates are highest among non-Hispanic white women (20.6%). Asian-American women have a c-section rate of 19.2%; African-American women, a rate of 18.9%, and Hispanic women, a rate of 13.9%.

Description

Regional anesthesia, either a spinal or epidural, is the preferred method of pain relief during a c-section. The benefits of regional anesthesia include allowing the mother to be awake during the surgery, avoiding the risks of general anesthesia, and allowing early contact between mother and child. Spinal anesthesia involves inserting a needle into a region between the vertebrae of the lower back and injecting numbing medications. An epidural is similar to a spinal except that a catheter is inserted so that numbing medications may be administered continuously. Some women experience a drop in blood pressure when a regional anesthetic is administered; this can be countered with fluids and/or medications.

In some instances, use of general anesthesia may be indicated. General anesthesia can be more rapidly administered in the case of an emergency (e.g., severe fetal distress). If the mother has a coagulation disorder that would be complicated by a drop in blood pressure (a risk with regional anesthesia), general anesthesia is an alternative. A major drawback of general anesthesia is that the procedure carries with it certain risks such as pulmonary aspiration and failed intubation. The baby may also be affected by the anesthetics since they cross the placenta; this effect is generally mild if delivery occurs within 10 minutes after anesthesia is administered.

Once the patient has received anesthesia, the abdomen is washed with an antibacterial solution and a portion of the pubic hair may be shaved. The first incision opens the abdomen. Infrequently, it will be vertical from just below the navel to the top of the pubic bone or, more commonly, it will be a horizontal incision across and above the pubic bone (informally called a "bikini cut").

The second incision opens the uterus. In most cases, a transverse incision is made. This is the favored type because it heals well and makes it possible for a woman to attempt a vaginal delivery in the future. The classical incision is vertical. Because it provides a larger opening

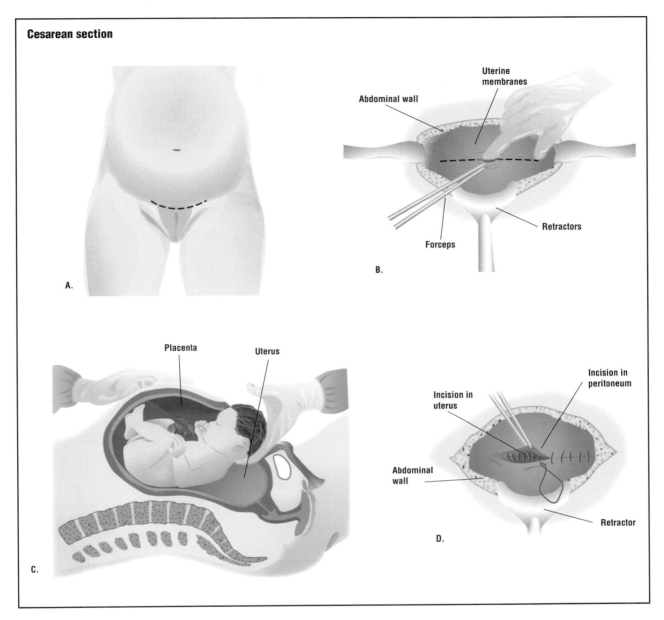

Cesarean section

A.

Abdominal wall
Uterine membranes
Forceps
Retractors
B.

Placenta
Uterus
C.

Incision in uterus
Incision in peritoneum
Abdominal wall
Retractor
D.

To remove a baby by cesarean section, an incision is made into the abdomen, usually just above the pubic hairline (A). The uterus is located and divided (B), allowing for delivery of the baby (C). After all the contents of the uterus are removed, the uterus is repaired, and the rest of the layers of the abdominal wall are closed (D). *(Illustration by GGS Inc.)*

than a low transverse incision, it is used in the most critical situations such as placenta previa. However, the classic incision causes more bleeding, a greater risk of abdominal infection, and a weaker scar.

Once the uterus is opened, the amniotic sac is ruptured and the baby is delivered. The time from the initial incision to birth is typically five minutes. The umbilical cord is clamped and cut, and the newborn is evaluated. The placenta is removed from the mother, and her uterus and abdomen are stitched closed (surgical staples may be

used instead in closing the outermost layer of the abdominal incision). From birth through suturing may take 30–40 minutes; the entire surgical procedure may be performed in less than one hour.

Diagnosis/Preparation

There are several ways that obstetricians and other doctors diagnose conditions that may make a c-section necessary. Ultrasound testing reveals the positions of the baby and the placenta and may be used to estimate the baby's size and gestational age. Fetal heart monitors, in use since the 1970s, transmit any signals of fetal distress. Oxygen deprivation may be determined by checking the amniotic fluid for meconium (feces); a lack of oxygen may cause an unborn baby to defecate. Oxygen deprivation may also be determined by testing the pH of a blood sample taken from the baby's scalp; a pH of 7.25 or higher is normal, between 7.2 and 7.25 is suspicious, and below 7.2 is a sign of trouble.

When a c-section becomes necessary, the mother is prepped for surgery. A catheter is inserted into her bladder and an intravenous (IV) line is inserted into her arm. Leads for monitoring the mother's heart rate, rhythm, and blood pressure are attached. In the **operating room**, the mother is given anesthesia, usually a regional anesthetic (epidural or spinal), making her numb from below her breasts to her toes. In some cases, a general anesthetic will be administered. Surgical drapes are placed over the body, except the head; these drapes block the direct view of the procedure.

Aftercare

A woman who undergoes a c-section requires both the care given to any new mother and the care given to any patient recovering from major surgery. She should be offered pain medication that does not interfere with breastfeeding. She should be encouraged to get out of bed and walk around eight to 24 hours after surgery to stimulate circulation (thus avoiding the formation of blood clots) and bowel movement. She should limit climbing stairs to once a day, and avoid lifting anything heavier than the baby. She should nap as often as the baby sleeps, and arrange for help with the housework, meals, and care of other children. She may resume driving after two weeks, although some doctors recommend waiting for six weeks, the typical recovery period from major surgery.

Risks

Because a c-section is a surgical procedure, it carries more risk to both the mother and the baby. The maternal death rate is less than 0.02%, but that is four times the maternal death rate associated with vaginal delivery. Complications occur in less than 10% of cases.

The mother is at risk for increased bleeding (a c-section may result in twice the blood loss of a vaginal delivery) from the two incisions, the placental attachment site, and possible damage to a uterine artery. The mother may develop infection of the incision, the urinary tract, or the tissue lining the uterus (endometritis); infections occur in approximately 7% of women after having a c-section. Less commonly, she may receive injury to the surrounding organs such as the bladder and bowel. When a general anesthesia is used, she may experience complications from the anesthesia. Very rarely, she may develop a wound hematoma at the site of either incision or other blood clots leading to pelvic thrombophlebitis (inflammation of the major vein running from the pelvis into the leg) or a pulmonary embolus (a blood clot lodging in the lung).

Undergoing a c-section may also inflict psychological distress on the mother, beyond hormonal mood swings and postpartum depression ("baby blues"). The woman may feel disappointment and a sense of failure for not experiencing a vaginal delivery. She may feel isolated if the father or birthing coach is not with her in the operating room, or if an unfamiliar doctor treats her rather than her own doctor or midwife. She may feel helpless from a loss of control over labor and delivery with no opportunity to actively participate. To overcome these feelings, the woman must understand why the c-section was necessary. She must accept that she could not control the unforeseen events that made the c-section the optimum means of delivery, and recognize that preserving the health and safety of both her and her child was more important than her delivering vaginally. Women who undergo a c-section should be encouraged to share their feelings with others. Hospitals can often recommend support groups for such mothers. Women should also be encouraged to seek professional help if negative emotions persist.

Normal results

The after-effects of a c-section vary, depending on the woman's age, physical fitness, and overall health. Following this procedure, a woman commonly experiences gas pains, incision pain, and uterine contractions (also common in vaginal delivery). Her hospital stay may be two to four days. Breastfeeding the baby is encouraged, taking care that it is in a position that keeps the baby from resting on the mother's incision. As the woman heals, she may gradually increase appropriate exercises to regain abdominal tone. Full recovery may be achieved in four to six weeks.

The prognosis for a successful vaginal birth after a cesarean (VBAC) may be at least 75%, especially when the c-section involved a low transverse incision in the uterus and there were no complications during or after delivery.

Morbidity and mortality rates

Surgical injuries to the ureter or bowel occur in approximately 0.1% of c-sections. The risk of infection to the incision ranges from 2.5% to 15%. Urinary tract infections occur in 2–16% of patients post-c-section. The risk for developing a deep-vein thrombosis is three to five times higher in patients undergoing c-section than vaginal delivery.

Of the hundreds of thousands of women in the United States who undergo a c-section each year, about 500 die from serious infections, hemorrhaging, or other complications. The overall maternal mortality rate is estimated to be between six and 22 deaths per 100,000 births; approximately one-third of maternal deaths that occur after c-section can be attributed to the procedure. These deaths may be related to the health conditions that made the operation necessary, and not simply to the operation itself.

Alternatives

When a c-section is being considered because labor is not progressing, the mother should first be encouraged to walk around to stimulate labor. Labor may also be stimulated with the drug oxytocin. A woman should receive regular prenatal care and be able to alert her doctor to the first signs of trouble. Once labor begins, she should be encouraged to move around and to urinate. The doctor should be conservative in diagnosing dystocia and fetal distress, taking a position of "watchful waiting" before deciding to operate.

Approximately 3–4% of babies present at term in the breech position. Before opting to perform an elective c-section, the doctor may first attempt to reposition the baby; this is called external cephalic version. The doctor may also try a vaginal breech delivery, depending on the size of the mother's pelvis, the size of the baby, and the type of breech position the baby is in. However, a c-section is safer than a vaginal delivery when the baby is 8 lb (3.6 kg) or larger, in a breech position with the feet crossed, or in a breech position with the head hyperextended.

A vaginal birth after cesarean (VBAC) is an option for women who have had previous c-sections and are in-

QUESTIONS TO ASK THE DOCTOR

- What is your medical training and how many c-sections have you performed?
- What percentage of women receive c-sections in your practice?
- If I have an elective c-section, what happens if I go into labor before the procedure is scheduled?
- What options are available to me for pain relief during and after the c-section?
- May a person of my choice remain with me during the procedure?
- When will I be able to hold/breastfeed my child?

terested in a trial of labor (TOL). TOL is a purposeful attempt to deliver vaginally. The success rate for VBAC in patients who have had a prior low transverse uterine incision is approximately 70%. The most severe risk associated with TOL is uterine rupture: 0.2–1.5% of attempted VBACs among women with a low transverse uterine scar will end in uterine rupture, compared to 12% of women with a classic uterine incision. To minimize this risk, the American College of Obstetricians and Gynecologists (ACOG) recommends that VBAC be limited to women with full-term pregnancies (37–40 weeks) who have only had one previous low transverse c-section.

Resources

BOOKS

Enkin, Murray, et al. *A Guide to Effective Care in Pregnancy and Childbirth,* 3rd ed. Oxford: Oxford University Press, 2000.

PERIODICALS

Harer, W. Benson. "Vaginal Birth After Cesarean Delivery: Current Status." *Journal of the American Medical Association* 287, no. 20 (May 2002).

Murphy, Deirdre, Rachel Liebling, Lisa Verity, Rebecca Swingler, and Roshni Patel. "Early Maternal and Neonatal Morbidity Associated with Operative Delivery in Second Stage of Labour: A Cohort Study." *The Lancet* 358 (October 13, 2001): 1203–07.

Wagner, Marsden. "Choosing Cesarean Section." *The Lancet* 356 (November 11, 2000): 1677–80.

Yokoe, Deborah, et al. "Epidemiology of and Surveillance for Postpartum Infections." *Emerging Infectious Diseases* 7, no. 5 (2001).

KEY TERMS

Breech presentation—The condition in which the baby enters the birth canal with its buttocks or feet first.

Cephalopelvic disproportion (CPD)—The condition in which the baby's head is too large to fit through the mother's pelvis.

Classic incision—In a cesarean section, an incision made vertically along the uterus.

Dystocia—Failure to progress in labor, either because the cervix will not dilate (expand) further or (after full dilation) the head does not descend through the mother's pelvis.

Hematoma—A collection of blood localized to an organ, tissue, or space of the body.

Low transverse incision—Incision made horizontally across the lower end of the uterus.

Placenta previa—The placenta totally or partially covers the cervix, preventing vaginal delivery.

Placental abruption—Separation of the placenta from the uterine wall before the baby is born, cutting off blood flow to the baby.

Preeclampsia—A pregnancy-related condition that causes high blood pressure and swelling.

Prolapsed cord—The umbilical cord is pushed into the vagina ahead of the baby and becomes compressed, cutting off blood flow to the baby.

Respiratory distress syndrome (RDS)—Difficulty breathing; found in infants with immature lungs.

Transverse presentation—The baby is laying sideways across the cervix instead of head first.

VBAC—Vaginal birth after cesarean.

ORGANIZATIONS

American Academy of Family Physicians. 8880 Ward Parkway, Kansas City, MO 64114. (816) 333-9700. <http://www.aafp.org>.

American Board of Obstetrics and Gynecology. 2915 Vine Street, Dallas, TX 75204. (214) 871-1619. <http://www.abog.org>.

American College of Obstetricians and Gynecologists. 409 12th St., SW, PO Box 96920, Washington, DC 20090-6920. <http://www.acog.org>.

International Cesarean Awareness Network. 1304 Kingsdale Ave., Redondo Beach, CA 90278. (310) 542-6400. <http://www.ican-online.org>.

OTHER

"Cesarean Birth." *American College of Obstetricians and Gynecologists,* March 1999 [cited February 26, 2003]. <http://www.medem.com>.

Duriseti, Ram. "Cesarean Section." *eMedicine,* August 29, 2001 [cited February 26, 2003]. <http://www.emedicine.com/aaem/topic99.htm>.

Sehdev, Harish. "Cesarean Delivery." *eMedicine,* February 22, 2002 [cited February 26, 2003]. <http://www.emedicine.com/med/topic3283.htm>.

Bethany Thivierge
Stephanie Dionne Sherk

Charts *see* **Medical charts**

Cheiloplasty *see* **Cleft lip repair**

Chemical debridement *see* **Debridement**

Chest radiography *see* **Chest x ray**

Chest surgery *see* **Thoracic surgery**

Chest tube insertion

Definition

A chest tube insertion is a procedure to place a flexible, hollow drainage tube into the chest in order to remove an abnormal collection of air or fluid from the pleural space (located between the inner and outer lining of the lung).

Purpose

Chest tube insertions are usually performed as an emergency procedure. Chest tubes are used to treat conditions that can cause the lung to collapse, which occurs because blood or air in the pleural space can hamper the ability of a patient to breath.

There are four common conditions than can require surgical chest tube insertion, including:

• pneumothorax (air leak from the lung into the chest)

• hemothorax (bleeding into the chest)

• empyema (lung abscess or pus in the chest)

• pneumothorax or hemothorax after surgery or from trauma to the chest

Demographics

There is no available data concerning the demographics of chest tube insertion since this is a common procedure performed in emergency rooms and surgical departments. However, pneumothorax seems to occur most often in males 25–40 years of age.

Description

The point of insertion in the chest most commonly occurs on the side (lateral thorax), at a line drawn from the armpit (anterior axillary line) to the side (lateral) of the nipple in males, or to the side (about 2 in [5 cm]) above the sternoxiphoid junction (lower junction of the sternum, or chest bone) in females. The skin is sterilized with antiseptic solution covering a wide area, and local anesthesia is administered to minimize discomfort. At the rib chosen for insertion, the skin over the rib is anesthetized with lidocaine (a local chemical anesthetic agent) using a 10-cc syringe and 25-gauge needle. At the rib below the rib chosen for pleural insertion, the tissues, muscles, bone, and lining covering the lung are also anesthetized using a 22-gauge needle.

All health-care providers will take precautions to keep the procedure sterile, including the usage of sterile gown, facemask, and eye protection. All equipment must be sterile as well and universal precautions are followed for blood and body fluids. Chest tube size is selected depending on the problem; an 18–20 F(rench) catheter is used for pneumothorax, a 32–26 F catheter for hemothorax, and trauma patients usually require a 38–40 F catheter size; children generally require smaller tube sizes.

The patient's arm is placed over the head with a restraint on the affected side. For an insertion line down the armpit (axillary line insertion), the patient's head is elevated from the bed 30–60°. Using the anesthetic needle and syringe, the physician will insert a needle (aspirate) into the pleural cavity to check for the presence of air or fluid. Then, an incision is made and a clamp is used to open the pleural cavity. At this stage, either air or fluid will rush out when the pleural cavity is opened. The chest tube is positioned for insertion with a clamp and attached to the suction-drain system. A silk suture is used to hold the tube firmly in place. The area is wrapped and an x ray is taken to visualize the status of the tube placement.

Diagnosis/Preparation

The diagnosis for chest tube insertion depends on the primary cause of fluid or air in the pleural cavity. For malignancy (cancer)-causing pleural effusion (fluid in the pleural space filled with malignant cells), the diagno-

sis can be established with positive cytopathology (cancer cell visualization and analysis) and a **chest x ray** that shows fluid accumulation.

The typical diagnostic signs and symptoms of empyema (lung infection) include fever, cough, and sputum discharge as well as the development of pleural effusion (causing chest pain and shortness of breath). This type of lung infection can progress to systemic disease with such signs as weakness, and loss of appetite (anorexia). Chest x rays can readily allow the clinician to view the pleural effusion and can also help to detect pneumothorax, since there is visual proof in the displacement of the tissues covering the lungs as a result of air in the pleural cavity. Additionally, during physical examinations, people with pnemothorax have diminished breath sounds, hyperesonance on percussion (a highly resonating sound when the physician taps gently on a patient's back), and diminished ability to expand the chest. Computed axial tomography (CAT) scans can be used to visualize and analyze complicated cases that may require chest tube insertion.

Aftercare

The chest tube typically remains secure and in place until imaging studies such as x rays show that air or fluid has been removed from the pleural cavity. This removal of air or fluid will allow the affected lung to fully re-expand, allowing for adequate or improved breathing. After chest tube insertion, the patient will stay in the hospital until the tube is removed. It is common to expect complete recovery from chest tube insertion and removal. During the stay, the medical and nursing staff will carefully and periodically monitor the chest tube for air leaks or if the patient is having breathing difficulties. Deep breathing and coughing after insertion can help with drainage and lung re-expansion.

Aftercare should also include chest tube removal and follow-up care. The patient is placed in the same po-

KEY TERMS

Clavicle—Also called the collar bone, it is a doubly curved long bone that connects the upper limb to the trunk.

Diminished breath sounds—A lack of breath sound due to fluid or air accumulation.

Diminished chest expansion—A decrease in the chest expansion due to an inability of the lungs to fully take in air.

Hyperesonance on percussion—A highly resonating sound when the physician taps gently on a patient's back; this is not a normal finding and should be investigated with an x ray.

Intercostal artery—Runs from the aorta.

Sternoxiphoid junction—The lower junction of the sternum or breast bone.

sition in which the tube was inserted. Using precautions to maintain a sterile field, the suture holding the tube in place is loosened and the chest is prepared for tying the insertion-point wound. The chest tube is then clamped to disconnect the suction system. At this point, the patient will be asked to hold his or her breath, and the clinician will remove the tube with a swift motion. After the suture is tied, dressing (gauze with antibiotic ointment) and tape is securely applied to close the wound. A chest x ray should be repeated soon after tube removal and, within 48 hours, a routine **wound care** clinic follow-up is advised to remove the dressing and to further assess the patient's medical status and condition.

Risks

Although chest tube insertion is a commonly used as a therapeutic measure, there are several complications that can develop, including:

- bleeding from an injured intercostal artery (running from the aorta)
- accidental injury to the heart, arteries, or lung resulting from the chest tube insertion
- a local or generalized infection from the procedure
- persistent or unexplained air leaks in the tube
- the tube can be dislodged or inserted incorrectly
- insertion of chest tube can cause open or tension pneumothorax

Normal results

Chest tube insertion is a commonly used procedure, and it is typical for patients to recover fully from insertion and removal. If no complications develop, the procedure can relieve air or fluid accumulation in the pleural cavity that caused breathing impairment. Breathing is usually improved, and follow-up within the immediate 48 hours after hospital discharge is advised so that the patient can be further assessed with x rays and in the wound care clinic.

Morbidity and mortality rates

Mortality and morbidity for chest tube insertion is not strongly associated with the procedure itself. The primary cause responsible for fluid or air accumulation in the pleural cavity is related to continued illness and outcome such as pleural effusions caused by cancer (malignant pleural effusions). Cancer, and not the insertion of a chest tube, determines a patient's sickness and outcome. Chest tube insertion may be problematic in persons affected with certain connective tissue diseases.

Alternatives

The diagnosis, indications, and procedure for chest tube insertion are specific and unambiguous. There is no other alternative to rapidly remove accumulation of fluid or air within the pleural cavity.

Resources

BOOKS

Pfenninger, John. *Procedures for Primary Care Physicians,* 1st Edition. St Louis: Mosby-Year Book, Inc., 1994.

Townsend, Courtney. *Sabiston Textbook of Surgery,* 16th Edition. St. Louis: W. B. Saunders Company, 2001.

ORGANIZATIONS

American Thoracic Society Homepage. <http://www.thoracic.org>.

Laith Farid Gulli, MD
Nicole Mallory, MS, PA-C
Alfredo Mori, MBBS

Chest x ray

Definition

A chest x ray is a procedure used to evaluate organs and structures within the chest for symptoms of disease. Chest x rays include views of the lungs, heart, small portions of the gastrointestinal tract, thyroid gland, and the bones of the chest area. X rays are a form of radiation that can penetrate the body and produce an image on an x-ray film. Another name for the film produced by x rays is radiograph.

Purpose

Chest x rays are ordered for a wide variety of diagnostic purposes. In fact, this is probably the most frequently performed type of x ray. In some cases, chest x rays are ordered for a single check of an organ's condition, and at other times, serial x rays are ordered to compare to previous studies. Some common reasons for chest x rays include the following.

Pulmonary disorders

Chest films are frequently ordered to diagnose or rule out pneumonia. One type, tuberculosis, can be observed on chest x rays, as can cardiac disease and damage to the ribs or lungs. Other pulmonary disorders such as pneumothorax (presence of air or gas in the chest cavity outside the lungs) or emphysema may be detected or evaluated through the use of chest x ray.

Cancer

A chest x ray may be ordered by a physician to check for possible tumors of the lungs, lymphoid tissue, or bones of the thorax. These may be primary tumors, or the areas in which cancer originates in the body. X rays also check for secondary spread of cancer from another organ to the chest.

Cardiac disorders

While less sensitive than **echocardiography**, chest x ray can be used to check for disorders such as congestive heart failure or pulmonary edema.

Other

Chest x rays are used to see foreign bodies that may have been swallowed or inhaled, and to evaluate response to treatment for various diseases. Often the chest x ray is also used to verify correct placement of chest tubes or catheters. Chest x rays can be used to check for fluid surrounding the lungs (pleural effusion).

A chest x ray of normal, healthy adult lungs. *(Photograph by John Smith, Custom Medical Stock Photo. Reproduced by permission.)*

Description

Routine chest x rays consist of two views, the frontal view (referred to as posterioranterior or PA) and the lateral (side) view. It is preferred that the patient stand for this exam, particularly when studying collection of fluid in the lungs.

During the actual time of exposure, the technologist will ask the patient to hold his or her breath. It is very important in taking a chest x ray to ensure there is no motion that could detract from the quality and sharpness of the film image. The procedure will only take a few minutes and the time patients must hold their breath is a matter of a few seconds.

The chest x ray may be performed in a physician's office or referred to an outpatient radiology facility or hospital radiology department. In some cases, particularly for patients who cannot get out of bed, a portable chest x ray may be taken. Portable films are sometimes

KEY TERMS

Bronchi—Plural of bronchus. The air passages in the lungs through which inhaled air passes on its way through the lungs.

Diaphragm—The large muscle that is located between the abdomen and the chest area. The diaphragm aids in breathing.

Gastrointestinal—The digestive organs and structures, including the stomach and intestines.

Interstitial lung disease—About 180 diseases fall into this category of breathing disorders. Injury or foreign substances in the lungs (such as asbestos fibers) as well as infections, cancers, or inherited disorders may cause the diseases. They can lead to breathing or heart failure.

Lymphoid—Tissues relating to the lymphatic system. A thin, yellowish fluid called lymph fluid, travels throughout the body. The lymphatic system helps control fluids in the body.

Portable chest x ray—An x ray procedure taken by equipment that can be brought to the patient. The resulting radiographs may not be as high in quality as stationary x-ray radiographs, but allow a technologist to come to the patient.

Pulmonary—Refers to the lungs and the breathing system and function.

Serial x rays—A number of x rays performed at set times in the disease progression or treatment intervals. The radiographs will be compared to one another to track changes.

Sternum—Also referred to as the breast bone, this is the long flat bone in the middle of the chest.

Thorax—The chest area, which runs between the abdomen and neck and is encased in the ribs.

X ray—A form of electromagnetic radiation with shorter wavelengths than normal light. X rays can penetrate most structures.

---

of poorer quality than those taken with permanent equipment, but are the best choice for some patients or situations when the patient cannot be moved or properly positioned for the chest x ray. Patients confined to bed may be placed in as upright a position as possible to get a clear picture, particularly of chest fluid.

Preparation

There is no advance preparation necessary for chest x rays. Once the patient arrives in the exam area, a hospital gown will replace all clothing on the upper body and all jewelry must be removed.

Aftercare

No aftercare is required by patients who have chest x rays.

Risks

The only risk associated with chest x ray is minimal exposure to radiation, particularly for pregnant women and children. Those patients should use protective lead aprons during the procedure. Technologists are cautioned to check carefully possible dislodging of any tubes or monitors in the chest area from the patient's placement during the exam.

Normal results

A radiologist, or physician specially trained in the technique and interpretation of x rays, will evaluate the results. A normal chest x ray will show normal structures for the age and medical history of the patient. Findings, whether normal or abnormal, will be provided to the referring physician in the form of a written report.

Abnormal findings on chest x rays are used in conjunction with a physician's physical exam findings, patient medical history, and other diagnostic tests including laboratory tests to reach a final diagnosis. For many diseases, chest x rays are more effective when compared to previous chest x-ray studies. The patient is asked to help the radiology facility in locating previous chest radiographs from other facilities.

Pulmonary disorders

Pneumonia shows up on radiographs as patches and irregular areas of density (from fluid in the lungs). If the bronchi (air passages in the lungs which are usually not visible) can be seen, a diagnosis of bronchial pneumonia may be made. Shifts or shadows in the hila (lung roots) may indicate enlarged lymph nodes of a malignancy. Widening of the spaces between ribs and increased lucency of the lung fields suggests emphysema. Other pulmonary diseases may also be detected or suspected through chest x ray.

Cancer

In nearly all patients with lung cancer, some sort of abnormality can be seen on a chest radiograph. Hilar masses (enlargements at that part of the lungs where vessels and nerves enter) are one of the more common symptoms as are abnormal masses and fluid buildup on the outside surface of the lungs or surrounding areas. Interstitial lung disease, which is a large category of disorders, many of which are related to exposure of substances (such as asbestos fibers), may be detected on a chest x ray as increased prominence of the interstitial pattern, often in the lower portions of the lungs.

Other

Congestive heart failure and other cardiac diseases may be indicated on the view of a heart and lung in a chest radiograph. Fractures of the sternum and ribs are sometimes detected as breaks on the chest x ray, though often dedicated bone films are needed. In some instances, the radiologist's view of the diaphragm may indicate an abdominal problem. Foreign bodies that may have been swallowed or inhaled can usually be located by the radiologist, as they will look different from any other tissue or structure in the chest. Serial chest x rays may be ordered to track changes over a period of time, usually to evaluate response to therapy of a malignancy.

Resources

ORGANIZATIONS

American Lung Association. 1740 Broadway, New York, NY 10019. (800) 586–4872. <http://www.lungusa.org>.

Emphysema Anonymous, Inc. P.O. Box 3224, Seminole FL 34642. (813) 391–9977.

National Heart, Lung and Blood Institute. P.O. Box 30105, Bethesda, MD 20824–0105. (301) 251–1222. <http://www.nhlbi.nih.gov>.

Teresa Norris, RN
Lee Shratter, MD

Children's surgery *see* **Pediatric surgery**
Chin cosmetic surgery *see* **Mentoplasty**
Chloride test *see* **Electrolyte tests**

Cholecystectomy

Definition

A cholecystectomy is the surgical removal of the gallbladder. The two basic types of this procedure are open cholecystectomy and the laparoscopic approach. It is estimated that the laparoscopic procedure is currently used for approximately 80% of cases.

Purpose

A cholecystectomy is performed to treat cholelithiasis and cholecystitis. In cholelithiasis, gallstones of varying shapes and sizes form from the solid components of bile. The presence of these stones, often referred to as gallbladder disease, may produce symptoms of excruciating right upper abdominal pain radiating to the right shoulder. The gallbladder may become the site of acute infection and inflammation, resulting in symptoms of upper right abdominal pain, nausea, and vomiting. This condition is referred to as cholecystitis. The surgical removal of the gallbladder can provide relief of these symptoms. Cholecystectomy is used to treat both acute and chronic cholecystitis when there are significant pain symptoms. The typical composition of gallstones is predominately cholesterol, or a compound called calcium bilirubinate.

Cholelithiasis

Most patients with cholelithiasis have no significant physical symptoms. Approximately 80% of gallstones do not cause significant discomfort. Patients who develop biliary colic generally do have some symptoms. When gallstones obstruct the cystic duct, intermittent, extreme, cramping pain typically develops in the right upper quadrant of the abdomen. This pain generally occurs at night and can last from a few minutes to several hours. An acute attack of cholecystitis is often associated with the consumption of a large, high-fat meal.

The medical management of gallstones depends to a great degree on the presentation of the patient. Patients with no symptoms generally do not require any medical treatment. The best treatment for patients with symptoms is usually surgery. Laparoscopic cholecystectomy is typically preferred over the open surgical approach because of the decreased recovery period. Patients who are not good candidates for either type of surgery can obtain some symptom relief with drugs, especially oral bile salts.

Cholecystitis

Cholecystitis is an inflammation of the gallbladder, both acute and chronic, that results after the development of gallstones in some individuals. The most common symptoms and physical findings associated with cholecystitis include:

- pain and tenderness in the upper right quadrant of the abdomen
- nausea
- vomiting

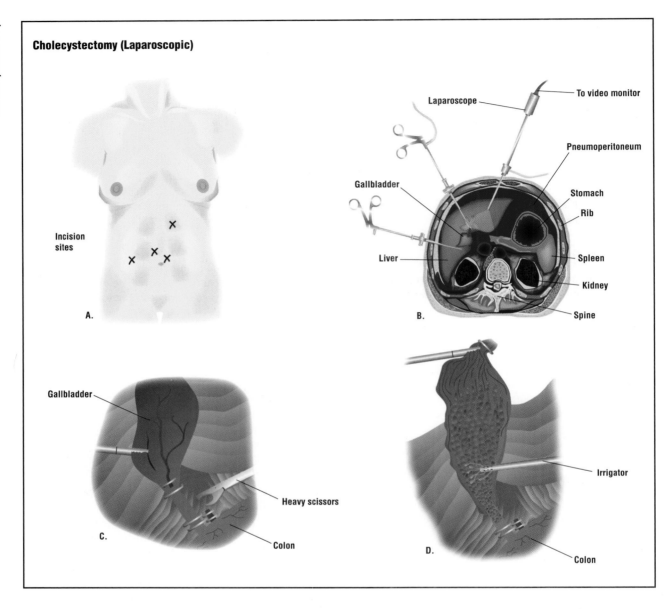

Cholecystectomy (Laparoscopic)

In a laparoscopic cholecystectomy, four small incisions are made in the abdomen (A). The abdomen is filled with carbon dioxide, and the surgeon views internal structures with a video monitor (B). The gallbladder is located and cut with laparoscopic scissors (C). It is then removed through an incision (D). *(Illustration by GGS Inc.)*

• fever

• jaundice

• history of pain after eating large, high-fat meals

Demographics

Overall, cholelithasis is found in about 20,000,000 Americans. An overwhelming majority of these individuals do not ever develop symptoms. Overall, about 500,000 to 600,000 (2–3%) are treated with cholecystectomies every year. Typically, the incidence of cholelithasis increases with age. The greatest incidence occurs in individuals between the ages of 40 and 60 years. The following groups are at an increased risk for developing choleliathiasis:

• pregnant women

• female sex

• family history of gallstones

• obesity

• certain types of intestinal disease

• age greater than 40 years

- oral contraceptive use

- diabetes mellitus

- estrogen replacement therapy

- rapid weight loss

Overall, patients with cholelathiasis have about a 20% chance of developing biliary colic (the extremely painful complication that usually requires surgery) over a 20-year period.

Acute cholecystitis develops most commonly in women between the ages of 40 and 60 years. Some ethnic groups such as Native Americans have a dramatically higher incidence of cholecystitis.

Description

The laparoscopic cholecystectomy involves the insertion of a long, narrow cylindrical tube with a camera on the end, through an approximately 0.4 in (1 cm) incision in the abdomen, which allows visualization of the internal organs and projection of this image onto a video monitor. Three smaller incisions allow for insertion of other instruments to perform the surgical procedure. A laser may be used for the incision and cautery (burning unwanted tissue to stop bleeding), in which case the procedure may be called laser laparoscopic cholecystectomy.

In a conventional or open cholecystectomy, the gallbladder is removed through a surgical incision high in the right abdomen, just beneath the ribs. A drain may be inserted to prevent accumulation of fluid at the surgical site.

Diagnosis/Preparation

The initial diagnosis of acute cholecystitis is based on the following symptoms:

- constant, dull upper right quadrant abdominal pain

- fever

- chills

- nausea

- vomiting

- pain aggravated by moving or coughing

Most patients have elevated leukocyte (white blood cells) levels. Leukocyte levels are determined using laboratory analysis of blood samples. Traditional x rays are not particularly useful in diagnosing cholecystitis. Ultrasonography of the gallbladder usually provides evidence of gallstones, if they are present. Ultrasonography can also help identify inflammation of the gallbladder. Nuclear imaging may also be used. This type of imaging cannot identify gallstones, but it can provide evidence of obstruction of the cystic and common bile ducts.

Cholelithiasis is initially diagnosed based on the following signs and symptoms:

- history of biliary colic or jaundice

- nausea

- vomiting

- sudden onset of extreme pain in the upper right quadrant of the abdomen

- fever

- chills

Laboratory blood analysis often finds evidence of elevated bilirubin, alkaline phosphatase, or aminotransferase levels. Ultrasonography, computed tomography (CT) scanning, and radionuclide imaging are able to detect the impaired functioning of bile flow and of the bile ducts.

As with any surgical procedure, the patient will be required to sign a consent form after the procedure is explained thoroughly. Food and fluids will be prohibited after midnight before the procedure. Enemas may be ordered to clean out the bowel. If nausea or vomiting are present, a suction tube to empty the stomach may be used, and for laparoscopic procedures, a urinary drainage catheter will also be used to decrease the risk of accidental puncture of the stomach or bladder with insertion of the trocar (a sharp, pointed instrument).

Aftercare

Postoperative care for the patient who has had an open cholecystectomy, as with those who have had any major surgery, involves monitoring of blood pressure, pulse, respiration, and temperature. Breathing tends to be shallow because of the effect of anesthesia, and the patient's reluctance to breathe deeply due to the pain caused by the proximity of the incision to the muscles used for respiration. The patient is shown how to support the operative site when breathing deeply and coughing and is given pain medication as necessary. Fluid intake and output is measured, and the operative site is observed for color and amount of wound drainage. Fluids are given intravenously for 24–48 hours, until the patient's diet is gradually advanced as bowel activity resumes. The patient is generally encouraged to walk eight hours after surgery and discharged from the hospital within three to five days, with return to work approximately four to six weeks after the procedure.

Care received immediately after laparoscopic cholecystectomy is similar to that of any patient undergoing surgery with general anesthesia. A unique postoperative pain may be experienced in the right shoulder related to pressure from carbon dioxide used in the laparoscopic tubes. This pain may be relieved by lying down on the left side with right knee and thigh drawn up to the chest. Walking will also help increase the body's reabsorption

of the gas. The patient is usually discharged the day after surgery and allowed to shower on the second postoperative day. The patient is advised to gradually resume normal activities over a three-day period, while avoiding heavy lifting for about 10 days.

Risks

Potential problems associated with open cholecystectomy include respiratory problems related to location of the incision, wound infection, or abscess formation. Possible complications of laparoscopic cholecystectomy include accidental puncture of the bowel or bladder and uncontrolled bleeding. Incomplete reabsorption of the carbon dioxide gas could irritate the muscles used in respiration and cause respiratory distress. While most patients with acute cholecystitis respond well to the laparoscopic technique, about 5–20% of these patients require a conversion to the open technique because of complications.

Normal results

The prognosis for cholecystitis and cholelithaisis patients who receive cholecystectomy is generally good. Overall, cholecystectomy relieves symptoms in about 95% of cases.

Morbidity and mortality rates

The complication rate is less than 0.5% with open cholecystectomy and about 1% with laparoscopic cholecystectomy. The primary complication with the open technique is infection, whereas bile leak and hemorrhage are the most common complications associated with the laparoscopic technique. The overall mortality rate associated with cholecystectomy is less than 1%. However, the rate of mortality in the elderly is higher.

In a small minority of cases, symptoms will persist in patients who receive cholecystectomy. This has been named the post-cholecystectomy syndrome and usually results from functional bowel disorder, errors in diagnosis, technical errors, overlooked common bile duct stones, recurrence of common bile duct stones, or the spasm of a structure called the sphincter of Oddi.

Alternatives

Acute cholecystitis usually improves following conservative therapy in most patients. This conservative therapy involves the withholding of oral feedings, the use of intravenous feedings, and the administration of **antibiotics** and **analgesics**. This is only a short-term alternative in hospitalized patients. Most of these patients should receive cholecystectomy within a few days to prevent recurrent attacks. In the short-term, patients often receive narcotic analgesics such as meperidine to relieve the intense pain associated with this condition. Patients who have evidence of gallbladder perforation or gangrene need to have an immediate cholecystectomy.

In patients with cholelithasis who are deemed unfit for surgery, alternative treatments are sometimes effective. These individuals often have symptom improvement after lifestyle changes and medical therapy. Lifestyle changes include dietary avoidance of foods high in polyunsaturated fats and gradual weight loss in obese individuals. Medical therapy includes the administration of oral bile salts. Patients with three or fewer gallstones of cholesterol composition and with a gallstone diameter less than 0.6 in (15 mm) are more likely to receive medical therapy and have positive results. The primary requirements for receiving medical therapy include the presence of a functioning gallbladder and the absence of calcification on computed tomography (CT) scans. Other non-surgical alternatives include using a solvent to dissolve the stones and using sound waves to breakup small stones. A major drawback to medical therapy is the high recurrence rate of stones in those treated.

Resources

BOOKS

"Cholecystitis," and ""Cholelithiasis." In *Ferri's Clinical Advisor*, edited by Fred F. Ferri. St. Louis: Mosby, 2001.

Current Surgical Diagnosis & Treatment. New York: McGraw-Hill, 2003.

"The Digestive System." *Conn's Current Therapy*. Philadelphia: W.B. Saunders, 2001.

"Diseases of the Liver, Gallbladder, and Bile Ducts." In *Cecil Textbook of Medicine*, edited by Lee Goldman, and J. Claude Bennett. Philadelphia: W.B. Saunders, 2000.

"Liver, Biliary Tract, & Pancreas." In *Current Medical Diagnosis & Treatment*. New York: McGraw-Hill, 2003.

Schwartz, Seymour I. (ed.) *Principles of Surgery*. New York: McGraw-Hill, 1999.

Mark Mitchell

Cholesterol tests *see* **Lipid tests**

Circulation support *see* **Mechanical circulation support**

Circumcision

Definition

The surgical removal of the foreskin of the penis, or prepuce of the clitoris.

Purpose

In the United States, circumcision in infant boys is performed for social, medical, or cultural/religious reasons. Once a routine operation urged by pediatricians and obstetricians for newborns in the middle of the twentieth century, circumcision has become an elective option that parents make for their sons on an individual basis. Families who practice Judaism or Islam may select to have their sons circumcised as a religious practice. Others choose circumcision for medical benefits.

Female circumcision (also known as female genital mutilation) is usually performed for cultural and social reasons by family members and others who are not members of the medical profession, with no anesthesia. Not only is the prepuce of the clitoris removed but often the vaginal opening is sewn to make it smaller. This practice is supposed to ensure the virginity of a bride on her wedding day. It also prevents the woman from achieving sexual pleasure during coitus. This practice is not universally approved by the medical profession and is considered by many to be a human rights violation.

Some of the medical reasons parents of male infants choose circumcision are to protect against infections of the urinary tract and the foreskin, prevent cancer, lower the risk of getting sexually transmitted diseases, and prevent phimosis (a tightening of the foreskin that may close the opening of the penis). Though studies indicate that un-

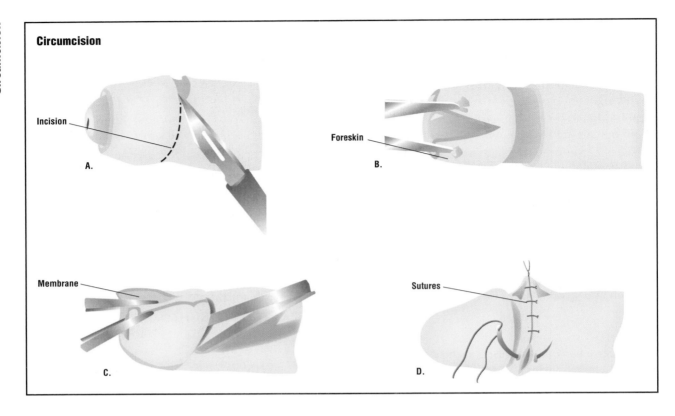

Circumcision

Incision — A.

Foreskin — B.

Membrane — C.

Sutures — D.

During a circumcision, the outer layer of the foreskin around the penis is cut (A). The foreskin is pulled away (B), and the remaining membrane is cut away (C). Sutures are used to stitch the area (D). *(Illustration by GGS Inc.)*

circumcised boys under the age of five are 20 times more likely than circumcised boys to have urinary tract infections (UTIs), the rate of incidence of UTIs is quite low and treatable with **antibiotics**. There are also indications that circumcised men are less likely to suffer from penile cancer, inflammation of the penis, or have many sexually transmitted diseases. Here again, there is a low rate of incidence. Good hygiene usually prevents most infections of the penis. Phimosis and penile cancer are very rare, even in men who have not been circumcised. Education and safe sex practices can prevent sexually transmitted diseases in ways that a surgical procedure cannot because these are diseases acquired through risky behaviors.

In 2002, however, new research indicated that circumcised men may be less at risk for contracting HIV infections than uncircumcised men, whose foreskins have higher concentrations of cells that are targeted specifically by HIV. Genital hygiene and safe sex practices are still crucial to preventing the spread of HIV.

Another study during that same year found that circumcised men who engaged in risky sexual behaviors were less likely to contract penile human papillomavirus (HPV), which has been implicated in the incidence of cervical cancer in women. There was little difference between circumcised and noncircumcised men's incidence of the virus if the men were in a monogomous relationship.

With these factors in mind, the American Academy of Pediatrics has issued a policy statement that maintains that though there is existing scientific evidence that indicates the medical benefits of circumcision, the benefits are not strong enough to recommended circumcision as a routine practice.

Demographics

Though the incidence of male circumcision has decreased from 90% in 1979 to 60% in 1999, it is still the most common surgical operation in the United States. Circumcision rates are much lower for the rest of the industrialized world. In Britain, it is only done for religious practices or to correct a specific medical condition of the penis.

Description

The foreskin of the penis protects the sensitivity of the glans and shields it from irritation by urine, feces, and foreign materials. It also protects the urinary opening against infection and incidental injury.

In circumcision of infants, the foreskin is pulled tightly into a specially designed clamp, which forces the foreskin away from the broadened tip of the penis. Pressure from the clamp stops bleeding from blood vessels that supplied the foreskin. In older boys or adults, an incision is made around the base of the foreskin, the foreskin is pulled back, and then it is cut away from the tip of the penis. Stitches are usually used to close the skin edges.

Circumcision should not be performed on infants with certain deformities of the penis that may require a portion of the foreskin for repair. The most common condition for surgery using the foreskin is hypospadias, a congenital deformity of the penis where the urinary tract opening is not at the tip of the glans. Also, infants with a large hydrocele, or hernia, may suffer complications through circumcision. Premature infants and infants with serious infections are also poor candidates to be circumcised, as are infants with hemophilia, other bleeding disorders, or whose mothers had taken anticoagulant drugs. In older boys or men, circumcision is a minor procedure and can be performed on virtually anyone without a serious illness or unusual deformity.

Diagnosis/Preparation

Despite a long-standing belief that infants do not experience serious pain from circumcision, physicians now believe that some form of local anesthesia is necessary. Over 80% of pediatric residents, 80% of family practice residents, and 60% of obstetric/gynecological residents are routinely given instruction on pain control for circumcisions. Local anesthesia is often injected at the base of the penis (dorsal penile nerve block) or under the skin around the penis (subcutaneous ring block). Both anesthetics block key nerves and provide significantly lowered perceived pain. EMLA cream (lidocaine 2.5% and prilocaine 2.5%) can also be used.

Aftercare

After circumcision, the wound should be washed daily. An antibiotic ointment or petroleum jelly may be applied to the site. If there is an incision, a wound dressing will be present and should be changed each time the diaper is changed. Sometimes a plastic ring is used instead of a bandage. The ring will usually fall off in five to eight days. The penis will heal in seven to 10 days.

Infants who undergo circumcision may be fussy for some hours afterward, so parents should be prepared for crying, feeding problems, and sleep problems. Generally, these go away within a day. In older boys, the penis may be painful, but this will go away gradually. A topical anesthetic ointment or spray may be used to relieve this temporary

---

WHO PERFORMS THE PROCEDURE AND WHERE IS IT PERFORMED?

Medical circumcisions are performed in the hospital by a pediatrician for an infant or child. For an adult, a general surgeon or urologist may perform a circumcision, especially if there are other urinary tract repairs to be made.

A Jewish religious circumcision, a *Bris Milah*, is performed when an infant male is eight days old. It is conducted by a trained *mohel*, with family and friends present, in a non-medical setting.

---

discomfort. There may also be a bruise on the penis, which typically disappears with no particular attention.

Risks

Complications following newborn circumcision appear in between two and six of every 1,000 procedures. Most complications are minor. Bleeding occurs in half of the complications and is usually easy to control. Infections are rare and occur at the circumcision site, the opening to the bladder, or at the tip of the penis as a result of contact with urine or feces. Infections are indicated by fever and signs of inflammation, and are treatable with antibiotics.

There may be injuries to the penis itself, and these may be difficult to repair. In 2000, there were reports that the surgical clamps used in circumcision were at fault in over 100 injuries reported between July 1996 and January 2000. In nearly all cases, the clamps were assumed to be in working order but had been repaired with replacement parts that were not of the manufacturer's specifications. Physicians were urged to inspect the clamps before use and ensure that their dimensions fit their infant patients.

Normal results

When an infant or an adult is circumcised, the surgical wound should heal quickly, with normal urinary function resuming immediately. An infant or older child should have no complications and should be able to pass through adolescence and eventual sexual activity normally. After a period of recovery, an adult male should be able to resume sexual intercourse normally.

Morbidity and mortality rates

Complications as a result of circumcision are usually minor if the physician is experienced and makes sure the Mogen or Gomco clamps that are used are in good working order. Severe penile injuries are rare, but they are serious, and include penile **amputation** (partial or total), laceration, hemorrhage, and damage to the urinary tract. Other serious complications such as meningitis, penile necrosis, necrotizing faciitis, and sepsis can occur. Some of these, like meningitis and sepsis, can even cause death.

Hidden complications also occur. Subcutaneous masses have been detected under the skin of the penis. These masses usually have no symptoms, but, left untreated, could lead more serious outcomes. Physicians should examine the penis at every well-baby checkup during the first year. If a mass is detected, it can easily be removed under a local anesthesia and sent to a pathology lab.

Alternatives

The only alternative to this surgery is to make an informed decision not to have an infant circumcised. Some Jewish parents are even electing not to hold a *Bris Milah*, a religious circumcision, for their sons, and choosing instead to hold a *Brit Shalom*, a naming ceremony, similar to that given for their infant daughters.

Resources

BOOKS

Gollaher, David L. *Circumcision: A History of the World's Most Controversial Surgery.* New York: Basic Books, 2000.

PERIODICALS

"Circumcision." *Harvard Men's Health Watch* 6, no. 3 (October 2001).

Imperio, Winnie Anne. "Circumcision Appears Safe, But Not Hugely Beneficial." *OB GYN News* 35, no. 7 (1 April 2000): 9.

"Link to Uncircumcised Males Found." *Women's Health Weekly* (May 9, 2002): 10.

Schmitt, B. D. "The Circumcision Descision: Pros and Cons." *Clinical Reference Systems* (2000): 1579.

OTHER

American Academy of Pediatrics. *New AAP Circumcision Policy Released (Press Release).* March 1, 1999. <http://www.aap.org/advocacy/archives/marcircum.htm>.

Janie F. Franz

Claw toe surgery *see* **Hammer, claw, and mallet toe surgery**

Cleft lip repair

Definition

Cleft lip repair (cheiloplasty) is surgical procedure to correct a groove-like defect in the lip.

Purpose

A cleft lip does not join together (fuse) properly during embryonic development. Surgical repair corrects the defect, preventing future problems with breathing, speaking, and eating, and improving the person's physical appearance.

Demographics

Cleft lip is the second most common embryonic (congenital) deformity. (Club foot is the most common

Infant in recovery from a cleft lip repair. *(Biophoto Associates/Science Source. Reproduced by permission.)*

congenital deformity.) Cleft lip occurs in approximately one in 750–1,000 live births. The highest incidence exists in North American Indians and Japanese (approximately one in 350 births). African Americans and Africans represent the lowest incidence of cleft lip deformity (approximately one in 1,500 births). There is a higher frequency of clefting in certain populations of Scandinavia and Middle European countries.

Cleft lip occurs more commonly in males, while cleft palate is more likely to occur in females. Cleft lip alone (without cleft palate) occurs in approximately 20% of cases across both genders. The majority of cases—80%—have both cleft lip and cleft palate. A unilateral cleft lip, commonly occurring on the left side, is more common than a bilateral cleft lip.

Potential causes

Most cases of cleft lip have no known cause. However, there is a strong genetic correlation. Other single gene defects that are associated with cleft lip include: Van der Woude syndrome, Opitz Syndrome, Aarskog syndrome, Fryns syndrome, Waardenburg syndrome, and Coffin-Siris syndrome. Approximately 5% of cleft conditions are associated with a genetic syndrome. Most of these syndromes do not include mental retardation.

Facial cleft has been implicated with maternal exposure to environmental causes, such as rubella or medications that can harm the developing embryo. These medications include steroids, antiseizure drugs, vitamin A, and oral anti-acne medications (such as Acutane) taken during the first three months of pregnancy. Cleft lip is also associated with fetal alcohol syndrome and maternal diabetes.

Risk of cleft lip increases with paternal age, especially over 30 years at the time of conception. Generally, the risk is higher when both parents are over 30 years of age. However, most cases seem to be isolated within the family with no obvious causation.

When the affected child has unilateral cleft lip and palate, the risk for subsequent children increases to 4.2%. Advances in high resolution ultrasonography (prenatal ultrasound exam) have made it possible to detect facial abnormalities in the developing embryo (in utero).

Description

Developmental anatomy

Important structures of the embryo's mouth form at four to seven weeks of gestation. Development during this period entails migration and fusion of mesenchymal cells with facial structures. If this migration and fusion is interrupted (usually by a combination of genetic and environmental factors), a cleft can develop along the lip. The type of clefting varies with the embryonic stage when its development occurred.

There are several types of cleft lip, ranging from a small groove on the border of the upper lip to a larger deformity that extends into the floor of the nostril and part of the maxilla (upper jawbone).

Cleft lip repair

The edges of the cleft between the lip and nose are cut (A and B). The bottom of the nostril is formed with suture (C). The upper part of the lip tissue is closed (D), and the stitches are extended down to close the opening entirely (E). *(Illustration by Argosy.)*

Unilateral cleft lip results from failure of the maxillary prominence on the affected side to fuse with medial nasal prominences. The result is called a persistant labial groove. The cells of the lip become stretched and the tissues in the persistent groove break down, resulting in a lip that is divided into medial (middle) and lateral (side) portions. In some cases, a bridge of tissue (simart band) joins together the two incomplete lip portions.

Bilateral cleft lip occurs in a fashion similar to the unilateral cleft. Patients with bilateral cleft lip may have varying degrees of deformity on each side of the defect. An anatomical structure (intermaxillary segment) pro-

jects to the front and hangs unattached. Defects associated with bilateral cleft lip are particularly problematic due to discontinuity of the muscle fibers of the orbicularis oris (primary muscle of the lip.) This deformity can result in closure of the mouth and pursing of the lip.

Classification

In addition to classification as unilateral or bilateral, cleft lips are further classified as complete or incomplete. A complete cleft involves the entire lip, and typically the alveolar arch. An incomplete cleft involves only part of the lip. The Iowa system (which also classifies cleft palate) classifies cleft lip in five groups:

- Group I—clefts of the lip only
- Group II—clefts of palate only
- Group III—clefts of lip, alveolus, and palate
- Group IV—clefts of lip and alveolus
- Group V—miscellaneous

Another widely accepted cleft lip classification is based on recommendations of the American Cleft Palate Association. This classification divides cleft lip into unilateral or bilateral (right, left or extent) in thirds— (i.e., one-third, two-thirds, three-thirds), or median cleft lip, the extent of which is also measured in thirds.

Surgical procedure

Cleft lip repair can be initiated at any age, but optimal results occur when the first operation is performed between two and six months of age. Surgery is usually scheduled during the third month of life.

While the patient is under general anesthesia, the anatomical landmarks and incisions are carefully demarcated with methylene blue ink. An endotracheal tube prevents aspiration of blood. The surgical field is injected with a local anesthestic to provide further numbing and blood vessel constriction (to limit bleeding). Myringotomy (incisions in one or both eardrums) is performed, and myringotomy tubes are inserted to permit fluid drainage.

There are several operative techniques for cleft lip reconstruction. The Millard rotation advancement (R-A) technique is the most widely accepted form of repair. This method involves rotation of the entire philtral dimple (groove in the upper lip) and Cupid's bow (double curve of the upper lip). The scar falls along the new philtral column (central section of the upper lip), and is adjusted as required since the procedure allows for flexibility.

The Millard procedure begins with an incision on the edge of the cleft side of the philtrum, and the cutting continues upward, medially, and to the side. A second incision extends to the buccal sulcus (top part of the upper jaw). The length of this incision depends on the size of the gap to be closed. In this second incision, the surgeon frees soft tissue, which allows him or her to completely lift the lip from the underlying bone. This dissection should be tested to ensure free advancement toward the middle (inadequate dissection is the root cause of poor results). Nasal deformity can be dealt with by a procedure known as the McComb nasal tip plasty, which elevates the depressed nasal dome and rim. Cartilage from the cleft side is freed from the opposite side, and is positioned and reshaped using nylon sutures.

Advantages of the Millard rotation advancement technique (include:

- It is the most common procedure (i.e., surgeons more familiar with it).
- The technique is adaptable and flexible.
- It permits construction of a normal-looking Cupid's bow.
- A minimal amount of tissue is discarded.
- The suture line is camouflaged.

The disadvantage of the Millard rotation advancement technique is the possible development of a vermilion notch (shortening of the entire lip in the vertical direction), resulting from contracture of the vertical scar. Cupid's bow is a critical part of the repair, making it very important to accurately determine the high point of Cupid's bow on the lateral lip.

Diagnosis/Preparation

Facial clefting has a wide range of clinical presentations, ranging from a simple microform cleft to the complete bilateral cleft involving the lip, palate, and nose. A comprehensive **physical examination** is performed immediately after birth, and the defect is usually evident by visual inspection and examination of the facial structures.

Care must be taken to diagnose other physical problems associated with a genetic syndrome. Weight, nutrition, growth, and development should be assessed and closely monitored.

Alveolar arch—An arch formed by the ridge of the alveolar process of the mandible (jawbone) or maxilla.

Alveolar part of the maxilla—The part of the bony upper jaw that contains teeth (the upper gum).

Bilateral cleft lip—Cleft that occurs on both sides of the lip.

Buccal sulcus—Groove in the upper part of the upper jaw (where there are teeth).

Cleft—Split or opening, which can occur in the lip or palate or both.

Columella—Outer portion of the nose that divides the nostrils.

Cupid's bow—Double curve of the upper lip.

Epithelium—Protective membranous layer of tissue, usually a single layer of cells very close together, which lines the cavities outside of an organism.

Flap—Anatomical section that is surgically cut using special incisions and moved (rotated/advanced) to repair a defect.

Inferior turbinate—Bony projections on each side of the nose.

Labial—Of or pertaining to the lips.

Lateral—Of or pertaining to a side (opposite of medial).

Maxilla—Bony upper jaw.

Medial—Toward the middle or center (i.e., the chest is medial to the arm).

Medial (or lateral) nasal prominence—The medial (toward the middle) or lateral (toward the sides) are anatomical structures that form and merge the nose of the developing embryo during weeks six to nine in utero.

Mesenchymal cells—Embryonic cells that develop into many structures, including the soft tissues in the lip.

Mixed dentition—A mix of both "baby teeth" and permanent teeth.

Myringotomy—A procedure that involves making a small incision in the eardrum to release pressure caused by excess fluid accumulation.

Orbicularis oris—Concentrically shaped muscle that surrounds the upper and lower lips.

Oropharynx—The part of the throat at the back of the mouth.

Palate—The roof of the mouth composed of two anatomical structures, the hard and soft palates.

Philtral units—Consists of several anatomical landmarks: the philtral dimple (the skin or depression below the nose extending to the upper lip in the midline); philtral columns (the skin columns on the right and left side of the philtral dimple); philtral tubercle (in the midline of the upper lip); white roll (a linear tissue prominence that joins the upper lip portion of the philtral dimple and vermilion—the dark pink tissue that makes up the lip); nasal columella (the outer portion of the nose that divides the nostrils).

Philtal dimple—The skin or depression below the nose, extending to the upper lip in the midline.

Septal mucosa—the epithelium in the nasal mucosa

Unilateral cleft lip—A cleft that occurs on either the right or left side of the lip.

Vermilion—The dark pink tissue that makes up the lip.

Presurgical tests include a variety of procedures, such as hemoglobin studies. It is important for the pateint's parents and physician to discuss the operation prior to surgery.

Aftercare

The postoperative focus is on ensuring proper nutrition, as well as lip care and monitoring the activity level. Breast milk or full-strength formula is encouraged immediately after surgery or shortly thereafter. Lip care for patients with sutures should include gentle cleansing of suture lines with cotton swabs and diluted hydrogen peroxide. Liberal application of topical antibiotic ointment several times a day for 10 days is recommended. There will be some scar contracture, redness, and firmness of the area for four to six weeks after surgery. Parents should gently massage the area, and avoid sunlight until the scar heals.

The patient's activities may be limited. Some surgeons use elbow immobilizers to minimize the risk of accidental injury to the lip. Immobilizers should be removed several times a day in a supervised setting, allowing the child to move the restricted limb(s).

Interaction between the orthodontist and surgeon as part of the treatment team begins in the neonatal period, and continues through the phases of mixed dentition.

Risks

There may be excessive scarring and contraction of the lips. Two types of scars, hypertrophic or keloid, may develop. Hypertrophic scars appear as raised and red areas that usually flatten, fade in color, and soften within a few months. Keloids form as a result of the accelerated growth of tissue in response to the surgery or trauma to the area. The keloid can cause itching and a burning sensation. Scratching must be avoided because it can lead to healing problems. Some patients require minimal revision surgery, but in most cases, the initial redness and contracture is part of the normal healing process.

Normal results

Ideal surgical results for cleft lip include symmetrically shaped nostrils, and lips that appear as natural as possible and have a functional muscle. Many characteristics of the natural lip can be achieved; however, the outcome ultimately depends on a number of factors, including the skill of the surgeon, accurate presurgery markings, alignment of bones within the affected area, uncomplicated healing of the initial repair, and the effect of normal growth on the repaired lip. Additional surgical correction to reconstruct nasal symmetry is sometimes necessary.

Morbidity and mortality rates

Generally, cleft lip repair is well-tolerated in healthy infants. There are no major health problems associated with this reconstructive surgery. Depending on the results, it may be necessary to perform additional operations to achieve desired functional and cosmetic outcomes.

Alternatives

There are no alternatives for this surgery. Obvious deformity and impairments of speech, hearing, eating, and breathing occur as a direct result of the malformation. These issues can not be corrected without surgery.

Resources

BOOKS

Aston, S.J., R.W. Beasley, C.H.M. Thorne, *Grabb and Smith's Plastic Surgery* 5th ed. Philadelphia, PA: Lippincott-Raven Publishers, 1997.

Bluestone, Charles. *Pediatric Otolaryngology.* Philadelphia, PA: Saunders, 2003.

Cohen, M. *Mastery of Plastic and Reconstructive Surgery.* Little, Brown & Company, Boston, MA: 1994.

Georgiade, N. *Pediatric Plastic Surgery.* C. V. Mosby, Co., St Louis, MO: 1984.

Millard, Ralph, D. *Principlization of Plastic Surgery.* Boston, MA: Little, Brown & Company, 1986.

Papel, Ira. *Facial Plastic and Reconstructive Surgery* 2nd ed. Thieme Medical Pub., 2002.

PERIODICALS

Byrd, H.S. "Selected Readings in Plastic Surgery: Cleft Lip I: Primary Deformities." *Baylor University Medical Center* 8 (1997): 221.

Salomon, J. and P.C. Hobar. "Selected Readings in Plastic Surgery: Cleft Lip II: Secondary Deformities." *Baylor University Medical Center* 2, no.22 (1997).

ORGANIZATIONS

American Board of Plastic Surgery,Inc. Seven Penn Center, Suite 400, 1635 Market Street, Philadelphia, PA 19103-2204. (215) 587-9322. <http://www.abplsurg.org>.

International Birth Defects Information Systems. <http://ibis-birthdefects.org/start/index.htm>.

The International Craniofacial Institute. <http://www.craniofacial.net/additional_services/additional_services.asp>.

OTHER

Wide Smiles. <http://www.communicationdisorder.net/Cleft Palate.html>.

Laith Farid Gulli, M.D.,M.S.
Robert Ramirez, B.S.
Randall J. Blazic, M.D.,D.D.S.
Bilal Nasser, ,M.D., M.S.

Closed fracture reduction *see* **Fracture repair**

Club foot repair

Definition

Club foot repair, also known as foot tendon release or club foot release, is the surgical repair of a birth defect of the foot and ankle called club foot.

Purpose

Club foot or *talipes equinovarus* is the most common birth defect of the lower extremity, characterized by the foot turning both downward and inward. The defect can range from mild to severe and the purpose of club foot repair is to provide the child with a functional foot that looks as normal as possible and that is painless, plantigrade, and flexible. Plantigrade means that the child is able to stand with the sole of the foot on the ground, and not on his heels or the outside of his foot.

Demographics

In the United States, club foot is a common birth defect, and occurs at a rate of one to four cases per 1,000 live births among whites. Severe forms of clubfoot affect some 5,000 babies (about one in 735) born in the United States each year. Boys are affected with severe forms of clubfoot twice as often as girls. The risk increases 30-fold in individuals who have a relative of the first-degree affected by the defects.

Description

A newborn baby's club foot is first treated with applying a cast because the tendons, ligaments, and bones are quite flexible and easy to reposition. The procedure involves stretching the foot into a more normal position and using a cast to maintain the corrected position. The cast is removed every week or two, so as to stretch the foot gradually into a correct position. Serial casting goes on for approximately three months.

In 30% of cases, manipulation and casting is successful, and the foot can be placed in a brace to maintain the correction. In about 70% of cases, manipulation and castings alone do not correct the deformity completely and a decision will be made concerning surgery.

The type of surgery depends on how severe the club foot is. The deformity features tight and short tendons around the foot and ankle. Surgery consists of releasing all the tight tendons and ligaments in the posterior (back) and medial (inside) aspects of the foot and repairing them in a lengthened position. Metal pins may also be used to maintain the bones in place for some six weeks. Surgery usually involves an overnight stay in hospital. After surgery, the foot is casted for some three months, followed by the use of a brace to hold the correction. The brace is worn for approximately six to 12 months after surgery.

Diagnosis/Preparation

Presurgical diagnosis requires radiography. The evaluation usually includes only the acquisition of weight-bearing images because the stress involved is reproducible. In babies, weight-bearing is simulated by the application of dorsal flexion stress.

Some surgeons prefer to wait until the child is about one year old before performing surgery, so that the foot may grow a little larger to facilitate surgery. Other surgeons operate as early as three months of age when it becomes clear that further castings will not achieve any more correction.

Aftercare

The patient usually stays in the hospital for two days after club foot repair. The foot is casted and kept elevated, with application of ice packs to reduce swelling and pain. Painkillers may also be prescribed to relieve pain. During the 48 hours following surgery, the skin near the cast and the toes are examined carefully to ensure that blood circulation, movement, and feeling are maintained. After leaving the hospital, the cast is usually left on for about three months. Skin irritations due to the cast or infections may occur. A course of physical therapy may be indicated after removal of the cast to help keep the foot in good position and improve its flexibility and to strengthen the muscles in the repaired foot. The well-treated clubfoot is no handicap and is fully compatible with a normal, active life. Most children who have undergone club foot repair develop normally and participate fully in any athletic or recreational activity that they choose.

Risks

The risks involved in club foot repair are the general risks associated with anesthesia and surgery.

Risks associated with anesthesia

• adverse reactions to medications
• breathing problems

Risks associated with surgery

• excessive bleeding
• infections

Normal results

If club foot repair is required, the foot usually becomes quite functional after surgery. In some cases, the foot and calf may remain smaller throughout the patient's life.

Morbidity and mortality rates

If left untreated, club foot will result in an abnormal gait, and further deformity may occur on side of the foot due to preferential weight bearing.

QUESTIONS TO ASK THE DOCTOR

- Is there any treatment needed to prevent the club foot from coming back after surgery?
- What are the chances that my child's club foot will get corrected?
- How long will it take to recover from the surgery?
- What procedures do you follow?
- How much club foot surgery do you perform each year?

Alternatives

The Ponseti non-surgical treatment

Dr. Ignacio Ponseti developed this method which consists of a weekly series of gentle manipulations followed by the application of casts which are placed from the toes to the upper thigh. Five to seven casts are applied every week. Before applying the last cast, which is worn for three weeks, the heel-cord is cut to finalize the correction of the foot. By the time the cast is removed the heel-cord has healed. After this two-month period of casting, a splint is worn full-time by the patient for a few months and is then worn only at night for two to four years. Special shoes also maintain the foot in the corrected position.

The French treatment

This method consists of daily physical therapy, featuring gentle and painless stretching of the foot. The foot is then taped to maintain the corrected position until just the next day's visit. At night, the taped foot is inserted into a continuous passive motion machine at home to maximize the amount of stretching. The tape is removed for a few hours each day to wash the foot, air the skin, and to perform exercises. Removable splints are also used to support the taped foot. The one-hour physical therapy sessions are conducted five days each week for approximately three months. Taping is stopped when the child starts walking.

Resources

BOOKS

Lehman, W. B. *The Clubfoot*. Philadelphia: Lippincott, Williams and Wilikins, 1980.
Ponseti, I. V. *Congenital Clubfoot. Fundamentals of Treatment*. Oxford: Oxford University Press, 1996.

KEY TERMS

Orthopedics—The branch of medicine that deals with bones and joints.

Simons, G. W. *The Clubfoot: The Present and a View of the Future* New York: Springer Verlag, 1994.

PERIODICALS

Aronson, J. and C. L. Puskarich. "Deformity and Disability from Treated Clubfoot." *Journal of Pediatrics and Orthopedics* 10 (1990): 109–112.
Cooper, D. M. and F. R. Dietz. "Treatment of Idiopathic Clubfoot. A Thirty Year Follow-up." *Journal of Bone and Joint Surgery* 77A (1995): 1477–1479.
Herzenberg, J. E., C. Radler, and N. Bor. "Ponseti Versus Traditional Methods of Casting for Idiopathic Clubfoot." *Journal of Pediatrics and Orthopedics* 22 (July-August 2002): 517–521.
Ideka, K. "Conservative Treatment of Idiopathic Clubfoot." *Journal of Pediatrics and Orthopedics* 12 (March-April 1992): 217–223.

ORGANIZATIONS

American Academy of Pediatrics. 141 Northwest Point Boulevard, Elk Grove Village, IL 60007-1098. (847) 434-4000. <http://www.aap.org>.
Shrine and Shriner's Hospitals. 2900 Rocky Point Dr., Tampa, FL 33607-1460. (813) 281-0300. <http://www.shriner-shq.org/index.html>

OTHER

American Academy of Pediatrics. "Club Foot." *Essentials of Musculoskeletal Care* [cited April 2003]. <http://www.aap.org/pubserv/essenexp.htm>.
The Club Foot Club [cited April 2003]. <http://home.ica.net/~maudefamily>.
"Help for Patients with Club Foot." *Shrine and Shriners Hospitals*. March 28, 2003 [cited April 2003]. <http://www.shrinershq.org/patientedu/clubfoot2.html>.
"List of Physicians Qualified in the Ponseti Method." *Virtual Children's Hospital* [cited April 2003]. <http://www.vh.org/pediatric/patient/orthopaedics/clubfeet/physicians.html>.
"Patient Guide to Club Foot." *John Hopkins Department of Orthopedic Surgery* [cited April 2003]. <http://www.hopkinsmedicine.org/orthopedicsurgery/peds/clubfoot_new.htm>.

Monique Laberge, Ph.D.

Coarctation of the aorta *see* **Heart surgery for congenital defects**

Cochlear implants

Definition

A cochlear implant is a small, complex electronic device used to treat severe to profound hearing loss. It is surgically implanted underneath the skin behind the patient's ear.

Purpose

A cochlear implant delivers useful auditory signals from the environment to the patient by electronically bypassing nonfunctional parts of the ear and directly stimulating the auditory nerve. Unlike a hearing aid, it does not merely amplify sound. Instead, an implant increases the amount of nervous response to sound. Although it does not restore normal hearing, the additional input provided by the implant often improves sound detection and increases speech understanding.

Description

Normal hearing occurs because sound travels from the outer ear into the ear canal and vibrates the eardrum. The vibration is carried through the middle ear by three small bones attached to the eardrum and on to a fluid-filled part of the inner ear called the cochlea. Movement in the cochlear fluid is transferred to hair fibers within the cochlea. The movement of these hair cells stimulates nerve cells called ganglion cells that send an electrical current to the auditory nerve. In turn, the nerve carries the current to the brain, where the electrical stimulation is recognized as sound.

A common cause of hearing loss is damage to the hair cells within the cochlea. This kind of deafness, called sensorineural deafness, can often be treated with cochlear implants. This is particularly true if damage to the hair cells is not accompanied by damage to the auditory nerve itself. As of 2002, it is estimated that over 35,000 individuals have received cochlear implants.

Cochlear implants consist of internal and external parts. The external parts include a microphone, a speech processor, and a transmitter. The internal parts include a receiver-stimulator and an electrode. Some models include a small headpiece that is worn just behind the ear and contains all the external parts while other models also use body-worn modules that are placed in a shoulder pouch, in a pocket, or worn on a belt. The convenience of the all-in-one headpiece is balanced by shorter life for the batteries used in the smaller units, although systems using rechargeable batteries do solve some of these issues.

Within the headpiece, the microphone picks up sound in the environment. The speech processor converts

these sounds into a digital signal. The content of the generated digital signal is determined by the programming of the processor and is complex. It includes information about the pitch, loudness, and timing of sound signals and attempts to filter out extraneous noise. The transmitter converts the digital signals into FM radio signals and sends them through the skin to the internal parts of the implant. The transmitter and the internal parts are kept in correct alignment by using magnets present in both the internal and external parts of the device.

The internal parts are those that are surgically implanted into the patient. The receiver-stimulator is disk-shaped and is about the size of a quarter. It receives the digital signals from the transmitter and converts them into electrical signals. A wire connects the receiver to a group of electrodes that are threaded into the cochlea when the implant is placed. As many as 24 electrodes, depending on the type of the implant, stimulate the ganglion cells in the cochlea. These cells transmit the signals to the brain through the auditory nerve. The brain then interprets the signals as sound.

The sounds heard through an implant are different from the normal hearing sounds and have been described as artificial or robot-like. This is because the implant's handful of electrodes cannot hope to match the complexity of a person's 15,000 hair cells. However, as more electrodes are added, electrode placement issues are solved, and the software for the implant speech processor takes into account more and more aspects of sound, the perceived results are moving closer to how speech and other sounds are naturally perceived.

Despite the benefits that the implant appears to offer, some hearing specialists and members of the deaf community believe that the benefits may not outweigh the risks and limitations of the device. Because the device must be surgically implanted, it carries some surgical risk. Manufacturers can not promise how well a person will hear with an implant. Moreover, after getting an implant, some people say they feel alienated from the

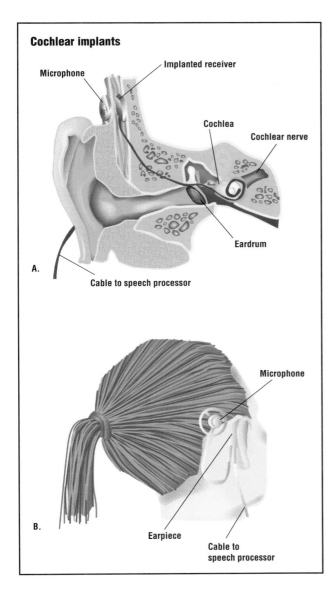

Cochlear implants

A. Microphone — Implanted receiver — Cochlea — Cochlear nerve — Eardrum — Cable to speech processor

B. Microphone — Earpiece — Cable to speech processor

A cochlear implant has a microphone outside the ear that transmits sounds to an implanted receiver. In turn, the receiver transmits electrical impulses to the cochlea and cochlear nerve, which is stimulated in normal hearing. *(Illustration by GGS Inc.)*

deaf community, while at the same time not feeling fully a part of the hearing world. The decision to undergo cochlear implant surgery is a complex one and a person should take into account the risks and realistic rewards of the device.

Surgical procedure

The procedure can be preformed on an outpatient basis for adult and adolescent patients. With children, it is often performed with a one-night stay in the hospital.

QUESTIONS TO ASK THE DOCTOR

- How "normal" will the implant make my/my child's hearing?
- What kind of training does the patient undergo to learn how to use the device?
- How do I care for the device?

The internal parts of the implant are placed under the skin behind the patient's ear. The area is shaved, although newer procedures allow for sterilization of the hair in the area so less shaving has to occur. Once the sterile field is established, the surgeon makes an 2–3 in (5–7.6 cm) incision behind the ear and opens the mastoid bone (the ridge on the skull behind the ear) leading into the middle ear. A depression is made in the bone next to the opening to allow the receiver-stimulator to sit flush with the skull surface. After seating, the receiver-stimulator is held in place with a long-lasting suture.

The surgeon then goes through the opening in the mastoid bone to create a new opening in the cochlea for the implant electrodes. The electrode is then very slowly and careful threaded through this new opening. Care is taken during the procedure, and the electrode structure itself is designed to align the electrodes as closely as possible to the ganglion cells, as this allows the electrical signals that function to be less powerful. Once in place, the device is tested to be certain it is working. If all is well, the surgeon then closes up the incision with absorbable sutures, so the area does not need to be revisited to remove the stitches.

The entire operation takes between one and two hours, although the procedure is more complex for younger patients due to the smaller size of their middle ear structures and tends to take longer.

Aftercare

For a short period of time after the surgery, a special bandage is worn on the head during sleep. After about one month, the surgical wounds are healed and the patient returns to the implant clinic to be fitted with the external parts of the device and to have the device turned on and mapped. Mapping involves fine tuning the speech processor and setting levels of stimulation for each electrode, from soft to loud.

The patient is then trained in how to interpret the sounds heard through the device. The length of the training varies from days to years, depending on how well the person can interpret the sounds heard through the device.

Risks

As with all operations, there are risks with this surgery. These include:

- infection at the incision site
- bleeding
- complications related to anesthesia
- transient dizziness
- facial paralysis (rarely)
- temporary taste disturbances
- additional hearing loss
- device failure

However, it should be noted that serious surgical complications have been observed at only one in 10,000 procedures of this type.

Some long-term risks of the implant include the unknown effects of electrical stimulation on the nervous system. It is also possible to damage the implant's internal components by a blow to the head, which will render the device unworkable.

A further consideration is that the use of **magnetic resonance imaging** (MRI) for patients with cochlear implants is not recommended because of the magnets present in the devices. Several companies have developed implants that do not use magnets or have altered the receiver-stimulator make up to make it easier to remove the magnets before testing. One fact that reduces the concern about MRI testing is that for many medical indications, MRI can be replaced with a computer assisted tomography scan (CAT or CT scan), which is not a problem for persons with cochlear implants.

Additionally, in July 2002, the Food and Drug Administration (FDA) issued a warning about a possible connection between increased incidence of meningitis and the presence of a cochlear implant. This warning included special vaccine recommendations for those with implants, as well as the voluntary removal from the market of certain devices. Specifically, those implants that included a positioner to hold the electrodes in place in the cochlea appear to be associated with an increased risk of the disease.

Normal results

Most profoundly deaf patients who receive an implant are able to discern medium and loud sounds, including speech, at comfortable listening levels. Many use sound clues from the implant, together with speech reading and other facial cues, to achieve understanding.

KEY TERMS

Auditory nerve—The nerve that carries electrical signals from the cochlea to the brain.

Cochlea—The hearing part of the inner ear. This snail-shaped structure contains fluid and thousands of microscopic hair cells tuned to various frequencies.

Hair cells—Sensory receptors in the inner ear that transform sound vibrations into messages that travel to the brain.

Inner ear—The interior section of the ear, where sound vibrations and information about balance are translated into nerve impulses.

Middle ear—The small cavity between the eardrum and the oval window that houses the three tiny bones of hearing.

Sensoineural deafness—Hearing loss due to the inability to convert sound from vibration to electrical signals. Often involves defects in the function of cochlear hair cells.

Almost all adults improve their communication skills when combining the implant with speech reading (lip reading), and some can understand spoken words without speech reading. More than half of adults who lost hearing after they learned to speak can understand some speech without speech reading. Especially with the use of accessory devices, the great majority can utilize the telephone with their implants.

Children who were born deaf or who lost their hearing before they could speak have the most difficulty in learning to use the implant. Research suggests, however, that most of these children are able to learn spoken language and understand speech using the implant. In general, the earlier the implant occurs the greater the chance of the implant providing sufficient sound input to provide speech understanding. As with the use of the telephone in adults, accessory devices such as special microphones often help the function of the implant in classroom settings.

Resources

BOOKS

Christiansen, John B. and Irene W. Leigh. *Cochlear Implants in Children: Ethics and Choices.* Washington, DC: Galladet University Press, 2002.

Niparko, John K., ed. *Cochlear Implants: Principles and Practices.* Philadelphia: Lippincott, Williams & Wilkins, 2000.

PERIODICALS

Cheng, Andre K., et al. "Cost-Utility Analysis of the Cochlear Implant in Children." *Journal of the American Medical Association* 284, no. 7 (August 16, 2000): 850–856.

"The Earlier the Implant, the Greater the Benefit." *The Hearing Journal* (February 2001).

Mraz, Stephen J. "Breaking the Wall of Silence." *Machine Design* (December 9, 1999).

ORGANIZATIONS

Alexander Graham Bell Association for the Deaf. 3417 Volta Place NW, Washington, DC 20007. (202) 337-5220. <http://www.agbell.org>.

Cochlear Implant Club International. 5335 Wisconsin Ave. NW, Suite 440, Washington, D.C. 20015-2052. (202) 895-2781. <http://www.cici.org>.

Hearing Loss Link. 2600 W. Peterson Ave., Ste. 202, Chicago, IL 60659. (312) 743-1032, (312) 743-1007 (TDD).

National Association for the Deaf. 814 Thayer Ave., Silver Spring, MD 20910. (301) 587-1788, (301) 587-1789 (TDD). <http://www.nad.org>.

OTHER

Cochlear Implant Recipients may be at Greater Risk for Meningitis. FDA Public Health Web Notification. October 17, 2002 [cited February 23, 2003]. <http://www.fda.gov/cdrh/safety/cochlear.html>.

Carol A. Turkington
Michelle L. Johnson

Colectomy *see* **Bowel resection**

Collagen periurethral injection

Definition

Collagen periurethral injection is a procedure in which collagen is injected around the urethra and bladder neck as a treatment for stress incontinence in women.

Purpose

The bladder and urethra are supported by muscles, ligaments, and connective tissues around the base of the bladder. This support prevents the leakage of urine, along with the watertight seal provided by the urethra. As a result of pregnancy, childbirth, and aging, or damage by scarring from surgery or radiotherapy, these structures may become damaged or weakened, thus causing stress incontinence, meaning an involuntary loss

of urine that occurs during physical activity such as coughing, sneezing, laughing, or **exercise**.

The injection of bulking agents such as collagen around the urethra aims to improve the lost support of the bladder and urethra. The substance most commonly used for injection is collagen; other bulking agents are being developed, for example, a silicon base suspended in a viscous gel called Macroplastique. Teflon paste, introduced in the 1970s, initially gave good results, but was discontinued after reported problems with excessive scarring and with the migration of Teflon particles to other tissues in the body. The collagen used in the procedure comes from the cartilage of cattle and has been extensively sterilized to produce a viscous paste for injection. There is no risk of bovine spongiform encephalopathy (BSE) transmission because the processing of the paste destroys any bacterial or viral particles.

Description

The collagen periurethral injection procedure is quick, and usually over within 15–20 minutes. No incisions are made, meaning that it can be carried out using a local anesthetic or a regional anesthetic such as an epidural. The surgeon uses a fine fiber-optic cystoscope to examine the inside of the urethra and bladder, and then inserts a fine needle to inject the collagen. Usually three injections are made around the urethra. The exact amount of collagen used depends on how much closure the urethra requires.

Aftercare

Since the procedure is very short and there is little discomfort afterwards, it is performed on an outpatient basis, and women can go home the same day. Recovery from the operation is very quick.

Risks

Periurethral injection is not associated with major complications. Urinary tract infection is common in up

KEY TERMS

Anesthetic—A drug that causes unconsciousness or a loss of general sensation.

Bladder—A membranous sac that serves as a reservoir for urine. Contraction of the bladder results in urination.

Catheterization—The placement of a catheter in a specific anatomic area most commonly for the purpose of treatment or diagnosis.

Collagen—The protein substance of the white fibres (collagenous fibres) of skin, tendon, bone, cartilage, and all other connective tissue.

Cystoscope—An instrument that allows the doctor to see inside the bladder and remove tissue samples.

Epidural—Located within the spinal canal, on or outside the dura mater, the tough membrane surrounding the spinal cord.

Incontinence—The inability to control excretory functions, as defecation (faecal incontinence) or urination (urinary incontinence).

Periurethral—Surrounding the urethra.

Stress incontinence—Involuntary loss of urine that occurs during physical activity such as coughing, sneezing, laughing, or exercise.

Urethra—The tube that passes urine from the bladder to the outside.

to a fifth of the women having undergone the procedure, but is usually quickly and easily treated with **antibiotics**. Some women experience difficulty urinating immediately after the procedure, but this is not unexpected following an operation involving the bladder and urethra that may easily lead to swelling and bruising of the tissues. It is a relatively uncommon problem after periurethral injection, but may occur. The condition usually settles quickly, but may require catheterization. Long-term problems are very rare.

Normal results

Since periurethral injection is so quick and easy with very few complications, it would appear to be an ideal treatment for stress incontinence. However, there is a problem with the longer-term results. Within three months after injection, good results are reported with at least 80% of women cured or improved. However, after two years, less than half of these women will still be cured. Longer-term studies are still being performed, but it is likely that the results will keep becoming poorer as time goes by. This is due to the injected collagen dispersing away from the urethra over time. Injections can be repeated and some women do require more than one injection before they are cured. Ongoing research into newer injection substances may improve these results. The results in younger, physically active women are also less successful, usually lasting for a shorter time. Repeated injections are not the simple solution they may seem, because collagen is very expensive and the long-term effects of repeated injections are unknown. Physicians thus tend to prefer one of the alternative operations if long-term cure of stress incontinence is the aim.

Alternatives

Other treatments are available to treat incontinence. They include:

- Physiotherapy. This treatment aims to increase the strength and support provided by the pelvic floor muscles.

- Surgical procedures. Operations such as colposuspension, sling procedures, needle-suspensions, and vaginal repair operations are all based on lifting and re-supporting the bladder and urethra.

Resources

BOOKS

Burgio, K. L., L. Pearce, A. J. Lucco, and K. F. Jeter. *Staying Dry: A Practical Guide to Bladder Control.* Baltimore: Johns Hopkins University Press, 1990.

Kaschak Newman, D. *Managing and Treating Urinary Incontinence.* Baltimore: Health Professions Press, 2002.

PERIODICALS

Block, C. A., C. S. Cooper, and C. E. Hawtrey. "Long-term Efficacy of Periurethral Collagen Injection for the Treatment of Urinary Incontinence Secondary to Myelomeningocele." *Journal of Urology* 169 (January 2003): 327–329.

Culligan, P. J., et al. "The Safety of Reusing Injectable Collagen: A Multicenter Microbiological Study." *International Urogynecological Journal of Pelvic Floor Dysfunction* 13 (2002): 232–234.

Dmochowski, R. R., and R. A. Appell. "Injectable Agents in the Treatment of Stress Urinary Incontinence in Women: Where Are We Now?" *Urology* 56 (December 2000): 32–40.

Kassouf. W., G. Capolicchio, G. Berardinucci, and J. Corcos. "Collagen Injection for Treatment of Urinary Incontinence in Children." *Journal of Urology* 165 (May 2001): 1666–1668.

ORGANIZATIONS

National Association for Women's Health. 300 W. Adams Street, Suite 328, Chicago, IL 60606-5101. (312) 786-1468. <http://www.nawh.org/>.

OTHER

National Women's Health Information Center. <www.4woman, org/>.

"Periurethral Injection Therapy for Incontinence." eMedicine. <www.emedicine.com/med/topic3049.htm>.

"Stress Incontinence." *MEDLINE Encyclopedia.* <www.nlm.nih.gov/medlineplus/ency/article/000891.htm >.

Monique Laberge, Ph.D.

Colon anastomosis *see* **Ileoanal anastomosis**

Colonoscopy

Definition

Colonoscopy is an endoscopic medical procedure that uses a long, flexible, lighted tubular instrument called a colonoscope to view the rectum and the entire inner lining of the colon (large intestine).

Purpose

A colonoscopy is generally recommended when the patient complains of rectal bleeding, has a change in bowel habits, and/or has other unexplained abdominal symptoms. The test is frequently used to look for colorectal cancer, especially when polyps or tumor-like growths have been detected by a **barium enema** examination and other diagnostic imaging tests. Polyps can be removed through the colonoscope, and samples of tissue (biopsies) can be taken to detect the presence of cancerous cells. In addition, colonoscopy can also be used to remove foreign bodies, control hemorrhaging, and excise tumors.

The test also enables physicians to check for bowel diseases such as ulcerative colitis and Crohn's disease and is an essential tool for monitoring patients who have a past history of polyps or colon cancer. Colonoscopy is being used increasingly as a screening tool in both asymptomatic patients and patients at risk for colon cancer. It has been recommended as a screening test in all people 50 years or older.

Description

Colonoscopy can be performed either in a physician's office or in an endoscopic procedure room of a hospital. For otherwise healthy patients, colonoscopy is generally performed by a gastroenterologist or surgeon in an office setting; when performed on patients with other medical conditions requiring hospitalization, it is often performed in the endoscopy department of a hospital, where more intensive physiologic monitoring and/or general anesthesia can be better provided.

An intravenous line is inserted into a vein in the patient's arm to administer, in most cases, a sedative and a painkiller.

During the colonoscopy, patients are asked to lie on their sides with their knees drawn up towards the abdomen. The doctor begins the procedure by inserting a lubricated, gloved finger into the anus to check for any abnormal masses or blockage. A thin, well-lubricated colonoscope is then inserted into the anus and gently advanced through the colon. The lining of the intestine is examined through the colonoscope. The physician views images on a television monitor, and the procedure can be documented using a video recorder. Still images can be recorded and saved on a computer disk or printed out. Occasionally, air may be pumped through the colonoscope to help clear the path or open the colon. If excessive secretions, stool, or blood obstructs the viewing, they are suctioned out through the scope. The doctor may press on the abdomen or ask the patient to change position in order to advance the scope through the colon.

The entire length of the large intestine can be examined in this manner. If suspicious growths are observed, tiny biopsy forceps or brushes can be inserted through the colon and tissue samples can be obtained. Small polyps or inflamed tissue can be removed using tiny instruments passed through the scope. For excising tumors or performing other types of surgery on the colon during

Endoscopic view of a colon polyp. *(G-I Associates/Custom Medical Stock Photo. Reproduced by permission.)*

colonoscopy, an electrosurgical device or laser system may be used in conjunction with the colonoscope. To stop bleeding in the colon, a laser, heater probe, or electrical probe is used, or special medicines are injected through the scope. After the procedure, the colonoscope is slowly withdrawn and the instilled air is allowed to escape. The anal area is then cleansed with tissues. Tissue samples taken by biopsy are sent to a clinical laboratory, where they are analyzed by a pathologist.

The procedure may take anywhere from 30 minutes to two hours depending on how easy it is to advance the scope through the colon. Colonoscopy can be a long and uncomfortable procedure, and the bowel-cleansing preparation may be tiring and can produce diarrhea and cramping. During the colonoscopy, the sedative and the pain medications will keep the patient drowsy and relaxed. Some patients complain of minor discomfort and pressure from the colonoscope. However, the sedative and pain medication usually cause most patients to dose off during the procedure.

Patients who regularly take **aspirin**, **nonsteroidal anti-inflammatory drugs** (NSAIDs), blood thinners, or insulin should be sure to inform the physician prior to the colonoscopy. Patients with severe active colitis, ex-

tremely dilated colon (toxic megacolon), or severely inflamed bowel may not be candidates for colonoscopy. Patients requiring continuous ambulatory peritoneal dialysis are generally not candidates for colonoscopy due to a higher risk of developing intraperitoneal bleeding.

Diagnosis/Preparation

The physician should be notified if the patient has allergies to any medications or anesthetics, bleeding problems, or is pregnant. The doctor should be informed of all the medications the patient is taking and if he or she has had a barium enema x-ray examination recently. If the patient has had heart valves replaced, the doctor should be informed so that appropriate **antibiotics** can be administered to prevent infection. The risks are explained to the patient beforehand, and the patient is asked to sign a consent form.

The colon must be thoroughly cleansed before performing colonoscopy. Consequently, for two or more days before the procedure, considerable preparation is necessary to clear the colon of all stool. The patient is asked to refrain from eating any solid food for 24–48 hours before the test. Only clear liquid such as juices, broth, and gelatin are allowed. Red or purple juices should be avoided, since they can cause coloring of the colon that may be misinterpreted during the colonoscopy. The patient is advised to drink plenty of water to avoid dehydration. A day or two before the colonoscopy, the patient is prescribed liquid, tablet, and/or suppository **laxatives** by the physician. In addition, commercial enemas may be prescribed. The patient is given specific instructions on how and when to use the laxatives and/or enemas.

On the morning of the colonoscopy, the patient is not to eat or drink anything. Unless otherwise instructed by the physician, the patient should continue to take all current medications. However, vitamins with iron, iron supplements, or iron preparations should be discontinued for a few weeks prior to the colonoscopy because iron residue in the colon can inhibit viewing during the procedure. These preparatory procedures are extremely important to ensure a thoroughly clean colon for examination.

After the procedure, the patient is kept under observation until the medications' effects wear off. The patient has to be driven home and can generally resume a normal diet and usual activities unless otherwise instructed. The patient is advised to drink plenty of fluids to replace those lost by laxatives and fasting.

For a few hours after the procedure, the patient may feel groggy. There may be some abdominal cramping and a considerable amount of gas may be passed. If a biopsy was performed or a polyp was removed, there may be small amounts of blood in the stool for a few days. If the patient experiences severe abdominal pain or has persistent and heavy bleeding, this information should be brought to the physician's attention immediately.

For patients with abnormal results such as polyps, the gastroenterologist will recommend another colonoscopy, usually in another year or so.

Risks

The procedure is virtually free of any complications and risks. Rarely, (two in 1,000 cases) a perforation (a hole) may occur in the intestinal wall. Heavy bleeding due to the removal of the polyp or from the biopsy site occurs infrequently (one in 1,000 cases). Some patients may have adverse reactions to the sedatives administered during the colonoscopy, but severe reactions are very rare. Infections due to a colonoscopy are also extremely rare. Patients with artificial or abnormal heart valves are usually given antibiotics before and after the procedure to prevent an infection.

Normal results

The results are normal if the lining of the colon is a pale reddish pink and there are no masses that appear abnormal in the lining.

Abnormal results indicate polyps or other suspicious masses in the lining of the intestine. Polyps can be removed during the procedure, and tissue samples can be taken by biopsy. If cancerous cells are detected in the tissue samples, then a diagnosis of colon cancer is made. A pathologist analyzes the tumor cells further to estimate the tumor's aggressiveness and the extent of the disease. This is crucial before deciding on the mode of treatment for the disease. Abnormal findings could also be due to inflammatory bowel diseases such as ulcerative colitis or Crohn's disease. A condition called diverticulosis, which causes many small finger-like pouches to protrude from the colon wall, may also contribute to an abnormal result in the colonoscopy.

Morbidity and mortality rates

In 2003, an estimated 57,100 people will die from colorectal cancer. Although screening could find precancerous growths (polyps), which lead to colorectal cancer, screening rates in the United States remain low. Removing polyps before they turn into cancer could prevent the disease and potentially reduce deaths. Scientific evidence shows that more than one-third of deaths from colorectal cancer could be avoided if people aged 50 years and older were screened regularly.

Despite recent advances in screening and treatment for colon cancer, it is still one of the most common cancers among men and women in the United States. According to a report in the *American Journal of Gastroenterology,* there has been no improvement in colon cancer survival in the United States since the 1980s. As well, the number of patients surviving five years after their cancer diagnosis did not improve.

Recent National Cancer Institute-funded clinical trials show that taking daily aspirin for as little as three years could reduce the development of colorectal polyps by 19–35% in people at high risk for colorectal cancer.

The Center for Disease Control and Prevention recommends that everyone 50 years of age and over have one or a combination of the four recommended screening tests: fecal occult blood test, **sigmoidoscopy**, colonoscopy, or barium enema.

Alternatives

New research suggests that a simple blood test may identify people at risk of colorectal cancer. The blood test detects a genetic alteration that may identify people who are likely to develop the disease and who would benefit from additional screening; however, further research has to be done before this test becomes available.

KEY TERMS

Barium enema—An x-ray test of the bowel after giving the patient an enema of a white chalky substance that outlines the colon and the rectum.

Biopsy—Removal of a tissue sample for examination under the microscope to check for cancer cells.

Computed tomography (CT) scan—A radiologic imaging modality that uses computer processing to generate an image of the tissue density; also called computerized axial tomography (CAT) and computerized transaxial tomography (CTAT).

Colonoscope—A thin, flexible, hollow, lighted tube that is inserted through the anus and rectum to the colon to enable the physician to view the entire lining of the colon.

Crohn's disease—A chronic inflammatory disease that generally starts in the gastrointestinal tract and causes the immune system to attack one's own body.

Diverticulosis—A condition that involves the development of sacs that bulge through the large intestine's muscular walls, but are not inflamed. It may cause bleeding, stomach distress, and excess gas.

Electrosurgical device—A medical device that uses electrical current to cauterize or coagulate tissue during surgical procedures; often used in conjunction with laparoscopy.

Endoscopic—To visualize a hollow organ's interior.

Fecal occult blood test—A blood test that chemically checks the stool for hidden (occult) blood.

Magnetic resonance imaging (MRI)—A test that provides pictures of organs and structures inside the body. In many cases, MRI provides information that cannot be obtained from x-ray tests.

Pathologist—A doctor who specializes in the diagnosis of disease by studying cells and tissues under a microscope.

Polyps—An abnormal growth that develops on the inside of a hollow organ such as the colon.

Sigmoidoscopy—A process of passing a long, hollow tubular instrument through the anus in order to permit inspection, diagnosis, treatment, and imaging, especially of the sigmoid flexure.

Ulcerative colitis—A chronic condition in which recurrent ulcers are found in the colon. It is manifested clinically by abdominal cramping and rectal bleeding.

Virtual colonoscopy—Two new techniques that provide views of the colon to screen for colon polyps and cancer. The images are produced by computerized manipulations rather than direct observation through the colonoscope; one technique uses the x-ray images from a CT scan, and the other uses magnetic images from an MRI scan.

Virtual colonoscopy is a new technique under development and evaluation for screening for colon polyps and cancer, and is undergoing continual improvement. One technique uses images from a **magnetic resonance imaging** (MRI) scan, and the other uses the x-ray images from a computerized tomography (CT) scan. They both provide views of the colon that are similar to those obtained in a colonoscopy. The images of the colon are produced by computerized manipulations rather than direct observation through the colonoscope.

While the CT scan technique is available in many radiology units, the MRI scan technique is still experimental. The colon is cleaned out using potent laxatives for both types of studies. A virtual image of the colon is formed after the scans are performed, and the images are analyzed and manipulated.

One benefit of the CT scan is that it can find polyps that occasionally are missed by colonoscopy because the polyps lie behind folds within the colon. Nevertheless, criticisms of the CT scan include:

• It cannot find small polyps (<0.2 in [5 mm] in size) that are easily seen in a colonoscopy.

• It is less able to find flat polyps compared to a colonoscopy.

• The procedure does not require patients to be sedated or put under anesthesia, and it can be performed in less than one minute, compared with about 30–60 minutes, plus recovery time required for standard colonoscopy.

• Small pieces of stool can look like polyps on the CT scan and lead to a diagnosis of polyp when there is none.

• If colonic polyps are found by virtual colonoscopy, then standard colonoscopy must be done to remove the polyps. As a result, the individual must undergo two procedures.

Although the CT scan is a good option for individuals who cannot or will not undergo standard colonoscopy, it has not been determined if it should be a primary screening tool for individuals at either normal risk or high risk for polyps or cancer.

Resources

BOOKS

Beers, Mark H. and Robert Berkow, eds. *Merck Manual of Diagnosis and Therapy,* 17th edition. Whitehouse Station, NJ: Merck & Co., 1999.

Dachman, Abraham H., (editor). *Atlas of Virtual Colonoscopy.* Berlin: Springer Verlag, 2003.

Dafnis, George. *Colonoscopy: Introduction and Development, Completion Rates, Complications and Cancer Detection (Comprehensive Summaries of Uppsala Dissertations from the Faculty of Medicine, 1039).* Uppsala, Sweden: Uppsala University, 2001.

Tierney, Lawrence M., Stephen J. McPhee, and Maxine A. Papadakis (editors). *Current Medical Diagnosis & Treatment 2003.* Stamford, CT: Appleton & Lange, 2002.

PERIODICALS

Dominitz, J. A., et al. "Complications of Colonoscopy." *Gastrointestinal Endoscopy* 57, no 4 (April 2003): 441–5.

Isenberg, G. A., et al. "Virtual Colonoscopy." *Gastrointestinal Endoscopy* 57, no 4 (April 2003): 451–4.

Rabeneck, Linda, Hashem B. El-Serag, Jessica A. Davila, and Robert S. Sandler. "Outcomes of Colorectal Cancer in the United States: No Change in Survival (1986–1997)." *The American Journal of Gastroenterology* 98, no 2 (February 2003): 471–477.

ORGANIZATIONS

American College of Gastroenterology (ACG). 4900-B South 31st Street, Arlington, VA 22206-1656. (703) 820-7400; Fax: (703) 931-4520. <http://www.acg.gi.org>.

Colorectal Cancer Network (CCNetwork). P.O. Box 182, Kensington, MD 20895-0182. (301) 879-1500; Fax: (301) 879-1901. <http://www.colorectal-cancer.net>.

International Foundation for Functional Gastrointestinal Disorders (IFFGD). P.O. Box 170864, Milwaukee, WI 53217. (888) 964-2001, (414) 964-1799; Fax: (414) 964-7176. Email: <iffgd@iffgd.org>. <http://www.iffgd. org>.

National Digestive Diseases Information Clearinghouse. 2 Information Way, Bethesda, MD 20892-3570. E-mail: <nddic@info.niddk.nih.gov>. <http://www. niddk.nih.gov>.

Society of American Gastrointestinal Endoscopic Surgeons (SAGES). 2716 Ocean Park Boulevard, Suite 3000, Santa Monica, CA 90405. (310) 314-2404; Fax: (310) 314-2585. <http://www.sages.org>.

Society of Gastroenterology Nurses and Associates Inc. 401 North Michigan Avenue, Chicago, IL 60611-4267. (800) 245-7462; Fax: (312) 527-6658. <http://www.sgna.org>.

OTHER

Centers for Disease Control and Prevention. United States Department of Health and Human Services. *Screen for Life. National Colorectal Cancer Action Campaign.* 2003 [cited April 9, 2003] <http://www.cdc.gov/cancer/screen forlife/>.

Mayo Foundation for Medical Education and Research. *Colorectal Cancer Screening Health Decision Guide.* 2003 [cited April 4, 2003] <http://www.mayoclinic.com/invoke.cfm?objectid=B487B5A5-4F52-40E1-A76587E33E 0DD676>.

PDR Health (Thompson Healthcare). *Colon Cancer: The Case For Early Detection.* 2003 [cited April 2, 2003] <http:// www.pdrhealth.com/content/lifelong_health/chapters/ fgac31.shtml >.

Society of American Gastrointestinal Endoscopic Surgeons. *Patient Information from Your Surgeon & SAGES.* 2002 [cited April 9, 2003] <http://www.sages.org/pi_colono scopy.html>.

Jennifer E. Sisk, MA
Crystal H. Kaczkowski, MSc

Colorectal surgery

Definition

Colorectal surgery repairs damage to the colon, rectum, and anus through a variety of procedures that may have little or great long-term consequence to the patient. It may also involve surgery to the pelvic floor to repair hernias.

Purpose

Colorectal surgery is performed to repair damage to the colon, rectum, and anus, caused by diseases of the lower digestive tract, such as cancer, diverticulitis, and inflammatory bowel disease (ulcerative colitis and Crohn's disease). Injury, obstruction, and ischemia (compromised blood supply) may require bowel surgery. Masses and scar tissue can grow within the rectum, causing blockages that prevent normal elimination of feces. Other diseases such as diverticulitis and ulcerative colitis can cause perforations in the rectum. Surgical removal of the damaged area or areas can return normal bowel function.

Demographics

Colorectal cancer affects 140,000 people annually, causing 60,000 deaths. Polypectomy (the removal of polyps in the colon), usually performed during a routine diagnostic test (colonscopy or flexible **sigmoidoscopy**), has been a factor in the declining incidence of this cancer. However, incidence of the disease, as reported in the Journal of the National Cancer Institute in 2001, differed among ethnic groups, with Hispanics having 10.2 cases per 100,000 people, to African Americans having 22.8 cases per 100,000. Surgery is the optimal treatment for colorectal cancer, resulting in cure in 80% of patients. Recurrence due to surgical failure is low, from 4% to 8%, when surgery is meticulously performed.

Crohn's disease and ulcerative colitis, both chronic inflammatory diseases of the colon, affect approximately 1,000,000 young adults. Surgery is recommended when medication fails patients with ulcerative colitis. Usually, surgery is drastic, removing the colon and rectum and creating an interior or exterior pouch to collect body wastes. Nearly three-fourths of all Crohn's patients face surgery to removed a diseased section of the intestine or rectum.

Diverticulosis, the growth of pouches in the walls of the intestine, occurs in nearly half of all Americans by the time they reach age 60 and in practically everyone over 80. Sometimes these diverticuli become infected and diverticulitis occurs. Diverticulitis may also require surgery to remove part of the colon if there have been recurrent episodes with complications or perforations.

Description

Colorectal surgery is a necessary treatment option for colorectal cancer, ulcerative colitis, Crohn's disease, and some cases of diverticulitis, often resulting in major reconstruction of the intestinal tract. Other bowel conditions that may require surgery to a lesser extent are hemorrhoids, anal fissures (tears in the lining of the anus), rectal prolapse, and bowel incontinence. Most of these surgeries repair tears, remove blockages, or tighten sphincter muscles. Patients with anal fissures, for example, experience immediate relief, with more than 90% of them never having the problem recur.

Some colorectal surgeons also treat pelvic floor disorders such as perineal hernia and rectocele (a bulging of the rectum toward the vagina).

Types of surgery

There are a variety of procedures a colorectal surgeon may use to treat intestinal disorders. Until 1990, all col-

orectal surgery was performed by making large incisions in the abdomen, opening up the intestinal cavity, and making the repair. Most of these repairs involved resection (cutting out the diseased or damaged portion) and anastomosis (attaching the cut ends of the intestine together). Some were tucks to tighten sphincter muscles or repair fissures, and others cut out hemorrhoids. Some colorectal surgeons perform a strictureplasty, a new procedure that widens the intestine instead of making it shorter; this is used with patients with extensive Crohn's disease.

Often colorectal surgery involves creating an ostomy, which is an opening from the inside of the body to the outside, usually to remove body wastes (feces or urine). There are several types of ostomy surgeries that colorectal surgeons do. A **colostomy** is a surgical procedure that brings a portion of the large intestine through the abdominal wall, creating an opening, or stoma, to carry feces out of the body to a pouch. An **ileostomy** removes the entire colon, the rectum, and the anus. The lower end of the small intestine (the ileum) becomes the stoma.

For all ostomies, a pouch will generally be placed around the stoma on the patient's abdomen during surgery. During the hospital stay, the patient and his or her caregivers will be educated on care of the stoma and the ostomy pouch. Determination of appropriate pouching supplies and a schedule of how often to change the pouch should be established. Regular assessment and meticulous care of the skin surrounding the stoma is important to maintain an adequate surface on which to attach the pouch. Some patients with colostomies are able to routinely irrigate the stoma, resulting in regulation of bowel function; rather than needing to wear a pouch, these patients may need only a dressing or cap over their stoma. Often, an enterostomal therapist will visit the patient in the hospital or at home after discharge to help the patient with stoma care.

Most colostomies and ileostomies are permanent. Temporary colostomies are created to divert stool from injured or diseased portions of the large intestine, allowing rest and healing. Although colorectal cancer is the most common indication for a permanent colostomy, only about 10–15% of patients with this diagnosis require a colostomy.

A new procedure called an **ileoanal anastomosis** creates an internal reservoir that is sewn to the anus and acts as an artificial rectum. It usually is not used with Crohn's disease patients because their disease often recurs.

Laparoscopic surgery is being used with many diseases of the intestinal tract, including initial cancers. For this surgery, the colon and rectal surgeon inserts a laparoscope (an instrument that has a tiny video camera attached) through a small incision in the abdomen. Other small incisions are made through which the surgeon inserts **surgical instruments**. This surgery often results in fewer complications, a shorter stay in the hospital, less postoperative pain, a quicker return to normal activities, and less scarring. It is not recommended for patients who have had extensive prior abdominal surgery, large tumors, previous cancer, or serious heart problems.

Diagnosis/Preparation

Some disease or conditions may require a minimally invasive surgery. Other diseases such as inflammatory bowel disease and colorectal cancer may require an ostomy, a more drastic procedure. Determining whether this surgery is necessary is a decision the physician makes based on a number of factors, including patient history, the amount of pain the patient is experiencing, and the results of several diagnostic tests. Due to the lifestyle impact of ostomy surgery, surgeons make that decision with careful input from the patient. Sometimes, though, an immediate decision may be necessary in emergency situations involving injuries or puncture wounds in the abdomen, or intestinal perforations related to diverticulear disease, ulcers, or cancer, which can be life-threatening.

Diagnostic tests

Colonoscopy, flexible sigmoidoscopy, and a lower GI (gastrointestinal) series help determine the condition of the intestinal tract. These tests can identify masses and perforations on bowel walls.

A lower GI series is a series of x rays of the colon and rectum, which can identify ulcers, cysts, polyps, diverticuli (pouches in the intestine), and cancer. The patient is given a **barium enema**; the barium coats the intestinal tract, making any signs of disease easier to see on x rays.

Flexible sigmoidoscopy, a flexible tube with a miniature camera, is inserted into the rectum so the physician can examine the lining of the rectum and the sigmoid colon, the last third of the intestinal tract. The sigmoidoscope can also remove polyps or tissue for biopsy.

A colonoscopy is a similar procedure to the flexible sigmoidoscopy, except the flexible tube looks at the entire intestinal tract. For the patient's comfort, a sedative is given.

Magnetic resonance imaging (MRI), used both prior to and during surgery, allows physicians to determine the precise margins for resections of the colon, so that they can eliminate all of the diseased tissue. MRI can also identify patients who could most benefit from adjuvant therapy such as chemotherapy or radiation.

Preoperative preparation

The doctor will outline the procedure, possible side effects, and what the patient may experience after

---

QUESTIONS TO ASK THE DOCTOR

- Am I a good candidate for laparoscopic surgery?
- What tests will you require?
- What drugs will be given for pain after the surgery?
- What will I need to do to prepare for surgery?
- What will my recovery time be and what restrictions will I have?
- How many of these procedures have you performed?
- What are my risks for this surgery?

---

surgery. As with any surgical procedure, the patient will be required to sign a consent form. Blood and urine studies, along with various x rays and an electrocardiograph (EKG), may be ordered. If necessary, an enterostomal therapist will be contacted to mark an appropriate place on the abdomen for the stoma and offer preoperative education on ostomy management.

In order to empty and cleanse the bowel, the patient may be placed on a restricted diet for several days prior to surgery. A liquid diet may be ordered for at least the day before surgery, with nothing by mouth after midnight. A series of enemas and/or oral preparations (GoLytely, Colyte, or senna) may be ordered to empty the bowel of stool. Oral anti-infectives (neomycin, erythromycin, or kanamycin sulfate) may be ordered to decrease bacteria in the intestine and help prevent postoperative infection.

Aftercare

Postoperative care involves monitoring blood pressure, pulse, respiration, and temperature. Breathing tends to be shallow because of the effect of the anesthesia and the patient's reluctance to breathe deeply and experience pain that is caused by the abdominal incision. The patient is instructed how to support the operative site during deep breathing and coughing, and given pain medication as necessary. Fluid intake and output is measured, and the operative site is observed for color and amount of wound drainage.

The patient is usually helped out of bed the evening of the surgery and allowed to sit in a chair. Most patients are discharged in two to four days.

The nasogastric tube will remain in place, attached to low, intermittent suction until bowel activity resumes. For the first 24–48 hours after surgery, the ostomy will drain bloody mucus. Fluids and electrolytes are given intravenously until the patient's diet can gradually be resumed, beginning with liquids only, then adding solids. Usually within 72 hours, passage of gas and stool through the stoma begins. Initially the stool is liquid, gradually thickening as the patient begins to take solid foods. The patient is usually out of bed in eight to 24 hours after surgery and discharged in two to four days.

Risks

Potential risks of colorectal surgery are those of any major surgery and usually occur while the patient is still in the hospital. The patient's general health prior to surgery will also be an indication of the potential for risk. Of special concern are cardiac problems and stressed immune systems.

Psychological complications may result from ostomy surgery because of the fear of the social stigma attached to wearing a colostomy bag. Patients may also be depressed and have feelings of low self-worth because of the change in their lifestyle and their appearance. Some patients may feel ugly and sexually unattractive and may worry that their spouse or significant other will no longer find them appealing. Counseling and education regarding surgery and the inherent lifestyle changes are often necessary.

Normal results

Complete healing is expected without complications. The period of time required for recovery from the surgery may vary, depending on the patient's overall health prior to surgery. Dietary changes may be encouraged to prevent future disorders or to manage a current disease.

Morbidity and mortality rates

Mortality has been decreased from nearly 28% to under 6% through the use of prophylactic **antibiotics** prescribed before and after surgery. Strong indicators of survival outcome or increased complications from surgery for elderly patients are underlying medical conditions. Therefore, the underlying medical conditions of at-risk patients should be controlled prior to a colorectal surgery.

Even among higher risk patients, mortality is about 16%. This rate is greatly reduced (between 0.8% and 3.8%) when the ostomies and resections for cancer are performed by a board-certified colon and rectal surgeon.

The physician and the nursing staff monitor the patient's **vital signs** and the surgical incision, alert for:

- excessive bleeding
- wound infection
- thrombophlebitis (inflammation and blood clot in the veins in the legs)
- pneumonia
- pulmonary embolism (blood clot or air bubble in the lungs' blood supply)
- cardiac stress due to allergic reaction to the general anesthetic

Symptoms that the patient should report, especially after discharge, include:

- increased pain, swelling, redness, drainage, or bleeding in the surgical area
- flu-like symptoms such as headache, muscle aches, dizziness, or fever
- increased abdominal pain or swelling, constipation, nausea or vomiting, or black, tarry stools

Stomal complications can also occur. They include:

- Death (necrosis) of stomal tissue. Caused by inadequate blood supply, this complication is usually visible 12–24 hours after the operation and may require additional surgery.
- Retraction (stoma is flush with the abdomen surface or has moved below it). Caused by insufficient stomal length, this complication may be managed by use of special pouching supplies; elective revision of the stoma is also an option.
- Prolapse (stoma increases length above the surface of the abdomen). Most often this results from an overly large opening in the abdominal wall or inadequate fixation of the bowel to the abdominal wall; surgical correction is required when blood supply is compromised.
- Stenosis (narrowing at the opening of the stoma). Often this is associated with infection around the stoma or scarring. Mild stenosis can be removed under local anesthesia; severe stenosis may require surgery for reshaping the stoma.
- Parastomal hernia (bowel-causing bulge in the abdominal wall next to the stoma). This occurs due to placement of the stoma where the abdominal wall is weak or an overly large opening in the abdominal wall is created. The use of an ostomy support belt and special pouching supplies may be adequate. If severe, the defect in the abdominal wall should be repaired and the stoma moved to another location.

Alternatives

When a colostomy is deemed necessary, there are usually no alternatives to the surgery, though there can

KEY TERMS

Adjuvant therapy—Treatment that is added to increase the effectiveness of surgery, usually chemotherapy or radiation used to kill any cancer cells that might be remaining.

Anastomosis—The surgical connection of two sections of tubes, ducts, or vessels.

Diverticuli—Pouches in the intestinal wall usually created from a diet low in fiber.

Embolism—Blockage of a blood vessel by any small piece of material traveling in the blood; the emboli may be caused by germs, air, blood clots, or fat.

Enema—Insertion of a tube into the rectum to infuse fluid into the bowel and encourage a bowel movement. Ordinary enemas contain tap water, mixtures of soap and water, glycerine and water, or other materials.

Intestine—Commonly called the bowels, divided into the small and large intestine. They extend from the stomach to the anus.

Ischemia—A compromise in blood supply delivered to body tissues that causes tissue damage or death.

Ostomy—A surgical procedure that creates an opening from the inside of the body to the outside, usually to remove body wastes (feces or urine).

Sigmoid colon—The last third of the intestinal tract that is attached to the rectum.

be alternatives in the type of surgery involved and adjuvant therapies related to the disease.

Resources

BOOKS

Johnston, Lorraine. *Colon & Rectal Cancer: A Comprehensive Guide for Patients and Families.* Sebastopol, CA: O'Reilly, 2000.

Levin, Bernard. *American Cancer Society Colorectal Cancer.* New York: Villard, 1999.

PERIODICALS

Beets-Tan, R. G. H., et al. "Accuracy of Maganetic Resonance Imaging in Prediction of Tumour-free Resection Margin in Rectal Cancer Surgery." *The Lancet* 357 (February 17, 2001): 497.

"Laparoscopy Could Offer Long-term Survival Benefit over Conventional Surgery." *Cancer Weekly* (July 30, 2002): 14.

Schwenk, Wolfgang. "Pulmonary Function Following Laparoscopic or Conventional Colorectal Resection: A Randomized Controlled Evaluation." *Journal of the American Medical Association,* 281 (April 7, 1999): 1154.

Senagore, A. J., and P. Erwin-Toth. "Care of the Laparoscopic Colectomy Patient." *Advances in Skin & Wound Care* 15 (November–December 2002): 277–284.

Walling, Anne D. "Follow-up after Resection for Colorectal Cancer Saves Lives. (Tips from Other Journals)." *American Family Physician,* 66 (August 1, 2002): 485.

ORGANIZATIONS

American Board of Colon and Rectal Surgery (ABCRS). 20600 Eureka Road, Suite 713, Taylor, MI 48180. (734) 282-9400. <www.fascrs.org>.

Mayo Clinic. 200 First St. S.W., Rochester, MN 55905. (507) 284-2511. <www.mayoclinic.org>.

United Ostomy Association, Inc. (UOA). 19772 MacArthur Blvd., Suite 200, Irvine, CA 92612-2405. (800) 826-0826. <http://www.uoa.org>.

Wound Ostomy and Continence Nurses Society. 2755 Bristol Street, Suite 110, Costa Mesa, CA 92626. (714) 476-0268. <http://www.wocn.org>.

OTHER

National Digestive Diseases Information Clearinghouse. *Ileostomy, Colostomy, and Ileoanal Reservoir Surgery.* (February 1, 2000): 1.

Janie F. Franz

Colostomy

Definition

A colostomy is a surgical procedure that brings a portion of the large intestine through the abdominal wall to carry feces out of the body.

Purpose

A colostomy is a means to treat various disorders of the large intestine, including cancer, obstruction, inflammatory bowel disease, ruptured diverticulum, ischemia (compromised blood supply), or traumatic injury. Temporary colostomies are created to divert stool from injured or diseased portions of the large intestine, allowing rest and healing. Permanent colostomies are performed when the distal bowel (at the farthest distance) must be removed or is blocked and inoperable. Although colorectal cancer is the most common indication for a permanent colostomy, only about 10–15% of patients with this diagnosis require a colostomy.

Colostomy

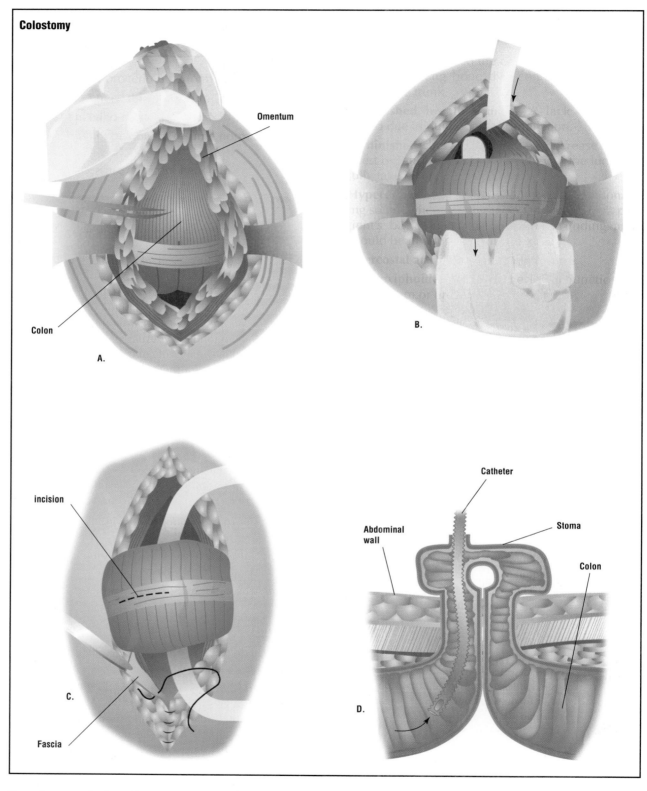

Omentum

Colon

A.

B.

incision

Fascia

C.

Catheter

Abdominal
wall

Stoma

Colon

D.

To perform a colostomy, the surgeon enters the abdomen and locates the colon, or large intestine (A). A loop of the colon is pulled through the abdominal incision (B); then the colon is cut to allow the insertion of a catheter (C). The skin and tissues are closed around the new opening, called a stoma (D). *(Illustration by GGS Inc.)*

Demographics

Estimates of all ostomy surgeries (those involving any opening from the abdomen for the removal of either feces or urine) range from 42,000 to 65,000 each year; about half are temporary. Emergency surgeries for bowel obstruction and/or perforation comprise 10–15% of all colorectal surgeries; a portion of these result in colostomy.

Description

Surgery will result in one of three types of colostomies:

- End colostomy. The functioning end of the intestine (the section of bowel that remains connected to the upper gastrointestinal tract) is brought out onto the surface of the abdomen, forming the stoma (artificial opening) by cuffing the intestine back on itself and suturing the end to the skin. The surface of the stoma is actually the lining of the intestine, usually appearing moist and pink. The distal portion of bowel (now connected only to the rectum) may be removed, or sutured closed and left in the abdomen. An end colostomy is usually a permanent ostomy, resulting from trauma, cancer, or another pathological condition.

- Double-barrel colostomy. This involves the creation of two separate stomas on the abdominal wall. The proximal (nearest) stoma is the functional end that is connected to the upper gastrointestinal tract and will drain stool; the distal stoma, connected to the rectum and also called a mucous fistula, drains small amounts of mucus material. This is most often a temporary colostomy performed to rest an area of bowel, and to be later closed.

- Loop colostomy. This surgery brings a loop of bowel through an incision in the abdominal wall. The loop is held in place outside the abdomen by a plastic rod slipped beneath it. An incision is made in the bowel to allow the passage of stool through the loop colostomy. The supporting rod is removed approximately seven to 10 days after surgery, when healing has occurred that will prevent the loop of bowel from retracting into the abdomen. A loop colostomy is most often performed for creation of a temporary stoma to divert stool away from an area of intestine that has been blocked or ruptured.

Diagnosis/Preparation

A number of diseases and injuries may require a colostomy. Among the diseases are inflammatory bowel disease and colorectal cancer. Determining whether this surgery is necessary is a decision the physician makes based on a number of factors, including patient history, amount of pain, and the results of tests such as

colonoscopy and lower G.I. (gastrointestinal) series. Due to lifestyle impact of the surgery, the decision is made after careful consultation with the patient. However, an immediate decision may be made in emergency situations involving injuries or puncture wounds in the abdomen or intestinal perforations related to diverticular disease, ulcers, or life-threatening cancer.

As with any surgical procedure, the patient will be required to sign a consent form after the procedure is explained thoroughly. Blood and urine studies, along with various x rays and an electrocardiograph (EKG), may be ordered as the doctor deems necessary. If possible, the patient should visit an enterostomal therapist, who will mark an appropriate place on the abdomen for the stoma and offer preoperative education on ostomy management.

In order to empty and cleanse the bowel, the patient may be placed on a low-residue diet for several days prior to surgery. A liquid diet may be ordered for at least the day before surgery, with nothing by mouth after midnight. A series of enemas and/or oral preparations (GoLytely or Colyte) may be ordered to empty the bowel of stool. Oral anti-infectives (neomycin, erythromycin, or kanamycin sulfate) may be ordered to decrease bacteria in the intestine and help prevent postoperative infection. A nasogastric tube is inserted from the nose to the stomach on the day of surgery or during surgery to remove gastric secretions and prevent nausea and vomiting. A urinary catheter (a thin plastic tube) may also be inserted to keep the bladder empty during surgery, giving more space in the surgical field and decreasing chances of accidental injury.

Aftercare

Postoperative care for the patient with a new colostomy, as with those who have had any major surgery, involves monitoring of blood pressure, pulse, respirations, and temperature. Breathing tends to be shallow because of the effect of anesthesia and the patient's reluctance to breathe deeply and experience pain that is caused by the abdominal incision. The patient is instructed how to support the operative site during deep breathing and coughing, and given pain medication as necessary. Fluid intake and output is measured, and the opera-

QUESTIONS TO ASK THE DOCTOR

- What kinds of preoperative tests will be required?
- What drugs will be given for pain after the surgery?
- What will I need to do to prepare for surgery?
- Is there an enterostomal therapist I can talk to before the surgery?
- What will my recovery time be and what restrictions will I have?
- Is there an ostomy support group at the hospital that I can attend?

tive site is observed for color and amount of wound drainage. The nasogastric tube will remain in place, attached to low, intermittent suction until bowel activity resumes. For the first 24–48 hours after surgery, the colostomy will drain bloody mucus. Fluids and electrolytes are infused intravenously until the patient's diet can gradually be resumed, beginning with liquids. Usually within 72 hours, passage of gas and stool through the stoma begins. Initially, the stool is liquid, gradually thickening as the patient begins to take solid foods. The patient is usually out of bed in eight to 24 hours after surgery and discharged in two to four days.

A colostomy pouch will generally have been placed on the patient's abdomen around the stoma during surgery. During the hospital stay, the patient and his or her caregivers will be educated on how to care for the colostomy. Determination of appropriate pouching supplies and a schedule of how often to change the pouch should be established. Regular assessment and meticulous care of the skin surrounding the stoma is important to maintain an adequate surface on which to attach the pouch. Some patients with colostomies are able to routinely irrigate the stoma, resulting in regulation of bowel function; rather than needing to wear a pouch, these patients may only need a dressing or cap over their stoma. Often, an enterostomal therapist will visit the patient in the hospital or at home after discharge to help the patient with stoma care.

Dietary counseling will be necessary for the patient to maintain normal bowel function and to avoid constipation, impaction, and other discomforts.

Risks

Potential complications of colostomy surgery include:

- excessive bleeding
- surgical wound infection
- thrombophlebitis (inflammation and blood clot to veins in the legs)
- pneumonia
- pulmonary embolism (blood clot or air bubble in the lungs' blood supply)

Psychological complications may result from colostomy surgery because of the fear of the perceived social stigma attached to wearing a colostomy bag. Patients may also be depressed and have feelings of low self-worth because of the change in their lifestyle and their appearance. Some patients may feel ugly and sexually unattractive and may worry that their spouse or significant other will no longer find them appealing. Counseling and education regarding surgery and the inherent lifestyle changes are often necessary.

Normal results

Complete healing is expected without complications. The period of time required for recovery from the surgery may vary depending on the patient's overall health prior to surgery and the patient's willingness to participate in stoma care. The colostomy patient without other medical complications should be able to resume all daily activities once recovered from the surgery. Adjustments in diet and daily personal care will need to be made.

Morbidity and mortality rates

Complications after colostomy surgery can occur. The doctor should be made aware of any of the following problems after surgery:

- increased pain, swelling, redness, drainage, or bleeding in the surgical area
- headache, muscle aches, dizziness, or fever
- increased abdominal pain or swelling, constipation, nausea or vomiting, or black, tarry stools

Stomal complications can also occur. They include:

- Death (necrosis) of stomal tissue. Caused by inadequate blood supply, this complication is usually visible 12–24 hours after the operation and may require additional surgery.
- Retraction (stoma is flush with the abdomen surface or has moved below it). Caused by insufficient stomal length, this complication may be managed by use of special pouching supplies. Elective revision of the stoma is also an option.

- Prolapse (stoma increases length above the surface of the abdomen). Most often this results from an overly large opening in the abdominal wall or inadequate fixation of the bowel to the abdominal wall. Surgical correction is required when blood supply is compromised.

- Stenosis (narrowing at the opening of the stoma). Often this is associated with infection around the stoma or scarring. Mild stenosis can be removed under local anesthesia; severe stenosis may require surgery for reshaping the stoma.

- Parastomal hernia (bowel causing bulge in the abdominal wall next to the stoma). This occurs due to placement of the stoma where the abdominal wall is weak or an overly large opening in the abdominal wall was made. The use of an ostomy support belt and special pouching supplies may be adequate. If severe, the defect in the abdominal wall should be repaired and the stoma moved to another location.

Mortality rates for colostomy patients vary according to the patient's general health upon admittance to the hospital. Even among higher risk patients, mortality is about 16%. This rate is greatly reduced (between 0.8% and 3.8%) when the colostomy is performed by a board-certified colon and rectal surgeon.

Alternatives

When a colostomy is deemed necessary, there are usually no alternatives to the surgery, though there can be alternatives in the type of surgery involved and adjuvant therapies related to the disease. For example, laparoscopic surgery is being used with many diseases of the intestinal tract, including initial cancers. For this surgery, the colon and rectal surgeon inserts a laparoscope (an instrument that has a tiny video camera attached) through a small incision in the abdomen. Other small incisions are made for the surgeon to insert laparoscopic instruments to use in creating the colostomy. This surgery often results in a shorter stay in the hospital, less postoperative pain, a quicker return to normal activities, and far less scarring. It is not recommended for patients who have had extensive prior abdominal surgery, large tumors, previous cancer, or serious heart problems.

Resources

BOOKS

Doughty, Dorothy. *Urinary and Fecal Incontinence.* St. Louis: Mosby-Year Book, Inc., 1991.

Hampton, Beverly, and Ruth Bryant. *Ostomies and Continent Diversions.* St. Louis: Mosby-Year Book, Inc., 1992.

Monahan, Frances. *Medical-Surgical Nursing.* Philadelphia: W. B. Saunders Co., 1998.

ORGANIZATIONS

United Ostomy Association, Inc. (UOA). 19772 MacArthur Blvd., Suite 200, Irvine, CA 92612-2405. (800) 826-0826. <http://www.uoa.org>.

Wound Ostomy and Continence Nurses Society. 2755 Bristol Street, Suite 110, Costa Mesa, CA 92626. (714) 476-0268. <http://www.wocn.org>.

OTHER

National Digestive Diseases Information Clearinghouse. *Ileostomy, Colostomy, and Ileoanal Reservoir Surgery.* (February 1, 2000): 1.

Janie F. Franz
Kathleen D. Wright, RN

Colporrhaphy

Definition

Colporrhaphy is the surgical repair of a defect in the vaginal wall, including a cystocele (when the bladder protrudes into the vagina) and a rectocele (when the rectum protrudes into the vagina).

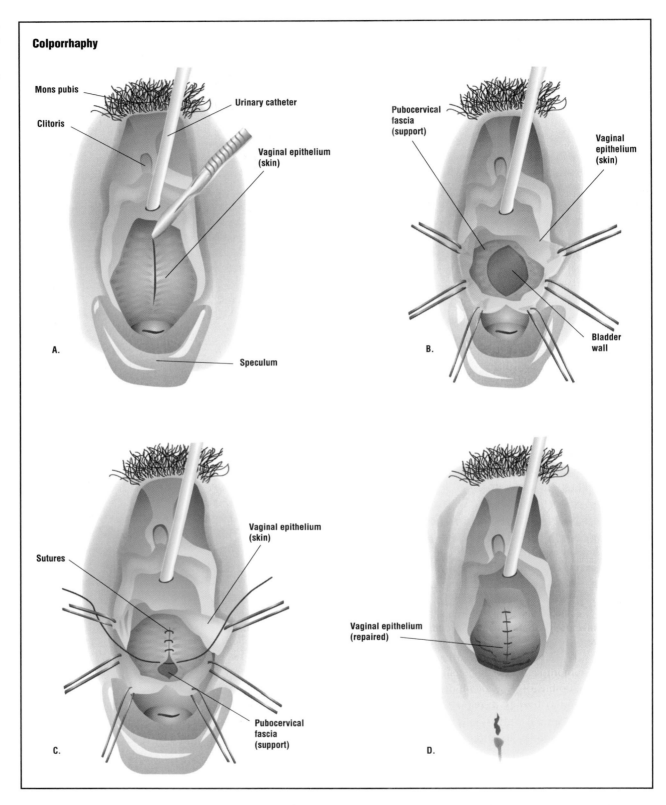

Colporrhaphy

A.
- Mons pubis
- Clitoris
- Urinary catheter
- Vaginal epithelium (skin)
- Speculum

B.
- Pubocervical fascia (support)
- Vaginal epithelium (skin)
- Bladder wall

C.
- Sutures
- Vaginal epithelium (skin)
- Pubocervical fascia (support)

D.
- Vaginal epithelium (repaired)

In this anterior colporrhaphy, a speculum is used to hold open the vagina, and the cystocele is visualized (A). The wall of the vagina is cut open to reveal an opening in the supporting structures, or fascia (B). The defect is closed (C), and the vaginal skin is repaired (D). *(Illustration by GGS Inc.)*

Purpose

A prolapse occurs when an organ falls or sinks out of its normal anatomical place. The pelvic organs normally have tissue (muscle, ligaments, etc.) holding them in place. Certain factors, however, may cause those tissues to weaken, leading to prolapse of the organs. A cystocele is defined as the protrusion or prolapse of the bladder into the vagina; a urethrocele is the prolapse of the urethra into the vagina. These are caused by a defect in the pubocervical fascia (fibrous tissue that separates the bladder and vagina). A rectocele occurs when the rectum prolapses into the vagina, caused by a defect in the rectovaginal fascia (fibrous tissue that separates the rectum and vagina). When a part of the small intestine prolapses into the vagina, it is called an enterocele. Uterine prolapse occurs when the uterus protrudes downward into the vagina.

Factors that are linked to pelvic organ prolapse include age, repeated childbirth, hormone deficiency, ongoing physical activity, and prior **hysterectomy**. Symptoms of pelvic organ prolapse include stress incontinence (inadvertent leakage of urine with physical activity), a vaginal bulge, painful sexual intercourse, back pain, and difficult urination or bowel movements.

Demographics

Approximately 50% of women report occasional urinary incontinence, with 10% reporting regular incontinence. This percentage increases with age; daily incontinence is experienced by 20% of women over the age of 75. According to a recent study, approximately 16% of women ages 45 to 55 experience mild pelvic organ prolapse, while only 3% experience prolapse severe enough to warrant surgical repair.

Description

Colporrhaphy may be performed on the anterior (front) and/or posterior (back) walls of the vagina. An anterior colporrhaphy treats a cystocele or urethrocele, while a posterior colporrhaphy treats a rectocele. Surgery is generally not performed unless the symptoms of the prolapse have begun to interfere with daily life.

The patient is first given general, regional, or local anesthesia. A speculum is inserted into the vagina to hold it open during the procedure. An incision is made into the vaginal skin and the defect in the underlying fascia is identified. The vaginal skin is separated from the fascia and the defect is folded over and sutured (stitched). Any excess vaginal skin is removed and the incision is closed with stitches.

WHO PERFORMS THE PROCEDURE AND WHERE IS IT PERFORMED?

Colporrhaphy is usually performed in a hospital **operating room** by a gynecologist or urologist. A gynecologist is a medical doctor who specializes in the areas of women's general and reproductive health, pregnancy, and labor and childbirth. A urologist is a medical doctor who specializes in the diagnosis and treatment of diseases of the urinary tract and genital organs.

Diagnosis/Preparation

Physical examination is most often used to diagnose prolapse of the pelvic organs. A speculum is inserted into the vagina, and the patient is asked to strain or sit in an upright position. The physician then inspects the anterior, posterior, upper (apex), and side (lateral) walls of the vagina for prolapse or bulging. In some cases, a physical examination cannot sufficiently diagnose pelvic prolapse. For example, cystogram may be used to determine the extent of a cystocele; the bladder is filled by urinary catheter with contrast medium and then x-rayed.

The patient will be asked to refrain from eating or drinking after midnight on the day of the procedure. The physician may request that an enema be administered the night before the procedure if posterior colporrhaphy will be performed.

Aftercare

A Foley catheter may remain for one to two days after surgery. The patient will be given a liquid diet until normal bowel function returns. The patient will be instructed to avoid activities for several weeks that will cause strain on the surgical site, including lifting, coughing, long periods of standing, sneezing, straining with bowel movements, and sexual intercourse.

Risks

Risks of colporrhaphy include potential complications associated with anesthesia, infection, bleeding, injury to other pelvic structures, dyspareunia (painful intercourse), recurrent prolapse, and failure to correct the defect. A fistula is a rare complication of colporrhaphy in which an opening develops between the vagina and bladder or the vagina and rectum.

Normal results

A woman will usually be able to resume normal activities, including sexual intercourse, about four weeks after the procedure. After successful colporrhaphy, the symptoms associated with cystocele or rectocele will recede, although a separate procedure may be needed to treat stress incontinence. Anterior colporrhaphy is approximately 66% successful at restoring urinary continence.

Morbidity and mortality rates

There is approximately a 1% risk of serious complications associated with colporrhaphy; the procedure is generally viewed to be safe with a very low rate of overall complications.

Alternatives

Surgery is generally reserved for more severe cases of pelvic organ prolapse. Milder cases may be treated by a number of medical interventions. The physician may recommend that the patient do Kegel exercises, a series of contractions and relaxations of the muscles in the perineal area. These exercises are thought to strengthen the pelvic floor and may help prevent urinary incontinence. One study showed an decrease of 62% in the amount of urine leakage among women ages 35 to 75 who performed Kegel exercises regularly for 16 weeks.

A pessary, a device that is inserted into the vagina to help support the pelvic organs, may be recommended. Pessaries come in different shapes and sizes and must be fitted to the patient by a physician. Hormone replacement therapy may also be prescribed if the woman has gone through menopause; hormones may improve the quality of the supporting tissues in the pelvis.

Resources

PERIODICALS

Cespedes, R. Duane, Cindy A. Cross, and Edward J. McGuire. "Pelvic Prolapse: Diagnosing and Treating Cystoceles, Rectoceles, and Enteroceles." *Medscape Women's Health eJournal* 3, no. 4 (1998).

Viera, Anthony, and Margaret Larkins-Pettigrew. "Practice Use of the Pessary." *American Family Physician* 61 (May 1, 2000): 2719–26.

ORGANIZATIONS

American Academy of Family Physicians. 8880 Ward Parkway, Kansas City, MO 64114. (816) 333-9700. <http://www.aafp.org>.

American Board of Obstetrics and Gynecology. 2915 Vine Street, Dallas, TX 75204. (214) 871-1619. <http://www.abog.org>.

American Urological Association. 1120 North Charles Street, Baltimore, MD 21201. (410) 727-1100. <http://www.auanet.org>.

OTHER

"Cystocele (Fallen Bladder)." *National Kidney and Urologic Diseases Information Clearinghouse,* March 2002 [cited March 20, 2003]. <http://www.niddk.nih.gov/health/urolog/summary/cystocel>.

Jelovsek, Frederick R. "Cystocoele, Rectocoele, and Pelvic Support Surgery." *Society of Gynecologic Surgeons,* 2001 [cited March 20, 2003]. <http://www.sgsonline.org/ed pro002.html>.

Miklos, John R., and Robert D. Moore. "Prolapse Treatment." *Atlanta Center for Laparoscopic Urogynecology,* 2002 [cited March 20, 2003]. <http://www.urogynecologychannel.com/pro_treat.shtml>.

Stendardo, Stef. "Urinary Incontinence: Assessment and Management in Family Practice." *American Academy of Family Physicians,* 2002 [cited March 20, 2003]. <http://www.aafp.org/PreBuilt/videocme/urinary_mono.pdf>.

"Surgical Treatment of Genuine Stress Incontinence." *Royal College of Obstetricians and Gynaecologists,* August

2002 [cited March 20, 2003]. <http://www.rcog.org.uk/resources/worddocs/incontinencedraft.doc>.

Stephanie Dionne Sherk

Colposcopy

Definition

Colposcopy is a procedure that allows a physician to examine a woman's cervix and vagina using a special microscope called a colposcope. It is used to check for precancerous or abnormal areas.

Purpose

Colposcopy is used to identify or rule out the existence of any precancerous conditions in the cervical tissue. If a Pap test shows abnormal cell growth, colposcopy is usually the first follow-up test performed. The physician will attempt to find the area that produced the abnormal cells and remove it for further study (biopsy) and diagnosis.

Colposcopy may also be performed if the cervix looks abnormal during a routine examination. It may be suggested for women with genital warts and for diethylstilbestrol (DES) daughters (women whose mothers took the anti-miscarriage drug DES when pregnant with them). Colposcopy is used in the emergency department to examine victims of sexual assault and abuse and document any physical evidence of vaginal injury.

Demographics

It is estimated that 30–44% of women fail to follow-up with colposcopy after an abnormal Pap test. Minority women, teenagers, and those of low socioeconomic status are at a greater risk of this.

Description

Colposcopy is usually performed in a physician's office and is similar to a regular gynecologic exam. An instrument called a speculum is inserted to hold the vagina open, and the gynecologist looks at the cervix and vagina using a colposcope, a low-power microscope designed to magnify the cervix 10–40 times its normal size. Most colposcopes are connected to a video monitor that displays the area of interest. Photographs are taken during the examination to document abnormal areas.

The colposcope is placed outside the patient's body and never touches the skin. The cervix and vagina are

WHO PERFORMS THE PROCEDURE AND WHERE IS IT PERFORMED?

Colposcopy may be performed by a gynecologist or other qualified health care provider in an outpatient setting. A gynecologist specializes in the areas of women's general health, pregnancy, labor and childbirth, prenatal testing, and genetics. In cases of sexual assault, a nurse practitioner or registered nurse may perform the procedure. If a biopsy is performed, a pathologist examines the tissue samples under a powerful microscope in the laboratory and sends the results to the health care provider who, in turn, informs the patient of the results.

swabbed with dilute acetic acid (vinegar). The solution highlights abnormal areas by turning them white (instead of a normal pink color). Abnormal areas can also be identified by looking for a characteristic pattern made by abnormal blood vessels.

If any abnormal areas are seen, the doctor will take a biopsy of the tissue, a common procedure that takes about 15 minutes. Several samples might be taken, depending on the size of the abnormal area. A biopsy may cause temporary discomfort and cramping, which usually go away within a few minutes. If the abnormal area appears to extend inside the cervical canal, a scraping of the canal may also be done. The biopsy results are usually available within a week.

If the tissue sample indicates abnormal growth (dysplasia) or is precancerous, and if the entire abnormal area can be seen, the doctor can destroy the tissue using one of several procedures, including ones that use high heat (diathermy), extreme cold (cryosurgery), or lasers. Another procedure, called a loop electrosurgical excision (LEEP), uses low-voltage, high-frequency radio waves to excise tissue. If any of the abnormal tissue is within the cervical canal, a **cone biopsy** (removal of a conical section of the cervix for inspection) will be needed.

Diagnosis/Preparation

Women who are pregnant, or who suspect that they are pregnant, must tell their doctor before the procedure begins. Pregnant women may undergo colposcopy if they have an abnormal Pap test; special precautions, however, must be taken during biopsy of the cervix.

Patients should be instructed not to douche, use tampons, or have sexual intercourse for 24 hours before colposcopy. Patients should empty their bladder and bowels before colposcopy for comfort. Colposcopy does not require any anesthetic medication because pain is minimal. If a biopsy is done, there may be mild cramps or a sharp pinching when the tissue is removed. To lessen this pain, the doctor may recommend ibuprofen (Motrin) taken the night before and the morning of the procedure (no later than 30 minutes before the appointment). Patients who are pregnant or allergic to **aspirin** or ibuprofen can instead take **acetaminophen** (Tylenol).

Aftercare

If a biopsy was done, there may be a dark vaginal discharge afterwards. After the sample is removed, the doctor applies Monsel's solution to the area to stop the bleeding. When this mixes with blood, it creates a black fluid that looks like coffee grounds. This fluid may be present for a couple of days after the procedure. It is also normal to have some spotting after colposcopy. Pain-relieving medication can be taken to lessen any postprocedural cramping.

Patients should not use tampons, douche, or have sex for at least a week after the procedure (or until the doctor says it is safe) because of the risk of infection.

Risks

Patients may have bleeding or infection after biopsy. Bleeding is usually controlled with a topical medication prescribed by the physician or health care provider. If colposcopy is performed on a pregnant patient, there is a risk of premature labor.

A patient should call her doctor right away if she notices any of the following symptoms:

- heavy vaginal bleeding (more than one sanitary pad an hour)
- fever, chills, or an unpleasant vaginal odor
- lower abdominal pain

Normal results

If visual inspection shows that the surface of the cervix is smooth and pink, this is considered normal. Areas that look abnormal may actually be normal variations; a biopsy will indicate whether the tissue is normal or abnormal.

Abnormal conditions that can be detected using colposcopy and biopsy include precancerous tissue changes (cervical dysplasia), cancer, and cervical warts caused by human papilloma virus.

Morbidity and mortality rates

Complications associated with colposcopy are extremely rare. There is a risk that the procedure will miss precancerous or cancerous tissues and thus prolong treatment until the cancer has become advanced. Of the 12,800 women who are diagnosed in the United States each year with cervical cancer, approximately 37.5% will die as a result of the disease.

Alternatives

While the Pap test is an effective screening test for abnormal cell growth of the cervix, it is an inadequate diagnostic alternative to colposcopy because of the potential for false negative results (10–50%). In some instances, a repeat Pap test may be recommended before performing colposcopy (e.g., in the case of inflammation or no previous abnormal Pap test).

Resources

BOOKS

Ryan, Kenneth J., Ross S. Berkowitz, and Robert L. Barbieri. *Kistner's Gynecology,* 7th ed. St. Louis: Mosby, 1999.

PERIODICALS

McKee, M. Diane, Joseph Lurio, Paul Marantz, William Burton, and Michael Mulvihill. "Barriers to Follow-up of Abnormal Papanicolaou Smears in an Urban Community Health Center." *Archives of Family Medicine* 8 (March/April 1999): 129–34.

ORGANIZATIONS

American College of Obstetricians and Gynecologists. 409 12th St., SW, PO Box 96920, Washington, DC 20090-6920. <http://www.acog.org>.

American Society for Colposcopy and Cervical Pathology. 20 W. Washington St., Ste. #1, Hagerstown, MD 21740. (301) 733-3640. <http://www.asccp.org>.

Association of Women's Health, Obstetric, and Neonatal Nurses. 2000 L St., NW, Ste. 740, Washington, DC 20036. (800) 673-8499. <http://www.awhonn.org>.

DES Action USA. 610 16th St., Ste. 301, Oakland, CA 94612. (510) 465-4011. <http://www.desaction.org>.

KEY TERMS

Biopsy—Removal of sample of abnormal tissue for more extensive examination under a microscope.

Cervix—The neck of the uterus.

Cryosurgery—Freezing and destroying abnormal cells.

Diathermy—Also called electrocautery, this is a procedure that heats and destroys abnormal cells.

Diethylstilbestrol (DES)—A synthetic form of estrogen that was widely prescribed to women from 1940 to 1970 to prevent complications during pregnancy, and linked to several serious birth defects and disorders of the reproductive system in daughters of women who took DES.

Dysplasia—Development of abnormal tissue.

Human papilloma virus (HPV)—A virus that causes common warts of the hands and feet, as well as lesions in the genital and vaginal area. More than 50 types of HPV have been identified, some of which are linked to cancerous and precancerous conditions, including cancer of the cervix.

Loop electrosurgical excision (LEEP)—A procedure that can help diagnose and treat cervical abnormalities using a thin wire loop that emits a low-voltage high-frequency radio wave that can excise tissue.

Monsel's solution—A solution used to stop bleeding.

Pap test—The common term for the Papanicolaou test, a simple smear method of examining stained cells to detect cancer of the cervix.

Speculum—A retractor used to separate the walls of the vagina to make visual examination easier.

Society of Gynecologic Oncologists. 401 North Michigan Ave., Chicago, IL 60611. (312) 644-6610. <http://www.sgo.org>.

OTHER

"Colposcopy (Position Paper)." *American Academy of Family Physicians,* [cited March 11, 2003]. <http://www.aafp.org/x6665.xml>.

Garcia, Agustin. "Cervical Cancer." *eMedicine,* April 17, 2002 [cited March 11, 2003]. <http://www.emedicine.com/med/topic324.htm>.

Mayeaux, E. J. "Colposcopy Atlas." *Louisiana State University Health Sciences Center Medical Library,* [cited March 11, 2003]. <http://lib-sh.lsumc.edu/fammed/atlases/colpo.html>.

Pattan, Charles. "Colposcopy." *eMedicine,* July 15, 2002 [cited March 11, 2003]. <http://www.emedicine.com/med/topic3298.htm>.

Jennifer E. Sisk, MA
Stephanie Dionne Sherk

Colpotomy

Definition

A colpotomy, also known as a vaginotomy, is a procedure by which an incision is made in the vagina.

Purpose

A colpotomy is performed either to visualize pelvic structures or to perform surgery on the fallopian tubes or ovaries.

Role of colpotomy in gynecologic surgery

Several gynecologic surgery protocols require a colpotomy as part of the overall surgical procedure. It is performed whenever the surgeon needs to access the vagina. Several of these surgeries include:

• Tubal sterilization. Sterilization is a procedure that can be performed using either abdominal or vaginal procedures. When a vaginal procedure is selected by the surgeon, he performs a colpotomy and may also insert a culdoscope to locate the tubes (culdoscopy), and close them off.

• Removal of myomas. Myomas are fibroid tumors of the muscle tissue of the uterus and they are sometimes removed vaginally by colpotomy.

• Removal of pelvic cysts and masses. In one treatment variant, patients may undergo a laparoscopy followed by a colpotomy for the vaginal extraction of the pelvic cyst or mass.

• **Hysterectomy**. One technique used to surgically remove the uterus combines three steps, an initial laparoscopic stage, followed by a vaginal stage, and a final laparoscopic stage. The colpotomy is performed during the second step to deliver the uterus into the vagina.

• Dysmenorrhea. Separation of the uterosacral ligaments via colpotomy is an approach that has been used for the relief of dysmenorrhea (painful menstruation).

• Complications in pregnancy and childbirth. Colpotomy may be used in the management of difficult pregnancies and childbirths.

Demographics

According to Professor V. Base-Smith at the University of Cincinnati College of Nursing, removal of the uterus is the second most commonly performed surgical procedure in the United States after cesarean delivery. Analysis of the demographics show that:

- 650,000 hysterectomies are performed annually, expected to reach approximately 834,000 by 2005.
- 6.1–8.6 per 1,000 women undergo hysterectomy per year.
- In the United States, the Northeast has the lowest hysterectomy rate, while the South has the highest rate.
- African-American women experience hysterectomy more frequently than European-American women.

The ratio of abdominal to vaginally performed hysterectomies is 3:1, meaning that colpotomy is performed in one out of four hysterectomy procedures.

Female sterilization is a common contraception method. About 20,000 female sterilizations are carried out each year in Canada and nearly 10% of North American women 30 years or older have been sterilized in a procedure that involved colpotomy.

Description

The patient is placed in a supine position on the operating table with her legs in stirrups and the incision site is prepared. An antiseptic solution, such as chlorhexidine, is applied to the skin using highly disinfected forceps and gauze swabs. The patient is covered with surgical drapes with the window positioned directly over the incision site. Throughout the procedure, the **vital signs** of the patient are monitored (blood pressure, pulse, respiratory rate) as well as her level of consciousness and blood loss. **Pain management** depends on the surgery that requires the colpotomy, and may involve local, regional, or general anesthesia. The incision is only made as large as necessary for the requirements of the overall surgery.

For example, when a decision has been made to remove a myoma by colpotomy, the procedure may proceed as follows:

- A small myoma screw is inserted into the myoma and a grasper with locking mechanism is placed on the lower edge of the wound.
- The myoma is directed toward the cul-de-sac using the myoma screw.
- A colpotomy is performed.
- The myoma is grasped and removed vaginally. During this part of the procedure, the surgeon examines whether the myoma extends into the uterine cavity.
- If it does, the uterus is guided to the colpotomy site. T-clamps are placed on the edges of the wounds and the fundus of the uterus is delivered, via the colpotomy incision, into the vagina.
- The uterus is sutured in three layers (endometrial, myometrial and serosal).
- The repaired uterus is returned to the abdominal cavity.
- The colpotomy incision is sutured.

Preparation

The procedure is explained to the patient within the broader context of the surgery that includes the colpotomy. Preoperative preparation includes whatever is required for the overall surgical procedure that will be performed.

Aftercare

Aftercare for colpotomy is associated with the overall surgery that required the colpotomy.

For example, if a colpotomy is performed for **tubal ligation** (female sterilization), the procedure takes only 15–30 minutes and women usually go home the same day. It may take a few days at home to recover. Sexual intercourse is usually postponed until the colpotomy in-

KEY TERMS

Anesthesia—A combination of drugs administered by a variety of techniques by trained professionals that provide sedation, amnesia, analgesia, and immobility adequate for the accomplishment of the surgical procedure with minimal discomfort, and without injury, to the patient.

Antiseptic—Substance preventing or stopping the growth of microorganisms.

Cul-de-sac—The closed end of a pouch.

Culdoscopy—Procedure by which a surgeon performs a colpotomy and inserts a culdoscope, an instrument with a light on the end, through the incision.

Culdocentesis—Removal of material from the pouch of Douglas, a deep peritoneal recess between the uterus and the upper vaginal wall, by means of puncture of the vaginal wall.

Cyst—A closed sac having a distinct membrane and developing abnormally in a body cavity or structure.

Dysmenorrhea—Painful menstruation.

Fallopian tubes—The pair of anatomical tubes that carry the egg from the ovary to the uterus.

Forceps—An instrument for grasping, holding firmly, or exerting traction upon objects especially for delicate operations.

Hysterectomy—Surgical removal of the uterus.

Laparoscopy—Visual examination of the inside of the abdomen by means of a laparoscope or surgery performed using a laparoscope.

Myoma—A tumor consisting of muscle tissue.

Ovary—One of the two essential female reproductive organs that produce eggs and sex hormones.

Pelvic—Located near the pelvis, the skeletal structure comprised of four bones that encloses the pelvic cavity.

Sterilization—To make sterile, meaning to deprive of the power of reproducing.

Uterus—The womb, an organ in females for containing and nourishing the young during development before to birth.

Vagina—A canal in the female body that leads from the cervix to the external orifice opening to the outside of the body.

Vulva—The external parts of the female genital organs that include the mons pubis, labia majora, labia minora, clitoris, vestibule of the vagina, bulb of the vestibule, and Bartholin's glands.

---

cision is completely healed, and as advised by the doctor. The healing process usually requires several weeks and there are no visible scars. In the case of a colpotomy performed for myoma removal, aftercare is more elaboate with the patient's vital signs monitored in the **recovery room** until she regains consciousness.

Risks

Complications such as bleeding, infection, or reaction to the anesthetic, may occur as with any type of gynecological surgery.

Normal results

Colpotomy results are considered normal when the incision performed allows the surgeon to meet the goal of the overall surgical protocol.

Morbidity and mortality rates

Colpotomy morbidity rates are not reported. This is because the procedure represents one surgical process in an operation that involves other surgical peocedures. In the case of colpotomy performed in the context of tubal sterilization, morbidity with tubal ligation is 5%; mortality is less than 4 in 100,000 cases.

As for hysterectomies, a higher morbidity and mortality rate is associated with abdominal than with vaginal hysterectomy surgery, the latter procedure being the only one to involve colpotomy.

Alternatives

In the case of colpotomy used for tubal ligation procedures, **laparoscopy** or laparotomy procedures are currently the preferred technique, since fewer and fewer U.S. surgeons are trained to use colpotomy as an approach for sterilization.

See also Laparotomy, exploratory.

Resources

BOOKS

Masterson, B. J. *Manual of Gynecologic Surgery (Comprehensive Manuals of Surgical Specialties)*. New York: Springer Verlag, 1986.

Reiffenstahl, G., W. Platzer, and P.-G. Knapstein. *Vaginal Operations*. Philadelphia: Lippincott, Williams & Wilkins, 1996.

Stewart, E. G., and P. Spencer. *The V Book: A Doctor's Guide to Complete Vulvovaginal Health*. New York: Bantam Doubleday Dell Publishers, 2002.

PERIODICALS

Diakomanolis, E., A. Rodolakis, Z. Boulgaris, G. Blachos, and S. Michalas. "Treatment of Vaginal Intraepithelial Neoplasia With Laser Ablation and Upper Vaginectomy." *Gynecologic and Obstetric Investigation* 54 (2002): 17-20, 419-427.

Ghezzi, F., L. Raio, M. D. Mueller, T. Gyr, M. Buttarelli, and M. Franchi. "Vaginal Extraction of Pelvic Masses Following Operative Laparoscopy." *Surgical Endoscopy* 16 (December 2002): 1691-1696.

Goodlin, R. C. "In Defense of the Anterior Vaginotomy." *Journal of Reproductive Medicine* 47 (August 2002): 693-694.

Gortzak-Uzan, L., A. Walfisch, Y. Gortzak, M. Katz, M. Mazor, and M. Hallak. "Accidental Vaginal Incision During Cesarean Section. A Report of Four Cases." *Journal of Reproductive Medicine* 46 (November 2001): 1017-1020.

Ou, C. S., A. Harper, Y. H. Liu, and R. Rowbotham. "Laparoscopic Myomectomy Technique. Use of Colpotomy and the Harmonic Scalpel." *Journal of Reproductive Medicine* 47 (October 2002): 849-853.

ORGANIZATIONS

American Association of Gynecological Laparoscopists. 13021 East Florence Avenue, Sante Fe Springs, CA 90670-4505. (800) 554-2245. <www.aagl.com/>.

American College of Obstetricians and Gynecologists. 409 12th Street, SW, Washington, DC 20024-2188. E-mail: resources@acog.org. <www.acog.org/>.

American Society for Colposcopy and Cervical Pathology. 20 West Washington Street, Suite 1, Hagerstown, MD 21740. (301) 733-3640 or (800) 787-7227. <www.asccp.org>.

National Association for Women's Health. 300 W. Adams Street, Suite 328, Chicago, IL 60606-5101. (312) 786-1468. <www.nawh.org/>.

OTHER

"Culdocentesis and Colpotomy." *Managing Complications of Pregnancy and Childbirth: A Guide for Midwives and Doctors*. World Health Organization. [cited May 14, 2003]. <http://www.who.int/reproductive-health/impac/Procedures/Culdocentesis_P69_P70.html>.

National Women's Health Information Center. U.S. Department of Health and Human Services. [cited May 14, 2003]. <http://www.4woman.org/>.

Monique Laberge, Ph.D.

Complete blood count

Definition

A complete blood count (CBC) is a series of tests used to evaluate the composition and concentration of the cellular components of blood. It consists of the following tests: red blood cell (RBC) count, white blood cell (WBC) count, and platelet count; measurement of hemoglobin and mean red cell volume; classification of white blood cells (WBC differential); and calculation of **hematocrit** and **red blood cell indices**. The hematocrit is the percentage of blood by volume that is occupied by the red cells (i.e., the packed red cell volume). Red blood cell indices are calculations derived from the red blood cell count, hemoglobin, and hematocrit that aid in the diagnosis and classification of anemia.

Purpose

The CBC provides valuable information about the blood and to some extent the bone marrow, which is the blood-forming tissue. The CBC is used for the following purposes:

- as a preoperative test to ensure both adequate oxygen carrying capacity and hemostasis
- to identify persons who may have an infection
- to diagnose anemia
- to identify acute and chronic illness, bleeding tendencies, and white blood cell disorders such as leukemia
- to monitor treatment for anemia and other blood diseases
- to determine the effects of chemotherapy and radiation therapy on blood cell production

Precautions

The CBC requires a sample of blood collected from a vein. The nurse or phlebotomist inserting the needle should clean the skin first. The tourniquet should be removed from the arm as soon as the blood flows. If a fingerstick is used to collect the blood, care must be taken to wipe away the first drop, and not to squeeze the finger excessively as this causes the blood to be diluted by tissue fluid. Many drugs affect the results by causing increased or decreased RBC, WBC, and/or platelet production. Medications should be taken into account when interpreting results.

Description

The CBC is commonly performed on an automated hematology analyzer using well mixed whole blood that is added to a chemical called EDTA to prevent clotting. A CBC is a group of tests used to quantify the number of RBCs, WBCs, and platelets, provide information about their size and shape, measure the hemoblobin content of RBCs, determine the percentage and absolute number of the five white blood cell types, and identify early and abnormal blood cells. These tests are performed simultaneously, (usually in less than one minute), using an automated hematology analyzer. When the performance limit of the automated hematology analyzer is exceeded, sample dilution or pretreatment, manual smear review, or manual cell counts may be required. Each laboratory has established rules for determining the need for manual smear review based upon specific CBC parameters. For example, a manual differential is always performed when nucleated immature red blood cells are found on an electronic cell count.

Electronic cell counting

Electronic blood cell counting is based upon the principle of impedance (i.e., resistance to current flow). Some hematology analyzers combine impedance counting with light scattering to measure platelets. A small sample of the blood is aspirated into a chamber (the WBC counting bath) and diluted with a balanced isotonic saline solution that is free of particles. The diluted blood sample is split into two parts, one for counting RBCs and platelets and the other for counting WBCs. The RBC portion is transferred to the RBC/platelet counting bath where it is diluted further. The other portion remains in the WBC bath and a detergent (lysing agent) is added to destroy (hemolyze) the red blood cells. A small portion of the diluted fluid in each bath is allowed to flow past a small aperture. An electrical current is produced in each aperture by two electrodes, one on the inside and the other on the outside of the aperture. The saline solution is responsible for conducting current between the electrodes. The cells move through the aperture one at a time. When a cell enters the aperture, it displaces a volume of electrolyte equal to its size. The cell acts as an electrical resistor, and impedes the flow of current. This produces a voltage pulse, the magnitude of which is proportional to the size of the cell. Instrument electronics are adjusted to discriminate voltage pulses produced by different cells. These adjustments are called thresholds. For example, the threshold for counting a RBC is equivalent to a cell volume of 36 femtoliters or higher. Voltage pulses that are equivalent to volumes of 2–20 femtoliters are counted as platelets. This process is repeated two more times so that the RBC, WBC, and platelet counts are performed in triplicate. Each time frame for counting is several seconds and many thousands of cells are counted. The computer processes the counting data first by determining the agreement between the three counts. If acceptable criteria are met, the counts are accepted and used to calculate the result.

The hemoglobin concentration is measured optically using the solution in the WBC bath. The lysing agent contains potassium cyanide that reacts with the hemoglobin to form cyanmethemoglobin. The optical density of the cyanmethemoglobin is proportional to hemoglobin concentration.

The voltage pulses produced by the white blood cells depend upon the size of the cell and its nuclear density. Therefore, the pulses may be analyzed to differentiate between the types of WBCs found. For example, lymphocytes are the smallest WBCs and comprise the lower end of the size scale. Monocytes, prolymphocytes, and immature granulocytes comprise the central area of the WBC histogram, and mature granulocytes comprise the upper end. In addition to cell sizing, automated instruments may use any of three other methods to distinguish between subpopulations. These are radio frequency conductance, forward and angular light scattering, and fluorescent staining.

Red blood cell count

The red cells, the most numerous of the cellular elements, carry oxygen from the lungs to the body's tissues. They are released from the bone marrow into the blood in an immature form called the reticulocyte that still retains much of the cellular RNA needed for hemoglobin production. Reticulocytes may be counted on some automated analyzers and are an index to recovery from anemia. The average life span of RBCs in the circulation is approximately 120 days.

The red blood cell (RBC) count determines the total number of red cells (erythrocytes) in a sample of blood. Most anemias are associated with a low RBC count, hemoglobin, and hematocrit. Common causes include excessive bleeding; a deficiency of iron, vitamin B_{12}, or folic acid; destruction of red cells by antibodies or mechanical trauma; bone marrow malignancy and fibrosis; and structurally abnormal hemoglobin. The RBC count is also decreased due to cancer, kidney diseases, and excessive IV fluids. An elevated RBC count may be caused by dehydration, hypoxia (decreased oxygen), or a disease called polycythemia vera. Hypoxia may result from high altitudes, chronic obstructive lung diseases, and congestive heart failure.

Hematocrit and cell indices

The hematocrit is a test that measures the volume of blood in percent that is comprised of the red blood cells. Automated cell counters calculate the hematocrit by multiplying the RBC count by the mean red cell volume. A decrease in the number or size of red cells also decreases the amount of space they occupy, resulting in a lower hematocrit. Conversely, an increase in the number or size of red cells increases the amount of space they occupy, resulting in a higher hematocrit. Thalassemia minor, a genetic cause of anemia, is an exception in that it usually causes an increase in the number of red blood cells, but because they are small, it results in a decreased hematocrit.

The three main RBC indices are used to determine the average size and hemoglobin content of the RBCs and they help determine the cause of anemia. The three indices are described below:

• Mean corpuscular volume (MCV)—the average size of the red blood cells expressed in femtoliters. MCV is calculated by dividing the hematocrit (as percent) by the RBC count in millions per microliter of blood, then multiplying by 10.

• Mean corpuscular hemoglobin (MCH)—the average amount of hemoglobin inside an RBC expressed in picograms. The MCH is calculated by dividing the hemoglobin concentration in grams per deciliter by the RBC count in millions per microliter, then multiplying by 10.

• Mean corpuscular hemoglobin concentration (MCHC)—the average concentration of hemoglobin in the RBCs expressed in percent. It is calculated by dividing the hemoglobin in grams per deciliter by the hematocrit, then multiplying by 100.

The mechanisms by which anemia occurs will alter the RBC indices in a predictable manner. Therefore, the RBC indices permit the physician to narrow down the possible causes of an anemia. The MCV is an index of the size of the RBCs. When the MCV is below normal, the RBCs will be smaller than normal and are described as microcytic. When the MCV is elevated, the RBCs will be larger than normal and are termed macrocytic. RBCs of normal size are termed normocytic. Failure to produce hemoglobin results in smaller than normal cells. This occurs in many diseases including iron deficiency anemia, thalassemia (an inherited disease in which globin chain production is deficient), and anemias associated with chronic infection or disease. Macrocytic cells occur when division of RBC precursor cells in the bone marrow is impaired. The most common causes of macrocytic anemia are vitamin B_{12} deficiency, folate deficiency, and liver disease. Normocytic anemia may be caused by decreased production (e.g., malignancy and other causes of bone marrow failure), increased destruction (hemolytic anemia), or blood loss. The RBC count is low, but the size and amount of hemoglobin in the cells is normal.

White blood cell count

The majority of CBCs include both a WBC count and an automated differential. A differential determines the percentage of each of the five types of mature white blood cells. An elevated WBC count occurs in infection, allergy, systemic illness, inflammation, tissue injury, and leukemia. A low WBC count may occur in some viral infections, immunodeficiency states, and bone marrow failure. The WBC count provides clues about certain illnesses, and helps physicians monitor a patient's recovery from others. The differential will reveal which WBC types are affected most. For example, an elevated WBC count with an absolute increase in lymphocytes having an atypical appearance is most often caused by infectious mononucleosis. The differential will also identify early WBCs that may be reactive (e.g., a response to acute infection) or the result of a leukemia.

When the electronic WBC count is abnormal or a cell population is flagged, meaning that one or more of the results is atypical, a manual differential is performed. In that case, a wedge smear is prepared. This is done by placing a drop of blood on a glass slide, and using a second slide to pull the blood over the first slide's surface. The smear is air dried, then stained with Wright stain and examined under a microscope using oil immersion (1000x magnification). One hundred white cells are counted and identified as either neutrophils, lymphocytes, monocytes, eosinophils, or basophils based on the shape and appearance of the nucleus, the color of cytoplasm, and the presence and color of granules. The purpose is to determine if these cells are present in a normal distribution, or if one cell type is increased or decreased. Any atypical or immature cells also are counted.

In addition to determining the percentage of each mature white blood cell, the following tests are performed as part of the differential:

• Evaluation of RBC morphology is performed. This includes grading of the variation in RBC size (anisocytosis) and shape (poikioocytosis); reporting the type and number of any abnormal RBCs such as target cells, sickle cells, stippled cells, etc.; reporting the presence of immature RBCs (polychromasia); and counting the number of nucleated RBCs per 100 WBCs.

• An estimate of the WBC count is made and compared to the automated or chamber WBC count. An estimate of the platelet count is made and compared to the automated or chamber platelet count. Abnormal platelets such as clumped platelets or excessively large platelets are noted on the report.

• Any immature white blood cells are included in the differential count of 100 cells, and any inclusions or abnormalities of the WBCs are reported.

WBCs consist of two main subpopulations, the mononuclear cells and the granulocytic cells. Mononuclear cells include lymphocytes and monocytes. Granulocytes include neutropohils (also called polymorphonuclear leukocytes or segmented neutrophils), eosinophils, and basophils. Each cell type is described below:

- Neutrophils are normally the most abundant WBCs. They measure 12–16 µm in diameter. The nucleus stains dark purple-blue, and is divided into several lobes (usually three or four) consisting of dense chromatin. A neutrophil just before the final stage of maturation will have an unsegmented nucleus in the shape of a band. These band neutrophils may be counted along with mature neutrophils or as a separate category. The cytoplasm of a neutrophil contains both primary (azurophilic) and secondary (specific) granules. The secondary granules are lilac in color and are more abundant, almost covering the pink cytoplasm. Neutrophils are phagocytic (able to engulf objects) cells and facilitate removal of bacteria and antibody-coated antigens. The neutrophilic granules are rich in peroxidase, and aid the cell in destroying bacteria and other ingested cells.

- Eosinophils are 14–16 µm in diameter and contain a blue nucleus that is segmented into two distinct lobes. The cytoplasm is filled with large refractile orange-red granules. The granules contain peroxidase, hydrolases, and basic proteins that aid in the destruction of phagocytized cells. Eosinophils are increased in allergic reactions and parasitic infections.

- Basophils, like eosinophils, are 14–16 µm in diameter and have a blue nucleus that is bilobed. The cytoplasm of the basophil is filled with large dark blue-black granules that may obscure the nucleus. These contain large amounts of histamine, heparin, and acid mucopolysaccharides. Basophils mediate the allergic response by releasing histamine.

- Lymphocytes are the second most abundant WBCs. They may be small (7–9 µm in diameter) or large (12–16 µm in diameter). The nucleus is dark blue and is nearly round or slightly indented and the chromatin is clumped and very dense. The cytoplasm is medium blue and usually agranular. An occasional lymphocyte will have a few azurophilic granules in the cytoplasm. Lymphocytes originate in the lymphoid tissues and are not phagocytic. They are responsible for initiating and regulating the immune response by the production of antibodies and cytokines.

- Monocytes are the largest WBCs, measuring 14–20 µm in diameter. They have a large irregularly shaped and folded blue nucleus with chromatin that is less dense than other WBCs. The cytoplasm is gray-blue, and is filled with fine dust-like lilac colored granules. Monocytes are phagocytic cells that process and present antigens to lymphocytes, an event required for lymphocyte activation.

Platelet count

Platelets are disk-shaped structures formed by the detachment of cytoplasm from megakaryocytes. They aid in the coagulation process by attaching or adhering to the walls of injured blood vessels, where they stick together to form the initial platelet plug. A low platelet count may occur in patients with AIDS, viral infections, lymphoma, and lupus erythematosus, or in patients taking certain drugs, most notably quinine and quinidine. Decreased platelet production is also a cause of thrombocytopenia, and may be due to aplastic anemia, leukemia, lymphoma, or bone marrow fibrosis. A low platelet count can occur due to increased destruction. This can result from antibody production that is often drug-induced (heparin treatment being a prominent cause). Increased destruction also results from autoantibody production as occurs in idiopathic thrombocytopenic purpura (ITP) and thrombotic episodes that consume platelets such as occur in thrombotic thrombocytopenic purpura (TTP), disseminated intravascular coagulation (DIC), and hemolytic-uremic syndrome (HUS). Inherited (congenital) thrombocytopenia can be caused by Glanzmann's thrombasthenia, Fanconi syndrome, and Wiskott-Aldrich syndrome.

Thrombocytosis, an increased platelet count, is most often caused by a reaction to injury or inflammation. In these cases the platelet count increases transiently and is usually within the range of 400,000–800,000 per microliter. Persistent or higher counts are usually associated with myeloproliferative disease (malignant disease involving blood forming cells) such as chronic granulocytic (myelogenous) leukemia, polycythemia vera, or primary (essential) thrombocythemia.

The platelet count is most often measured by impedance counting but is performed manually when the platelet count is very low, platelet clumping is observed, or abnormally large (giant) platelets are present. Often these abnormalities and others such as cryoglobulinemia, cell fragmentation (hemolysis), and microcytic RBCs are signaled by abnormal RBC and platelet indices and abnormal population flags. An abnormal mean platelet volume or platelet histogram indicates that morphological platelet abnormalities are present and the platelets should be observed from a stained blood film to characterize the abnormality. The platelet count can be estimated using the Wright-stained blood smear used for a differential WBC count by multiplying the average number of platelets per oil immersion field by 20,000. Platelet estimates should correlate with actual counts. When they disagree, the platelet count should be repeated and a manual count performed if necessary.

Preparation

The CBC does not require fasting or any special preparation.

KEY TERMS

Anemia—A diminished oxygen carrying capacity caused by a decrease in the size, number, or function of red blood cells.

Capillaries—The smallest of the blood vessels that bring oxygenated blood to tissues.

Cytoplasm—The part of a cell that is outside the nucleus, like the white of an egg.

EDTA—A colorless compound used to keep blood samples from clotting. Its chemical name is ethylenediaminetetraacetic acid. EDTA functions by binding the calcium in the blood sample.

Hematocrit—The volume of blood occupied by the red blood cells expressed in percent.

Hemoglobin—A protein inside red blood cells that carries oxygen to body tissues.

Hypochromic—A descriptive term applied to a red blood cell with a decreased concentration of hemoglobin.

Macrocytic—A descriptive term applied to a larger than normal red blood cell.

Mean corpuscular hemoglobin (MCH)—A measurement of the average weight of hemoglobin in a red blood cell.

Mean corpuscular hemoglobin concentration (MCHC)—The measurement of the average concentration of hemoglobin in a red blood cell.

Mean corpuscular volume (MCV)—A measure of the average volume of a red blood cell.

Mean platelet volume (MPV)—A measure of the average volume of a platelet.

Microcytic—A descriptive term applied to a smaller than normal red blood cell.

Normochromic—A descriptive term applied to a red blood cell with a normal concentration of hemoglobin.

Normocytic—A descriptive term applied to a red blood cell of normal size.

Nucleus—The part of a cell that has DNA, like an egg yolk.

Red blood cell indices—Measurements that describe the size and hemoglobin content of red blood cells.

Red cell distribution width (RDW)—A measure of the variation in size of red blood cells.

Thalassemia—Any of a group of inherited disorders of hemoglobin metabolism in which there is impaired synthesis of one or more of the polypeptide chains of globin; several genetic types exist.

Thrombocyte—Another name for platelet.

Thrombocytopenia—An abnormally low platelet count.

Thrombocytosis—An abnormally high platelet count. It occurs in polycythemia vera and other disorders in which the bone marrow produces too many platelets.

Aftercare

Discomfort or bruising may occur at the puncture site. Applying pressure to the puncture site until the bleeding stops helps to reduce bruising; warm packs relieve discomfort. Some people feel dizzy or faint after blood has been drawn and should be treated by resting awhile.

Risks

Other than potential bruising at the puncture site, and/or dizziness, there are no complications associated with this test.

Normal results

CBC values vary by age and sex. Normal values are ultimately determined by the laboratory performing the test. As a guide, the normal values for men and non-pregnant women are as follows:

- WBCs: 4,500–11,000 per microliter for women and men, with neutrophils representing 50–70%, lymphocytes 25–35%, monocytes 4–6%, eosinophils 1–3%, basophils 0.4–1%, and bands 0–5%.

- RBCs: 4.2–5.0 million per microliter for women; 4.5–6.2 million per microliter for men.

- Hemoglobin: 12–15 g/dL for women; 13.6–17.2 g/dL for men.

- Hematocrit: 35–47% for women; 42–52% for men.

- Platelets: 150,000 and 350,000 per microliter.

- Reticulocyte count: 0.5–1.5%.

Normal adult results for red blood cell indices are as follows:

- MCV: 80–98 fl (femtoliters)

- MCHC: 32–36%

- MCH: 27–31 pg (picograms)

- RDW: 11.5–14.5%

In addition to normal values, critical values (alert, panic values) are established for hemoglobin (and hematocrit), WBC count, and platelet count. Precipitously low hemoglobin is associated with hypoxia that can have life-threatening complications. Extremely low WBCs indicates an inability to fight infection and a high risk of sepsis. A severely reduced platelet count predisposes the patient to spontaneous internal bleeding. Representative critical values are shown below.

- Hemoglobin: less than 5.0 g/dL

- Hematocrit: less than 15%

- Platelet count: less than 30,000 per microliter

- WBC count: less than 2,500 per microliter and greater than 30,000 per microliter

Abnormal blood count results are seen in a variety of conditions. One of the most common is anemia, which is characterized by a low RBC count, hemoglobin, and hematocrit. The category into which a person's anemia is placed is in part based upon the red blood cell indices provided. The indices provide a significant clue as to the cause of the anemia, but further testing is needed to confirm a specific diagnosis. The most common causes of macrocytic anemia (high MCV) are vitamin B_{12} and folic acid deficiencies. Lack of iron in the diet, thalassemia (a type of hereditary anemia), and chronic illness are the most common causes of microcytic anemia (low MCV). Normocytic anemia (normal MCV) can be caused by kidney and liver disease, bone marrow disorders, leukemia, excessive bleeding, or hemolysis of the red blood cells. Iron deficiency and thalassemia are the most common causes of hypochromic anemia (low MCHC). Normocytic anemias are usually also normochromic and share the same causes. The red cell distribution width (RDW) is increased in anemias caused by deficiencies of iron, vitamin B_{12}, or folic acid. Abnormal hemoglobins, such as in sickle cell anemia, can change the shape of red blood cells as well as cause them to hemolyze, or rupture. The abnormal shape and the cell fragments resulting from hemolysis increase the RDW. Conditions that cause more immature cells to be released into the bloodstream, such as severe blood loss, will increase the RDW. The larger size of immature cells creates a distinct size variation.

Infections and leukemias are associated with increased numbers of WBCs. Increases or decreases in the percentage of each white cell can be associated with a number of diseases or conditions, including cancer, leukemia, anemia, multiple sclerosis, allergies, parasitic and viral diseases, infections, and tissue damage.

Resources

BOOKS

Chernecky, Cynthia C. and Barbara J. Berger. *Laboratory Tests and Diagnostic Procedures.* 3rd ed. Philadelphia, PA: W. B. Saunders, 2001.

Henry, John B. *Clinical Diagnosis and Management by Laboratory Methods.* Philadelphia: W. B. Saunders, 2001.

Kee, Joyce LeFever. *Handbook of Laboratory and Diagnostic Tests.* 4th ed. Upper Saddle River, NJ: Prentice Hall, 2001.

Wallach, Jacques. *Interpretation of Diagnostic Tests.* 7th ed. Philadelphia, PA: Lippincott Williams & Wilkins, 2000.

Victoria E. DeMoranville
Mark A. Best

Computerized axial tomography *see*
CT scans

Cone biopsy

Definition

A cone biopsy is a surgical procedure in which a cone-shaped tissue sample from the cervix is removed for examination. Also called cervical conization, a cone biopsy is done to diagnose cervical cancer or to remove cancerous or precancerous tissue.

Purpose

The cervix is the neck-shaped opening at the lower part of the uterus. The American Cancer Society estimated that in 2003, approximately 12,200 women would be diagnosed with cancer of the cervix and 4,100 women

---

WHO PERFORMS THE PROCEDURE AND WHERE IS IT PERFORMED?

A cone biopsy is usually performed by a gynecologist who specializes in the areas of women's general and reproductive health, pregnancy, labor and delivery, and prenatal testing. Tissue samples are analyzed by a pathologist who specializes in the diagnosis of diseases from microscopic analysis of cells and tissues. The procedure is generally done on an outpatient basis in a hospital or doctor's office.

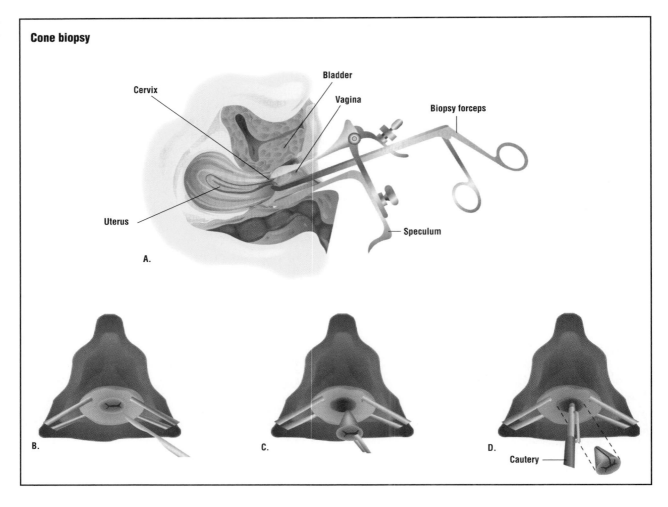

Cone biopsy

Bladder

Cervix

Vagina

Biopsy forceps

Uterus

Speculum

A.

B.

C.

D.

Cautery

In a cone biopsy, the patient lies on her back, and a speculum is inserted into the vagina (A). The cervix is visualized, and a cone-shaped piece of the cervix is removed (B and C). A cauterizing tool is used to stop any bleeding (D). *(Illustration by GGS Inc.)*

would die of the disease. When cervical cancer is detected and treated in its early stages, however, the long-term rate of survival is almost 100%.

A cone biopsy is performed to diagnose cancer of the cervix or to detect precancerous changes. The procedure is often recommended if a Pap test indicates the presence of abnormal cells. In some cases, a cone biopsy may be used as a conservative treatment for cervical cancer for women who wish to avoid a **hysterectomy** (surgical removal of the uterus).

Demographics

The risk of developing cervical cancer increases with age through a woman's 20s and 30s; the risk remains about the same for women over the age of 40. Minority women and women of low socioeconomic status have higher rates of cervical cancer and an increased

mortality rate. According to the Centers for Disease Control and Prevention (CDC), African-American, Asian-American, and Hispanic women have a higher-than-average incidence of the disease, while African-American and Hispanic women have a higher rate of cervical cancer-related death.

Description

The procedure is performed with the patient lying on her back with her legs in stirrups. General anesthesia is commonly used, although regional (spinal or epidural) or local anesthesia may also be used. A speculum is inserted into the vagina to hold it open during surgery.

There are several different methods that may be used to perform a cone biopsy. Cold-knife conization is the removal of a cone-shaped wedge of tissue with a scalpel (surgical knife). The tissue may also be removed using a carbon dioxide laser (called laser conization). A loop electrosurgical excision procedure (LEEP) uses low-voltage, high-frequency radio waves to excise the tissue. Some surgeons choose to cover the open cervical tissue with flaps of tissue stitched into place.

The tissue sample will then be examined under a microscope for the presence of cancerous cells. If abnormal cells are found around the edge of the biopsy, then further surgery will be required to excise any remaining cancer. If there is evidence of invasive cancer (i.e., the cancer has spread to surrounding tissues), then other treatments (more extensive surgery, chemotherapy, and/or radiation) may be recommended.

Diagnosis/Preparation

A number of tests may be performed prior to cone biopsy to determine if precancerous or cancerous cells exist. A Pap test involves scraping the cervix for a sample of cells and then staining and examining the cells for any abnormalities. **Colposcopy** is a procedure that allows a physician to examine a woman's cervix and vagina using a special microscope called a colposcope. A cervical biopsy involves the extraction of a smaller tissue sample and is less invasive than a cone biopsy. Based on the results of these tests, a cone biopsy may be indicated if moderate to severe cell abnormalities are found.

As cone biopsy is commonly performed under general anesthesia, the patient is usually instructed to refrain from eating and drinking after midnight on the day of surgery.

Aftercare

After the procedure, the patient may experience some cramping, discomfort, or mild to moderate bleeding. The biopsy site may take up to six weeks to completely heal. The patient will be instructed to avoid intercourse, tampons, and douches for at least three weeks following the procedure.

Risks

Bleeding during and after cone biopsy is the most common complication. Rarely, uncontrolled bleeding during the procedure may result in an emergency hysterectomy. Other potential complications include reaction to the anesthesia, infection of the biopsy site, injury to the uterus or other tissues, cervical stenosis (when the cervical canal narrows or becomes closed), and failure to remove all cancerous tissue. If too much tissue is removed during a cone biopsy so that the internal opening of the cervix to the uterus (called the internal os) is affected, a woman may have difficulty carrying a pregnancy to term, increasing her risk of miscarriage or premature birth.

> ## QUESTIONS TO ASK THE DOCTOR
>
> - Why is a cone biopsy recommended in my case?
> - How will the biopsy be removed?
> - How long will the procedure take?
> - When will I find out the results?
> - What will happen if the results are positive for cancer or another abnormality?

Normal results

Numerous studies have indicated that cone biopsy is successful in excising all cancerous tissue in 90% of patients with cervical cancer.

Morbidity and mortality rates

Two to 8% of women who undergo a cone biopsy will experience bleeding for up to two weeks. One study found that cervical stenosis occurs at a rate of 3–8%, depending on the method of conization.

Alternatives

Cryotherapy (freezing and destroying of abnormal cells) or laser vaporization (using a laser to destroy abnormal cells) may be used to treat early-stage cancer. A hysterectomy may be necessary to remove more invasive cancer. In a subtotal hysterectomy, only the uterus is removed. In a radical hysterectomy, the uterus, cervix, ovaries, fallopian tubes, lymph nodes, and lymph channels are removed. The type of hysterectomy performed depends on how far the cancer has spread. In all cases, menstruation stops and a woman loses the ability to bear children.

Resources

PERIODICALS

Brun, J. L., A. Youbi, and C. Hocke. "Complications, Sequellae and Outcome of Cervical Conizations: Evaluation of Three Surgical Techniques." *Journal of Gynecology and Obstetrics and Reproductive Biology* 31, no. 6 (January 10, 2002): 558–64.

Canavan, Timothy, and Nipa Doshi. "Cervical Cancer." *American Family Physician* 61 (March 1, 2000): 1369–76.

Soutter, W. P., et al. "Is Conservative Treatment for Adenocarcinoma In Situ of the Cervix Safe?" *British Journal of Obstetrics and Gynaecology* 108, no. 11 (November 2001): 1184–9.

ORGANIZATIONS

American Cancer Society. 1599 Clifton Road NE, Atlanta, GA 30329. (800) ACS-2345. <http://www.cancer.org>.

American College of Obstetricians and Gynecologists. 409 12th St., S.W., PO Box 96920, Washington, D.C. 20090-6920. <http://www.acog.org>.

OTHER

"All About Cervical Cancer: Overview." *American Cancer Society,* 2003 [March 18, 2003]. <http://www.cancer.org/docroot/CRI/CRI_2_1x.asp>.

"Cone Biopsy (Conization) for Abnormal Pap Test." *National Cervical Cancer Coalition,* May 23, 2002 [cited March 18, 2003]. <http://www.nccc-online.org/news_052302_9.asp>.

Nyirjesy, Istvan. "Conization of Cervix." *eMedicine,* June 28, 2002 [cited March 18, 2003]. <http://www.emedicine.com/med/topic3338.htm>.

Ries, L. A., et al., (eds). "SEER Cancer Statistics Review, 1973–1999." *National Cancer Institute,* 2002 [cited March 18, 2003]. <http://seer.cancer.gov/csr/1973_1999>.

Stephanie Dionne Sherk

Confidentiality *see* **Patient confidentiality**

Congenital glaucoma surgery *see* **Goniotomy**

Conization *see* **Cone biopsy**

Conscious sedation *see* **Sedation, conscious**

Continent ileostomy *see* **Ileoanal reservoir surgery**

Corneal keratoplasty *see* **Corneal transplantation**

Corneal transplantation

Definition

In corneal transplant, also known as keratoplasty, a patient's damaged cornea is replaced by the cornea from the eye of a human cadaver. This is the most common type of human **transplant surgery** and has the highest success rate. Eye banks acquire and store eyes from donors to supply the need for transplant corneas.

Purpose

Corneal transplant is used when vision is lost because the cornea has been damaged by disease or traumatic injury, and there are no other viable options.

WHO PERFORMS THE PROCEDURE AND WHERE IS IT PERFORMED?

Corneal transplants are performed by an ophthalmologist, who is a corneal specialist and is expert at transplants and corneal diseases. Patients might be referred to a corneal specialist by their ophthalmologist or optometrist.

Surgery is performed in a hospital setting, usually on an outpatient basis. Some surgeons may also perform the procedure at an ambulatory surgery center designed for outpatient procedures.

Some of the conditions that might require corneal transplant include the bulging outward of the cornea (keratoconus), a malfunction of the cornea's inner layer (Fuchs' dystrophy), and painful corneal swelling (pseudophakic bullous keratopathy). Other conditions that might make a corneal transplant necessary are tissue growth on the cornea (pterygium) and Stevens-Johnson syndrome, a skin disorder that can affect the eyes. Some of these conditions cause cloudiness of the cornea; others alter its natural curvature, which also can reduce vision quality.

Injury to the cornea can occur because of chemical burns, mechanical trauma, or infection by viruses, bacteria, fungi, or protozoa. The herpes virus produces one of the more common infections leading to corneal transplant.

Corneal transplants are used only when damage to the cornea is too severe to be treated with corrective lenses. Occasionally, corneal transplant is combined with other eye surgery such as cataract surgery to solve multiple eye problems with one procedure.

Demographics

The Eye Bank Association of America reported that corneal transplant recipients range in age from nine days to 103 years. More than 40,000 corneal transplants are performed in the United States each year. The cost is usually covered in part by **Medicare** and health insurers, although the patient might be required to incur part of the cost for the procedure. All eye tissue is donated. It is illegal to buy or sell human tissue.

Description

The cornea is the transparent layer of tissue at the front of the eye. It is composed almost entirely of a spe-

Corneal transplant

In a corneal transplant, the eye is held open with a speculum (A). A laser is used to make an initial cut in the existing cornea (B). The surgeon uses scissors to remove it (C), and a donor cornea is placed (D). It is stitched with very fine sutures (E). *(Illustration by GGS Inc.)*

cial type of collagen. It normally contains no blood vessels, but because it contains nerve endings, cornea damage can be very painful.

In a corneal transplant, a disc of tissue is removed from the center of the eye and replaced by a corresponding disc from a donor eye. The circular incision is made using an instrument called a trephine, which resembles a cookie cutter. In one form of corneal transplant, penetrating keratoplasty (PK), the disc removed is the entire thickness of the cornea and so is the replacement disc.

The donor cornea is attached with extremely fine sutures. Surgery can be performed under anesthesia that is confined to one area of the body while the patient is awake (local anesthesia) or under anesthesia that places the entire body of the patient in a state of unconsciousness (general anesthesia). Surgery requires 30–90 minutes.

Over 90% of all corneal transplants in the United States are PK. In lamellar keratoplasty (LK), only the outer layer of the cornea is removed and replaced. LK has many advantages, including early suture removal and decreased infection risk. It is not as widely used as PK,

however, because it is more time consuming and requires much greater technical ability by the surgeon.

A less common but related procedure called epikeratophakia involves suturing the donor cornea directly onto the surface of the existing host cornea. The only tissue removed from the host is the extremely thin epithelial cell layer on the outside of the host cornea. There is no permanent damage to the host cornea, and this procedure can be reversed. This procedure is mostly performed on children. In adults, the use of contact lenses can usually achieve the same goals.

Diagnosis/Preparation

Surgeons may discuss the need for corneal transplants after other viable options to remedy corneal trauma or disease have been discussed. No special preparation for corneal transplant is needed. Some ophthalmologists may request that the patient have a complete **physical examination** before surgery. Any active eye infection or eye inflammation usually needs to be brought under control before surgery. The patient may also be asked to skip breakfast on the day of surgery.

Aftercare

Corneal transplant is often performed on an outpatient basis, although some patients need brief hospitalization after surgery. The patient will wear an eye patch at least overnight. An eye shield or glasses must be worn to protect the eye until the surgical wound has healed. Eye drops will be prescribed for the patient to use for several weeks after surgery. Some patients require medication for at least a year. These drops include **antibiotics** to prevent infection as well as **corticosteroids** to reduce inflammation and prevent graft rejection.

For the first few days after surgery, the eye may feel scratchy and irritated. Vision will be somewhat blurry for as long as several months.

Sutures are often left in place for six months, and occasionally for as long as two years. Some surgeons may prescribe rigid contact lenses to reduce corneal astigmatism that follows corneal transplant.

Risks

Corneal transplants are highly successful, with over 90% of the operations in United States achieving restoration of sight. However, there is always some risk associated with any surgery. Complications that can occur include infection, glaucoma, retinal detachment, cataract formation, and rejection.

Graft rejection occurs in 5–30% of patients, a complication possible with any procedure involving tissue transplantation from another person (allograft). Allograft rejection results from a reaction of the patient's immune system to the donor tissue. Cell surface proteins called histo-compatibility antigens trigger this reaction. These antigens are often associated with vascular tissue (blood vessels) within the graft tissue. Because the cornea normally contains no blood vessels, it experiences a very low rate of rejection. Generally, blood typing and tissue typing are not needed in corneal transplants, and no close match between donor and recipient is required. However, the Collaborative Corneal Transplantation Study found that patients at high risk for rejection could benefit from receiving corneas from a donor with a matching blood type.

Symptoms of rejection include persistent discomfort, sensitivity to light, redness, or a change in vision. If a rejection reaction does occur, it can usually be blocked by steroid treatment. Rejection reactions may become noticeable within weeks after surgery, but may not occur until 10 or even 20 years after the transplant. When full rejection does occur, the surgery will usually need to be repeated.

Although the cornea is not normally vascular, some corneal diseases cause vascularization (the growth of blood vessels) into the cornea. In patients with these conditions, careful testing of both donor and recipient is performed just as in transplantation of other organs and tissues such as hearts, kidneys, and bone marrow. In such patients, repeated surgery is sometimes necessary in order to achieve a successful transplant.

Normal results

Patients can expect restored vision after the healing process is complete. In some patients, this might take as long as a year. Patients with keratoconus, corneal scars, early bullous keratopathy, or corneal stromal dystrophies have the highest rate of transplant success. Corneal transplants for keratoconus patients have a success rate of more than 90%.

Morbidity and mortality rates

While there is risk involved with any surgery, corneal transplants are relatively safe. In 2001, there was some concern about cornea donors transmitting Creutzfeldt-Jakob disease, a fatal bone-deteriorating disease, after questions of infection arose in Europe. A study showed the risk of transmission in the United States was small, as was any infection risk from cornea donors. Currently, cornea donors are screened using medical standards of the Eye Bank Association of America. These guidelines restrict donors who died from unknown causes, or suffered from immune deficiency diseases, hepatitis, and other infectious diseases.

Transplant recipients may have to receive another transplant if the first is unsuccessful or if, after a number of years, the disease returns.

KEY TERMS

Cadaver—The human body after death.

Cataract—A condition of cloudiness of the lens of the eye.

Cornea—The transparent layer of tissue at the very front of the eye.

Corticosteroids—Synthetic hormones widely used to fight inflammation.

Epikeratophakia—A procedure in which the donor cornea is attached directly onto the host cornea.

Epithelial cells—Cells that form a thin surface coating on the outside of a body structure.

Fibrous connective tissue—Dense tissue found in various parts of the body containing very few living cells.

Fuchs' dystrophy—A hereditary disease of the inner layer of the cornea.

Glaucoma—A vision defect caused when excessive fluid pressure within the eye damages the optic nerve.

Histocompatibility antigens—Proteins scattered throughout body tissues that are unique for almost every individual.

Keratoconus—An eye condition in which the cornea bulges outward, interfering with normal vision; usually both eyes are affected.

Pseudophakic bullous keratopathy (PBK)—Painful swelling of the cornea occasionally occurring after surgery to implant an artificial lens in place of a lens affected by cataract.

Retinal detachment—A serious vision disorder in which the light-detecting layer of cells inside the eye (retina) is separated from its normal support tissue and no longer functions properly.

Trephine—A small surgical instrument that is rotated to cut a circular incision.

Alternatives

An increasingly popular alternative to corneal transplants is phototherapeutic keratectomy (PTK). This technique is now used to treat corneal scars and dystrophies, and some infections. Surgeons use an excimer laser and a computer to vaporize diseased tissue, leaving a smooth surface. New tissue begins growing immediately and recovery takes only a few days. Patients must be carefully selected, however, and success is greatest if damage is restricted to the cornea's top layer.

Intrastromal corneal rings are implantable devices that could be used for some keratoconus patients. The rings are implanted and the procedure is reversible. However, not much is known about long-term stability. Some companies also are developing synthetic corneas that are implanted using synthetic penetrating keratoplasty. This procedure may become more widely used for high-risk patients and those with severe chemical burns.

Resources

BOOKS

Boruchoff, S. Arthur, and Richard A. Thoft. "Keratoplasty: Lamellar and Penetrating." In *The Cornea,* edited by Gilbert Smolin and Richard A. Thoft. Boston: Little, Brown and Co., 1994.

Brightbill, Frederick S., ed. *Corneal Surgery.* St. Louis: Mosby, 1993.

Bruner, William E., Walter J. Stark, and A. Edward Maumenee. *Manual of Corneal Surgery.* New York: Churchill Livingstone, 1987.

Miller, Stephen J. H. *Parsons' Diseases of the Eye,* 18th ed. New York: Churchill Livingstone, 1990.

Vaughan, Daniel, ed. *General Ophthalmology,* 14th ed. Stamford: Appleton & Lange, 1995.

PERIODICALS

Kennedy, R. H., et al. "Eye Banking and Screening for Creutzfeldt-Jakob Disease." *Archives of Ophthalmology* 119 (May 2001): 721–6.

Watson, B. C., and G. L. White Jr. "Corneal Transplantation." *American Family Physician* 54 (Nov. 1996): 1945–48.

ORGANIZATIONS

American Academy of Ophthalmology. 655 Beach Street, P.O. Box 7424, San Francisco, CA 94120-7424. <http://www.aao.org>.

Eye Bank Association of America. 1015 Eighteenth Street NW, Suite 1010, Washington, D.C. 20036. (202) 775-4999. <http://www.restoresight.org>.

OTHER

Asbell, Penny A., and Syed M. Ahmad. "New Techniques in Corneal Transplant." *Review of Ophthalmology,* May 15, 2002 [cited February 20, 2003]. <www.revophth.com/index.asp?page=1_94.htm>.

Cimberle, Michela. "New Type of Artificial Cornea Performs Better than Donor Grafts in High-Risk Cases." *Ocular Surgery News,* June 1, 2002 [cited February 23, 2003]. <www.osnsupersite.com/view.asp?ID=2346>.

Coronary artery bypass graft surgery

"Collaborative Corneal Transplantation Studies." *National Eye Institute,* October 21, 1999 [cited February 25, 2003]. <www.nei.nih.gov/neitrials/statics/study36.htm>.

"Corneal Transplantation." *Merck Manual of Diagnosis and Therapy,* [cited February 25, 2003]. <www.merck.com/pubs/mmanual/section8/chapter96/96l.htm>.

"Facts About the Cornea and Corneal Disease." *National Eye Institute,* June 2001 [cited March 4, 2003]. <www.nei.nih.gov/health/cornealdisease/index.htm>.

Victor Leipzig, PhD
Mary Bekker

Coronary artery bypass graft surgery

Definition

Coronary artery bypass graft surgery is a surgical procedure in which one or more blocked coronary arteries are bypassed by a blood vessel graft to restore normal blood flow to the heart. These grafts usually come from the patient's own arteries and veins located in the leg, arm, or chest.

Purpose

Coronary artery bypass graft surgery (also called coronary artery bypass surgery [CABG] and bypass operation) is performed to restore blood flow to the heart. This relieves chest pain and ischemia, improves the patient's quality of life, and, in some cases, prolongs the patient's life. The goals of the procedure are to relieve symptoms of coronary artery disease, enable the patient to resume a normal lifestyle, and to lower the risk of a heart attack or other heart problems.

According to the American Heart Association, appropriate candidates for coronary artery bypass graft surgery include patients who:

• have blockages in at least two to three major coronary arteries, especially if the blockages are in arteries that feed the heart's left ventricle or in the left anterior descending artery

• have angina so severe that even mild exertion causes chest pain

• have poor left ventricular function

• cannot tolerate percutaneous transluminal coronary **angioplasty** and do not respond well to drug therapy

Demographics

Coronary artery bypass graft surgery is widely performed in the United States. It is estimated that more than 800,000 coronary artery bypass graft surgeries are performed worldwide every year. The American Heart Association reports that 519,000 coronary artery bypass graft surgeries were performed in the United States in 2000, of which 371,000 were performed on men and 148,000 on women.

Description

Coronary artery bypass graft surgery builds a detour around one or more blocked coronary arteries with a graft from a healthy vein or artery. The graft goes around the clogged artery (or arteries) to create new pathways for oxygen-rich blood to flow to the heart.

Procedure

After general anesthesia is administered, the surgeon removes the veins or prepares the arteries for grafting. If the saphenous vein is to be used for the graft, a series of incisions are made in the patient's thigh or calf. If the radial artery is to be used for the graft, incisions are made in the patient's forearm. It is important to note that the removal of veins or arteries for grafting does not deprive the area of adequate blood flow.

More commonly, a segment of the internal mammary artery is used for the graft, and the incisions are made in the chest wall. The internal mammary arteries are most commonly used because they have shown the best long-term results. Because they have their own oxygen-rich blood supply, the internal mammary arteries can usually be kept intact at their origin, then sewn to the coronary artery below the site of blockage.

The surgeon decides which grafts to use, depending on the location of the blockage, the amount of the blockage, and the size of the patient's coronary arteries.

In traditional coronary artery bypass surgery, the surgeon makes an incision down the center of the patient's chest, cuts through the breastbone, and retracts the rib cage open to expose the heart. The patient is connected to a heart-lung bypass machine, also called a cardiopulmonary bypass pump, that takes over for the heart and lungs during the surgery. During this "on-pump" procedure, the heart-lung machine removes carbon dioxide from the blood and replaces it with oxygen. A tube is inserted into the aorta to carry the oxygenated blood from the bypass machine to the aorta for circulation to the body. The heart-lung machine allows the heart's beating to be stopped, so the surgeon can operate on a still heart. Aortic clamps are used to restrict blood flow to the area of the heart where grafts will be placed so the heart is blood-free during the surgery. The clamps remain until the grafts are in place.

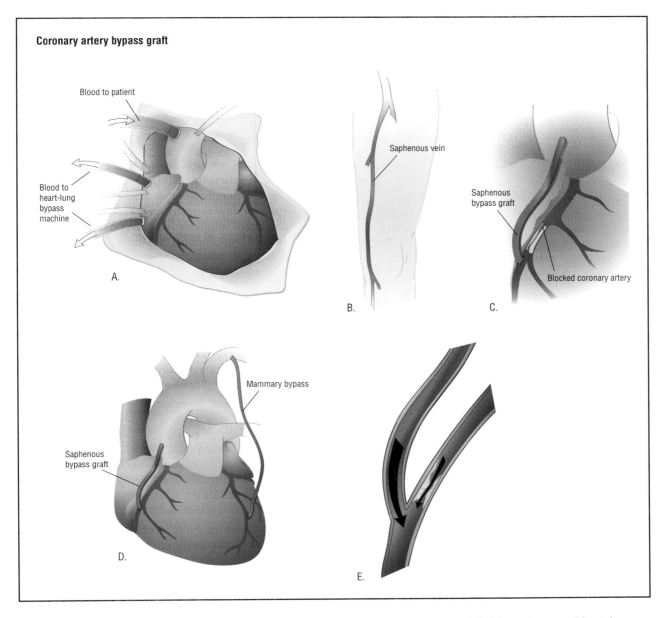

Coronary artery bypass graft

A.
Blood to patient
Blood to heart-lung bypass machine

B.
Saphenous vein

C.
Saphenous bypass graft
Blocked coronary artery

D.
Mammary bypass
Saphenous bypass graft

E.

During a coronary artery bypass graft (CABG), the chest is opened to visualize the heart (A). A heart-lung machine takes over the function of the heart during the procedure. A portion of the saphenous vein of the leg is removed (B). This vessel is used to bypass a blockage of the coronary artery. It is attached from the aorta past the point of blockage (C). Another option is to bypass a blockage with the mammary artery (D). The bypass increases blood flow to the area served by the coronary artery (E). *(Illustration by Argosy.)*

Some patients may be candidates for minimally invasive coronary artery bypass surgery or for off-pump bypass surgery. During minimally invasive surgery, smaller chest and graft removal incisions are used, promoting a quicker recovery and less risk of infection. Off-pump bypass surgery, also called beating heart surgery, is a surgical technique performed while the heart is still beating. The surgeon uses advanced equipment to stabilize portions of the heart and bypass the blocked artery while the rest of the heart keeps pumping and circulating blood through the body.

After the grafts are prepared, a small opening is made just below the blockage in the diseased coronary artery. Blood will be redirected through this opening once the graft is sewn in place. If a leg or arm vein is used, one end is connected to the coronary artery and the other to the aorta; if a mammary artery is used, one end is connected to the coronary artery while the other remains attached to the aorta. The procedure is repeated on as many coronary arteries as necessary. On average, three or four coronary arteries are bypassed during surgery. Blood flow is checked to assure the graft supplies adequate blood to the heart.

If the procedure was done "on-pump," electric shocks start the heart pumping again after the grafts have been completed. The heart-lung machine is turned off and the blood slowly returns to normal body temperature. After implanting pacing wires and inserting a chest tube to drain fluid, the surgeon closes the chest cavity. Sometimes a temporary pacemaker is attached to the pacing wires to regulate the heart rhythm until the patient's condition improves. After surgery, the patient is transferred to an **intensive care unit** for close monitoring.

Diagnosis/Preparation

Diagnosis

The diagnosis of coronary artery disease is made after the patient's medical history is carefully reviewed, a physical exam is performed, and the patient's symptoms are evaluated. Tests used to diagnose coronary artery disease include:

• electrocardiogram

• stress tests

• cardiac catheterization

• imaging tests such as a **chest x ray**, **echocardiography**, or computed tomography (CT)

• blood tests to measure blood cholesterol, triglycerides, and other substances

Preparation

The individual should quit smoking or using tobacco products before the surgery. The individual needs to make the commitment to be a nonsmoker after the surgery. There are several **smoking cessation** programs available in the community. The individual can ask a health care provider for more information about quitting smoking.

Coronary artery bypass graft surgery should ideally be postponed for three months after a heart attack. Patients should be medically stable before the surgery, if possible.

During a preoperative appointment, usually scheduled within one to two weeks before surgery, the patient will receive information about what to expect during the surgery and the recovery period. The patient will usually meet the cardiologist, anesthesiologist, nurse clinicians, and surgeon during this appointment or just before the procedure.

If the patient develops a cold, fever, or sore throat within a few days before the surgery, he or she should notify the surgeon's office.

The evening before the surgery, the patient showers with antiseptic soap provided by the surgeon's office. After midnight, the patient should not eat or drink anything.

The patient is usually admitted to the hospital the same day the surgery is scheduled. The patient should bring a list of current medications, allergies, and appropriate medical records upon **admission to the hospital**.

Before the surgery, the patient is given a blood-thinning drug—usually heparin—that helps to prevent blood clots. A sedative is given the morning of surgery. The chest and the area from where the graft will be taken are shaved.

Coronary **angiography** will have been previously performed to show the surgeon where the arteries are blocked and where the grafts might best be positioned. Heart monitoring is initiated. The patient is given general anesthesia before the procedure.

The length of the procedure depends upon the number of arteries being bypassed, but it generally takes from three to five hours—sometimes longer.

Aftercare

Recovery in the hospital

The patient recovers in a surgical intensive care unit for one to two days after the surgery. The patient will be connected to chest and breathing tubes, a mechanical ventilator, a heart monitor, and other monitoring equipment. A urinary catheter will be in place to drain urine. The breathing tube and ventilator are usually removed about six hours after surgery, but the other tubes usually remain in place as long as the patient is in the intensive care unit.

Drugs are prescribed to control pain and to prevent unwanted blood clotting. Daily doses of **aspirin** are started within six to 24 hours after the procedure.

The patient is closely monitored during the recovery period. **Vital signs** and other parameters such as heart sounds, oxygen, and carbon dioxide levels in arterial blood are checked frequently. The chest tube is checked to ensure that it is draining properly. The patient may be fed intravenously for the first day or two.

Chest physiotherapy is started after the ventilator and breathing tubes are removed. The therapy includes coughing, turning frequently, and taking deep breaths. Sometimes oxygen is delivered via a mask to help loosen and clear secretions from the lungs. Other exercises will be encouraged to improve the patient's circulation and prevent complications due to prolonged bed rest.

If there are no complications, the patient begins to resume a normal routine on the second day, including eating regular food, sitting up, and walking around a bit. Before being discharged from the hospital, the patient usually spends a few days under observation in a non-surgical unit. During this time, counseling is usually provided on eating right and starting a light **exercise** program to keep the heart healthy.

The average hospital stay after coronary artery bypass graft surgery is five to seven days.

Recovery at home

INCISION AND SKIN CARE. The incision should be kept clean and dry. When the skin is healed, the incision should be washed with soapy water. The scar should not be bumped, scratched, or otherwise disturbed. Ointments, lotions, and dressings should not be applied to the incision unless specific instructions have been given.

DISCOMFORT. While the incision scar heals, which takes one to two months, it may be sore. Itching, tightness, or numbness along the incision are common. Muscle or incision discomfort may occur in the chest during activity.

Swelling or aching may occur in the legs if the saphenous vein was used for the graft. Special support stockings may be needed to decrease leg swelling after surgery. While sitting, the patient should not cross the legs and the feet should be elevated. Walking daily, even if the legs are swollen, will help improve circulation and reduce swelling.

LIFESTYLE CHANGES. The patient needs to make several lifestyle changes after surgery, including:

• Quitting smoking. Smoking causes damage to the bypass grafts and other blood vessels, increases the patient's blood pressure and heart rate, and decreases the amount of oxygen available in the blood.

• Managing weight. Maintaining a healthy weight, by watching portion sizes and exercising, is important. Being overweight increases the work of the heart.

• Participating in an exercise program. The exercise program is usually tailored for the patient, who will be encouraged to participate in a cardiac rehabilitation program supervised by exercise professionals.

• Making dietary changes. Patients should eat a lot of fruits, vegetables, grains, and non-fat or low-fat dairy products, and reduce fats to less than 30% of all calories.

WHO PERFORMS THE PROCEDURE AND WHERE IS IT PERFORMED?

The surgery team for coronary artery bypass graft surgery includes the cardiovascular surgeon, assisting surgeons, a cardiovascular anesthesiologist, a perfusion technologist (who operates the heart-lung machine), and specially trained nurses. The surgery is performed in a hospital.

• Taking medications as prescribed. Aspirin and other heart medications may be prescribed, and the patient may need to take these medications for life.

• Following up with health care providers. The patient must schedule follow-up visits to determine how effective the surgery was, to confirm that progressive exercise is safe, and to monitor his or her recovery and control risk factors.

Risks

Coronary artery bypass graft surgery is major surgery and patients may experience any of the normal complications associated with major surgery and anesthesia, such as the risk of bleeding, pneumonia, or infection. Possible complications include:

• graft closure or blockage

• development of blockages in other arteries

• damage to the aorta

• long-term development of atherosclerotic disease of saphenous vein grafts

• abnormal heart rhythms

• high or low blood pressure

• recurrence of angina

• blood clots that can lead to a stroke or heart attack

• kidney failure

• depression or severe mood swings

• possible short-term memory loss, difficulty thinking clearly, and problems concentrating for long periods (These effects generally subside within six months after surgery.)

There is a higher risk for complications in patients who:

• are heavy smokers

• have a history of lung, kidney, or metabolic diseases

QUESTIONS TO ASK THE DOCTOR

- Why is this surgery being performed?
- Am I a candidate for minimally invasive coronary artery bypass surgery?
- Which technique will be used during the surgery, the "on-pump" or "off-pump" technique?
- Who will be performing the surgery? How many years of experience does this surgeon have? How many other coronary artery bypass graft surgeries has this surgeon performed?
- Should I take my medications the day of the surgery?
- How long will I have to stay in the hospital after the surgery?
- After I go home from the hospital, how long will it take me to recover from surgery?
- What should I do if I experience chest discomfort or other symptoms similar to those I felt before surgery?

- What types of symptoms should I report to my doctor?
- How should I care for my incision?
- What types of medications will I have to take after surgery?
- When will I be able to resume my normal activities?
- If I have had the surgery once, can I have it again to correct future blockages?
- Are there any medications, foods, or activities I should avoid to prevent my symptoms from recurring?
- What lifestyle changes (including diet, **weight management**, exercise, and activity changes) are recommended after the procedure to improve my heart health?
- How often do I need to see my doctor for follow-up visits after the surgery?

- have diabetes
- have had a recent heart attack
- have a history of angina, ventricular arrhythmias, congestive heart failure, cerebrovascular disease, or mitral regurgitation

Normal results

Full recovery from coronary artery bypass graft surgery takes two to three months and is a gradual process. Upon release from the hospital, the patient will feel weak because of the extended bed rest in the hospital. Within a few weeks, the patient should begin to feel stronger.

Most patients are able to drive in about three to eight weeks, after receiving approval from their physician. Sexual activity can generally be resumed in three to four weeks, depending on the patient's rate of recovery.

It takes about six to eight weeks for the sternum to heal. During this time, the patient should not perform activities that cause pressure or weight on the breastbone or tension on the arms and chest. Pushing and pulling heavy objects (as in mowing the lawn) should be avoided and lifting objects more than 20 lbs (9 kg) is not permitted. The patient should not hold his or her arms above shoulder level for a long period of time, such as when doing household chores. The patient should try not to stand in one place for longer than 15 minutes. Stair climbing is permitted unless other instructions have been given.

Within four to six weeks, people with sedentary office jobs can return to work; people with physical jobs such as construction work or jobs requiring heavy lifting must wait longer (up to 12 weeks) or may have to change careers.

About 90% of patients experience significant improvements after coronary artery bypass graft surgery. Patients experience full relief from chest pain and resume their normal activities in about 70% of the cases; the remaining 20% experience partial relief.

For most people, the graft remains open for about 10–15 years.

Coronary artery bypass surgery does not prevent coronary artery disease from recurring. Therefore, lifestyle changes are strongly recommended and medications are prescribed to reduce this risk. About 40% of patients have a new blockage within 10 years after surgery and require a second bypass, change in medication, or an interventional procedure.

Morbidity and mortality rates

The risk of death during coronary artery bypass graft surgery is 2–3%.

In 5–10% of coronary artery bypass graft surgeries, the bypass graft stops supplying blood to the bypassed

KEY TERMS

Angiotensin-converting enzyme (ACE) inhibitor—A drug that lowers blood pressure by interfering with the breakdown of a protein-like substance involved in blood pressure regulation.

Angina—Also called angina pectoris, chest pain or discomfort that occurs when diseased blood vessels restrict blood flow to the heart.

Aorta—The main artery that carries blood from the heart to the rest of the body; the aorta is the largest artery in the body.

Artery—A vessel that carries oxygen-rich blood to the body.

Atherectomy—A non-surgical technique for treating diseased arteries with a rotating device that cuts or shaves away obstructing material inside the artery.

Atria—The right and left upper chambers of the heart.

Beta blocker—An anti-hypertensive drug that limits the activity of epinephrine, a hormone that increases blood pressure.

Brachytherapy—The use of radiation during angioplasty to prevent the artery from narrowing again (a process called restenosis).

Calcium channel blocker—A drug that lowers blood pressure by regulating calcium-related electrical activity in the heart.

Cardiac rehabilitation—A structured program of education and activity offered by hospitals and other organizations.

Coronary artery disease—Also called atherosclerosis, it is a build-up of fatty matter and debris in the coronary artery wall that causes narrowing of the artery.

Echocardiogram—An imaging procedure used to create a picture of the heart's movement, valves, and chambers.

Graft—To implant living tissue surgically.

Homocysteine—An amino acid normally found in small amounts in the blood.

Ischemia—Decreased blood flow to an organ, usually caused by constriction or obstruction of an artery.

Lipoproteins—Substances that carry fat through the blood vessels for use or storage in other parts of the body.

Mammary artery—A chest wall artery that descends from the aorta and is commonly used for bypass grafts.

Radial artery—An artery located in the arm and used for bypass grafts.

Rotoblation—A non-surgical technique for treating diseased arteries.

Saphenous vein—A long vein in the thigh or calf commonly used for bypass grafts.

Stent—A device made of expandable, metal mesh that is placed (by using a balloon catheter) at the site of a narrowing artery; the stent stays in place to keep the artery open.

Sternum—Also called the breastbone, the sternum is the bone in the chest that is separated during open heart surgery.

Stress test—A test used to determine how the heart responds to stress.

Vein—A blood vessel that returns oxygen-depleted blood from various parts of the body to the heart.

Ventricles—The lower pumping chambers of the heart.

artery within one year. Younger people who are healthy except for the heart disease achieve good results with bypass surgery. Patients who have poorer results from coronary artery bypass graft surgery include those over the age of 70, those who have poor left ventricular function, are undergoing a repeat surgery or other procedures concurrently, and those who continue smoking, do not treat high cholesterol or other coronary risk factors, or have another debilitating disease.

Over the long term, symptoms recur in only about 3–4% of patients per year. Five years after coronary artery bypass graft surgery, survival expectancy is 90%, at 10 years it is about 85%, at 15 years it is about 55%, and at 20 years it is about 40%.

Angina recurs in about 40% of patients after 10 years. In most cases, it is less severe than before the surgery and can be controlled with drug therapy. In patients who have had vein grafts, 40% of the grafts are severely obstructed 10 years after the procedure. Repeat coronary artery bypass graft surgery may be necessary, and is usually less successful than the first surgery.

Alternatives

All patients with coronary artery disease can help improve their condition by making lifestyle changes such as quitting smoking, losing weight if they are overweight, eating healthy foods, reducing blood cholesterol, exercising regularly, and controlling diabetes and high blood pressure.

All patients with coronary artery disease should be prescribed medications to treat their condition. Antiplatelet medications such as aspirin or clopidogrel (Plavix) are usually recommended. Other medications used to treat angina may include beta blockers, nitrates, and angiotensin-converting enzyme (ACE) inhibitors. Medications may also be prescribed to lower lipoprotein levels, since elevated lipoprotein levels have been associated with an increased risk of cardiovascular problems.

Treatment with vitamin E is not recommended because it does not lower the rate of cardiovascular events in people with coronary artery disease. Although antioxidants such as vitamin C, beta-carotene, and probucol show promising results, they are not recommended for routine use. Treatment with folic acid and vitamins B_6 and B_{12} lowers homocysteine levels (reducing the risk for cardiovascular problems), but more studies are needed to determine if lowered homocysteine levels correlate with a reduced rate of cardiovascular problems in treated patients.

Less invasive, nonsurgical interventional procedures—such as balloon angioplasty, stent placement, rotoblation, atherectomy, or brachytherapy—can be performed to open a blocked artery. These procedures may be the appropriate treatment for some patients before coronary artery bypass graft surgery is considered.

Enhanced external counterpulsation (EECP) may be a treatment option for patients who are not candidates for interventional procedures or coronary artery bypass graft surgery. During EECP, a set of cuffs is wrapped around the patient's calves, thighs, and buttocks. These cuffs gently but firmly compress the blood vessels in the lower limbs to increase blood flow to the heart. The inflation and deflation of the cuffs are electronically synchronized with the heartbeat and blood pressure using **electrocardiography** and blood pressure monitors. EECP may encourage blood vessels to open small channels to eventually bypass blocked vessels and improve blood flow to the heart. Not all patients are candidates for this procedure, and treatments, lasting one to two hours, must be repeated about five times a week for up to seven weeks.

Resources

BOOKS

American Heart Association. "Considering Surgery or Other Interventions." In *Guide to Heart Attack Treatment, Recovery, Prevention.* New York: Time Books, 1996.

Barry, Frank. *The Healthy Heart Formula: The Powerful, New, Commonsense Approach to Preventing and Reversing Heart Disease.* New York: John Wiley & Sons, 1998.

DeBakey, Michael E., and Antonio M. Gotto Jr. "Surgical Treatment of Coronary Artery Disease." In *The New Living Heart.* Holbrook, MA: Adams Media Corporation, 1997.

McGoon, Michael D., and Bernard J. Gersh. *Mayo Clinic Heart Book: The Ultimate Guide to Heart Health, Second Edition.* New York: William Morrow and Co., Inc., 2000.

Texas Heart Institute. "Heart Surgery." In *Texas Heart Institute Heart Owner's Handbook.* New York: John Wiley & Sons, 1995.

Topol, Eric J. *Cleveland Clinic Heart Book: The Definitive Guide for the Entire Family from the Nation's Leading Heart Center.* New York: Hyperion, 2000.

Trout, Darrell, and Ellen Welch. *Surviving with Heart: Taking Charge of Your Heart Care.* Golden, CO: Fulcrum Publishing, 2002.

PERIODICALS

Eagle, K. A., et al. "ACC/AHA Guidelines for Coronary Artery Bypass Graft Surgery: Executive Summary and Recommendations: A Report of the American College of Cardiology/American Heart Association Task Force on Practice Guidelines (Committee to Revise the 1991 Guidelines for Coronary Artery Bypass Graft Surgery)." *Circulation* 100 (1999): 1464–1480.

Mullany, Charles J. "Coronary Artery Bypass Surgery." *Circulation* 107 (2003): e21–e22.

Sabik, Joseph. *Off-Pump Bypass Surgery: Improving Outcomes for Coronary Artery Bypass Surgery.* Cleveland Clinic Heart Center, The Cleveland Clinic Foundation. November 2001.

ORGANIZATIONS

American College of Cardiology. Heart House. 9111 Old Georgetown Rd., Bethesda, MD 20814-1699. (800) 253-4636, ext. 694, or (301) 897-5400. <http://www.acc.org>.

American Heart Association. 7272 Greenville Ave., Dallas, TX 75231. (800) 242-8721 or (214) 373-6300. <http://www.americanheart.org>.

The Cleveland Clinic Heart Center, The Cleveland Clinic Foundation. 9500 Euclid Avenue, F25, Cleveland, Ohio, 44195. (800) 223-2273, ext. 46697, or (216) 444-6697. <http://www.clevelandclinic.org/heartcenter>.

National Heart, Lung, and Blood Institute. National Institutes of Health. Building 1. 1 Center Dr., Bethesda, MD 20892. E-mail: NHLBIinfo@rover.nhlbi. <http://www.nhlbi.nih.gov>.

Texas Heart Institute. Heart Information Service. P.O. Box 20345, Houston, TX 77225-0345. <http://www.tmc.edu/thi>.

OTHER

The Heart: An Online Exploration. The Franklin Institute Science Museum. 222 North 20th Street, Philadelphia, PA, 19103. (215) 448-1200. <http://sln2.fi.edu/biosci/heart.html>.

HeartCenterOnline. <http://www.heartcenteronline.com>.

Heart Information Network. <http://www.heartinfo.org>.
Heart Surgeon.com. <http://www.heartsurgeon.com>.

Lori De Milto
Angela M. Costello

Coronary stenting

Definition

A coronary stent is an artificial support device placed in the coronary artery to keep the vessel open after treatment for coronary artery disease. Also called atherosclerosis, coronary artery disease is a build-up of fatty matter and debris on the walls of the arteries. Over time, this buildup narrows the arteries and reduces blood supply to the heart.

The stent is usually a stainless steel mesh tube that is available in various sizes to match the size of the artery and hold it open after the blockage in the artery has been treated.

Purpose

The coronary stent is used to keep coronary arteries expanded, usually following a balloon **angioplasty** or other interventional procedure. Balloon angioplasty (also called percutaneous transluminal coronary angioplasty, or PTCA) and other interventional procedures are performed to open narrowed coronary arteries and improve blood flow to the heart. By forming a rigid support, the stent can prevent the vessel from reclosing (a process called restenosis) and reduce the need for coronary bypass surgery.

Demographics

According to the American Heart Association, 1,025,000 angioplasties were performed in the United States in 2000; of these, 561,000 were balloon angioplasties. There were 655,000 men and 370,000 women who had angioplasties in 2000. Stent placement is part of more than 70% of interventional procedures.

Description

Coronary stenting usually follows balloon angioplasty. After the patient receives a local anesthetic to numb the area, a **cardiac catheterization** procedure is performed in which a long, narrow tube (catheter) is passed through a sheath placed within a small incision in the femoral artery in the upper thigh. Sometimes, the catheter is placed in an artery in the arm.

A catheter with a small balloon at the tip is guided to the point of narrowing in the coronary artery. Contrast material is injected through the catheter so the physician can view the site where the artery is narrowed on a special monitor. When the balloon catheter is positioned at the location of the blockage in the coronary artery, it is slowly inflated to widen that artery and compress the blockage or fatty area into the artery wall and stretch the artery open.

The stent is inserted into the artery with the balloon-tip catheter. When the stent is correctly positioned in the coronary artery, the balloon is inflated, expanding the stent against the walls of the coronary artery. The balloon catheter is deflated and removed, leaving the stent permanently in place to hold the coronary artery open.

Stents coated with drugs to decrease clotting or narrowing at the site are currently under investigation. These coated stents have significantly reduced restenosis rates—down to 3%—in some clinical studies. One coated stent brand, the Cordis CYPHER, became the first coated stent approved by the FDA in April 2003.

A cardiac **angiography** will follow to ensure that the stent is keeping the artery open.

Diagnosis/Preparation

Diagnosis

The diagnosis of coronary artery disease is made after the patient's medical history is carefully reviewed, a physical exam is performed and the patient's symptoms are evaluated. Tests used to diagnose coronary artery disease include:

- electrocardiogram
- stress tests
- cardiac catheterization
- imaging tests such as a **chest x ray**, **echocardiography**, or computed tomography (CT)
- blood tests to measure blood cholesterol, triglycerides, and other substances

Preparation

The patient should quit smoking or using tobacco products before the procedure, and needs to make the commitment to be a nonsmoker after the surgery. There are several **smoking cessation** programs available in the community. The patient can ask a health care provider for more information about quitting smoking.

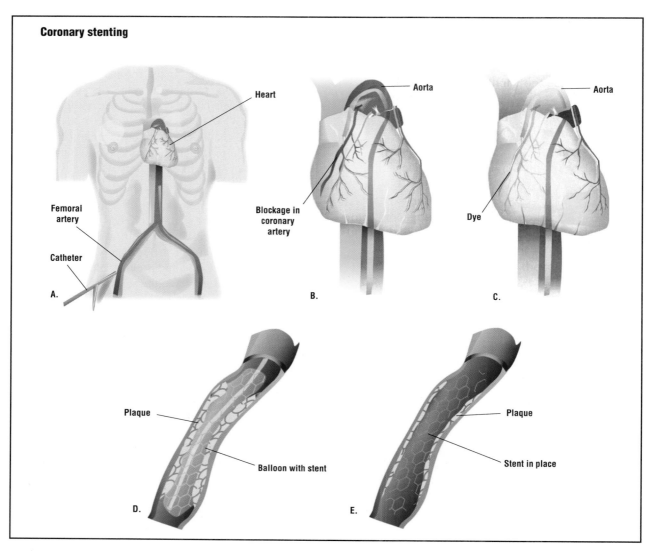

Coronary stenting

Heart

Aorta

Aorta

Femoral artery

Catheter

Blockage in coronary artery

Dye

A.

B.

C.

Plaque

Balloon with stent

Plaque

Stent in place

D.

E.

During coronary stenting, a catheter is fed into the femoral artery of the upper leg (A). The catheter is fed up to coronary arteries to an area of blockage (B). A dye is released, allowing visualization of the blockage (C). A stent is placed on the balloon-tipped catheter. The balloon is inflated, opening the artery (D). The stent holds the artery open after the catheter is removed (E). *(Illustration by GGS Inc.)*

The patient is usually instructed to take **aspirin** or another blood-thinning medication for several days before the procedure. Aspirin can help decrease the possibility of blood clots forming at the stent.

It is advisable for the patient to arrange for transportation home, because drowsiness may last several hours and driving is not permitted after the procedure.

After midnight the night before the procedure, the patient should not eat or drink anything.

The patient usually goes to the hospital the same day the procedure is scheduled, and should bring a list of current medications, allergies, and appropriate medical records upon **admission to the hospital**.

An intravenous needle will be inserted into a vein in the arm to deliver medications and fluids during the procedure. The catheter insertion site may be shaved. A sedative is given to make the patient drowsy and relaxed, but the patient will not be completely asleep during the procedure.

Aftercare

The procedure generally takes from 90 minutes to two hours to perform, but the preparation and recovery time add several hours to the overall procedure time. Although patients often go home the same day or the evening of the procedure, they should plan to stay at the hospital most of the day.

Recovery in the hospital

The patient is instructed to stay flat in bed without bending the legs so that the artery can heal from the insertion of the catheter. A stitch or collagen plug may be placed at the site of the catheter insertion to seal the wound and firm pressure may be applied to the area. A flat position is required for two to six hours after the procedure. A health care provider will help the patient get out of bed for the first time when the doctor approves it. The patient will be allowed to eat after he or she is able to get out of bed.

The patient is closely monitored during the recovery period. **Vital signs** and other parameters such as the heart's rhythm and electrical activity as well as oxygen and carbon dioxide levels in arterial blood are checked frequently. A catheter may be placed to drain urine during the recovery period.

A blood thinner may be given to the patient intravenously for the first few hours after the procedure to prevent clotting.

Recovery at home

Medications are prescribed to control pain. Minor chest discomfort is common after the procedure. However, the patient should notify the health care provider if severe chest, arm, or back discomfort is experienced. Some bleeding and bruising near the catheter insertion site are also common after the procedure. However, severe bleeding should be reported to a health care provider immediately. If bleeding occurs, the patient should contact 9-1-1 and lay down immediately. The dressing covering the area should be removed and firm pressure should be applied to the area until help arrives.

Ointments, lotions, and dressings should not be applied to the catheter insertion site unless specific instructions have been given.

Medications are prescribed to prevent unwanted blood clotting. Daily doses of aspirin or other anticoagulant medications are started after the procedure and are continued after the patient goes home.

The patient should not have any **magnetic resonance imaging** (MRI) tests for six months after the procedure, because the magnetic field may move the stent.

LIFESTYLE CHANGES. The patient needs to make several lifestyle changes after surgery, including:

- Quitting smoking. Smoking causes damage to blood vessels, increases the patient's blood pressure and heart rate, and decreases the amount of oxygen available in the blood.

- Managing weight. Maintaining a healthy weight by watching portion sizes and exercising is important. Being overweight increases the work of the heart.
- Participating in an **exercise** program. The exercise program is usually tailored for the patient, who will be encouraged to participate in a cardiac rehabilitation program supervised by exercise professionals.
- Making dietary changes. Patients should eat a lot of fruits, vegetables, grains, and non-fat or low-fat dairy products, and reduce fats to less than 30% of all calories. A diet low in cholesterol and vitamin K (to prevent interference with the anticoagulant medication) may be recommended.
- Taking medications as prescribed. Aspirin and other heart medications may be prescribed, and the patient may need to take these medications for life.
- Managing other health conditions such as diabetes or high blood pressure. Taking medications as prescribed and following the doctor's guidelines are very important ways for the patient to manage his or her health.
- Following up with health care providers. The patient needs to regularly see the physician to monitor his or her recovery and control risk factors. Routine stress testing is a part of the follow-up treatment to detect restenosis that may occur without symptoms.

Risks

Although coronary stents greatly reduce the risk of restenosis following balloon angioplasty, there is still some risk that the stented artery may close.

Serious complications are uncommon, but may include infection, damage to the heart or blood vessels, and blood clots. Anticlotting medication is given after stent placement to prevent the risk of blood clots. Less serious complications include bleeding, swelling, or bruising where the catheter was placed.

Normal results

The patient usually goes home the day or evening of the procedure, but sometimes an overnight stay in the hospital is necessary so monitoring can be continued. Patients should have someone to take them home after the procedure; driving is not recommended for at least 24 hours after the procedure.

Fatigue and weakness are common after the procedure. The patient should limit activities for the first two days after the procedure and can gradually resume normal activities by the end of the week.

For the first week after the procedure, pushing and pulling heavy objects (as in mowing the lawn) should be avoided, and lifting objects more than 20 lbs (9 kg) is not permitted. Stair climbing is permitted unless other instructions have been given.

Balloon angioplasty and the placement of a stent do not prevent coronary artery disease from recurring; therefore, lifestyle changes are strongly recommended and medications are prescribed to further reduce this risk.

Morbidity and mortality rates

Death is very rare (1%) as a result of the stent placement procedure.

Sometimes a blockage returns to the treated coronary artery (restenosis). If restenosis occurs, it usually happens within the first six months after the procedure. If the patient has previously experienced restenosis, there is an increased risk that it will recur. Repeat blockages can be treated with other interventional procedures; **coronary artery bypass graft surgery** may be needed.

Alternatives

All patients with coronary artery disease can help improve their condition by making lifestyle changes such as quitting smoking, losing weight if they are overweight, eating healthy foods, reducing blood cholesterol, exercising regularly, and controlling diabetes and high blood pressure.

All patients with coronary artery disease should be prescribed medications to treat their condition. Antiplatelet medications such as aspirin or clopidogrel (Plavix) are usually recommended. Medications may also be prescribed to lower lipoprotein levels, since elevated lipoprotein levels have been associated with an increased risk of cardiovascular problems.

Treatment with vitamin E is not recommended because it does not lower the rate of cardiovascular events in people with coronary artery disease. Although antioxidants such as vitamin C, beta-carotene, and probucol show promising results, they are not recommended for routine use. Treatment with folic acid and vitamins B_6 and B_{12} lowers homocysteine levels (reducing the risk for cardiovascular problems), but more studies are needed to determine if lowered homocysteine levels correlate with a reduced rate of cardiovascular problems in treated patients.

Other interventional procedures used to open a blocked artery include rotoblation, brachytherapy, and atherectomy.

Coronary artery bypass graft surgery is a treatment option that is considered when medications and interventional therapies do not adequately treat coronary artery disease. During coronary artery bypass graft surgery, a blood vessel graft to restore normal blood flow to the heart is used to bypass one or more blocked coronary arteries. These grafts usually come from the patient's own arteries and veins located in the leg, arm, or chest.

KEY TERMS

Angina—Also called angina pectoris, chest pain or discomfort that occurs when diseased blood vessels restrict blood flow to the heart.

Anticoagulant—A medication, also called a blood thinner, that prevents blood from clotting.

Atherectomy—A non-surgical technique for treating diseased arteries with a rotating device that cuts or shaves away obstructing material inside the artery.

Brachytherapy—The use of radiation during angioplasty to prevent the artery from narrowing again (a process called restenosis).

Cardiac angiography—A procedure used to visualize blood vessels of the heart.

Catheter—A long, thin flexible tube that can be inserted into the body; in this case, it is threaded to the heart.

Echocardiogram—An imaging procedure used to create a picture of the heart's movement, valves, and chambers.

Electrocardiogram (ECG, EKG)—A test that records the electrical activity of the heart.

Homocysteine—An amino acid normally found in small amounts in the blood.

Restenosis—The narrowing of a blood vessel after it has been opened, usually by balloon angioplasty.

Stress test—A test used to determine how the heart responds to stress.

Thrombosis—The development of a blood clot in the vessels, which may clog a blood vessel and stop the flow of blood.

Enhanced external counterpulsation (EECP) may be a treatment option for patients who are not candidates for interventional procedures or coronary artery bypass graft surgery. During EECP, a set of cuffs is wrapped around the patient's calves, thighs, and buttocks. These cuffs gently but firmly compress the blood vessels in the lower limbs to increase blood flow to the heart. The inflation and deflation of the cuffs are electronically synchronized with the heartbeat and blood pressure using **electrocardiography** and blood pressure monitors. EECP may encourage blood vessels to open small channels to eventually bypass blocked vessels and improve blood flow to the heart. Not all patients are candidates for this procedure, and treatments, lasting one to two hours, must be repeated about five times a week for up to seven weeks.

Resources

BOOKS

American Heart Association. "Considering Surgery or Other Interventions." In *Guide to Heart Attack Treatment, Recovery, Prevention.* New York: Time Books, 1996.

Barry, Frank. *The Healthy Heart Formula: The Powerful, New, Commonsense Approach to Preventing and Reversing Heart Disease.* New York: John Wiley & Sons, 1998.

Garratt, Kirk N., Guy S. Reeder, and David R. Holmes Jr. "Cardiac Catheterization and Angiography." In *Mayo Clinic Practice of Cardiology,* edited by Emilio R. Giuliani, et al. St. Louis: Mosby Publishing, 1996.

McGoon, Michael D., and Bernard J. Gersh. *Mayo Clinic Heart Book: The Ultimate Guide to Heart Health, Second Edition.* New York: William Morrow and Co., Inc., 2000.

Texas Heart Institute. *Texas Heart Institute Heart Owner's Handbook.* New York: John Wiley & Sons, 1995.

Topol, Eric J. *Cleveland Clinic Heart Book: The Definitive Guide for the Entire Family from the Nation's Leading Heart Center.* New York: Hyperion, 2000.

Trout, Darrell, and Ellen Welch. *Surviving with Heart: Charge of Your Heart Care.* Golden, CO: Fulcrum Publishing, 2002.

PERIODICALS

Dangas, George, and Frank Keupper. "Restenosis: Repeat Narrowing of a Coronary Artery." *Circulation* 105 (2002): 2586–2587.

Michaels, Andrew D., and Kanu Chatterjee. "Angioplasty versus Bypass Surgery for Coronary Artery Disease." *Circulation* 106 (2002): e187–e190.

ORGANIZATIONS

American College of Cardiology. Heart House. 9111 Old Georgetown Rd., Bethesda, MD 20814-1699. (800) 253-4636, ext. 694, or (301) 897-5400. <http://www.acc.org>.

American Heart Association. 7272 Greenville Ave. Dallas, TX 75231. (800) 242-8721 or (214) 373-6300. <http://www.americanheart.org>.

The Cleveland Clinic Heart Center, The Cleveland Clinic Foundation. 9500 Euclid Avenue, F25, Cleveland, Ohio, 44195. (800) 223-2273, ext. 46697, or (216) 444-6697. <http://www.clevelandclinic.org/heartcenter>.

National Heart, Lung and Blood Institute. National Institutes of Health. Building 1. 1 Center Dr., Bethesda, MD 20892. E-mail: NHLBIinfo@rover.nhlbi. <http://www.nhlbi.nih.gov>.

OTHER

The Heart: An Online Exploration. The Franklin Institute Science Museum. 222 North 20th Street, Philadelphia, PA, 19103. (215) 448-1200. <http://sln2.fi.edu/biosci/heart.html>.

Heart Information Network. <http://www.heartinfo.org>.

HeartCenterOnline. <http://www.heartcenteronline.com>.

Cindy L. A. Jones, PhD
Angela M. Costello

Corpus callosotomy

Definition

Corpus callosotomy is a treatment for epilepsy, in which a group of fibers connecting the two sides of the brain, called the corpus callosum, is cut.

Purpose

Corpus callosotomy is used to treat epilepsy that is unresponsive to drug treatments. A person with epilepsy may be considered a good candidate for one type of epilepsy surgery or another if he or she has seizures that are not adequately controlled by drug therapy, and has tried at least two (perhaps more, depending on the treatment center's guidelines) different anti-epileptic drugs.

The seizures of epilepsy are due to unregulated spreading of electrical activity from one part of the brain to other parts. In many people with epilepsy, this activity begins from a well-defined focal point, which can be identified by electrical testing. Surgical treatment of focal-origin seizures involves removal of the brain region containing the focal point, usually in a procedure called temporal lobectomy. In other people, no focal point is found, or there may be too many to remove individually. These patients are most likely to receive corpus callosotomy.

The purpose of a corpus callosotomy is to prevent spreading of seizure activity from one half of the brain to the other. The brain is divided into two halves, or hemispheres, that are connected by a thick bundle of nerve fibers, the corpus callosum. When these fibers are cut, a seizure that begins in one hemisphere is less likely to spread to the other. This can reduce the frequency of seizures significantly.

The initial surgery may cut the forward two-thirds of the corpus callosum, leaving the rest intact. If this does not provide sufficient seizure control, the remaining portion may be cut.

Demographics

Corpus callosotomy is most often performed for children with "drop attacks," or atonic seizures, in which a sudden loss of muscle tone causes the child to fall to the floor. It is also performed in people with uncontrolled generalized tonic-clonic, or grand mal, seizures, or with massive jerking movements. Of the 20,000 to 70,000 people in the United States considered candidates for any type of epilepsy surgery, approximately 5,000 receive surgery per year. Between 1985 and 1990, more than 800 corpus callosotomies were performed, and the number has increased since then. Corpus callosotomy is

WHO PERFORMS THE PROCEDURE AND WHERE IS IT PERFORMED?

Corpus callosotomy is performed by a neurosurgeon in a hospital **operating room**.

performed by a special neurosurgical team, at a regional epilepsy treatment center.

Description

During corpus callosotomy, the patient is under general anesthesia, lying on the back. The head is fixed in place with blunt pins attached to a rigid structure. The head is shaved either before or during the procedure.

Incisions are made in the top of the skull to remove a flap of bone, exposing the brain. The outer covering is cut, and the two hemispheres are pulled slightly apart to expose the corpus callosum. The fibers of the corpus callosum are cut, taking care to avoid nearby arteries and ventricles (fluid-filled cavities in the brain).

Once the cut is made and any bleeding is controlled, the brain covering, bone, and scalp are closed and stitched.

Diagnosis/Preparation

The candidate for any type of epilepsy surgery will have had a wide range of tests prior to surgery. These include **electroencephalography** (EEG), in which electrodes are placed on the scalp, on the brain surface, or within the brain to record electrical activity. EEG is used to attempt to locate the focal point(s) of the seizure activity.

Several neuroimaging procedures are used to obtain images of the brain. These may reveal structural abnormalities that the neurosurgeon must be aware of. These procedures may include **magnetic resonance imaging** (MRI), x rays, computed tomography (CT) scans, or **positron emission tomography (PET)** imaging.

Neuropsychological tests may be done to provide a baseline against which the results of the surgery are measured. A Wada test may also be performed. In this test, a drug is injected into the artery leading to one half of the brain, putting it to sleep, allowing the neurologist to determine where language and other functions in the brain are localized, which may be useful for predicting the result of the surgery.

Aftercare

The patient remains in the hospital for about a week, possibly more depending on any complications that have occurred during surgery and on the health of the patient. There may be some discomfort afterwards. Tylenol with codeine may be prescribed for pain. Bending over should be avoided if possible, as it may lead to headache in the week or so after the procedure. Ice packs may be useful for pain and itchiness of the sutures on the head. Another several weeks of convalescence at home are required before the patient can resume normal activities. Heavy lifting or straining may continue to cause headaches or nausea, and should be avoided until the doctor approves. A diet rich in fiber can help avoid constipation, which may occur following surgery. Patients remain on anti-seizure medication at least for the short term, and may continue to require medication.

Risks

There is a slight risk of infection or hemorrhage from the surgery, usually less than 1%. Disconnection of the two hemispheres of the brain can cause some neuropsychological impairments such as decreased spontaneity of speech (it may be difficult to bring the right words into one's mind) and decreased use of the nondominant hand. These problems usually improve over time. Complete cutting of the corpus callosotomy produces more long-lasting, but very subtle deficits in connecting words with images. These are usually not significant, or even noticed, by the patient.

Normal results

Patients typically experience a marked reduction in number and severity of seizures, with a small percentage of people becoming seizure free. Drop attacks may be eliminated completely in approximately 70% of patients. Other types of seizure are also reduced by 50% or more from corpus callosotomy surgery.

Morbidity and mortality rates

Serious morbidity or mortality occurs in 1% or less of patients. Combined major and minor complication rates are approximately 20%.

Alternatives

Newer anti-seizure medications have partially replaced corpus callosotomy. Focal epilepsy is treated with focal surgery such as temporal lobectomy or **hemispherectomy**. Vagus nerve stimulation is an alternative for some patients.

See also Hemispherectomy; Vagal nerve stimulation.

Resources

BOOKS

Devinsky, O. *A Guide to Understanding and Living with Epilepsy.* Philadelphia: EA Davis, 1994.

ORGANIZATIONS

Epilepsy Foundation. <www.epilepsyfoundation.org>.

Richard Robinson

Corticosteroids

Definition

Corticosteroids are a group of natural and synthetic analogs (chemical cousins) of the hormones secreted by the pituitary gland, also known as the hypothalamic-anterior pituitary-adrenocortical (HPA) axis. These analogs include glucocorticoids, which are anti-inflammatory agents with a large number of other functions; mineralocorticoids, which control salt and water balance primarily through action on the kidneys; and corticotropins, which control secretion of hormones by the pituitary gland.

Purpose

Glucocorticoids have multiple effects, and are used for a large number of conditions. They affect glucose utilization and fat metabolism, bone development, and are potent anti-inflammatory agents. They may be used for replacement of natural hormones in patients with pituitary deficiency (Addison's disease), as well as for a wide number of other conditions including arthritis, asthma, anemia, various cancers, and skin inflammations. Additional uses include inhibition of nausea and vomiting after chemotherapy, treatment of septic shock, treatment of spinal cord injuries, and treatment of hirsutism (excessive hair growth). The choice of drug will vary with the condition.

Cortisone and hydrocortisone, which have both glucocorticoid and mineralocorticoid effects, are the drugs of choice for replacement therapy of natural hormone deficiency. Synthetic compounds, which have greater anti-inflammatory effects and less effect on salt and water balance, are usually preferred for other purposes. These compounds include dexamethasone, which is almost exclusively glucocorticoid in its actions, as well as prednisone, prednisolone, betamethasone, trimacinolone, and others. Glucocorticoids are formulated in oral dosage forms, topical creams and ointments, oral and nasal inhalations, rectal foams, and ear and eye drops.

Mineralocorticoids control the retention of sodium in the kidneys. In mineralocorticoid deficiency, there is excessive loss of sodium through the kidneys, with resulting water loss. Fludrocortisone (Florinef) is the only drug available for treatment of mineralocorticoid deficiency, and is available only in an oral form.

Corticotropin (ACTH, adrenocorticotropic hormone) stimulates the pituitary gland to release cortisone. A deficiency of corticotropic hormone will have the same effects as a deficiency of cortisone. The hormone, which is available under the brand names Acthar and Actrel, is used for diagnostic testing to determine the cause of a glucocorticoid deficiency. It is rarely used for replacement therapy, however, since direct administration of glucocorticoids may be easier and offers better control over dosages.

Recommended dosage

Dosage of glucocorticoids varies with drug, route of administration, condition being treated, and patient.

Fludrocortisone, for use in replacement therapy, is normally dosed at 0.1 mg/day. Some patients require higher doses. It should normally be taken in conjunction with cortisone or hydrocortisone.

ACTH, when used for diagnostic purposes, is given as 10 to 25 units by intravenous solution over eight hours. A long-acting form, which may be used for replacement therapy, is given by subcutaneous (SC) or intramuscular (IM) injection at a dose of 40 to 80 units every 24–72 hours.

Precautions

The most significant risk associated with administration of glucocorticoids is suppression of natural corticosteroid secretion. When the hormones are administered, they suppress the secretion of ACTH, which in turn reduces the secretion of the natural hormones. The extent of suppression varies with dose, drug potency, duration of treatment, and individual patient response. While suppression is seen primarily with drugs administered systemically, it can also occur with topical drugs such as creams and ointments, or drugs administered by

inhalation. Abrupt cessation of corticosteroids may result in acute adrenal crisis (Addisonian crisis) which is marked by dehydration with severe vomiting and diarrhea, hypotension, and loss of consciousness. Acute adrenal crisis is potentially fatal.

Chronic overdose of glucocorticoids leads to Cushingoid syndrome, which is clinically identical to Cushing's syndrome. The only difference is that in Cushingoid, the excessive steroids are from drug therapy rather than excessive glandular secretion. Symptoms vary, but most people have upper body obesity, rounded face, increased fat around the neck, and thinning arms and legs. In its later stages, this condition leads to weakening of bones and muscles with rib and spinal column fractures.

The short-term adverse effects of corticosteroids are generally mild, and include indigestion, increased appetite, insomnia, and nervousness. There are also a very large number of infrequent adverse reactions, the most significant of which is drug-induced paranoia. Delirium, depression, menstrual irregularity, and increased hair growth are also possible.

Long-term use of topical glucocorticoids can result in thinning of the skin. Oral steroid inhalations may cause fungal overgrowth in the oral cavity. Patients must be instructed to rinse their mouths carefully after each dose.

Corticosteroids are included in pregnancy category C. The pregnancy category system classifies drugs according to their established risks for use during pregnancy. Corticosteroids have caused congenital malformations in animal studies, including cleft palate. Breastfeeding while taking these medications should be avoided.

Because fludrocortisone has glucocorticoid activity as well as mineralocorticoid action, the same hazards and precautions apply to fludrocortisone as to the glucocorticoids. Overdose of fludrocortisone may also cause edema (swelling), hypertension, and congestive heart failure.

Corticotropin has all the same risks as the glucocorticoids. Prolonged use may cause reduced response to the stimulatory effects of corticotropin.

Warnings

Patients with the following conditions should use corticosteroids with caution:

• osteoporosis or any other bone disease

• current or past tuberculosis

• glaucoma or cataracts

• infections of any type (virus, bacteria, fungus, amoeba)

• sores in the nose or recent nose surgery (if using nasal spray forms of corticosteroids)

KEY TERMS

Hallucination—A false or distorted perception of objects, sounds, or events that seems real. Hallucinations usually result from drugs or mental disorders.

Hormone—A substance that is produced in one part of the body, then travels through the bloodstream to another part of the body where it has its effect.

Hypertension—High blood pressure.

Hypotension—Low blood pressure.

Inflammation—Pain, redness, swelling, and heat that usually develop in response to injury or illness.

Ointment—A thick, spreadable substance that contains medicine and is meant to be used on the outside of the body.

Pregnancy category—A system of classifying drugs according to their established risks for use during pregnancy. Category A: Controlled human studies have demonstrated no fetal risk. Category B: Animal studies indicate no fetal risk, but no human studies; or adverse effects in animals, but not in well-controlled human studies. Category C: No adequate human or animal studies; or adverse fetal effects in animal studies, but no available human data. Category D: Evidence of fetal risk, but benefits outweigh risks. Category X: Evidence of fetal risk. Risks outweigh any benefits.

- underactive or overactive thyroid
- liver disease
- stomach or intestine problems
- diabetes
- heart disease
- high blood pressure
- high cholesterol
- kidney disease or kidney stones
- myasthenia gravis
- systemic lupus erythematosus (SLE)
- emotional problems
- skin conditions that cause the skin to be thinner and bruise more easily

Interactions

Corticosteroids interact with many other drugs a patient might take. Patients should inform their doctor about all other medications (both prescription and over-the-counter) they take, and discuss possible interactions.

Resources

BOOKS

Brody, T. M., J. Larner, K. P. Minneman, and H. C. Neu. *Human Pharmacology: Molecular to Clinical,* 2nd ed. St. Louis: Mosby Year-Book, 1998.

Griffith, H. W., and S. Moore. *2001 Complete Guide to Prescription and Nonprescription Drugs.* New York: Berkely Publishing Group, 2001.

ORGANIZATIONS

American Academy of Allergy, Asthma and Immunology. 611 East Wells Street, Milwaukee, WI 53202. Telephone: (414) 272–6071. Web site: <http://www.aaaai.org>.

Asthma and Allergy Foundation of America. 1125 15th Street NW, Suite 502, Washington, DC 20005. Telephone: (800) 727–8462. Web site: <http://www.aafa.org>.

National Heart, Lung and Blood Institute. National Institutes of Health, P.O. Box 30105, Bethesda, MD 20824-0105. Telephone: (301) 251–1222. <http://www.nhlbi.nih.gov/nhlbi/nhlbi.htm>.

Samuel Uretsky, PharmD

Cosmetic surgery *see* **Plastic, reconstructive, and cosmetic surgery**

Cotrel-Dubousset spinal instrumentation *see* **Spinal instrumentation**

CPR *see* **Cardiopulmonary resuscitation**

Craniofacial reconstruction

Definition

Craniofacial reconstruction refers to a group of procedures used to repair or reshape the face and skull of a living person, or to create a replica of the head and face of a dead or missing person. The word "craniofacial" is a combination of "cranium," which is the medical word for the upper portion of the skull, and facial. Craniofacial reconstruction is sometimes called orbital-craniofacial surgery; "orbital" refers to the name of the bony cavity in the face that surrounds the eyeball.

Purpose

Craniofacial reconstruction has several different purposes depending on the group of patients or persons

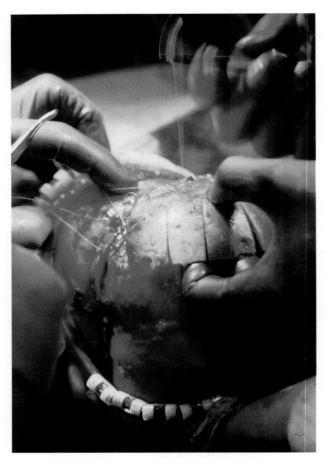

A child undergoing surgery on the skull. *(Photograph by Alexander Tsiaras. Science Source/Photo Researchers. Reproduced by permission.)*

in question. In children, craniofacial reconstruction is done to repair abnormalities in the shape of the child's skull and facial features resulting from birth defects or genetic disorders. It is also done to repair traumatic injuries resulting from accidents or child abuse. Craniofacial reconstruction in children requires special techniques and planning because the surgeon must allow for future growth of the child's facial bones and skull.

In adults, craniofacial reconstruction is most commonly done following head or facial trauma, but it is also performed on cancer patients who have lost part of the bony structures or soft tissue of the face following tumor surgery. In both adults and children, the reconstruction is intended to restore the functioning of the patient's mouth, jaw, and sensory organs as well as improve his or her appearance. Craniofacial reconstruction is a complicated procedure because the surgeon is operating on a part of the body that contains the brain and upper part of the spinal cord, the eyes, and other sensory organs, and the opening of the patient's airway—all within a small space.

The third major application of craniofacial reconstruction is in forensic medicine and anthropology. Forensic is a term that refers to legal matters. Physicians who specialize in forensic science study the remains of people who have died to establish not only the cause of death but in some cases, the identity of the dead person. Craniofacial reconstruction is one approach to this identification. Anthropologists, the scientists who study the origins and cultural development of humans, make use of craniofacial reconstruction to understand what prehistoric people looked like and to compare them with present-day humans.

Demographics

Birth defects and genetic disorders

About 7%, or 227,500, of the children born each year in the United States are affected by birth defects of the head and face. According to the American Society of Plastic Surgeons, 37,732 procedures were performed to repair birth defects in 2001, an increase of 2% over the number of surgeries in 2000.

The demographics of specific birth defects affecting the head and face vary; some are considered rare disorders. Figures for some of the disorders most likely to be treated surgically include:

• Cleft palate. Cleft lip or palate is the fourth most common birth defect affecting American children, one in every 700 newborns. The male:female ratio is 2:1 in children of all races. Asian-American children have a higher than average incidence of cleft palate, while African-American children have a lower than average incidence.

• Down syndrome. Down syndrome is the most common congenital disorder caused by a chromosomal abnormality; it occurs in one in every 900 infants. Children with Down syndrome have facial characteristics that typically include slanted eyes, a flattened nasal bridge, small rounded ears, and a large protruding tongue. There are about 350,000 people in the United States with Down syndrome.

• Treacher Collins syndrome. This congenital disorder is caused by a mutation on human chromosome 5 that can arise spontaneously or be inherited from the parents. The craniofacial abnormalities in Treacher Collins include an abnormally small jaw and airway that can cause breathing problems; the ears may also be malformed or missing. Treacher Collins syndrome affects one in every 10,000 infants.

• Apert and Crouzon syndromes. These two disorders are sometimes grouped together because they are both characterized by craniosynostosis, which is the medical term for premature closing of the sutures (seams) in the bones at the top of the skull. Children with these syndromes have misshapen heads and a sunken-in appearance to the face. They also have breathing problems and malpositioning of the teeth caused by deformed facial bones. Apert syndrome is very rare, affecting only one child in every 150,000. Crouzon syndrome occurs in one out of every 25,000 infants.

Traumatic injuries

Traumatic injuries to the face and head can include blunt trauma, lacerations (tears), and burns. Heat, chemicals, or electricity may cause burns. According to the American Burn Institute, there are 1.1 million burn injuries each year in the United States that are serious enough to require medical treatment. In 2001, 16,879 adults needed plastic surgery to repair burn injuries, while 24,298 required maxillofacial surgery for injuries to the face and jaw.

Prior to the early 1980s, when more rigorous seat belt laws were passed, most severe facial injuries in the United States resulted from automobile accidents. As of 2003, however, 70% of facial injuries treated in urban hospitals are caused by assaults; at least 10% of fractured facial bones in women are the result of domestic violence. Falls cause a significant number of facial injuries in small children and the elderly. Another common source of facial trauma in children is animal bites.

Cancer patients

Cancers of the head and neck affect about 55,000 Americans each year; about 13,000 of these patients die. These cancers include cancers of the skin of the face, the esophagus, the larynx (voice box), the mouth, and the nasal passages. Most of these cancers are preventable because they result from prolonged exposure to either sunlight (facial skin) or tobacco (mouth, throat, nose, and larynx). Men are two to four times as likely to develop cancers of the mouth and throat as women.

Description

General background

Craniofacial reconstruction dates back to the late nineteenth century, when doctors in Germany and France first used it to produce more accurate images of the faces of certain famous people who had died before the invention of photography. Early craniofacial reconstructions included those of Bach, Dante, Kant, and Raphael. The technique was then applied to reconstructing the appearance of prehistoric humans for museums and research institutions. An important contribution to the field was the

WHO PERFORMS THE PROCEDURE AND WHERE IS IT PERFORMED?

Craniofacial reconstruction of congenital abnormalities requires a team of medical specialists, including plastic surgeons, maxillofacial surgeons, neurosurgeons, dentists, ophthalmologists, and psychiatrists. These procedures can be done in a department of plastic surgery in a teaching hospital; increasingly, however, they are being performed in separate clinics or institutes that specialize in craniofacial reconstruction in children.

Craniofacial reconstruction following trauma is started as soon as possible once the patient's general condition is stable. Although at one time surgeons delayed the treatment of disfiguring injuries for several weeks, recent studies have found that early treatment gives better results as well as minimizing the need for revision plastic surgery. These procedures can be started in a hospital emergency room or done in a specialized trauma center. Facial injuries resulting from burns or electrical trauma may be treated at special burn centers.

Craniofacial reconstruction following cancer treatment is done in specialized departments of plastic and reconstructive surgery within larger hospitals. Many of these are teaching hospitals associated with major medical schools.

Forensic craniofacial reconstruction is done in specialized facilities in university departments of anthropology or in laboratories related to the criminal justice system.

publication in 1901 of three major papers on the classification of facial fractures by René Le Fort, a French surgeon. Le Fort identified the lines of weakness in the facial bones where fractures are most likely to occur. Traumatic injuries of the facial bones are still classified as Le Fort I, II, and III fractures. A Le Fort I fracture runs across the maxilla, or upper jaw; a Le Fort II fracture is pyramidal in shape, breaking the cheekbone below the orbit (eye socket) and running across the bridge of the nose; a Le Fort III fracture separates the frontal bone behind the forehead from the zygoma (cheekbone) as well as breaking the nasal bridge. A Le Fort III fracture is sometimes called a craniofacial separation.

Craniofacial reconstruction

Frontal bone

Nasal bone

Fractures

Maxilla

Mandible

A.

Incision

B.

C.

Plates and screws

D.   Repaired fracture

To repair severe fractures around the nasal bone (A), an incision is made into the patient's skin at the top of the head (B). The skin is pulled off the face to expose the fracture (C), which then can be repaired with plates and screws (D). *(Illustration by GGS Inc.)*

In the 1920s, British physicians pioneered the application of facial reconstruction to unsolved criminal cases and to treating World War I veterans who had been disfigured in combat. Prior to the invention of the computer, craniofacial reconstruction was done either by applying soft clay to the skull (or a cast of the skull) to recreate the person's features, or by making a two-dimensional drawing over a photograph or x-ray picture of the skull. It was difficult for surgeons operating on mutilated patients to predict the outcome of the operation from these two-dimensional sketches.

The first attempts at craniofacial reconstruction in children with congenital abnormalities were made in the late 1940s by Sir Harold Gillies, a British plastic surgeon who had treated disfigured World War II veterans. More recent advances in craniofacial reconstruction include improved understanding of the soft tissues of the face and better surgical techniques for repairing injuries to these tissues; the invention of surgical plastics that can be used instead of bone grafts to fill in missing pieces of bone; new techniques for fixing the facial bones in place during the healing process; and computerized imaging programs that help the surgeon analyze the patient's facial abnormality or injury. Some of these programs allow doctors to download data directly from x rays, computed tomography (CT) scans, or other diagnostic imaging programs in order to plan the operation and have a clearer picture of the results. In the case of children, computer imaging can be used to estimate the future growth lines of a child's skull and facial bones as well as his or her present condition. Orthodontists and other dental specialists have developed additional imaging programs that provide more details about the mouth and jaw area than can be obtained from **CT scans** and x-ray studies.

Craniofacial reconstruction of birth defects and genetic abnormalities

Craniofacial reconstruction in children with congenital abnormalities of the head and face is preceded by a consultation between the surgeon, other specialists, and the child's parents. It is important to determine the exact cause of the child's deformities, since some abnormalities may be found in as many as 150 different genetic disorders. Following the diagnosis, a comprehensive treatment plan is made that includes long-term psychosocial as well as surgical follow-up. Craniofacial reconstruction in children is complex because the surgeon must allow for changes in the proportions of the child's face and skull as he or she matures as well as attempt to make the facial features look as normal as possible. It is difficult to provide a general description of craniofacial surgery in children because there are many variables among children diagnosed with the same disorder as

well as a large number of different disorders requiring craniofacial reconstruction. Reconstructions in children, however, are always done under general anesthesia and usually take between three and six hours to complete.

Craniofacial reconstruction following trauma or surgery

Craniofacial reconstruction following trauma is a highly individualized process, depending on the nature and location of the patient's injuries. Emergency workers are trained to evaluate and clear the patient's airway before treating facial injuries as such; severe injuries to the midface and lower face frequently result in airway blockage caused by blood, loose teeth or bone fragments, or the tongue falling backward toward the windpipe. The trauma team may have to intubate the patient or perform an emergency **cricothyroidotomy** in order to help the patient breathe. The second priority in treating traumatic facial injuries is controlling severe bleeding.

Imaging studies of craniofacial injuries may need to be postponed for 24–72 hours in order to treat injuries to other organ systems. Over 60% of patients with severe facial trauma have other serious injuries in the head, chest, or abdomen; this high rate reflects the tremendous forces needed to fracture the human frontal bone, zygoma, and maxilla. In particular, a doctor who is examining a patient with severe facial trauma will be particularly concerned about damage to the brain, the spinal column in the neck region, and the eyes. All Le Fort II and III fractures have the potential for permanent damage to the eyes. There are specific maneuvers that the doctor can perform to assess the location and severity of bone fractures, possible dislocation of the jaw, and injury to the eyes and nose before taking an x ray or CT scan.

When the patient is out of immediate danger, x-ray studies and computed tomography (CT) scans are taken of the craniofacial injuries. Three-dimensional scans assist the surgeon in analyzing the fractures and the condition of the other structures in the face and head. Imaging studies can be used to generate computer images for plastic or metal implants to be matched to the patient's injuries for filling in sections of missing bone.

Surgery following facial trauma may take as long as four to 14 hours, as the goal is to repair as much as possible in one operation. The surgeon may use bone grafts, taking bone from other parts of the body to repair the facial bones, or fill in smaller areas of missing bone with hydroxyapatite cement or polymer implants. Broken facial bones are held in place with titanium miniplates and surgical screws. This technique is called rigid fixation; it often does away with the need to wire the jaws in place, and it speeds the patient's recovery. Lacerations (tears) in the

QUESTIONS TO ASK
THE DOCTOR

- Am I likely to need further surgery after recovery from craniofacial reconstruction?
- How normal can I expect to look at the end of the process?
- What are the risks of permanent damage to my eyesight or hearing?
- Does the hospital or clinic have a support group for people who have undergone craniofacial reconstruction?

skin are usually simply closed with stitches, although the surgeon will be careful to minimize scarring. If large areas of skin are missing, the surgeon will cut a flap, which is a section of living tissue carrying its own blood supply, from another area of the patient's body and transplant it to the face. Some facial injuries may require the assistance of a neurosurgeon, oral surgeon, or ophthalmologist.

Cancers on the skin of the face are usually removed and closed with a few stitches, although skin flaps may be required if the area of the face that is affected is large. Cancers of the head or neck may require bone grafts as well as skin flaps after the tumor has been removed. Reconstructive surgery after cancer treatment may involve the use of a microscope and special instruments to rejoin the facial blood vessels and nerve fibers. This technique, which is known as **microsurgery**, is done to preserve the function of the muscles in the face as well as restoring the patient's appearance as much as possible.

Diagnosis/Preparation

Diagnosis of the need for craniofacial reconstruction depends on the cause of the abnormality, injury, or disfigurement. The obstetrician or the child's pediatrician will often make the diagnosis of craniofacial abnormalities in children at the time of delivery. Some genetic disorders that are associated with congenital facial abnormalities, including Down syndrome and Treacher Collins syndrome, can be detected before birth by chromosomal analysis. In adults, the diagnosis is usually made by trauma surgeons in the emergency room or by physicians who have treated the patient for cancer.

Imaging studies, including x-ray photographs, CT scans, and **magnetic resonance imaging** (MRI), are used to analyze the patient's abnormalities or injuries before the operation in order to plan the surgery. The surgeon may also consult a neurosurgeon or ophthalmolo-

gist if the abnormality or injury involves the functioning of the patient's brain, spinal cord, or eyes.

Aftercare

Medical and surgical

Children who have had reconstructive surgery for congenital abnormalities are usually taken to a pediatric **intensive care unit** for a day or two, and remain in the hospital for a total of four to five days. Adults who have had reconstructive surgery following trauma may be monitored in an intensive care unit for one to two days after the operation, particularly if they required special treatment for airway problems. The total length of the hospital stay varies according to the severity of the patient's other injuries; some burn victims may be hospitalized for several months.

Short-term aftercare includes medications for pain, changes of surgical dressings, breathing exercises, and **antibiotics** to reduce the possibility of infection. Patients with injuries to the jaw or mouth may be given special semi-liquid or soft diets. Children are restricted from swimming for two months after reconstructive surgery and from more active sports for six months.

Long-term follow-up may include revision surgery six to 12 months after facial trauma. In the case of children, the patient will be followed until his or her growth is complete; most will need periodic consultations with an orthodontist as well as with the plastic surgeon. A dentist or an oral surgeon should check on patients who have had craniofacial surgery following trauma during their recovery to make sure that the teeth and jawbones are in proper alignment. All Le Fort fractures (I, II, and III) involve damage to the patient's normal occlusion (bite pattern).

Some patients may choose to have cosmetic surgery to remove or minimize facial scars after healing is complete, usually about six months after the reconstructive operation.

Psychological

The psychological aftereffects of a disfiguring congenital abnormality or post-traumatic injury are often problematic. Craniofacial reconstruction in children with congenital syndromes typically includes ongoing psychological assessment and counseling to help the parents as well as the child cope with feelings of guilt as well as deal with teasing or ridicule from others. Many parents blame themselves for their child's condition if it is associated with a genetic disorder. Children who have had a disfiguring injury often develop post-traumatic stress disorder (PTSD), depression, or anxiety. One study found that 98% of children between the ages of three and 12 who had been disfigured by accidents

KEY TERMS

Cleft palate—A birth defect in which the roof of the mouth is open because the two sides of the palate failed to join together during fetal development.

Congenital—Present at the time of birth.

Craniosynostosis—Premature closing of the sutures joining the skull bones.

Cranium—The large, rounded upper part of the skull that encloses the brain.

Down syndrome—A congenital disorder caused by a mutation of human chromosome 21 in which there are three chromosomes (trisomy) instead of the usual pair.

Flap—A piece of tissue used for grafting that has kept its own blood supply.

Forensic—Referring to legal or courtroom proceedings.

Frontal bone—The part of the skull that lies behind the forehead.

Le Fort fracture—A term that refers to a system for classifying fractures of the facial bones into three groups according to the region affected.

Mandible—The horseshoe-shaped bone that forms the lower jaw.

Maxilla—The facial bone that forms the upper jaw and holds the upper teeth.

Microsurgery—Surgery performed under a microscope on nerves and other very small structures with the help of special instruments.

Orbit—The bony cavity in the face that surrounds and protects the eyeball.

Suture—A type of body joint that is found only in the skull; the surfaces of the bones in the skull are held together by a thin layer of fibrous connective tissue.

Treacher Collins syndrome—A disorder that affects facial development and hearing, thought to be caused by a gene mutation on human chromosome 5; sometimes called mandibulofacial dysotosis.

Zygoma—The cheek bone in the front of the face below the eye socket, it is connected to the frontal bone of the forehead and the maxilla (upper jaw); sometimes called the os zygomaticum or zygomatic bone.

---

or dog bites had symptoms of PTSD within five days of the traumatic event. A year later, 44% of the children still had symptoms, and 21% met the full diagnostic criteria for PTSD. Psychiatric symptoms in children are often intensified as the youngsters reach adolescence and become even more preoccupied with their appearance.

Adult patients also have high rates of depression, PTSD, or anxiety disorders following craniofacial reconstruction. Support groups as well as individual psychotherapy appear to be effective in helping people learn to live with disfiguring injuries or the aftermath of cancer surgery. Specific concerns include coping with awkward social situations as well as internal feelings of guilt or anger. Some researchers have reported that men find it harder to adjust to facial disfigurement than women, possibly because males in Western societies are not encouraged to discuss concerns about their appearance.

Risks

Some of the risks of craniofacial reconstruction are common to all surgical procedures done under general anesthesia. These include bleeding, breathing problems, bruises underneath the skin, reactions to the anesthesia, and infection.

Risks that are specific to craniofacial reconstruction include damage to the nerves in the face and head; visible scarring; bone graft failure; and the need for further surgery.

Risk factors that can affect the results of craniofacial reconstruction include:

- poor nutrition
- HIV infection
- a weakened immune system
- damage to the skin from radiation therapy
- a connective tissue disease, such as lupus or scleroderma
- smoking
- time elapsed between a traumatic injury and surgical treatment
- poor blood circulation in the affected area

Normal results

Normal results of craniofacial reconstruction vary, depending on the type of injury or defect. Good results include improvement or restoration of the general shape of the patient's head or face; improving or maintaining the functioning of the eyes, ears, nose, mouth, and teeth; and a more nearly normal appearance to the face.

Morbidity and mortality rates

Morbidity and mortality rates vary widely, depending on the patient's age, general health, and the cause of the injury or abnormality.

Alternatives

There are no mainstream alternatives to craniofacial reconstruction in the treatment of birth defects, traumatic injuries, or disfigurement resulting from cancer surgery.

DNA analysis can be used together with craniofacial reconstruction to help identify badly disfigured or damaged human remains.

See also Cleft lip repair; Fracture repair.

Resources

BOOKS

"Chromosomal Abnormalities." In Section 19, Chapter 261 in *The Merck Manual of Diagnosis and Therapy,* edited by Mark H. Beers, and Robert Berkow. Whitehouse Station, NJ: Merck Research Laboratories, 1999.

Colucciello, Stephen A., MD. "Maxillofacial Trauma." In Chapter 138 in *The Emergency Medicine Reports Textbook of Adult and Pediatric Emergency Medicine,* edited by Gideon Bosker. Atlanta, GA: American Health Consultants, 2000.

"Musculoskeletal Abnormalities." In Section 19, Chapter 261 in *The Merck Manual of Diagnosis and Therapy,* edited by Mark H. Beers, and Robert Berkow. Whitehouse Station, NJ: Merck Research Laboratories, 1999.

Nafte, Myriam. *Flesh and Bone: An Introduction to Forensic Anthropology,* Chapter 7, "Reconstructing Identity." Durham, NC: Carolina Academic Press, 2000.

Sargent, Larry. *The Craniofacial Surgery Book.* Chattanooga, TN: Erlanger Health System, 2000.

PERIODICALS

Cordeiro, P. G., and J. J. Disa. "Challenges in Midface Reconstruction." *Seminars in Surgical Oncology,* 19 (October–November 2000): 218–225.

Eppley, B. L. "Craniofacial Reconstruction with Computer-Generated HTR Patient-matched Implants: Use in Primary Bony Tumor Excision." *Journal of Craniofacial Surgery,* 13 (September 2002): 650–657.

Eufinger, H., and M. Wehmoller. "Microsurgical Tissue Transfer and Individual Computer-aided Designed and Manufactured Prefabricated Titanium Implants for Complex Craniofacial Reconstruction." *Scandinavian Journal of Plastic and Reconstructive Surgery and Hand Surgery,* 36 (2002): 326–331.

Girotto, J. A., et al. "Long-term Physical Impairment and Functional Outcomes After Complex Facial Fractures." *Plastic and Reconstructive Surgery,* 108 (August 2001): 312–327.

Hunt, J. A., and P. C. Hobar. "Common Craniofacial Anomalies: The Facial Dysostoses." *Plastic and Reconstructive Surgery,* 110 (December 2002): 1714–1725.

Kos, M., et al. "Midfacial Fractures in Children." *European Journal of Pediatric Surgery,* 12 (August 2002): 218–225.

Leong, K., C. L. Nastala, and P. T. Wang. "Cosmetic Aspects of Cranial Reconstruction." *Neurosurgery Clinics of North America,* 13 (October 2002): 491–503.

Lorenz, R. R., et al. "Hydroxyapatite Cement Reconstruction in the Growing Craniofacial Skeleton: An Experimental Model." *Journal of Craniofacial Surgery,* 13 (November 2002): 802–808.

Moreira-Gonzalez, A., et al. "Clinical Outcome in Cranioplasty: Critical Review in Long-term Follow-up." *Journal of Craniofacial Surgery,* 14 (March 2003): 144–153.

Papadoupoulos, M. A., et al. "Three-dimensional Craniofacial Reconstruction Imaging." *Oral Surgery, Oral Medicine, Oral Pathology, Oral Radiology, and Endodontics,* 93 (April 2002): 382–393.

Parsa, Tatiana, Arthur Adamo, and Yvette Calderon. "Initial Evaluation and Management of Maxillofacial Injuries." *eMedicine,* August 28, 2002 [March 8, 2003].

Rusch, M. D., et al. "Psychological Adjustment in Children After Traumatic Disfiguring Injuries: A 12-month Follow-up." *Plastic and Reconstructive Surgery,* 106 (December 2000): 1451–1458.

Sarwer, D. B., and C. E. Crerand. "Psychological Issues in Patient Outcomes." *Facial Plastic Surgery: FPS,* 18 (May 2002): 125–133.

Strumas, N., O. Antonyshyn, C. B. Caldwell, and J. Mainprize. "Multimodality Imaging for Precise Localization of Craniofacial Osteomyelitis." *Journal of Craniofacial Surgery,* 14 (March 2003): 215–219.

Thompson, A., and G. Kent. "Adjusting to Disfigurement: Processes Involved in Dealing with Being Visibly Different." *Clinical Psychology Review,* 21 (July 2001): 663–682.

Vanezis, M., and P. Vanezis. "Cranio-Facial Reconstruction in Forensic Identification—Historical Development and a Review of Current Practice." *Medicine, Science, and the Law,* 40 (July 2000): 197–205.

Yucel, A., et al. "Malignant Tumors Requiring Maxillectomy." *Journal of Craniofacial Surgery,* 11 (September 2000): 418–429.

ORGANIZATIONS

American Burn Association. 625 North Michigan Avenue, Suite 1530, Chicago, IL 60611. (312) 642-9260. <www.ameriburn.org>.

American Cleft Palate-Craniofacial Association. 104 South Estes Drive, Suite 204, Chapel Hill, NC 27514. (919) 933-9044. <www.cleftline.org>.

American Society of Plastic Surgeons (ASPS). 444 East Algonquin Road, Arlington Heights, IL 60005. (847) 228-9900. <www.plasticsurgery.org>.

FACES: The National Craniofacial Association. P. O. Box 11082, Chattanooga, TN 37401. (800) 332-2373. <www.faces-cranio.org>.

Federal Bureau of Investigation (FBI), Laboratory Division. J. Edgar Hoover Building, 935 Pennsylvania Avenue, NW, Washington, DC 20535-0001. <www.fbi.gov/hq/lab/lab-home.htm>.

National Down Syndrome Society (NDSS). 666 Broadway, New York, NY 10012. (212) 460-9330 or (800) 221-4602. <www.ndss.org>.

National Organization for Rare Disorders (NORD). 55 Kenosia Avenue, P. O. Box 1968, Danbury, CT 06813-1968. (203) 744-0100. <www.rarediseases.org>.

University of Maryland Medical Center, R. Adams Cowley Shock Trauma Center. 22 South Greene Street, Baltimore, MD 21201. (410) 328-2757 or (800) 373-4111. <www.umm.edu/shocktrauma>.

OTHER

Tuncay, Orhan C., M. Nuveen, C. X. Nguyen, and J. Slattery. "The Development of a System for Three-Dimensional Imaging and Animation of the Craniofacial Complex." *Greater Philadelphia Society of Orthodontists Newsletter,* June 2000 [March 24, 2003]. <www.gpso.org/newsletter/3d_imaging.html>.

Rebecca Frey, PhD

Craniotomy

Definition

A craniotomy is a procedure to remove a lesion in the brain through an opening in the skull (cranium).

Purpose

A craniotomy is a type of brain surgery. It is the most commonly performed surgery for brain **tumor removal**. It also may be done to remove a blood clot (hematoma), to control hemorrhage from a weak, leaking blood vessel (cerebral aneurysm), to repair arteriovenous malformations (abnormal connections of blood vessels), to drain a brain abscess, to relieve pressure inside the skull, to perform a biopsy, or to inspect the brain.

Demographics

Because craniotomy is a procedure that is utilized for several conditions and diseases, statistical information for the procedure itself is not available. However, because craniotomy is most commonly performed to remove a brain tumor, statistics concerning this condition are given. Approximately 90% of primary brain cancers

WHO PERFORMS THE PROCEDURE AND WHERE IS IT PERFORMED?

The procedure is performed in a hospital with a **neurosurgery** department and an **intensive care unit**. The procedure is performed by a board certified neurosurgeon, who has completed two years of **general surgery** training and five years of neurosurgical training.

occur in adults, more commonly in males between 55 and 65 years of age. Tumors in children peak between the ages of three and 12. Brain tumors are presently the most common cancer in children (four out of 100,000).

Description

There are two methods commonly utilized by surgeons to open the skull. Either an incision is made at the nape of the neck around the bone at the back (occipital bone) or a curving incision is made in front of the ear that arches above the eye. The incision penetrates as far as the thin membrane covering the skull bone. During skin incision the surgeon must seal off many small blood vessels because the scalp has a rich blood supply.

The scalp tissue is then folded back to expose the bone. Using a high-speed drill, the surgeon drills a pattern of holes through the cranium (skull) and uses a fine wire saw to connect the holes until a segment of bone (bone flap) can be removed. This gives the surgeon access to the inside of the skill and allows him to proceed with surgery inside the brain. After removal of the internal brain lesion or other procedure is completed, the bone is replaced and secured into position with soft wire. Membranes, muscle, and skin are sutured into position. If the lesion is an aneurysm, the affected artery is sealed at the leak. If there is a tumor, as much of it as possible is resected (removed). For arteriovenous malformations, the abnormality is clipped and the repair redirects the blood flow to normal vessels.

Diagnosis/Preparation

Since the lesion is in the brain, the surgeon uses imaging studies to definitively identify it. Neuroimaging is usually accomplished by the following:

- CT (computed tomography, uses x-rays and injection of an intravenous dye to visualize the lesion)

- MRI (**magnetic resonance imaging**, uses magnetic fields and radio waves to visualize a lesion)

Craniotomy

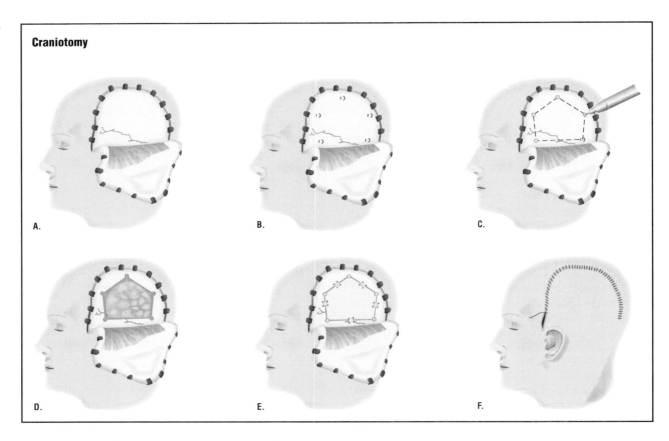

A.

B.

C.

D.

E.

F.

In a craniotomy, the skin over a part of the skull is cut and pulled back (A). Small holes are drilled into the skull (B), and a special saw is used to cut the bone between the holes (C). The bone is removed, and a tumor or other defect is visualized and repaired (D). The bone is replaced (E), and the skin closed (F). *(Illustration by GGS Inc.)*

• arteriogram (an x-ray of blood vessels injected with a dye to visualize a tumor or cerebral aneurysm)

Before surgery the patient may be given medication to ease anxiety and to decrease the risk of seizures, swelling, and infection after surgery. Blood thinners (Coumadin, heparin, **aspirin**) and **nonsteroidal anti-inflammatory drugs** (ibuprofen, Motrin, Advil, aspirin, Naprosyn, Daypro) have been correlated with an increase in blood clot formation after surgery. These medications must be discontinued at least seven days before the surgery to reverse any blood thinning effects. Additionally, the surgeon will order routine or special laboratory tests as needed. The patient should not eat or drink after midnight the day of surgery. The patient's scalp is shaved in the **operating room** just before the surgery begins.

Aftercare

Craniotomy is a major surgical procedure performed under general anesthesia. Immediately after surgery, the patient's pupil reactions are tested, mental status is assessed after anesthesia, and movement of the limbs (arms/legs) is evaluated. Shortly after surgery, breathing exercises are started to clear the lungs. Typically, after surgery patients are given medications to control pain, swelling, and seizures. Codeine may be prescribed to relive headache. Special leg stockings are used to prevent blood clot formation after surgery. Patients can usually get out of bed in about a day after surgery and usually are hospitalized for five to 14 days after surgery. The bandages on the skull are be removed and replaced regularly. The sutures closing the scalp are removed by the surgeon, but the soft wires used to reattach the portion of the skull that was removed are permanent and require no further attention. Patients should keep the scalp dry until the sutures are removed. If required (depending on area of brain involved), occupational therapists and physical therapist assess the patient's status postoperatively and help the patient improve strength, daily living skills and capabilities, and speech. Full recovery may take up to two months, since it is common for patients to feel fatigued for up to eight weeks after surgery.

Risks

The surgeon will discuss potential risks associated with the procedure. Neurosurgical procedures may result

QUESTIONS TO ASK
THE DOCTOR

- How is this procedure done?
- What kinds of tests and preparation are necessary before surgery?
- What risks are associated with the procedure?
- How often is normal brain tissue damaged during this type of surgery?
- What is the expected outcome of the surgery?
- What complications may result from this type of surgery?
- What is the recovery time?
- How many of these procedures have you done in the past year?

KEY TERMS

Abscess—A localized collection of pus or infection that is walled off from the rest of the body.

Arteriogram—An x-ray study of an artery that has been injected with a contrast dye.

Arteriovenous malformation—Abnormal, direct connection between the arteries and veins. Arteriovenous malformations can range from very small to large.

Cerebral aneurysm—An abnormal, localized bulge in a blood vessel that is usually caused by a congenital weakness in the wall of the vessel.

Cranium—Skull; the bony framework that holds the brain.

Computed tomography (CT)—An imaging technique that produces three-dimensional pictures of organs and structures inside the body using a 360° x-ray beam.

Edema—An accumulation of watery fluid that causes swelling of the affected tissue.

Hematoma—An accumulation of blood, often clotted, in a body tissue or organ, usually caused by a break or tear in a blood vessel.

Hemorrhage—Very severe, massive bleeding that is difficult to control.

Magnetic resonance imaging (MRI)—An imaging technique that uses magnetic fields and radio waves to create detailed images of internal body organs and structures, including the brain.

in bleeding, blood clots, retention of fluid causing swelling (edema), or unintended injury to normal nerve tissues. Some patients may develop infections. Damage to normal brain tissue may cause damage to an area and subsequent loss of brain function. Loss of function in specific areas can cause memory impairment. Some other examples of potential damage that may result from this procedure include deafness, double vision, numbness, paralysis, blindness, or loss of the sense of smell.

Normal results

Normal results depend on the cause for surgery and the patient's overall health status and age. If the operation was successful and uncomplicated recovery is quick, since there is a rich blood supply to the area. Recovery could take up to eight weeks, but patients are usually fully functioning in less time.

Morbidity and mortality rates

There is no information about the rates of diseases and death specifically related to craniotomy. The operation is performed as a neurosurgical intervention for several different diseases and conditions.

Alternatives

There are no alternative treatments if a neurosurgeon deems this procedure as necessary.

Resources

BOOKS

Connolly, E. Sanders, ed. *Fundamentals of Operative Techniques in Neurosurgery.* New York: Thieme Medical Publishers, 2002.

Greenberg, Mark S. *Handbook of Neurosurgery.* 5th ed. New York: Thieme Medical Publishers, 2000.

Miller, R. *Anesthesia.* 5th ed. Philadelphia, PA: Churchill Livingstone, 2000.

PERIODICALS

Gebel, J. M., and W. J. Powers. "Emergency Craniotomy for Intracerebral Hemorrhage: When Doesn't It Help and Does It Ever Help?" *Neurology* 58 (May 14, 2002): 1325-1326.

Mamminen, P., and T. K. Tan. "Postoperative Nausea and Vomiting After Craniotomy for Tumor Surgery: A Comparison Between Awake Craniotomy and General Anesthesia." *Journal of Clinical Anesthesia* 14 (June 2002): 279-283.

Osguthorpe, J. D., and S. Patel, eds. "Skull Base Tumor Surgery." *Otolaryngologic Clinics of North America* 34 (December 2001).

Rabinstein, A. A., J. L. Atkinson, and E. F. M. Wijdicks. "Emergency Craniotomy in Patients Worsening Due to

Expanded Cerebral Hematoma: To What Purpose?" *Neurology* 58 (May 14, 2002): 1367-1372.

ORGANIZATIONS

American Association of Neurological Surgeons. 5550 Meadowbrook Drive, Rolling Meadows, IL 60008. (888) 566-AANS (2267). Fax: (847) 378-0600. E-mail: info@aans. org. <http://www.neurosurgery.org/aans/index.asp>.

Laith Farid Gulli, M.D., M.S.
Nicole Mallory, M.S., PA-C
Robert Ramirez, B.S.

Creatine kinase test *see* **Cardiac marker tests**

Creatinine test *see* **Kidney function tests**

Cricothyroidotomy

Definition

Cricothyroidotomy is usually regarded as an emergency surgical procedure in which a surgeon or other trained person cuts a hole through a membrane in the patient's neck into the windpipe in order to allow air into the lungs. Cricothyroidotomy is a subtype of surgical procedure known as a **tracheotomy**; in some situations, it is considered an elective alternative to other types of tracheotomy.

Purpose

The primary purpose of a cricothyroidotomy is to provide an emergency breathing passage for a patient whose airway is closed by traumatic injury to the neck; by burn inhalation injuries; by closing of the airway due to an allergic reaction to bee or wasp stings; or by unconsciousness. It may also be performed in some seriously ill patients with structural abnormalities in the neck. Some surgeons consider a cricothyroidotomy to be preferable to a standard tracheotomy in treating patients in an **intensive care unit**.

Demographics

The demographics of cricothyroidotomies are difficult to establish because the procedure is relatively uncommon in the general population, even in emergency situations. In the emergency room, the incidence varied between 1.7% and 2.7%. A study found that nine of a group of 1,560 patients admitted for blunt or penetrating

---

**WHO PERFORMS
THE PROCEDURE AND
WHERE IS IT PERFORMED?**

Under ideal circumstances, a cricothyroidotomy would be performed in a hospital emergency room, ICU, or trauma center by a general surgeon, otolaryngologist, or anesthesiologist. Because it is an emergency procedure, however, a medical student, physician's assistant, paramedic, or nurse may also perform cricothyroidotomies. Many trauma centers require paramedics and nurses specializing in emergency medicine to practice performing cricothyroidotomies at least twice a year in a clinical laboratory in order to keep their skill level high. Since the procedure is risky but uncommon, it is important for emergency personnel to feel comfortable with the equipment and techniques required.

Military personnel are trained to perform emergency cricothyroidotomies in combat situations. There are also cases reported of cricothyroidotomies being done in emergencies by civilian bystanders with some medical training.

---

injuries of the neck required emergency cricothyroidotomies, or about 0.5%.

Another study found that the most important single cause of injuries requiring emergency cricothyroidotomy was traffic accidents (51%), followed by gunshot and knife wounds (29%); falls (5%); and criminal assault (5%).

Most cricothyroidotomies are performed on adolescent and young adult males, because this group accounts for the majority of cases of neck trauma in the United States. It is estimated that injuries to the neck account for 5–10% of all serious traumatic injuries.

Description

There are two basic types of cricothyroidotomy: needle cricothyroidotomy and surgical cricothyroidotomy.

Needle cricothyroidotomy

In a needle cricothyroidotomy, a syringe with a needle attached is used to make a puncture hole through the cricothyroid membrane that overlies the trachea. After the needle has reached the trachea, a catheter is passed over the needle into the windpipe and attached to a bag-valve device.

Cricothyroidotomy

Cricoid cartilage

Thyroid cartilage

Thyroid

Trachea

A.

Incision line

B.

Endotracheal tube

C.

D.

To perform a cricothyroidotomy, the surgeon makes an incision into the cricoid cartilage of the throat (B). The incision is held open while an endotracheal tube is inserted (C). The tube is secured in the trachea to maintain an airway for the patient (D). *(Illustration by GGS Inc.)*

Surgical cricothyroidotomy

In a surgical cricothyroidotomy, the doctor or other emergency worker makes an incision through the cricothyroid membrane into the trachea in order to insert a piece of tubing for ventilating the patient.

Diagnosis/Preparation

The primary concerns in emergency medical treatment are sometimes known as the ABCs: Airway patency (openness), Breathing, and Circulation. Keeping the airway patent is critical to an injured person's survival. The signs of a blocked airway in people are obvious, including a bluish complexion (cyanosis); noisy breathing, unusual breath sounds, or choking; emotional agitation or panic; and often loss of consciousness.

In an emergency situation, the following are considered reasons for performing a cricothyroidotomy first rather than attempting to open or clear the patient's airway by other methods:

• Major injuries to the face or jaw, such as multiple fractures of the jawbone or severe fractures of the patient's midface. In many cases of facial injury, the airway is blocked by broken teeth or fragments of bone from the jaw and cheekbones.

• Burns in or around the mouth.

• A neurological disorder or damage that has caused the patient's teeth to clamp shut.

• Fractured larynx. Fractures of the larynx most commonly result from automobile or motorcycle accidents, but also occur in cases of strangulation or attempted suicide by hanging.

• Larynx swollen shut by allergic reaction to bee or wasp venom.

Preparation

The first steps in preparation are the same for needle and surgical cricothyroidotomies. The patient is positioned lying on the back with a towel under the shoulders and the neck stretched backward (hyperextended). If the patient is conscious, he or she is given a local anesthetic. The doctor then palpates, or feels, the patient's throat for the thyroid cartilage, or Adam's apple. This piece of cartilage is an anatomical landmark for this procedure, which means that it is a structure that is relatively easy to identify and serves as a reference point for other structures. In men, the Adam's apple is easy to find by running the finger down the center of the neck. In women, however, the thyroid cartilage is less prominent. Below the thyroid cartilage is a softer area about the width of a finger; this is the cricothyroid membrane, which is a

piece of tissue lying between the thyroid cartilage above it and the cricoid cartilage below it.

When the doctor has located the cricothyroid membrane, he or she will scrub the skin over it with a povidone-iodine solution to prevent infection.

Needle cricothyroidotomy

In a needle cricothyroidotomy, the doctor uses a 12- or 14-gauge catheter and needle assembly. The needle is advanced through the cricothyroid cartilage at a 45-degree angle until the trachea is reached. When the doctor is able to withdraw air through the syringe, he or she knows that the catheter is in the correct spot. The catheter is then pushed forward over the needle, which is then removed. An endotracheal tube connector is then fitted onto the end of the catheter and connected to a bag-valve unit with an oxygen reservoir.

A needle cricothyroidotomy will supply the patient with enough oxygen for about 40–45 minutes; it is a time-limited technique because it does not allow the efficient escape of carbon dioxide from the bloodstream. It will, however, help to ventilate the patient until he or she can be taken to a hospital or trauma center.

Needle cricothyroidotomy is the only form of this procedure that can be done in children under 12 years of age. The reason for this restriction is that the upper part of the trachea is not fully developed in children, and a surgical incision through the cricothyroid membrane increases the risk of the child's developing subglottic stenosis, which is a condition in which the trachea is abnormally narrow below the level of the vocal cords due to an overgrowth of soft tissue. It is often seen in children who were intubated as infants.

Surgical cricothyroidotomy

In a surgical cricothyroidotomy, the doctor steadies the patient's thyroid cartilage with one hand and makes a horizontal (transverse) incision across the cricothyroid membrane. The incision is deepened until the airway is reached. The doctor then rotates the edge of the scalpel 90° in order to open the incision to receive an endotracheal or tracheotomy tube. A hemostat or surgical clamp may be used to hold the incision open while the doctor prepares to insert the tube through the opening into the trachea. After checking the tube to make certain that it is in the proper location, the doctor tapes it in place. If necessary, the doctor may use suction to clear the patient's airway.

In some emergency situations, the doctor or other medical professional may not have an antiseptic available to cleanse the skin over the patient's throat, and may have to use any sharp-edged implement that is handy to make the incision. Emergency cricothyroidotomies have been performed with scissors, hunting or pocketknives, razor blades, broken glass, and the jagged edges of a lid from a tin can. The airway has been held open with such objects as paper clips, nail clippers, the plastic barrel from a ballpoint pen, and a piece of plastic straw from a sports water bottle.

Aftercare

Needle cricothyroidotomy

A needle cricothyroidotomy must be replaced by a formal surgical tracheotomy or other means of ventilating the patient within 45 minutes.

Surgical cricothyroidotomy

A surgical cricothyroidotomy can be left in place for about 24 hours, but should be replaced within that time period by a formal tracheotomy performed in a hospital **operating room**.

Other aspects of aftercare depend on the cause of the airway blockage and the nature of the patient's injuries. The head and neck contain major blood vessels, a large portion of the central nervous system, the organs of sight, smell, hearing, and taste, and the central airway—all within a relatively small area. Injuries to the face and neck often require treatment by specialists in neurology, trauma surgery, otolaryngology, ophthalmology, and plastic surgery as well as by specialists in emergency medicine.

Risks

Needle cricothyroidotomy

The risks of a needle cricothyroidotomy include:

• external scar from needle puncture
• bleeding
• accidental perforation of the esophagus
• hypercarbia (overly high levels of carbon dioxide in the blood)

Surgical cricothyroidotomy

The risks of surgical cricothyroidotomy include:

• large visible external scar from the incision
• subglottic stenosis
• bleeding
• accidental perforation of the esophagus
• fracture of the larynx
• pneumothorax, which is a condition in which air has entered the space around the lungs

• damage to the vocal cords resulting in hoarseness or a changed voice

Normal results

Needle cricothyroidotomy

Normal results for a needle cricothyroidotomy would be adequate ventilation of a patient with a blocked airway for a brief period of time of about 45 minutes.

Surgical cricothyroidotomy

Normal results of a surgical cricothyroidotomy would be adequate ventilation in emergency circumstances of a patient with a blocked airway for a period of about 24 hours.

Morbidity and mortality rates

In general, cricothyroiditomy has a very low mortality rate, even when performed outside a hospital. By contrast, the mortality rate for patients who lose airway patency is 33%. Overall, emergency cricothyroidotomy is considered an effective way to create an emergency surgical airway with low overall morbidity.

Alternatives

Cricothyroidotomy is generally considered a procedure of last resort, to be performed when other ways of opening the patient's airway have failed or are unavailable. It is frequently done if **endotracheal intubation** has been attempted and failed, or if intubation cannot be performed due to the nature of the patient's injuries. Endotracheal intubation is a procedure in which a breathing tube is introduced directly into the trachea through the patient's mouth or nose with the help of a laryngoscope. It is most commonly done during general anesthesia, but can also be performed to help the patient breathe.

One alternative to cricothyroidotomy is a technique known as transtracheal jet ventilation (TTJV). In TTJV, a syringe is used to introduce a catheter through the patient's cricothyroid membrane. The catheter is connected to a high-pressure oxygen supply. In hospital settings,

KEY TERMS

Airway—The passageway through the mouth, nose, and throat that allows air to enter and leave the lungs; the term can also refer to a tube or other artificial device used to create an air passageway into and out of the lungs when the patient is under general anesthesia or unable to breathe properly.

Cricoid cartilage—A ring-shaped piece of cartilage that forms the lower and rear parts of the voice box or larynx; it is sometimes called the annular cartilage because of its shape.

Cricothyroid membrane—The piece of connective tissue that lies between the thyroid and cricoid cartilages.

Cyanosis—A bluish discoloration of the skin, caused by a loss of oxygen content in the blood.

Endotracheal intubation—A procedure in which a tube is inserted into the trachea in order to administer anesthesia or ventilate the patient.

Hypercarbia—An excess of carbon dioxide in the blood.

Patency—Being wide open, as in a patient's airway.

Pneumothorax—A condition in which air or gas has accumulated in the space in the chest around the lungs.

Subglottic stenosis—An abnormal narrowing of the trachea below the level of the vocal cords.

Thyroid cartilage—The largest cartilage in the human larynx, or voice box. It is sometimes called the Adam's apple.

Trachea—The windpipe.

Tracheotomy—The surgical creation of an opening into the windpipe through the neck; it is also called a tracheostomy.

Transtracheal jet ventilation (TTJV)—A technique for ventilating a patient that involves passing oxygen under pressure through a catheter that has been passed through the patient's cricothyroid membrane.

Ventilate—To assist a patient's breathing by use of a mechanical device or surgical procedure.

TTJV has about the same rate of complications as a surgical cricothyroidotomy. Its disadvantages are that it cannot be used outside a hospital setting and it takes longer to perform. A surgical cricothyroidotomy can be performed in 30 seconds to two minutes; TTJV takes twice to three times as long to perform.

See also Endotracheal intubation; Tracheotomy.

Resources

BOOKS

Gomella, Leonard G., and Alan T. Lefor. *Surgery On Call,* 3rd ed. New York: McGraw-Hill/Appleton & Lange, 2001.

PERIODICALS

Adams, B. D., and W. L. Whitlock. "Bystander Cricothyroidotomy Performed with an Improvised Airway." *Military Medicine,* 167 (January 2002): 76–78.

Bennett, John D. C. "Securing the Airway in Burns." *Journal of Burns,* 1 (2002): 1 [March 8, 23]. <www.journalofburns. com>.

Flynn, Sean. "How to Save a Soldier." *New York Times Magazine,* March 16, 2003. <www.nytimes.com/2003/03/16/magazine/16BATTLE.html>.

Francois, B., et al. "Complications of Tracheostomy Performed in the ICU: Subthyroid Tracheostomy vs Surgical Cricothyroidotomy." *Chest,* 123 (January 2003): 151–158.

Gillespie, M. B., and D. W. Eisele. "Outcomes of Emergency Surgical Airway Procedures in a Hospital-wide Setting." *Laryngoscope,* 109 (November 1999): 1766–1769.

Hayden, S. R., and E. A. Panacek. "Procedural Competency in Emergency Medicine: The Current Range of Resident Experience." *Academic Emergency Medicine,* 6 (July 1999): 728–735.

Janson, Paul, and Richard Iseke. "Hymenoptera Stings." *eMedicine,* July 26, 2002 [March 9, 2003]. <www.emedicine. com/med/topic1058.htm>.

Levy, David, and Robert Buckman. "Neck Trauma." *eMedicine,* June 21, 2001 [March 8, 2003]. <www.emedicine. com/emerg/topic331.htm>.

Parsa, Tatiana, Arthur Adamo, and Yvette Calderon. "Initial Evaluation and Management of Maxillofacial Injuries." *eMedicine,* August 28, 2002 [March 8, 2003]. <www. emedicine.com/med/topic3222.htm>.

Rehm, C. G., et al. "Cricothyroidotomy for Elective Airway Management in Critically Ill Trauma Patients with Technically Challenging Neck Anatomy." *Critical Care,* 6 (December 2002): 531–535.

Torres, Manuel. "Case Study: Airway and Facial Trauma." *Stat Page: Newsletter of the Center for Emergency Medicine,* 8 (February 1997): 6–7.

Vassiliu, P., et al. "Aerodigestive Injuries of the Neck." *American Surgeon,* 67 (January 2001): 75–79.

ORGANIZATIONS

Center for Emergency Medicine. 230 McKee Place, Suite 500, Pittsburgh, PA 15213. (412) 647-5300. <www.centerem. com>.

National Association of Emergency Medical Technicians (NAEMT). P. O. Box 1400, Clinton, MS 39060-1400. (800) 34-NAEMT. <www.naemt.org>.

University of Maryland Medical Center, R. Adams Cowley Shock Trauma Center. 22 South Greene Street, Baltimore, MD 21201. (410) 328-2757 or (800) 373-4111. <www. umm.edu/shocktrauma>.

OTHER

Jaberi, Mahmood, Kimberley Mitchell, and Colin Mackenzie. *Cricothyroidotomy: Good, Bad, or Ugly?* Third Place Scientific Award, 14th Trauma Anesthesia and Critical Care Symposium, San Diego, CA, May 17, 2001.

Rebecca Frey, PhD

Cryosurgery *see* **Cryotherapy**

Cryosurgery for retinal detachment *see* **Retinal cryopexy**

Cryotherapy

Definition

Cryotherapy is a technique that uses an extremely cold liquid or instrument to freeze and destroy abnormal skin cells that require removal. The technique has been in use since the turn of the century, but modern techniques have made it widely available to dermatologists and primary care doctors. The technique is also known as cryocautery or cryosurgery.

Purpose

Cryotherapy is used to destroy a variety of benign skin growths, such as warts, pre-cancerous lesions (actinic keratoses), and malignant lesions (basal cell and squamous cell cancers). It has been used at several medical centers for tumors of the prostate, liver, lung, breast, and brain as well as for cataracts, gynecological problems, and other diseases. The goal of cryotherapy is to freeze and destroy targeted skin growths while preserving the surrounding skin from injury.

Description

In dermatology applications, there are three main techniques used in cryotherapy. In the simplest tech-

nique, usually reserved for warts and other benign skin growths, the physician dips a cotton swab or other applicator into a cup containing a "cryogen" such as liquid nitrogen and applies it directly to the skin growth to freeze it. At a temperature of $-320°F$ $(-196°C)$, liquid nitrogen is the coldest cryogen available. The goal is to freeze the skin growth as quickly as possible, and then let it thaw slowly to cause maximum destruction of the skin cells. A second application may be necessary depending on the size of the growth. In another approach, a device is used to direct a small spray of liquid nitrogen or other cryogen directly onto the skin growth. Freezing may last from five to 20 seconds, depending on the size of the lesion. A second freeze-thaw cycle may be required. Sometimes, the physician inserts a small needle connected to a thermometer into the lesion to make certain the lesion is cooled to a temperature low enough to guarantee maximum destruction. In a third option, liquid nitrogen or another cryogen is circulated through a probe to cool it to low temperatures. The probe is then brought into direct contact with the skin lesion to freeze it. The freeze time can take two to three times longer than with the spray technique.

When used for cancer treatment, cryotherapy is usually performed as follows: for external tumors, liquid nitrogen is applied directly to the cancer cells with a cotton swab or spraying device; for internal tumors, liquid nitrogen is circulated through an instrument called a cryoprobe that is placed in contact with the tumor. To guide the cryoprobe and to monitor the freezing of the cells, the treating physician uses ultrasound to guide his work and spare nearby healthy tissue.

Preparation

No extensive preparation is required prior to cryotherapy. The area to be treated should be clean and dry, but sterile preparation is not necessary. Patients should know that they will experience some pain at the time of the freezing, but local anesthesia is usually not required. In dermatology applications, the physician may want to reduce the size of certain growths such as warts prior to the cryotherapy procedure, and may have patients apply salicylic acid preparations to the growth over several weeks. Sometimes, the physician will pare away some of the tissue using a device called a curette or a scalpel. In the case of **cervical cryotherapy**, the procedure is not performed during, or from two to three days before, the menstrual period.

Aftercare

In dermatology applications, redness, swelling, and the formation of a blister at the site of cryotherapy are all expected results of the treatment. A gauze dressing is applied, and patients should wash the site three or four times daily while fluid continues to ooze from the wound, usually for five to 14 days. A dry crust will form that falls off by itself. Wounds on the head and neck may take four to six weeks to heal, but those on the body, arms, and legs can take longer. Some patients experience pain at the site following the treatment. This can usually be eased with **acetaminophen** (Tylenol), though in some cases a stronger pain reliever may be required.

Risks

In dermatology applications, cryotherapy poses little risk and can be well tolerated by elderly and other patients who are not good candidates for other surgical procedures. As with other surgical procedures, there is some risk of scarring, infection, and damage to underlying skin and tissue. These risks are generally minimal in the hands of experienced physicians.

Care should be taken, however, in subjecting people with diabetes or certain circulation problems to cryotherapy for growths located on their lower legs, ankles, and feet. In these patients, healing can be poor and the risk of infection can be higher than for other patients.

Although cryotherapy is a relatively low-risk procedure, some side effects may occur as a result of the treatment. They include:

- Infection. Though uncommon, infection is more likely on the lower legs where healing can take several months.

- Pigmentary changes. Both hypopigmentation (lightening of the skin) and hyperpigmentation (darkening of the skin) are possible after cryotherapy. Both generally last a few months, but can be longer lasting.

- Nerve damage. Though rare, damage to nerves is possible, particularly in areas where they lie closer to the surface of the skin, such as the fingers, the wrist, and the area behind the ear. Reports suggest this will disappear within several months.

In cancer treatment, cryosurgery does have side effects, although they may be less severe than those associated with conventional surgery or radiation therapy. Cryosurgery of the liver may cause damage to the bile ducts or major blood vessels, which can lead to heavy bleeding or infection. Cryosurgery for prostate cancer may affect the urinary system. It also may cause incontinence (lack of control over urine flow) and impotence (loss of sexual function), although these side effects are often temporary. Cryosurgery for cervical tumors has not been shown to affect fertility, but this possibility is under study. More studies must be conducted to determine the long-term effects of cryosurgery as a cancer treatment approach.

Normal results

Some redness, swelling, blistering, and oozing of fluid are all common results of cryotherapy. Healing time can vary by the site treated and the cryotherapy technique used. When cryogen is applied directly to the growth, healing may occur in three weeks. Growths treated on the head and neck with the spray technique may take four to six weeks to heal, while growths treated on other areas of the body may take considerably longer. Cryotherapy boasts high success rates in permanently removing skin growths; even for malignant lesions such as squamous cell and basal cell cancers, studies have shown a cure rate of up to 98%. For certain types of growths such as some forms of warts, repeat treatments over several weeks are necessary to prevent the growth's return.

Alternatives

Alternatives to cryotherapy depend on the specific medical condition being treated. A general alternative is the use of conventional surgical procedures.

KEY TERMS

Actinic keratosis—A crusty, scaly pre-cancerous skin lesion caused by damage from the sun; frequently treated with cryotherapy.

Basal cell cancer—The most common form of skin cancer that usually appears as one or several nodules having a central depression; it rarely spreads (metasticizes), but is locally invasive.

Cervical cryotherapy—Surgery performed after a biopsy has confirmed abnormal cervical cells (dysplasia).

Cryogen—A substance with a very low boiling point, such as liquid nitrogen, used in cryotherapy treatment.

Melanoma—The most dangerous form of skin cancer.

Squamous cell cancer—A form of skin cancer that usually originates in sun-damaged areas or pre-existing lesions; at first local and superficial, it may later spread to other areas of the body.

Ultrasound—Imaging technique by which computerized moving pictures of the body are generated by high-frequency sound waves.

See also Cervical cryotherapy; Cryotherapy for cataracts.

Resources

BOOKS

Dawber, R., G. Colver, A. Jackson, and F. Pringle. *Cutaneous Cryosurgery: Principles and Clinical Practice,* 2nd ed. Oxford: Blackwell Science Inc., 1996.

Korpan, N. N. *Basics of Cryosurgery.* New York: Springer Verlag, 2002.

Lynch, Peter J., and W. Mitchell Sams Jr. *Principles and Practice of Dermatology,* 2nd ed. New York: Churchill Livingstone, 1996.

Roenigk, Randall K., and Henry H. Roenigk Jr. *Roenigk and Roenigk's Dermatologic Surgery: Principles and Practice.* New York: Marcel Dekker, 1996.

PERIODICALS

Housman, T. S., and J. L. Jorizzo. "Anecdotal Reports of Three Cases Illustrating a Spectrum of Resistant Common Warts Treated with Cryotherapy Followed by Topical Imiquimod and Salicylic Acid." *Journal of the American Academy of Dermatology* 47 (October 2002): 1501–1505.

Otte, J. W., M. A. Merrick, C. D. Ingersoll, and M. L. Cordova. "Subcutaneous Adipose Tissue Thickness Alters Cooling Time during Cryotherapy." *Archives of Physical and Medical Rehabilitation* 83 (November 2002): 1501–1505.

Palner, E. A., et al. "Cryotherapy for Retinopathy of Prematurity Cooperative Group. Multicenter Trial of Cryotherapy for Retinopathy of Prematurity: Ophthalmological Outcomes at 10 Years." *Archives of Ophthalmology* 119 (2001): 1110–1118.

Uchio, Y., M. Ochi, A. Fujihara, N. Adachi, J. Iwasa, and Y. Sakai. "Cryotherapy Influences Joint Laxity and Position Sense of the Healthy Knee Joint." *Archives of Physical and Medical Rehabilitation* 84 (January 2003): 131–135.

Wozniacka, A., A. Omulecki, and J. D. Torzecka. "Cryotherapy in the Treatment of Angiolymphoid Hyperplasia with Eosinophilia." *Medical Science Monitor* 9 (January 2003): CS1–CS4.

ORGANIZATIONS

American Academy of Dermatology. 930 N. Meacham Road, P.O. Box 4014, Schaumburg, IL 60168-4014. (847) 330-0230. Fax: (847) 330-0050. <http://www.aad.org>.

American Society for Dermatologic Surgery. 930 N. Meacham Road, PO Box 4014, Schaumburg, IL 60168-4014. (847) 330-9830. <http://www.asds-net.org>.

OTHER

"Cryotherapy." *Family Practice Notebook.* <www.fpnotebook.com/DER233.htm.>.

Richard H. Camer
Monique Laberge, PhD

Cryotherapy for cataracts

Definition

Cryosurgery, or cryotherapy, is a technique that destroys abnormal tissue by freezing the cells. Cryotherapy can be used in the treatment of cataracts.

Purpose

The procedure is used to treat cataracts. A cataract is a form of clouding that develops in the lens of the eye. The crystalline lens consists mainly of protein matter and water. Normally, the protein is packed so as to allow light to pass through the lens. A cataract forms when protein molecules start aggregating and clump together, eventually clouding the lens and blocking light. If left untreated, cataracts may eventually cause blindness. **Cryotherapy** is performed to remove the clouding protein matter from the lens.

Demographics

In the United States, approximately 50% of people between the ages 65 and 74, and 70% of those over age 75 have a cataract, with women affected more often than men. African Americans experience impaired vision from both cataracts and glaucoma at twice the rate of Caucasian Americans, primarily due to lack of treatment.

Description

Cryotherapy involves the application of a very cold probe to the outside of the eye, which, because of the thin nature of the eye wall (sclera), transmits the freezing temperature to the retina. The intense cold stimulation to the retina can seal abnormal leaky retinal blood vessels. This technique is indicated for the treatment of cataracts that obscure the passage of light into the eye, thus limiting the effectiveness of techniques such as laser therapy.

Cryotherapy uses a cryogenic substance, such as liquid nitrogen, to freeze the cataract. At a temperature of -320°F (-196°C), liquid nitrogen is the coldest cryogenic substance available. The ophthalmologist uses a device to direct a small spray of liquid nitrogen directly onto the cataract. Freezing may last from five to 20 seconds, depending on the size of the cataract. A second freeze-thaw cycle may be required. Sometimes, the ophthalmologist will insert a small needle connected to a thermometer to make certain the cataract is cooled to a low enough temperature to guarantee destruction. In another option, liquid nitrogen or another cryogen is circulated through a probe to cool it to low temperatures. The probe is then brought into direct contact with the cataract to freeze it. The freeze time can take two to three times longer than with the spray technique.

Diagnosis/Preparation

In order to see the back of the eye properly, the examining ophthalmologist uses two powerful microscopes, the slit lamp and ophthalmoscope. Eye drops are also often used to make the pupil bigger, so that the back of the eye can be seen more clearly. The effect of these drops wears off after a few hours. Once a cataract has been diagnosed to the point that it is interfering with daily activities and normal lifestyle, an appointment is made to treat the cataract.

For cryotherapy, the patient may be asked to skip breakfast, depending on the time of surgery. Upon arrival for cryotherapy, he or she is given eye drops, and perhaps medications to help relax. A local or topical anesthetic is used to make the procedure painless. The patient may see light and movement, but will not be able to see the cryotherapy when it is performed. The skin around the eye is thoroughly cleansed, and sterile coverings are placed around the patient's head.

Aftercare

After cryotherapy, a patch is placed over the operated eye and the patient is asked to rest for a while. The attending physician checks to see if there are any problems, such as bleeding. Most people who have cataract cryotherapy go home the same day. They need to make arrangements for a ride since they can not drive. After the procedure, the doctor schedules exams to check the progress of the vision. Eyedrops or pills may be given to help healing and to control pressure inside the eye. The patient is also asked to wear an eye shield or eyeglasses to help protect the eye, and he or she is told to avoid rubbing or pressing the eye, and to not lift heavy objects because bending increases pressure in the eye. Walking, climbing stairs, and light household chores can be performed.

Risks

Narcotic analgesia may be required after the procedure to relieve pain. Cryotherapy also causes significant swelling of the eye and eyelid, which makes postoperative assessment difficult. Problems after cryotherapy are rare, but can occur and may include infection, bleeding, inflammation (pain, redness, swelling), loss of vision, or light flashes. With careful medical attention, these problems usually can be treated successfully.

Normal results

Surgical treatment for cataracts usually results in excellent vision. However, if other problems are present besides the cataract, as for example degeneration of the retina or optic nerve, results will not be as favorable.

Alternatives

The alternative treatment for cataracts is surgical cataract removal, which is one of the most common surgical procedures performed in the United States. Approximately 90% of patients who undergo this surgery experience improved vision. Two procedures are commonly used to surgically remove a cataract: phacoemulsification and extracapsular surgery. There are no medications, dietary supplements, exercises, or optical devices that have been shown to prevent or cure cataracts.

See also Cryotherapy; Phacoemulsification for cataracts.

Resources

BOOKS

Buettner, H., ed. *Mayo Clinic on Vision and Eye Health: Practical Answers on Glaucoma, Cataracts, Macular Degeneration & Other Conditions*. Rochester: Mayo Clinic, 2002.

Parker, J. N., ed. *The Official Patient's Sourcebook on Cataracts*. San Diego: ICON Health Publications, 2002.

Shulman, J. *Cataracts*. New York: St. Martin's Press, 1995.

PERIODICALS

Palner, E. A., et al. "Cryotherapy for Retinopathy of Prematurity Cooperative Group. Multicenter Trial of Cryotherapy for Retinopathy of Prematurity: Ophthalmological Outcomes at 10 Years." *Archives of Ophthalmology* 119 (2001): 1110–1118.

ORGANIZATIONS

American Academy of Ophthalmology. P.O. Box 7424, San Francisco, CA 94120-7424. (415) 561-8500. <http://www.aao.org/index.html>

New England Ophthalmological Society (NEOS). P.O. Box 9165, Boston, MA 02114. (617) 227-6484. <http://www.neos-eyes.org>

OTHER

American Academy of Ophthalmology. *Cataract Brochure 051084*. 2002.

American Academy of Ophthalmology. *Cataract Surgery, Better than Ever*. August 14, 2001 [cited April 2003]. <http://www.aao.org/aao/news/release/081401.cfm>.

Monique Laberge, Ph.D.

Cryotherapy for the cervix *see* **Cervical cryotherapy**

CSF analysis *see* **Cerebrospinal fluid (CSF) analysis**

CT-myelogram *see* **Myelography**

CT scans

Definition

Computed tomography (CT) scans are completed with the use of a 360-degree x-ray beam and computer production of images. These scans allow for cross-sectional views of body organs and tissues. Computed tomography is also known as computerized axial tomography or CAT scan.

Purpose

CT scans are used to image a wide variety of body structures and internal organs. Since the 1990s, CT

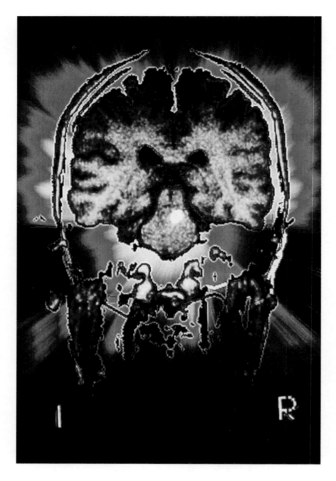

A CT scan of the human brain. *(Custom Medical Stock Photo. Reproduced by permission.)*

equipment has become more affordable and available. In some diagnoses, CT scans have become the first imaging exam of choice. Because the computerized image is so sharp, focused, and three-dimensional, many tissues can be better differentiated than on standard x rays. Common CT indications include:

- Sinus studies. The CT scan can show details of sinusitis and bone fractures. Physicians may order a CT scan of the sinuses to provide an accurate map for surgery.

- Brain studies. Brain scans can detect tumors, strokes, and hematomas (collections of blood that have escaped from the vessels). The introduction of CT scanning, especially spiral CT, has helped reduce the need for more invasive procedures such as cerebral angiography.

- Body scans. CT scans of the body will often be used to observe abdominal organs, such as the liver, kidneys, adrenal glands, spleen, pancreas, biliary tree and lymph nodes, and extremities.

- Aorta scans. CT scans can focus on the thoracic or abdominal sections of the aorta to locate aneurysms and other possible aortic diseases.

- Chest scans. CT scans of the chest are useful in distinguishing tumors and in detailing accumulation of fluid in chest infections.

Description

Computed tomography is a combination of focused x-ray beams, a detector array, and computerized production of an image. Introduced in the early 1970s, this radiologic procedure has advanced rapidly and is now widely used, sometimes in the place of standard x rays.

CT equipment

A CT scan may be performed in a hospital or outpatient imaging center. Although the equipment looks large and intimidating, it is very sophisticated and fairly comfortable. The patient is asked to lie on a narrow table that slides into the center of the scanner, called the gantry. The scanner looks like a square doughnut with a round opening in the middle, which allows the x-ray beam to rotate around the patient. The scanner's gantry section may also be tilted slightly to allow for certain cross-sectional angles.

CT procedure

The patient will feel the table move very slightly as the precise adjustments for each sectional image are made. A technologist watches the procedure from a window and views the images on a monitor.

It is essential that the patient lie very still during the procedure to prevent motion blurring. In some studies, such as chest CTs, the patient will be asked to hold his or her breath during image capture.

Following the procedure, films of the images are usually printed for the radiologist and referring physician to review. A radiologist can also interpret CT exams on a special viewing console. The procedure time will vary in length depending on the area being imaged. Average study times are from 30 to 60 minutes. Some patients may be concerned about claustrophobia, but the width of the gantry portion of the scanner is wide enough to preclude problems with claustrophobia, in most instances.

The CT image

Traditional x rays image organs in two dimensions, with the possibility that organs in the front of the body are superimposed over those in the back. CT scans allow for a more three-dimensional effect. Some have compared CT images to slices in a loaf of bread. Precise sections of the body can be located and imaged as cross-sectional views. The technologist's console displays a computerized image of each section captured by the x-ray beam and detector array. Thus, various densities of tissue can be easily distinguished.

Contrast agents

Contrast agents are often used in CT exams and in other radiology procedures to demonstrate certain anatomic details that, otherwise, may not be seen easily. Some contrast agents are natural, such as air or water. Other times, a water-based contrast agent is administered for specific diagnostic purposes. Barium sulfate is commonly used in gastrointestinal procedures. The patient may drink this contrast medium, or receive it in an enema. Oral and rectal contrasts are usually given when examining the abdomen or gastrointestinal tract, and not used when scanning the brain or chest. Iodine-based contrast media are the most widely used intravenous contrast agents and are usually administered through an antecubital (in front of the elbow) vein.

If contrast agents are used in the CT exam, these will be administered several minutes before the study begins. Abdominal CT patients may be asked to drink a contrast medium. Some patients may experience a salty taste, flushing of the face, warmth, slight nausea, or hives from an intravenous contrast injection. Technologists and radiologists have equipment and training to help patients through these minor reactions and to handle more severe reactions. Severe reactions to contrast are rare, but do occur.

Spiral CT

Spiral CT, also called helical CT, is a newer version of CT scanning that is continuous in motion and allows for three-dimensional re-creation of images. For example, traditional CT allows the technologist to take slices at very small and precise intervals one after the other. Spiral CT allows for a continuous flow of images, without stopping the scanner to move to the next image slice. A major advantage of spiral CT is higher resolution and the ability to reconstruct images anywhere along the length of the study area. The procedure also speeds up the imaging process, meaning less time for the patient to lie still. The ability to image the contrast medium more rapidly after it is injected and when it is at its highest level, is another advantage of spiral CT's high speed.

Some facilities have both spiral and conventional CT available. Although spiral is more advantageous for many applications, conventional CT is still a superior and precise method for imaging many tissues and structures. The physician will evaluate which type of CT works best for the specific exam purpose.

Preparation

If a contrast medium must be administered, the patient may be asked to fast from about four to six hours prior to the procedure. This is so if a patient experiences nausea, vomiting will not occur. Patients will usually be given a gown (like a typical hospital gown) to be worn during the procedure. All metal and jewelry should be removed to avoid artifacts on the film. Pregnant women or those who could possibly be pregnant should not have a CT scan unless the diagnostic benefits outweigh the risks. Contrast agents are often used in CT exams and the use of these agents should be discussed with the medical professional prior to the procedure. Patients should be asked to sign a consent form concerning the administration of contrast media. One common ingredient in contrast agents, iodine, can cause allergic reactions. Patients who are known to be allergic to iodine (or shellfish) should inform the physician prior to the CT scan.

Aftercare

No aftercare is generally required following a CT scan. Immediately following the exam, the technologist will continue to watch the patient for possible adverse contrast reactions. Patients are instructed to advise the technologist of any symptoms, particularly respiratory difficulty. The site of contrast injection will be bandaged and may feel tender following the exam. Hives may develop later and usually do not require treatment.

Risks

Radiation exposure from a CT scan is similar to, though higher than, that of a conventional x ray. Although this is a risk to pregnant women, the exposure to other adults is minimal and should produce no effects. Although severe contrast reactions are rare, they are a risk of many CT procedures. There is also a small risk of renal failure in high-risk patients.

Normal results

Normal findings on a CT exam show bone, the most dense tissue, as white areas. Tissues and fluid will show as various shades of gray, and fat will be dark gray or black. Air will also look black and darker than fat tissue. Intravenous, oral, and rectal contrast appear as white areas. The radiologist can determine if tissues and organs appear normal by the different gradations of the gray scale. In CT, the images that can cut through a section of tissue or organ provide three-dimensional viewing for the radiologist and referring physician.

Abnormal results may show different characteristics of tissues within organs. Accumulations of blood or other fluids where they do not belong may be detected. Radiologists can differentiate among types of tumors throughout the body by viewing details of their makeup.

Sinus studies

The increasing availability and lowered cost of CT scanning has led to its increased use in sinus studies, either as a replacement for a sinus x ray or as a follow-up to an abnormal sinus radiograph. The sensitivity of CT allows for location of areas of sinus infection, particularly chronic infection, and is useful for planning prior to functional **endoscopic sinus surgery**. CT scans can show the extent and location of tiny fractures of the sinus and nasal bones. Foreign bodies in the sinus and nasal area are also easily detected by CT. CT imaging of the sinuses is important in evaluating trauma or disease of the sphenoid bone (the wedge-shaped bone at the base of the skull). Sinus tumors will show as shades of gray indicating the difference in their density from that of normal tissues in the area.

Brain studies

The precise differences in density allowed by CT scanning can clearly show tumors, strokes, or other lesions in the brain area as altered densities. These lighter or darker areas on the image may indicate a tumor or hemorrhage within the brain. Different types of tumors can be identified by the presence of edema, by the tissue's density, or by abnormal contrast enhancement. Congenital abnormalities in children, such as hydrocephalus, may also be confirmed with CT. Hydrocephalus is suggested by enlargement of the fluid structures, called ventricles, of the brain.

Body scans

The body scan can identify abnormal body structures and organs. Throughout the body, a CT scan may indicate tumors or cysts; enlarged lymph nodes; abnormal collections of fluid, blood, or fat; and metastasis of cancer. Fractures or damage to soft tissues can be more easily seen on the sensitive images produced by CT scanning. Liver conditions, such as cirrhosis, abscess, and fatty liver, may be observed with a CT body scan.

CT of the aorta

CT provides the ability to visualize and measure the thickness of the aorta, which is very helpful in diagnosing

---

KEY TERMS

Aneurysm—The bulging of the blood vessel wall. Aortic aneurysms are the most dangerous. Aneurysms can break and cause bleeding.

Contrast (agent, medium)—A substance injected into the body that delineates certain structures that would otherwise be hard or impossible to see on the radiograph (film).

Gantry—A name for the portion of a CT scanner which houses the x-ray tube and detector array used to capture image information and send it to the computer.

Hematoma—A collection of blood that has escaped from the vessels. It may clot and harden, causing pain to the patient.

Hydrocephalus—Abnormal dilatation of fluid-containing ventricles in the brain.

Metastasis—Secondary cancer, or cancer that has spread from one body organ or tissue to another.

Radiologist—A medical doctor specially trained in radiology (x ray) interpretation and its use in the diagnosis of disease and injury.

Spiral CT—Also referred to as helical CT, this method allows for continuous 360-degree x-ray image capture.

Thoracic—Refers to the chest area. The thorax runs between the abdomen and neck and is encased in the ribs.

---

aortic aneurysms. The use of contrast will help define details within the aorta. In addition, increased areas of density can identify calcification, which helps differentiate between acute and chronic problems. An abnormal CT scan may indicate signs of aortic clots. Aortic rupture is suggested by signs, such as a hematoma around the aorta or the escape of blood or contrast from its cavity.

Chest scans

In addition to those findings which may indicate aortic aneurysms, chest CT studies can show other problems in the heart and lungs. The computer will not only show differences between air, water, tissues, and bone, but will also assign numerical values to the various densities. Mass lesions in the lungs may be indicative of tuberculosis or tumors. CT will help distinguish between the two. Enlarged lymph nodes in the chest area may indicate lymphoma. Spiral CT is particularly effective at identifying pulmonary emboli (clots in the lung's blood vessels).

Resources

BOOKS

Springhouse Corporation. *Illustrated Guide to Diagnostic Tests.* Springhouse, PA: Springhouse Corporation, 1998.

PERIODICALS

Beauchamp, N. "Imaging of Acute Cerebral Ischemia." *Radiology* 307 (August 1999).

Papatheofanis, Frank J. "Helical CT and Pulmonary Disease." *Decisions in Imaging Economics* (January/February 1997): 61–63.

ORGANIZATIONS

American College of Radiology. 1891 Preston White Drive, Reston, VA 20191-4397. (800) ACR–LINE. <http://www.acr.org>.

Stephen John Hage, AAAS, RT(R), FAHRA
Lee Alan Shratter, MD

Curettage and electrosurgery

Definition

Curettage is the surgical removal of growths or tissue from the wall of a body cavity or other surface, using a spoon-like instrument with a sharp edge called a curette. Electrosurgery is a procedure that cuts, destroys, or cauterizes tissue using a high-frequency electric current applied locally with a pencil-shaped metal instrument or needle. When the two procedures are combined, the surgery is referred to as curettage and electrosurgery.

Purpose

The general purpose of curettage is to scrape an area free of undesirable tissue. The purposes of electrosurgery are to destroy benign and malignant lesions, control bleeding, and cut or excise tissue.

Specifically, a curettage and electrosurgery procedure is used to treat the following conditions:

- benign skin lesions, such as angiomas, nevis, and warts
- actinic keratoses (AKs), which are premalignant skin lesions
- skin cancers, chiefly basal cell carcinoma (BCC) and cutaneous squamous cell carcinoma (SCC)
- genital warts that result from human papillomavirus (HPV) infection

Demographics

Curettage—with or without electrosurgery—is the second most commonly used treatment in the United

---

WHO PERFORMS THE PROCEDURE AND WHERE IS IT PERFORMED?

Curettage and electrosurgery is done in a hospital or clinic, although most physicians have small electrosurgical units in their offices to treat benign lesions. The procedure is usually performed by a dermatologist or dermatologic surgeon. The American Academy of Family Physicians and several private organizations offer basic training sessions in electrosurgery.

States. (Cryosurgery is the most commonly used treatment in the United States.)

Approximately 15% of actinic keratoses develop into squamous cell carcinoma. Based on current demographics in the United States, the incidence of actinic keratoses is expected to increase. Older individuals are more likely than younger ones to have actinic keratoses, because cumulative sun exposure increases with age. A survey of older Americans found keratoses in more than half of all men and more than a third of women between the ages of 65 and 74 who had a high degree of lifetime sun exposure. Some medical experts believe that the majority of people who live to the age of 80 have AKs.

Basal cell carcinoma is the most common form of skin cancer and the most common of all types of cancer. It affects about 800,000 individuals in the United States each year. BCC is primarily caused by chronic exposure to sunlight and until recently those most often affected were older, especially older men who worked outdoors. In the last several decades, the incidence of BCC among younger people has increased. So has the number of cases in women. However, many more men are still affected by BCC than women.

Squamous cell carcinoma is the second most common form of skin cancer, affecting more than 200,000 Americans each year. It too is most often caused by chronic exposure to sunlight.

Genital human papillomavirus infection is the most common sexually transmitted disease in the United States with about 55 million new cases reported each year. Genital warts are the most easily recognized sign of HPV infection, but many people with HPV infection never develop genital warts. Both drugs and surgery are used to treat genital warts, but the warts often come back after treatment because the treatment only removes the warts and does not cure the underlying infection.

Description

In the case of AK, the procedure is carried out under local anesthesia to reduce discomfort during curettage. First, the surgeon uses a curette to scrape off the undesirable AK cells down to the level of uninvolved tissue. This is followed by electrosurgery to widen the area of AK cell destruction and removal, and to cauterize the wound to limit bleeding.

In the treatment of skin cancers, curettage is used to scrape away the tumor cells and then an extra margin of surrounding tissue is destroyed by electrosurgery. These steps may be repeated several times in the same treatment session. Curettage and electrosurgery are considered suitable for small primary lesions on sun-exposed skin. It is less effective in the case of recurrent lesions that have attendant scar tissue. Tumors that have spread into subcutaneous tissues or subcutaneous fat are less likely to be cured when treated with this procedure.

The major techniques that may be involved in the electrosurgery step include electrodesiccation (removal of water), fulguration (production of a spark to destroy tissue), electrocoagulation (forming blood clots to stop bleeding), and electrosection (cutting). Electrosurgery can be used to incise, to shave, and to remove lesions. The correct output power is determined by starting at low power and increasing the power level until the desired result is achieved (destruction, coagulation, or cutting).

Diagnosis/Preparation

Skin biopsies and histologic examination confirm diagnoses for AKs and skin cancers such as basal cell carcinoma. A recommendation for curettage and electrosurgery is made following patient evaluation.

Injectable lidocaine is administered before most curettage and electrosurgical procedures. Lidocaine is often used together with epinephrine to further reduce blood loss. Anesthesia may not be necessary when small lesions are being treated. Another alternative is to use a mixture of local anesthetics, containing 2.5% lidocaine and 2.5% prilocaine, in a cream base. The cream is applied to the skin at least one hour before the procedure to achieve topical anesthesia.

Aftercare

After the procedure, the patient is advised to keep the wound clean and dry. The healing process takes at least several weeks or longer, depending on the size of the wound and other factors. Electrosurgery produces two types of skin wounds—partial- and full-thickness wounds. Partial-thickness wounds result from the electrodesiccation of skin lesions and the curettage and desiccation of basal cell carcinomas. These wounds may be cleansed daily and then covered with an antibiotic ointment that provides a moist environment for new tissue growth. The wound may then be covered with common adhesive bandages. Full-thickness wounds require closure with sutures.

Risks

As with every type of surgical procedure, there is a risk of infection. **Antibiotics** are not routinely given, but some physicians believe they may minimize the risk. Other potential risks include:

- Subcutaneous bleeding. If it occurs, subcutaneous bleeding may create a hematoma and require the wound to be reopened and drained.
- Temporary or permanent nerve damage. This may result from excision in an area with extensive nerves.
- Wounds that reopen. If this occurs, the risk of infection and scarring increases.
- Scarring.

Normal results

Curettage and electrosurgery results in the removal of the targeted skin lesion, AK, skin cancer, or genital wart and in the formation of a minor wound that heals rapidly after the procedure.

Alternatives

Alternative treatment for AKs include:

- cryosurgery, the most common method of treating AKs in the United States

KEY TERMS

Anesthesia—A combination of drugs administered by a variety of techniques by trained professionals that provide sedation, amnesia, analgesia, and immobility adequate for the accomplishment of the surgical procedure with minimal discomfort, and without injury, to the patient.

Anesthetics—Drugs or methodologies used to make a body area free of sensation or pain.

Basal cell carcinoma—Basal cell carcinoma is the most common malignant tumor, affecting more than 800,000 people annually in the United States.

Curettage—Procedure performed with a curette, a spoon-shaped instrument used to scrape tissue.

Cutaneous squamous cell carcinoma—Malignant skin tumor of the epidermis or its appendages.

- dermabrasion, a procedure performed with an instrument that removes skin with a rapidly rotating brush

- laser removal, a treatment that uses the infrared beam of a carbon dioxide laser to destroy AK cells

- surgical excision, an uncommon treatment for AKs, used only if the lesions are very thick or difficult to remove by other means

Alternative treatment for skin cancers include:

- cryosurgery, a treatment that uses subfreezing temperature to destroy the tumor

- surgical excision, a procedure useful for both primary and recurrent tumors

- Mohs micrographic surgery, a treatment used to deal with some recurrent lesions

- laser surgery, a procedure that uses a laser to excise or destroy the tumor

- radiation therapy, a treatment that is useful for definitive treatment of primary tumors and some recurrent cancers

- interferon therapy, a drug therapy that prevents the growth of cancerous cells

- photodynamic therapy, a treatment in which the patient is given a photoactive compound followed by photoirradiation

Resources

BOOKS

Duffy, S., and G. V. Cobb. *Practical Electrosurgery.* Philadelphia: Lippincott, Williams and Wilkins, 1994.

PERIODICALS

Gonzalez, D. I., C. M. Zahn, M. G. Retzloff, W. F. Moore, E. R. Kost, and R. R. Snyder. "Recurrence of Dysplasia After Loop Electrosurgical Excision Procedures With Long-term Follow-up." *American Journal of Obstetrics and Gynecology* 184 (February 2001): 315–321.

Moniak, C. W., S. Kutzner, E. Adam, J. Harden, and R. H. Kaufman. "Endocervical Curettage in Evaluating Abnormal Cervical Cytology." *Journal of Reproductive Medicine* 45 (April 2000): 285–292.

Sheridan, A. T., and R. P. Dawber. "Curettage, Electrosurgery and Skin Cancer." *Australasian Journal of Dermatology* 41 (February 2000): 19–30.

Werlinger, K. D., G. Upton, and A. Y. Moore. "Recurrence Rates of Primary Nonmelanoma Skin Cancers Treated by Surgical Excision Compared to Electrodesiccation-curettage in a Private Dermatological Practice." *Dermatology and Surgery* 28 (December 2002): 1138–1142.

Williams, D. L., C. Dietrich, and J. McBroom. "Endocervical Curettage when Colposcopic Examination is Satisfactory and Normal." *Obstetrics and Gynecology* 95 (June 2000): 801–803.

ORGANIZATIONS

American Academy of Dermatology Association. 1350 I Street NW, Suite 880, Washington, DC 20005. (202) 842-3555. <http://www.aadassociation.org/>.

American College of Obstetricians and Gynecologists. 409 12th St., S.W., PO Box 96920 Washington, D.C. 20090-6920. (312) 786-1468. <http://www.acog.com/>.

American Society for Dermatologic Surgery (ASDS). 5550 Meadowbrook Dr., Suite 120, Rolling Meadows, IL 60008. (847) 956-0900. <http://www.asds-net.org>.

National Association for Women's Health. 300 W. Adams Street, Suite 328, Chicago, IL 60606-5101. (312) 786-1468. <http://www.nawh.org/>.

OTHER

CANCERLIT: NIH Cancer Information Center. [cited May 14, 2003]. <http://www.cancer.gov/CancerInformation/cancer literature>.

National Women's Health Information Center. [cited May 14, 2003]. <http://www.4woman,org/>.

The Skin Cancer Foundation. [cited May 14, 2003]. <http://www.skincancer.org/>.

Monique Laberge, Ph.D.

Cyclocryotherapy

Definition

Cyclocryotherapy (CCT) is a procedure that employs temperatures as low as -112°F (-80°C) to destroy the ciliary body, an organ in the anterior chamber of the eye be-

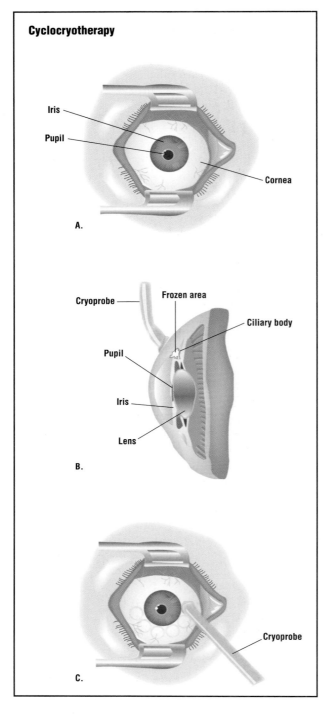

Cyclocryotherapy

A.

Iris

Pupil

Cornea

B.

Cryoprobe

Frozen area

Ciliary body

Pupil

Iris

Lens

C.

Cryoprobe

For cyclocryotherapy, the patient's eyelids are first retracted (A). A cryoprobe is applied to the outside of the eyeball in the area surrounding the iris (B). The probe freezes ciliary bodies in 50-60 seconds. The probe is applied to adjoining sites in a semicircle around the iris during one treatment (C). *(Illustration by GGS Inc.)*

hind the iris, which produces aqueous fluid. A certain amount of fluid is required to maintain the integrity of the eye, but an increase in intraocular fluid leads to an elevation in intraocular pressure (IOP); elevated IOP is a major cause of glaucoma. Ablation, or destruction, of part of the ciliary body lowers the IOP by decreasing the fluid or aqueous humor within the eye and thus helping to control glaucoma. The main purpose of CCT is to treat uncontrolled or refractory glaucoma. It is also used to reduce ocular pain in some patients with end-stage glaucoma.

Glaucoma is a general term used to describe a group of potentially blinding diseases, the main sign of which is a relatively high intraocular pressure. This increase in IOP causes damage to the optic nerve and the surrounding retinal tissue. In end-stage glaucoma, a patient's visual field is severely restricted. The increased intraocular pressure usually is caused by increased aqueous fluid in the eye. Treatment of glaucoma involves medical or surgical strategies to either increase the outflow of fluid from the eye, or to decrease the production of fluid in the eye, in an attempt to lower the IOP. The objective of glaucoma treatment is to attain an intraocular fluid level low enough such that damage to the optic nerve does not occur, yet is high enough such that the integrity of the eye is not sacrificed.

CCT is a last-resort treatment for patients in whom conventional medical and surgical techniques to control glaucoma have failed. Medical treatment involves the use of eyedrops that may be administered from one to four times a day. Surgical techniques are used to treat glaucoma when the number of eyedrops becomes cumbersome to the patient, or if patient compliance with medical therapy is difficult, or if medical therapy is not effective in lowering the IOP. One non-cyclodestructive surgical technique is filtration surgery, a procedure in which an outlet for the aqueous fluid is made through the sclera, the white fibrous covering of the anterior part of the eye. Another such procedure is argon laser trabeculoplasty, in which laser burns are made on the trabecular meshwork, the major drainage system to increase the number of drainage ports from the eye. Both these procedures promote outward flow of the intraocular fluid, decreasing the IOP.

In congenital glaucoma, other procedures that open up the fluid flow within the eye such as **goniotomy** or trabeculotomy are performed. Many patients with congenital glaucoma, due to a defect in the interior structure of the eye, have a limited ability to drain the aqueous fluid sufficiently. For pediatric patients, trabeculoplasty is not successful because the maturing eye will attempt to close the outlet. CCT may be performed on patients for which cyclophotocoagulation, another method of cyclodestruction, is not an option or not available. Many patients on whom this technique is employed have neovascular glaucoma, a type of glaucoma that is a result of uncontrolled diabetes or hypertension.

Purpose

The main purpose of CCT is to treat uncontrolled or refractory glaucoma. It is also used to reduce pain in some patients with end-stage glaucoma. This procedure lowers the intraocular pressure by destroying the source of intraocular fluid, the ciliary body, and subsequently lowering the intraocular pressure, as well as decreasing the pain of patients with some glaucomas, the most notable of which is neovascular glaucoma.

Demographics

Patients who undergo CCT are patients for whom certain techniques such as filtration surgery are contraindicated or for which other medical and surgical procedures have not been successful. Patients with neovascular glaucoma and congenital glaucoma make up a large percentage of the patients who undergo CCT. Because of the risks involved, cyclocryotherapy should not be performed on patients who have the potential for good vision, or on individuals who have had cataract surgery with intraocular lens implantation. CCT is a last-resort technique employed on patients for whom all other strategies have failed.

Description

Cyclocryotherapy is usually performed while the patient is awake and supine (laying down on the back). Prior to doing CCT, the doctor will inject an anesthetic into the posterior part of the eye; however, CCT may be performed under general anesthesia for anxious adults and for children. In performing the procedure, the surgeon locates the ciliary body with a lighted instrument and then applies a cryoprobe with a temperature of -112°F (-80°C) to the sclera of the eye. This probe is applied to the eye several times in a clockwise manner, using moderate pressure, carefully avoiding the area of the eye where the extraocular muscles, which control movement of the eye, attach to the eye. Each application by the probe lasts 50–60 seconds and usually only half of the eye is treated during the initial attempt; for less severe glaucoma and in older patients who respond better to this treatment, only a quarter of the eye will be treated. The surgeon leaves at least one quadrant of the eye untreated.

Immediately after surgery, a steroid is injected into the eye to reduce inflammation, and an eyedrop or ointment such as atropine is applied to the eye to maintain dilation of the eye. Some surgeons may inject into the eye an anesthetic that numbs the entire eye, including the

muscles. This injection has many risks associated with it, such as a droopy eyelid and an increased risk of corneal ulcers.

Diagnosis/Preparation

Cyclocryotherapy is a procedure of last resort in glaucoma patients. When all other therapies available to the patient have failed, CCT is considered, especially if the patient's vision is poor, i.e., less than 20/200, since there is a high risk of vision loss associated with this procedure. Patients and/or legal guardians of the patient are informed of the inherent risks and benefits, and CCT is performed only after **informed consent**. In preparation for CCT, the patient continues with all glaucoma medications up to the day of the procedure.

Aftercare

It is important that the patient continue with most topical glaucoma medications after surgery because a significant spike in IOP is expected after cyclocryotherapy. Glaucoma medications that should not be continued include miotics, which constrict the pupil and thus act in opposition to atropine, and drops derived from prostaglandins, which have very limited effect in some forms of glaucoma, especially neovascular glaucoma. Steroids are administered to the eye to reduce the risk of inflammation. Atropine, which dilates or enlarges the pupil and decreases post-operative discomfort, may be used a few times a day. Atropine and steroids are continued for a month after surgery.

As the retrobulbar anesthesia wears off, usually within 12 hours, **acetaminophen** (Tylenol) may be required for pain. In patients for whom the potential for good vision is unlikely and in whom the CCT is done to eliminate pain, the doctor may inject alcohol into the eye for continued pain relief.

Patients are seen for follow-up visits at a minimum of one day, one week, and one month after surgery.

QUESTIONS TO ASK THE DOCTOR

- How many of these procedures have you performed?
- Do you have advanced training in glaucoma surgery?
- Is CCT the best surgical procedure to treat my glaucoma or that of my child?
- What will vision be like after surgery?

Sometimes the procedure needs to be repeated and, if this is the case, it should be done no sooner than one month after the first attempt. The area that was treated initially is treated again and may be expanded to include a third quadrant.

Risks

The risks of this procedure are greater than for other types of glaucoma treatment. The most common side effect is pain after the procedure. A common risk of CCT is hypotony, which is a low level of fluid in the eye that can lead to phthisis bulbi, a condition in which the fluid level in the eye reaches a dangerously low level, such that the integrity of the eye is compromised. Other risks to consider are retinal detachment, inflammation of the iris, cataract formation, macular edema, and swelling of the cornea. The risk of inflammation within the eye is greater for diabetics. Loss of visual acuity, including total vision loss, is an associated risk of any of the previously mentioned risks and occurs in up to 67% of patients.

Patients with darker irises will have more side effects from this procedure, and pediatric patients with aniridia, or no iris, also have an increased rate of complications. Individuals who are aphakic, meaning they have had cataract extraction without a subsequent intraocular lens implantation, have fewer complications than patients with an intact lens.

Normal results

Normal results of cyclocryotherapy would be a reduction in the IOP and decreased intraocular pain. The overall success rate of CCT to reduce IOP in glaucoma patients is reported to be from 34% to 92%. Approximately 70% of patients with neovascular glaucoma have an IOP reduction of at least 50%. A determination of whether or not the surgery has been effective may not be clear until a month after CCT is performed; retreatment is required in up to one-third of adult patients. Repeated procedures increase the success of the surgery. CCT is successful in 90% of patients after a second surgery and in 95% after the third treatment. Among pediatric patients who undergo CCT, the success rate is only 30–44%, as the ciliary body of the child is more resistant to damage by **cryotherapy,** and thus repeat applications are more common.

Morbidity and mortality rates

Within four years of treatment, hypotony will occur in up to 12% of all patients who undergo CCT, but is seen in up to 40% of patients with neovascular glaucoma. Up to two-thirds of patients will lose some visual acuity after CCT; many of them will have vision worse than 20/400. About 20% of patients who have had cyclocryotherapy will develop cataracts.

Alternatives

An alternative to cyclocryotherapy is cyclophotocoagulation. This is another cyclodestructive procedure that employs the thermal energy of a laser instead of the freezing temperature of cryotherapy to ablate, or destroy, a part of the ciliary body. Cyclophotocoagulation is performed with the patient seated at the slit lamp biomicroscope. The eye is anesthetized prior to performing the procedure. In one type of cyclophotocoagulation, a fiberoptic laser endoscope is passed into the eye to help the surgeon visualize the interior of the eye. The energy of a laser passes through the endoscope and destroys the ciliary body directly. In another type of cyclodestruction, the energy of a diode laser is applied to the ciliary body through the sclera without the use of an endoscope.

Cyclophotocoagulation is as effective as CCT without as many of the complications inherent in CCT. The risks of transient elevation of intraocular inflammation and intraocular inflammation itself are decreased with this procedure over CCT for adult patients, but the risks associated with this procedure for pediatric patients are comparable to CCT. The cyclophotocoagulation procedure is not as painful as CCT.

Surgical removal of the part of the ciliary body is another alternative that is not often used. It is effective in lowering IOP, but the rate of complications such as hemorrhages in the vitreous, hypotony, and retinal detachment is high.

Therapeutic ultrasound can also be used to reduce the IOP in glaucoma patients, though the mechanism in which the IOP is lowered in this procedure is not clear.

In end-stage neovascular glaucoma patients who have no useful vision, medical treatment of pain control

KEY TERMS

Ciliary body—The part of the eye, located behind the iris, that makes the intraocular aqueous fluid.

Cyclocryotherapy—The use of subfreezing temperatures to treat glaucoma.

Glaucoma—A group of ocular diseases with which an increase in intraocular pressure causes a restriction in visual field and can lead to blindness.

Intraocular pressure (IOP)—The pressure inside the eye as measured by tonometry.

Ophthalmologist—A medical doctor with advanced training in the diagnosis and treatment of eye disease.

Neovascular glaucoma—A form of glaucoma that results from uncontrolled diabetes or hypertension.

Sclera—The white fibrous covering of the anterior part of the eye; it surrounds the cornea.

may sometimes be attained with the use of atropine and topical steroids alone. Retrobulbar injection of alcohol is sometimes necessary and, as a last resort in painful eyes without useful vision, enucleation, or removal, of the eye is required.

Resources

BOOKS

Albert, Daniel M. *Principles and Practice of Ophthalmology,* 2nd Ed. Philadelphia, PA: W.B. Saunders Company, 2000.

Azuara-Blanco, Augusto. *Handbook of Glaucoma.* London: Martin Dunitz Ltd., 2002.

Epstein, Daniel, et al. *Glaucoma.* Baltimore, MD: Williams and Wilkins, 1997.

Jaffe, Norman S. *Atlas of Ophthalmic Surgery,* London: Mosby-Wolfe, 1996.

Kanski, Jack. *Glaucoma: A Colour Manual of Diagnosis and Treatment,* 2nd Ed. Oxford: Butterworth Heinemann, 1996.

Ritch, Robert, et.al *The Glaucomas,* Vol. 2 Clinical Sciences. St Louis, MO: Mosby Yearbook, 1996.

Ritch, Robert, et.al *The Glaucomas,* Vol.3 Glaucoma Therapies. St Louis, MO: Mosby Yearbook, 1996.

PERIODICALS

Deepak, Gupta. "Surgical Update, Part III The Fallback Options When IOP Won't Drop." *Review of Optometry* (February 15, 2003): 79–86.

Sivak-Calcott, M. D., et al. "Evidence-based Recommendations for the Diagnosis and Treatment of Neovascular Glaucoma." *Ophthalmology* 108 (October 2001): 1767–1778.

Wagle, Nikhil. "Long-term Outcome of Cyclocryotherapy for Refractory Pediatric Glaucoma." *Ophthalmology* 105 (October 1998): 1921–7.

OTHER

Cyclotherapy for Endstage Glaucoma. <http.wills-glaucoma.org/cyclo.htm>.

Pediatric Glaucoma. <http://www.childrens.org/MSO/dept/lnav/view.asp?nav+554>.

Martha Reilly, OD

Cyclosporine *see* **Immunosuppressant drugs**

Cyst removal *see* **Ganglion cyst removal**

Cystectomy

Definition

Cystectomy is a surgical procedure that removes all or part of the urinary bladder, the muscular organ that collects urine from the kidneys for excretion at a later time. Partial or segmental cystectomy removes part of the bladder; simple cystectomy removes the entire bladder; and radical cystectomy removes the bladder as well as other pelvic organs or structures.

Purpose

Cystectomy is most commonly performed to treat cancer of the bladder. Once a patient has been diagnosed with bladder cancer, a staging system is used to indicate how far the cancer has spread and determine appropriate treatments. Superficial tumors isolated to the inner lining of the bladder (stage 0 or I) may be treated with non-surgical therapies such as chemotherapy or radiation, or with partial or simple cystectomy. Radical cystectomy is the standard treatment for cancer that has invaded the bladder muscle (Stage II, III, or IV). Muscle-invasive cancer accounts for 90% of all bladder cancers.

Other conditions that may require cystectomy include interstitial cystitis (chronic inflammation of the bladder), endometriosis that has spread to the bladder, severe urinary dysfunction, damage to the bladder from radiation or other treatments, or excessive bleeding from the bladder.

Demographics

Approximately 56,500 cases of urinary bladder cancer are diagnosed in the United States annually, with approximately 12,600 men and women dying of the disease each year. Men are more often diagnosed with bladder cancer (2.6 men for each woman diagnosed), and they also have a higher mortality rate (two men for each woman that dies). The average age that the disease is diagnosed is 65 years.

More cases of bladder cancer are found among white men and women. The Centers for Disease Control and Prevention (CDC) reported that from 1992–1999, whites were diagnosed with bladder cancer at a rate of 21.9 per 100,000 persons, while African Americans had a rate of only 12.4 per 100,000. The mortality rate, however, is similar among white and African-American patients (4.5 and 4.1 per 100,000 persons), respectively.

Description

Partial cystectomy

During partial or segmental cystectomy, only the area of the bladder where the cancer is found is removed. This allows for most of the bladder to be preserved. Because the cancer must not have spread to the bladder muscle and must be isolated to one area, partial cystectomy is only used infrequently for the patients who meet these select criteria.

The patient is first placed under general anesthesia. After an incision is made into the lower abdomen, the bladder is identified and isolated. The surgeon may choose to perform the operation with the bladder remaining inside the abdominal cavity (transperitoneal approach) or with the bladder lifted outside of the abdominal cavity (extraperitoneal approach). The cancerous area is excised (cut out) with a 0.8 in (2 cm) margin to ensure that all abnormal cells are removed. The bladder is then closed with stitches. The pelvic lymph nodes may also be removed during the procedure. After the cancerous tissue is removed, it is examined by a pathologist to determine if the margins of the tissue are clear of abnormal cells.

Simple or radical cystectomy

While partial cystectomy is considered a bladder-conserving surgery, simple and radical cystectomy involves the removal of the entire bladder. In the case of radical cystectomy, other pelvic organs and structures are also removed because of the tendency of bladder cancer to spread to nearby tissues. After the patient is placed under general anesthesia, an incision is made into the lower abdomen. Blood vessels leading to and from the bladder are ligated (tied off), and the bladder is divided from the urethra, ureters, and other tissues holding it in place. The bladder may then be removed.

The surgical procedure for radical cystectomy differs between male and female patients. In men, the prostate, seminal vesicles, and pelvic lymph nodes are removed with the bladder. In women, the uterus, fallopian tubes, ovaries, anterior (front) part of the vagina, and pelvic lymph nodes

are removed with the bladder. If the surgery is being performed as a treatment for cancer, the removed tissues may be examined for the presence of abnormal cells.

Urinary diversion

Once the bladder is removed, a new method for excreting urine must be created. One commonly used approach is the ileal conduit. A piece of the small intestine is removed, cleaned, and tied at one end to form a tube. The other end is used to form a stoma, an opening through the abdominal wall to the outside. The ureters are then connected to the tube. Urine produced by the kidneys flows down the ureters, into the tube, and through the stoma. The patient wears a bag to collect the urine.

For continent cutaneous diversion, a pouch is constructed out of portions of the small and large intestine; the ureters are connected to the pouch and a stoma is created through the abdominal wall. Urine is removed by inserting a thin tube (catheter) into the stoma when the pouch is full. Alternatively, a similar pouch called a neobladder may be created, attached to both the ureters and the urethra, in an attempt to preserve as close to normal bladder function as possible.

Diagnosis/Preparation

The medical team will discuss the procedure and tell the patient where the stoma will appear and what it will look like. The patient will receive instruction on caring for a stoma and bag. A period of fasting and an enema may be required.

Aftercare

After the operation, the patient is given fluid-based nutrition until the intestines begin to function normally again. **Antibiotics** are given to prevent infection. The nature of cystectomy means that there will be major lifestyle changes for the person undergoing the operation. Men may become impotent if nerves controlling pe-

Cystectomy

In a cystectomy with ileal conduit, an incision is made in the patient's lower abdomen (A). The ureters are disconnected from the bladder, which is then removed (B). They are then attached to a section of ileum (small intestine) that has been removed and refashioned for that purpose (C). A stoma, or hole in the abdominal wall, is created at the site to allow drainage of the urine (D). *(Illustration by GGS Inc.)*

nile erection are cut during removal of the bladder. Infertility is a consequence for women undergoing radical cystectomy because the ovaries and uterus are removed. Most women who undergo cystectomy, however, are postmenopausal and past their childbearing years.

Patients are fitted with an external bag that connects to the stoma and collects the urine. The bag is generally worn around the waist under the clothing. It takes a period of adjustment to get used to wearing the bag. Because there is no bladder, urine is excreted as it is produced.

QUESTIONS TO ASK THE DOCTOR

- Why is cystectomy recommended in my case?
- In the case of radical cystectomy, what other organs/structures will be removed?
- What method of urinary diversion will be performed?
- What non-surgical options are available to me?
- How long after surgery may I resume normal activity?

KEY TERMS

Endometriosis—A condition in which cells from the inner lining of the uterus grow elsewhere in the body.

Lymph nodes—Small organs located throughout the body that can filter out cancer cells and bacteria.

Ureters—Tubes that connect the kidneys to the bladder; urine produced by the kidneys passes through the ureters to the bladder.

The stoma must be treated properly to ensure that it does not become infected or blocked. Patients must be trained to care for their stoma. Often, there is a period of psychological adjustment to the major change in lifestyle created by the stoma and bag. Patients should be prepared for this by their physician.

Risks

As with any major surgery, there is a risk of infection; in this case, infection of the intestine is especially dangerous as it can lead to peritonitis (inflammation of the membrane lining the abdomen). In the case of partial cystectomy, there is a risk of urine leakage from the bladder incision site. Other risks include injury to nearby organs, complications associated with general anesthesia (such as respiratory distress), excessive blood loss, sexual dysfunction, or urinary incontinence (inadvertent leakage of urine).

Normal results

During a successful partial cystectomy, the cancerous or damaged area of the bladder is removed and the patient retains urinary control. A successful simple or radical cystectomy results in the removal of the bladder and the creation of a urinary diversion, with little or no effect on sexual function. Intestinal function returns to normal and the patient learns proper care of the stoma and bag. He or she adjusts to lifestyle changes and returns to a normal routine of work and recreation.

Morbidity and mortality rates

The overall rate of complications associated with radical cystectomy may be as high as 25–35%; major complications occur at a rate of 5%. The rate of radical cystectomy-related deaths is 1–3%. Partial cystectomy has a complication rate of 11–29%. Some studies have placed the rate of cancer reoccurrence after partial cystectomy at 40–80%.

Alternatives

Transurethral resection (TUR) is one method that may be used to treat superficial bladder tumors. A cystoscope (a thin, tubular instrument used to visualize the interior of the bladder) is inserted into the bladder through the urethra and used to remove any cancerous tissue. Non-surgical options include chemotherapy and radiation.

Resources

BOOKS

Walsh, Patrick C., et al., editors. *Campbell's Urology,* 8th edition. Philadelphia: Elsevier Science, 2002.

PERIODICALS

"Bladder Cancer, Part III: Treatment Approaches in Current Practice and in Evaluation." *Future Oncology* 6, no. 5 (April 30, 2001): 1322–40.

Carrion, Rafael, and John Seigne. "Surgical Management of Bladder Carcinoma." *Cancer Control: Journal of the Moffitt Cancer Center* 9, no. 4 (October 31, 2002): 284–92.

ORGANIZATIONS

American Cancer Society. 1599 Clifton Road NE, Atlanta, GA 30329. (800) ACS-2345. <http://www.cancer.org>.

Cancer Information Service, National Cancer Institute. Building 31, Room 10A19, 9000 Rockville Pike, Bethesda, MD 20892. (800) 4-CANCER. <http://www.nci.nih.gov/cancerinfo/index.html>.

OTHER

"All About Bladder Cancer." *American Cancer Society,* 2003 [cited April 4, 2003] <http://www.cancer.org/docroot/CRI/CRI_2x.asp>.

"Cancer Facts and Figures, 2002." *American Cancer Society,* 2002 [cited April 4, 2003] <http://www.cancer.org/downloads/STT/CancerFacts&Figures2002TM.pdf>.

Eggner, Scott, and Steven Campbell. "Cystectomy, Radical." *eMedicine,* August 1, 2001 [cited April 4, 2003] <http://www.emedicine.com/med/topic3061.htm>.

Feng, Adrian H. "Cystectomy, Partial." *eMedicine,* February 8, 2002 [cited April 4, 2003] <http://www.emedicine.com/med/topic3043.htm>.

Ries, L. A. G., et al., eds. "SEER Cancer Statistics Review." *National Cancer Institute,* 2002 [cited April 4, 2003] <http://seer.cancer.gov/csr/1973_1999>.

John T. Lohr, PhD
Stephanie Dionne Sherk

Cystocele repair

Definition

A cystocele is the protrusion or prolapse of the bladder into the vagina. A number of surgical interventions are available to treat cystoceles.

Purpose

A prolapse occurs when an organ falls out of its normal anatomical position. The pelvic organs normally have tissue (muscle, ligaments, etc.) holding them in place. Certain factors, however, may cause those tissues to weaken, leading to prolapse of the organs. A cystocele may be the result of a central or lateral (side) defect. A central defect occurs when the bladder protrudes into the center of the anterior (front) wall of the vagina due to a defect in the pubocervical fascia (fibrous tissue that separates the bladder and vagina). The pubocervical fascia is also attached on each side to tough connective tissue called the arcus tendineus; if a defect occurs close to this attachment, it is called a lateral or paravaginal defect. A central and lateral defect may be present simultaneously. The location of the defect determines what surgical procedure is performed.

Factors that are linked to cystocele development include age, repeated childbirth, hormone deficiency, menopause, constipation, ongoing physical activity, heavy lifting, and prior **hysterectomy**. Symptoms of bladder prolapse include stress incontinence (inadvertent leakage of urine with physical activity), urinary frequency, difficult urination, a vaginal bulge, vaginal pressure or pain, painful sexual intercourse, and lower back pain. Urinary incontinence is the most common symptom of a cystocele.

Surgery is generally not performed unless the symptoms of the prolapse have begun to interfere with daily life. A staging system is used to grade the severity of a cystocele. A stage I, II, or III prolapse descends to progressively lower areas of the vagina. A stage IV prolapse descends to

or protrudes through the vaginal opening. Surgery is generally reserved for stage III and IV cystoceles.

Demographics

Approximately 22.7 out of every 10,000 women will undergo pelvic prolapse surgery. The rate is highest among women between 60 and 69 years of age (42 per 10,000); the mean age of patients is 54.6. White women undergo pelvic prolapse surgery at a rate of 19.6 per 10,000 and a mean age of 54.3, while 6.4 per 10,000 African American women have surgery at a mean age of 49.3.

A 2002 study indicated cystocele repair accounts for 8% of all prolapse repair surgeries; in 1997, approximately 18,500 cystocele repairs were performed. Cystocele repair was combined with **rectal prolapse repair** in 10% of prolapse surgeries, with hysterectomy (surgical removal of the uterus) in 6%, and with both procedures in 16%.

Description

The goals of cystocele repair are to relieve a patient's symptoms, to improve or maintain urinary and sexual function, to return pelvic structures to their original position, and to prevent the formation of new defects. The anatomical structures involved in a cystocele may be approached vaginally, abdominally, or laparoscopically.

Vaginal repair

Anterior **colporrhaphy** is the most common procedure to repair a central defect. The patient is first given general or regional anesthesia. A speculum is inserted into the vagina to hold it open during the procedure. An incision is made into the vaginal skin and the defect in the underlying fascia is identified. The vaginal skin is separated from the fascia and the defect is folded over

Cystocele repair

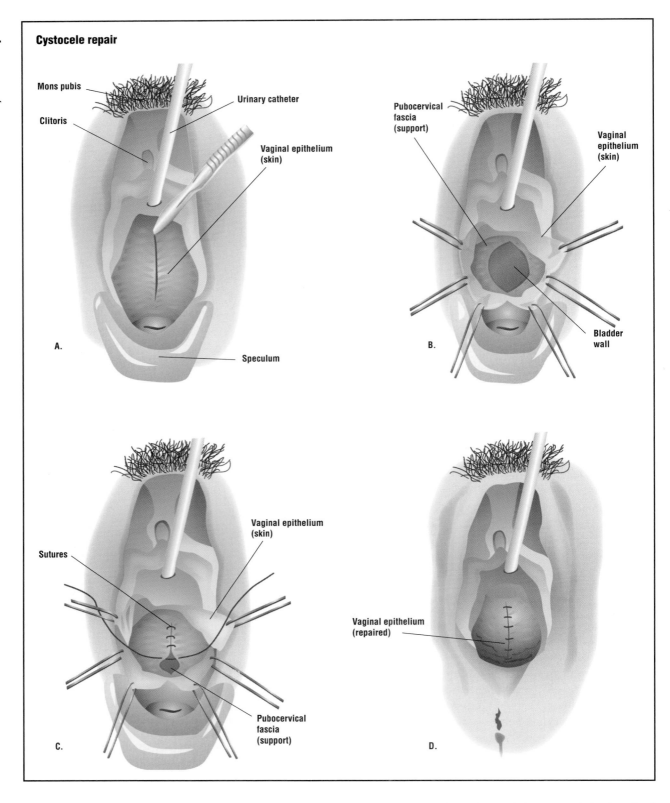

A.

Mons pubis

Clitoris

Urinary catheter

Vaginal epithelium (skin)

Speculum

B.

Pubocervical fascia (support)

Vaginal epithelium (skin)

Bladder wall

C.

Sutures

Vaginal epithelium (skin)

Pubocervical fascia (support)

D.

Vaginal epithelium (repaired)

In this cystocele repair by anterior colporrhaphy, a speculum is used to hold open the vagina, and the cystocele is visualized (A). The wall of the vagina is cut open to reveal an opening in the supporting structures, or fascia (B). The defect is closed (C), and the vaginal skin is repaired (D). *(Illustration by GGS Inc.)*

and sutured (stitched). Any excess vaginal skin is removed and the incision is closed with stitches.

Lateral defects may be repaired vaginally or abdominally. During a vaginal paravaginal repair, the approach and initial incision are similar to anterior colporrhaphy. The defect to the fascia is located and reattached to the arcus tendineus using sutures. The incision may then be stitched closed.

Abdominal and laparoscopic repair

A cystocele caused by a lateral defect may be treated through an abdominal incision made transversely (from side to side) just above the pubic hairline. The space between the pubic bone and bladder is identified and opened and the pubocervical fascia reattached to the arcus tendineus using methods similar to the vaginal paravaginal repair. In some cases, a retropubic colposuspension is performed during the same surgery. Also called a Burch procedure, colposuspension treats urinary incontinence by suspending the bladder neck to nearby ligaments with sutures. Other surgical treatments for incontinence may be combined with paravaginal repair.

A lateral defect may also be repaired by **laparoscopy**, a surgical procedure in which a laparoscope (a thin, lighted tube) and various instruments are inserted into the abdomen through small incisions. A patient's recovery time following laparoscopic surgery is shorter and less painful than following a traditional laparotomy (a larger surgical incision into the abdominal cavity).

Diagnosis/Preparation

Physical examination is most often used to diagnose a cystocele. A speculum is inserted into the vagina and the patient is asked to strain or sit in an upright position; this increase in intra-abdominal pressure maximizes the degree of prolapse and aids in diagnosis. The physician then inspects the walls of the vagina for prolapse or bulging.

In some cases, a physical examination cannot sufficiently diagnose pelvic prolapse. For example, cystography may be used to determine the extent of a cystocele; the bladder is filled by urinary catheter with contrast medium and then x rayed. Ultrasound or **magnetic resonance imaging** may also be used to visualize the pelvic structures.

Women who have gone through menopause may be given six weeks of estrogen therapy prior to surgery; this is thought to improve circulation to the vaginal walls and thus improve recovery time. **Antibiotics** may be administered to decrease the risk of postsurgical infection. An

intravenous (IV) line is placed and a Foley catheter is inserted into the bladder directly preceding surgery.

Aftercare

A Foley catheter may remain for one to two days after surgery. The patient is given a liquid diet until normal bowel function returns. The patient also is instructed to avoid activities for several weeks that cause strain on the surgical site; these include lifting, coughing, long periods of standing, sneezing, straining with bowel movements, and sexual intercourse.

Risks

Risks of cystocele repair include potential complications associated with anesthesia, infection, bleeding, injury to other pelvic structures, dyspareunia (painful intercourse), recurrent prolapse, and failure to correct the defect.

Normal results

A woman usually is able to resume normal activities, including sexual intercourse, in about four weeks after the procedure. After successful cystocele repair, symptoms recede, although a separate procedure may be needed to treat stress incontinence.

Morbidity and mortality rates

The risk of cystocele recurrence following surgical repair depends on the procedure used to treat it. Anterior colporrhaphy is associated with a 0–20% rate of recurrence; this rate is higher when colporrhaphy is combined with other surgical procedures. Abdominal paravaginal repair results in a 5% chance of recurrence, while vaginal paravaginal repair has the highest recurrence rate (7–22%).

KEY TERMS

Burch procedure—A surgical procedure, also called retropubic colposuspension, in which the neck of the bladder is suspended from nearby ligaments with sutures. It is performed to treat urinary incontinence.

Colporrhapy—A surgical procedure in which the vagina is sutured.

Ligaments—Tough fibrous connective tissue.

Magnetic resonance imaging—A specialized imaging technique used to visualize internal structures; it is considered superior to the standard x ray.

Pubocervical fascia—Fibrous tissue that separates the vagina and the bladder.

Ultrasound—A procedure that uses high-frequency sound waves to visualize structures in the human body.

Speculum—A retractor used to separate the walls of the vagina and aid in visual examination.

Alternatives

Surgery is generally reserved for more severe cystoceles. Milder cases may be treated by a number of medical interventions. The physician may recommend that the patient do Kegel exercises, a series of contractions and relaxations of the muscles in the perineal area. These exercises are thought to strengthen the pelvic floor and may help prevent urinary incontinence.

A pessary, a device that is inserted into the vagina to help support the pelvic organs, may be recommended. Pessaries come in different shapes and sizes and must be fitted to the patient by a physician. Hormone replacement therapy may also be prescribed if the woman has gone through menopause; hormones may improve the quality of the supporting tissues in the pelvis.

Resources

BOOKS

Ryan, Kenneth J., et al. *Kistner's Gynecology and Women's Health.* 7th ed. St. Louis, MO: Mosby, Inc., 1999.

Walsh, Patrick C., et al. *Campbell's Urology.* 8th ed. Philadelphia: Elsevier Science, 2002.

PERIODICALS

Brown, Jeanette S., L. Elaine Waetjen, Leslee L. Subak, David H. Thom, Stephen Van Den Eeden, and Eric Vittinghoff. "Pelvic Organ Prolapse Surgery in the United States, 1997." *American Journal of Obstetrics and Gynecology* 186 (April 2002): 712–6.

Cespedes, R. Duane, Cindy A. Cross, and Edward J. McGuire. "Pelvic Prolapse: Diagnosing and Treating Cystoceles, Rectoceles, and Enteroceles." *Medscape Women's Health eJournal* 3 (1998).

Viera, Anthony, and Margaret Larkins-Pettigrew. "Practice Use of the Pessary." *American Family Physician* 61 (May 1, 2000): 2719–2726.

ORGANIZATIONS

American Board of Obstetrics and Gynecology. 2915 Vine Street, Dallas, TX 75204. (214) 871-1619. <http://www.abog.org>.

American Urological Association. 1120 North Charles Street, Baltimore, MD 21201. (410) 727-1100. <http://www.auanet.org>.

OTHER

"Cystocele (Fallen Bladder)." *National Kidney and Urologic Diseases Information Clearinghouse.* March 2002 [cited April 11, 2003]. <http://www.niddk.nih.gov/health/urolog/summary/cystocel>.

Miklos, John. "Vaginal Prolapse Relaxation." *OBGYN.net.* 2002 [cited April 11, 2003]. <http://www.obgyn.net/urogyn/urogyn.asp?page=/urogyn/articles/miklos-vagprolapse>.

Stephanie Dionne Sherk

Cystoscopy

Definition

Cystoscopy (cystourethroscopy) is a diagnostic procedure that uses a cystoscope, which is an endoscope especially designed for urological use to examine the bladder, lower urinary tract, and prostate gland. It can also be used to collect urine samples, perform biopsies, and remove small stones.

Purpose

Cystoscopy is performed by urologists to examine the entire bladder lining and take biopsies of any questionable areas. Cystoscopy may be prescribed for patients who display the following conditions:

• blood in the urine (hematuria)
• inability to control urination (incontinence)
• urinary tract infection
• signs of congenital abnormalities in the urinary tract
• suspected tumors in the bladder
• bladder or kidney stones
• signs or symptoms of an enlarged prostate

- pain or difficulty urinating (dysuria)
- disorders of or injuries to the urinary tract
- symptoms of interstitial cystitis

Blood and urine studies, in addition to x rays of the kidneys, ureters, and bladder, may be performed before a cystoscopy to obtain as much diagnostic information as possible. During the cystoscopy, a retrograde pyelogram may also be performed to examine the kidneys and ureters.

Description

There are two types of cystoscopes used to carry out the procedure, a rigid type and a flexible type. Both types are used for the same purposes and differ only in their method of insertion. The rigid type requires that the patient adopt the lithotomy position, meaning that the patient lies on his or her back with knees up and apart. The flexible cystoscope does not require the lithotomy position.

A cystoscopy typically lasts from 10–40 minutes. The patient is asked to urinate before surgery and advised that relaxing pelvic muscles will help make this part of the procedure easier. A well-lubricated flexible or rigid cystoscope (urethroscope) is passed through the urethra into the bladder where a urine sample is taken. There may be some discomfort as the instrument is inserted. Fluid is then injected to inflate the bladder and allow the urologist to examine the entire bladder wall.

The cystoscope uses a lighted tip for guidance and enables biopsies to be taken or small stones to be removed through a hollow channel in the cystoscope.

During a cystoscopy, the urologist may remove bladder stones or kidney stones, gather tissue samples, and perform x-ray studies. To remove stones, an instrument that looks like a tiny basket or grasper is inserted through the cystoscope so that small stones can be extracted through the scope's channel. For a biopsy, special forceps are inserted through the cystoscope to pinch off a tissue sample. Alternatively, a small brush-like instrument may be inserted to scrape off some tissue. To perform x-ray studies such as a retrograde pyelogram, a dye is injected into the ureter by way of a catheter passed through the cystoscope. After completion of all required tests, the cystoscope is removed.

Preparation

Patients may be asked to give a urine sample before cytoscopy to check for infection and to avoid urinating for an hour before this part of the procedure. They wear a hospital gown during the procedure and the lower part of the body is covered with a sterile drape. A sedative may be given about one hour prior to the operation to help the patient relax. The region of the urethra is cleansed and a local anesthetic is applied. Spinal or general anesthesia may also be used for the procedure. Distension of the bladder with fluid is particularly painful, and if it needs to be done, as in the case of evaluating interstitial cystitis, general anesthesia is required. A signed consent form is necessary for this procedure.

Aftercare

After removal of the cystoscope, the urethra is usually sore, and patients should expect to feel a burning sensation while urinating for one to two days following

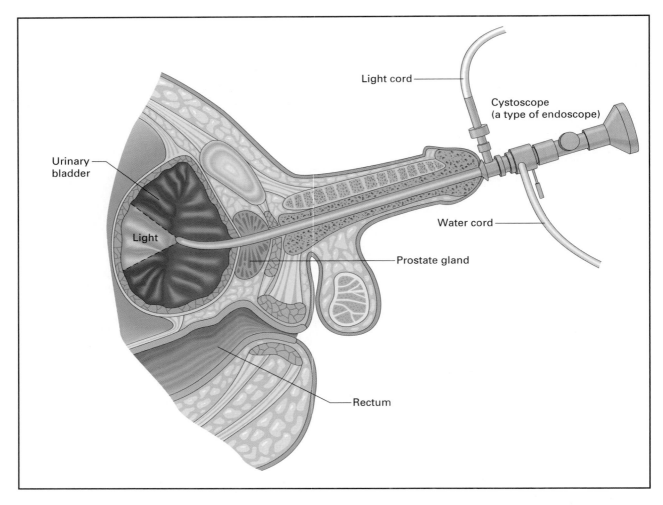

Illustration of cytoscopy procedure. *(From Fundamentals of Nursing, Standards & Practice, 1st edition by DELAUNE. (c) 1998. Reprinted with permission of Delmar Learning, a division of Thomson Learning: www.thomsonrights.com. Fax: 800-730-2215.)*

the procedure. To alleviate discomfort or pain, patients may be prescribed pain medication, and **antibiotics** may also be required to prevent infection. Minor pain may also be treated with over-the-counter, nonprescription drugs such as **acetaminophen**. To relieve discomfort, patients may be advised to drink two 8-oz glasses of water each hour for two hours and to take a warm bath to relieve the burning feeling. If not able to bathe, they may be advised to hold a warm, damp washcloth over the urethral opening.

Patients who have undergone a cystoscopy are instructed to:

• Take warm baths to relieve pain.

• Rest and refrain from driving for several days, especially if general anesthesia was used.

• Expect any blood in the urine to clear up in one to two days.

• Avoid strenuous **exercise** during recovery.

• Postpone sexual relations until the urologist determines that healing is complete.

Risks

As with any surgical procedure, there are some risks involved with a cystoscopy. Complications may include profuse bleeding, a damaged urethra, a perforated bladder, a urinary tract infection, or an injured penis.

Patients should contact their physician if they experience any of the following symptoms after the procedure, including pain, redness, swelling, drainage, or bleeding from the surgical site; signs of generalized infection, which may include headache, muscle aches, dizziness, or an overall ill feeling and fever; nausea or vomiting; or difficult or painful urination.

KEY TERMS

Anesthetic—A drug that causes loss of sensation. It is used to lessen the pain of surgery and medical procedures.

Bladder—The bladder is located in the lower part of the abdomen; it is a structure like a small balloon that collects urine for temporary storage and is emptied from time to time by urinating.

Catheter—A tubular, flexible surgical instrument for withdrawing fluids from (or introducing fluids into) a body cavity, especially one for introduction into the bladder through the urethra for the withdrawal of urine.

Cystoscope—Endoscope especially designed for urological use to examine the bladder, lower urinary tract, and prostate gland.

Diverticula—A pouch or sac occurring normally or from a herniation or defect in a membrane.

Endoscope—A highly flexible, thin viewing instrument used to see inside body cavities.

Endoscopy—A minimally invasive procedure that involves examination of body organs or cavities using an endoscope.

Interstitial cystitis—A chronic inflammatory condition of the bladder involving symptoms of bladder pain, frequent urination, and burning during urination.

Retrograde pyelogram—A pyelography or x-ray technique in which a dye is injected into the kidneys through the ureters.

Ureter—The tube that carries urine from each kidney to the bladder.

Urethra—The tube that carries urine from the bladder to outside the body. In females, the urethral opening is between the vagina and clitoris; in males, the urethra travels through the penis, opening at the tip.

Urogynecologist—A physician that specializes in female medical conditions concerning the urinary and reproductive systems.

Uroradiologist—A radiologist who specializes in diagnostic imaging of the urinary tract and kidneys.

Cystoscopy is a commonly performed procedure, but it is an invasive technique that involves small yet significant risk. If anesthesia is required, there is additional risk, particularly for people who are obese, smoke, or are in poor health. Those undergoing anesthesia must inform the doctor of any medications they are taking.

Normal results

A successful cystoscopy includes a thorough examination of the bladder and collection of urine samples for cultures. If no abnormalities are seen, the results are indicated as normal. In this case, the bladder wall appears smooth and the bladder is seen to be of normal size, shape, and position, without obstructions, growths, or stones.

The treating physician can tell the patient what was seen inside the bladder right after the procedure. If a biopsy sample was taken, this will take several days to be examined and tested.

Cystoscopy allows the urologist to detect inflammation of the bladder lining, prostatic enlargement, or tumors. If these are seen, further evaluation or biopsies may be needed. Cystoscopy with bladder distention can also evaluate interstitial cystitis. Bladder stones, urethral strictures, diverticula, or congenital abnormalities can also be detected.

Alternatives

There are procedures that can provide some information about the lining of the bladder, for example, x rays; however, none of these provide as much information to the doctor as a cystoscopy.

Resources

BOOKS

Buckman, Robert. "Bladder." In *What You Really Need To Know About Cancer: A Comprehensive Guide for Patients and Their Families.* Baltimore, MD: The Johns Hopkins University Press, 1997.

Miller, B. E., ed. *An Atlas of Sigmoidoscopy and Cystoscopy.* Boca Raton: CRC Press-Parthenon Publishers, 2001.

Segen, Joseph C., and Joseph Stauffer. "Cystoscopy." In *The Patient's Guide To Medical Tests: Everything You Need To Know About The Tests Your Doctor Prescribes.* New York: Facts On File, 1998.

Tierney, Lawrence M. Jr., Stephen J. McPhee, and Maxine A. Papadakis, eds. "Urology." In *Current Medical Diagnosis and Treatment.* Stamford, CT: Appleton & Lange, 1996.

PERIODICALS

Fraczyk, L., H. Godfrey, and R. Feneley. "Flexible Cystoscopy: Outpatients or Domiciliary?" *British Journal of Community Nursing* 7 (February 2002): 69–74.

Jabs, C. F., and H. P. Drutz. "The Role of Intraoperative Cystoscopy in Prolapse and Incontinence Surgery." *American Journal of Obstetrics and Gynecology* 185 (December 2001): 1368–1371.

Kwon, C. H., R. Goldberg, S. Koduri, and P. K. Sand. "The Use of Intraoperative Cystoscopy in Major Vaginal and Urogynecologic Surgeries." *American Journal of Obstetrics and Gynecology* 187 (December 2002): 1471–1472.

Payne, D. A., and R. C. Kockelbergh. "Improving the View at Flexible Cystoscopy." *Annals of The Royal College of Surgeons of England* 85 (March 2003): 132–138.

Sant, Grannum R., and Philip M. Hanno. "Interstitial Cystitis: Current Issues and Controversies in Diagnosis." *Urology* 57, Supplement 6A (June 2001): 82–88.

Satoh, E., N. Miyao, H. Tachiki, and Y. Fujisawa. "Prediction of Muscle Invasion of Bladder Cancer by Cystoscopy." *European Urology* 41 (February 2002): 178–181.

ORGANIZATIONS

American Urological Association. 1120 North Charles Street, Baltimore, MD 21201. (410) 727-1100. <http://www.auanet.org>.

American Foundation for Urologic Disease. 1128 North Charles Street, Baltimore, MD 21201. (800) 242-2383. <http://www.afud.org>.

Interstitial Cystitis Association. 51 Monroe Street, Suite 1402, Rockville, MD 20850. (301) 610-5300. <http://www.ichelp.org>.

Society of Urologic Nurses and Associates. East Holly Avenue, Box 56, Pitman, NJ 08071-0056. (609) 256-2335. <http://suna.inurse.com/>.

OTHER

"Cystoscopy." *Harvard Medical School.* <www.health.harvard.edu/fhg/diagnostics/cysto/cystoWhat.shtml>.

"Cystoscopy." *Medline Plus.* <www.nlm.nih.gov/medlineplus/ency/article/003903.htm>.

"What Is IC? Interstitial Cystitis Fact Sheet." *Interstitial Cystitis Association.* <http://www.ichelp.org/whatisic/ICFActSheet.html>.

Jennifer E. Sisk
Monique Laberge, PhD

D & C *see* **Dilatation and curettage**

Death and dying

Definition

Death is the end of life, a permanent cessation of all vital functions. Dying refers to the body's preparation for death, which may be very short in the case of accidental death, or can last weeks or months in some patients such as those with cancer.

Description

Risks of surgery

Specific risks vary from surgery to surgery and should be discussed with a physician. All surgeries and every administration of anesthesia have some risks; they are dependent upon many factors including the type of surgery and the medical condition of the patient. The patient should ask the anesthesiologist about any risks that may be associated with the anesthesia. Specific standards are set by the American Society of Anesthesiologists to enhance the safety and quality of anesthesia before surgery, basic methods of monitoring patients during surgery, and the best patient care during recovery.

Overwhelming data compiled in 2001 has confirmed that albumin is an effective marker of general nutrition; low albumin levels can increase the likelihood of post-surgery complications such as pneumonia, infection, and the inability to wean from a ventilator, by as much as 50%. In a national study of 54,000 surgery patients (average age of 61 years old), it was found that only one in five surgical patients were tested for low albumin before their operations.

In a study of 2,989 hospitalized patients admitted for more than one day, risk factors such as cholesterol levels (primarily low levels of high-density lipoprotein, HDL) and low serum albumin were associated with in-hospital death, infection, and length of stay. During the study follow-up, 62 (2%) of the patients died, 382 (13%) developed a nosocomial infection, and 257 (9%) developed a surgical site infection.

The National Veterans Affairs Surgical Risk Study was conducted in 44 Veterans Affairs Medical Centers and included 87,078 major noncardiac operations performed under general, spinal, or epidural anesthesia. Patient risk factors predictive of postoperative death included serum albumin level, American Society of Anesthesia class, emergency operation, and 31 additional preoperative variables.

Other factors related to death during surgery are: increasing age, **emergency surgery**, and general postoperative complications including cardiac, renal, and pulmonary complications. Age-related changes in the immune system play a significant role in the increased risk of infection, decreased ability to fight diseases, and slower wound healing after surgery. An aging body is more susceptible to subsequent infections because of previous illness or surgery and the subsequent weakening of the immune system. The anti-inflammatory medications (e.g., to control conditions such as arthritis) that many older people take are also known to slow wound healing.

One study found that risk of death during **coronary artery bypass graft surgery** is associated with hospital volume, i.e., the number of surgeries performed. High volume hospitals had a lower mortality rate during surgery. Mortality decreased with increasing volume of surgeries performed (3.6% in low [less than 500 cases], 3% in moderate [500-1,000 cases], and 2% in high [over 1,000 cases] volume hospitals). Thus, the volume of surgeries performed may be an important consideration when selecting a hospital.

Complications of surgery

The most common complications to surgery that can prove fatal are infection, bleeding, and complications of anesthesia.

The Joint Commission's Board of Commissioners reviewed 64 cases related to operative and post-operative complications since the late 1990s. Of the events reviewed, 84% of the complications resulted in patient deaths, while 16% resulted in a serious injury. All of the cases occurred in acute care hospitals; cases directly related to medication errors or to the administration of anesthesia were excluded. Of these complications, 58% occurred during the postoperative procedure period, 23% during intraoperative procedures, 13% during post-anesthesia recovery, and 6% during anesthesia induction.

The following types of procedures were most frequently associated with these reported complications:

- endoscopy and/or interventional imaging
- catheter or tube insertion
- open abdominal surgery
- head and neck surgery
- thoracic surgery
- orthopedic surgery

Of the 64 cases reviewed, 90% occurred in relation to non-emergent (elective or scheduled) procedures. The most frequent complications by type of procedure included the following:

- Naso-gastric/feeding tube insertion into the trachea or a bronchus.
- Massive fluid overload from absorption of irrigation fluids during genito-urinary/gynecological procedures.
- Endoscopic procedures (including non-gastrointestinal procedures) with perforation of adjacent organs. Of all abdominal and thoracic endoscopic surgery, liver lacerations were among the most common complications.
- Central venous catheter insertion into an artery.
- Burns from electrocautery used with a flammable prep solution.
- Open orthopedic procedures associated with acute respiratory failure, including cardiac arrest in the operating room.
- Imaging-directed percutaneous biopsy or tube placement resulting in liver laceration, peritonitis, or respiratory arrest while temporarily off prescribed oxygen.

Complications associated with misplacement of tubes or catheters usually involved a failure to confirm the position of the tube or catheter, a failure to communicate the results of the confirmation procedure, or misinterpretation of the radiographic image by a non-radiologist.

Preparing for death or incapacitation legally

An advance directive is a way to allow caregivers to know a patient's wishes, should the patient become un-able to make a medical decision. The hospital must be told about a patient's advance directive at the time of admission. Description of the type of care for different levels of illness should be in an advance directive. For instance, a patient may wish to have or not to have a certain type of care in the case of terminal or critical illness or unconsciousness. An advance directive will protect the patient's wishes in these matters.

A **living will** is one type of advance directive and may take effect when a patient has been deemed terminally ill. Terminal illness in general assumes a life span of six months or less. A living will allows a patient to outline treatment options without interference from an outside party.

A durable **power of attorney** for health care (DPA) is similar to a living will; however, it takes effect any time unconsciousness or inability to make informed medical decisions is present. A family member or friend is stipulated in the DPA to make medical decisions on behalf of the patient.

While both living wills and DPAs are legal in most states, there are some states that do not officially recognize these documents. However, they may still be used to guide families and doctors in treatment wishes.

Do-not-resuscitate (**DNR**) orders can be incorporated into an advance directive or by informing hospital staff. Unless instructions for a DNR are in effect, hospital staff will make every effort to help patients whose hearts have stopped or who have stopped breathing. DNR orders are recognized in all states and will be incorporated into a patient's medical chart if requested. Patients who benefit from a DNR order are those who have terminal or other debilitating illnesses. It is recommended that a patient who has not already been considered unable to make sound medical decisions discuss this option with his or her physician.

None of the above documents are complicated. They may be simple statements of desires for medical care options. If they are not completed by an attorney, they should be notarized and a copy should be given to the doctor, as well as to a trusted family member.

Mourning and grieving among cultures

The death of a loved one is a severe trauma, and the grief that follows is a natural and important part of life. No two people grieve exactly the same way, and cultural differences play a significant part in the grieving process. For many, however, the most immediate response is shock, numbness, and disbelief. Physical reactions may include shortness of breath, heart palpitations, sweating, and dizziness. At other times, there may be reactions such as loss of energy, sleeplessness or increase in sleep, changes in appetite, or stomach aches. Susceptibility to common illnesses, nightmares, and dreams about the deceased are not unusual during the grieving period.

Emotional reactions are as individual as physical reactions. A preoccupation with the image of the deceased, feelings of fear, hostility, apathy, emptiness, and even fear of one's own death, may occur. Depression, diminished sex drive, sadness, and anger at the deceased may occur. Bereavement may cause short- or long-term changes in the family unit and other relationships of the bereaved.

It is important for the bereaved to work through their feelings and not avoid their emotions. If emotions and feelings are not discussed with family members, friends, or primary support groups, then a therapist should be consulted to assist with the process.

Various cultures and religions view death in different manners and conduct mourning rituals according to their own traditions. In most cultures, visitors often come to express their condolences to the family and to bid farewell to the deceased. At times, funeral services are private. Various ethnic groups host a gathering after the funeral for those who attended. It is common for these events to become a celebration of the life of the deceased, which also helps the bereaved to begin the mourning process positively. Memories are often exchanged and toasts made in memory of the deceased. Knowing how much a loved one is cherished and remembered by friends and family is a comfort to those who experience the loss. Other methods of condolences include sending flowers to the home or the funeral parlor; sending a mass card, sending a donation to a charity that the family has chosen; or bringing a meal to the family during the weeks after the death.

Resources

BOOKS

Beauchamp, Daniel R., Mark B. Evers, Kenneth L. Mattox, Courtney M. Townsend, and David C. Sabiston, eds. *Sabiston Textbook of Surgery: The Biological Basis of Modern Surgical Practice.* 16th ed. London: W. B. Saunders Co., 2001.

Coberly, Margaret. *Sacred Passage: How to Provide Fearless, Compassionate Care for the Dying.* Boston: Shambhala Publications, 2002.

Heffner, John E., Ira R. Byock, and Lra Byock, eds. *Palliative and End-of-Life Pearls.* Philadelphia: Hanley and Belfus, Inc., 2002.

Kubler-Ross, Elisabeth, and David Kessler. *Life Lessons: Two Experts on Death and Dying Teach Us About the Mysteries of Life and Living.* New York: Scribner, 2000.

Soto, Gary. *The Afterlife.* Orlando, FL: Harcourt Children's Books, 2003.

KEY TERMS

Anesthesia—Loss of sensation and usually of consciousness without loss of vital functions artificially produced by the administration of one or more agents that block the passage of pain impulses along nerve pathways to the brain.

Anesthesiologist—A physician specializing in administering anesthesia.

Electrocautery—The use of a low-voltage electrified probe used to remove tissue through cauterization (burning).

Endoscopic—Of, relating to, or performed by means of an endoscope or endoscopy.

Euthanasia—To bring about the death of another person who has an incurable disease or condition.

High-density lipoprotein—A cholesterol-poor, protein-rich lipoprotein of blood plasma correlated with reduced risk of atherosclerosis.

Nosocomial—Originating or taking place in a hospital.

Serum albumin—A crystallizable albumin or mixture of albumins that normally constitutes more than half of the protein in blood serum and serves to maintain the osmotic pressure of the blood.

Percutaneous—Effected or performed through the skin.

Staton, Jana, Roger Shuy, and Ira Byock. *A Few Months to Live: Different Paths to Life's End* Baltimore, MD: Georgetown University Press, 2001.

Sweitzer, Bobbie Jean, ed. *Handbook of Preoperative Assessment and Management.* Philadelphia: Lippincott Williams & Wilkins, 2000.

PERIODICALS

Byock, Ira, and Steven H. Miles. "Hospice Benefits and Phase I Cancer Trials." *Annals of Internal Medicine* 138, no. 4 (February 2003): 335–337.

Smykowski, L., and W. Rodriguez. "The Post Anesthesia Care Unit Experience: A Family-centered Approach." *Journal of Nursing Care Quality* 18, no. 1 (January-March 2003): 5–15.

ORGANIZATIONS

American College of Physicians—American Society of Internal Medicine, 190 N. Independence Mall West, Philadelphia, PA 19106-1572. Washington Office: 2011 Pennsylvania Avenue NW, Suite 800, Washington, DC 20006-1837. (202) 261-4500 or (800) 338-2746. <http://www.acponline.org>.

Hospice Foundation of America, 2001 S Street, NW, Suite 300, Washington, DC 20009. (800) 854-3402 or (202) 638-5419. Fax: (202) 638-5312. E-mail: jon@hospicefoundation.org. <www.hospicefoundation.org>.

Inter-Institutional Collaborating Network On End-of-life Care (IICN). (415) 863-3045. <http://www.growthhouse.org>.

National Institutes of Health, 9000 Rockville Pike, Bethesda, MD 20892. (301) 496-4000. E-mail: NIHInfo@od. nih.gov. <http://www.nih.gov/>.

Promoting Excellence in End of Life Care, RWJ Foundation National Program Office, c/o The Practical Ethics Center, The University of Montana, 1000 East Beckwith Avenue, Missoula, MT 59812. (406) 243-6601. Fax: (406) 243-6633. E-mail: excell@selway.umt.edu. <http://www.promotingexcellence.org>.

Washington Home Center for Palliative Care Studies (CPCS), 4200 Wisconsin Avenue, NW, 4th Floor, Washington, DC 20016. (202) 895-2625. Fax: (202) 966-5410. E-mail: info@medicaring.org. <http://www.medicaring.org>.

OTHER

American College of Physicians. "How to Help During the Final Weeks of Life." *ACP Home Care Guide for Advanced Cancer.* [cited March 2, 2003]. <http://www.acponline.org/public/h_care/7-final.htm>.

American College of Physicians. "What to Do Before and After the Moment of Death." *ACP Home Care Guide.* [cited March 2, 2003]. <http://www.acponline.org/public/h_care/8-moment.htm>.

Byock, Ira, M.D. *DyingWell.org.* [cited March 2, 2003]. <http://www.dyingwell.org/default.htm>.

Kubler-Ross, Elisabeth, and Carol Bilger. *On Death and Dying: What the Dying Have to Teach Doctors, Nurses, Clergy, and Their Own Family.* (Audio Cassette, Abridged edition.) New York: Audio Renaissance, 2000.

Jacqueline N. Martin, M.S.
Crystal H. Kaczkowski, M.Sc.

Debridement

Definition

Debridement is the process of removing dead (necrotic) tissue or foreign material from and around a wound to expose healthy tissue.

Purpose

An open wound or ulcer can not be properly evaluated until the dead tissue or foreign matter is removed. Wounds that contain necrotic and ischemic (low oxygen content) tissue take longer to close and heal. This is because necrotic tissue provides an ideal growth medium

---

WHO PERFORMS THE PROCEDURE AND WHERE IS IT PERFORMED?

Debridement is performed by physicians such as plastic surgeons, dermatologists or surgeons, depending on the condition requiring the procedure. General physicians and surgeons are all trained in debridement techniques and they usually perform debridement procedures. Nurses specializing in **wound care** are prepared to perform conservative sharp wound debridement once they have satisfactorily completed didactic and clinical instruction in the sharp debridement procedure from an accredited agency, wound management specialty course, or an approved course in debridement.

Surgical debridement is usually performed on an outpatient basis or at the bedside. If the target tissue is deep or close to another organ, however, or if the patient is experiencing extreme pain, the procedure may be done in an **operating room**.

---

for bacteria, especially for *Bacteroides* spp. and *Clostridium perfringens* that causes the gas gangrene so feared in military medical practice. Though a wound may not necessarily be infected, the bacteria can cause inflammation and strain the body's ability to fight infection. Debridement is also used to treat pockets of pus called abscesses. Abscesses can develop into a general infection that may invade the bloodstream (sepsis) and lead to **amputation** and even death. Burned tissue or tissue exposed to corrosive substances tends to form a hard black crust, called an eschar, while deeper tissue remains moist and white, yellow and soft, or flimsy and inflamed. Eschars may also require debridement to promote healing.

Description

The four major debridement techniques are surgical, mechanical, chemical, and autolytic.

Surgical debridement

Surgical debridement (also known as sharp debridement) uses a scalpel, scissors, or other instrument to cut necrotic tissue from a wound. It is the quickest and most efficient method of debridement. It is the preferred method if there is rapidly developing inflammation of the body's connective tissues (cellulitis) or a more generalized infection (sepsis) that has entered the bloodstream. The physician starts by flushing the area with a saline (salt water) solution, and then applies a topical anesthetic or antalgic gel to the edges of the wound to minimize pain. Using forceps to grip the dead tissue, the physician cuts it away bit by bit with a scalpel or scissors. Sometimes it is necessary to leave some dead tissue behind rather than disturb living tissue. The physician may repeat the process again at another session.

Mechanical debridement

In mechanical debridement, a saline-moistened dressing is allowed to dry overnight and adhere to the dead tissue. When the dressing is removed, the dead tissue is pulled away too. This process is one of the oldest methods of debridement. It can be very painful because the dressing can adhere to living as well as nonliving tissue. Because mechanical debridement cannot select between good and bad tissue, it is an unacceptable debridement method for clean wounds where a new layer of healing cells is already developing.

Chemical debridement

Chemical debridement makes use of certain enzymes and other compounds to dissolve necrotic tissue. It is more selective than mechanical debridement. In fact, the body makes its own enzyme, collagenase, to break down collagen, one of the major building blocks of skin. A pharmaceutical version of collagenase is available and is highly effective as a debridement agent. As with other debridement techniques, the area first is flushed with saline. Any crust of dead tissue is etched in a cross-hatched pattern to allow the enzyme to penetrate. A topical antibiotic is also applied to prevent introducing infection into the bloodstream. A moist dressing is then placed over the wound.

Autolytic debridement

Autolytic debridement takes advantage of the body's own ability to dissolve dead tissue. The key to the technique is keeping the wound moist, which can be accomplished with a variety of dressings. These dressings help to trap wound fluid that contains growth factors, enzymes, and immune cells that promote wound healing. Autolytic debridement is more selective than any other debridement method, but it also takes the longest to work. It is inappropriate for wounds that have become infected.

Biological debridement

Maggot therapy is a form of biological debridement known since antiquity. The larvae of *Lucilia sericata*

(greenbottle fly) are applied to the wound as these organisms can digest necrotic tissue and pathogenic bacteria. The method is rapid and selective, although patients are usually reluctant to submit to the procedure.

Diagnosis/Preparation

The physician or nurse will begin by assessing the need for debridement. The wound will be examined, frequently by inserting a gloved finger into the wound to estimate the depth of dead tissue and evaluate whether it lies close to other organs, bone, or important body features. The assessment addresses the following points:

- the nature of the necrotic or ischaemic tissue and the best debridement procedure to follow
- the risk of spreading infection and the use of antibiotics
- the presence of underlying medical conditions causing the wound
- the extent of ischaemia in the wound tissues
- the location of the wound in the body
- the type of **pain management** to be used during the procedure

Before surgical or mechanical debridement, the area may be flushed with a saline solution, and an antalgic cream or injection may be applied. If the antalgic cream is used, it is usually applied over the exposed area some 90 minutes before the procedure.

Aftercare

After surgical debridement, the wound is usually packed with a dry dressing for a day to control bleeding. Afterward, moist dressings are applied to promote wound healing. Moist dressings are also used after mechanical, chemical, and autolytic debridement. Many factors contribute to wound healing, which frequently can take considerable time. Debridement may need to be repeated.

KEY TERMS

Abscess—A localized collection of pus buried in tissues or organs that may or may not discharge and usually results from an infectious process.

Anaerobic—Pertaining to a microorganism that either does not use oxygen or actually cannot live in the presence of oxygen.

Antalgic—Medication that alleviates pain.

Bacteroides—A family of anaerobic, rod-shaped bacteria. Its organisms are normal inhabitants of the oral, respiratory, intestinal, and urogenital cavities of humans, animals, and insects. Some species are infectious agents.

Eschar—A hardened dry crust that forms on skin exposed to burns or corrosive agents.

Gangrene—Death of tissue, usually in considerable mass and generally associated with loss of blood supply and followed by bacterial infection and decomposition.

Gas gangrene—A severe form of gangrene caused by *Clostridium* infection.

Hypoxia—Reduction of oxygen supply to tissues below physiological requirements despite adequate perfusion of the tissue by blood.

Ischemic—Tissue that has a low oxygen supply due to obstruction of the arterial blood supply or inadequate blood flow.

Necrotic—Affected with necrosis (cell death).

Pressure ulcer—Also known as a decubitus ulcer, pressure ulcers are open wounds that form whenever prolonged pressure is applied to skin covering bony outcrops of the body. Patients who are bedridden are at risk of developing pressure ulcers, commonly known as bedsores.

Sepsis—A severe systemic infection in which bacteria have entered the bloodstream.

Risks

It is possible that underlying tendons, blood vessels or other structures may be damaged during the examination of the wound and during surgical debridement. Surface bacteria may also be introduced deeper into the body, causing infection.

Normal results

Removal of dead tissue from pressure ulcers and other wounds speeds healing. Although these procedures cause some pain, they are generally well tolerated by patients and can be managed more aggressively. It is not uncommon to debride a wound again in a subsequent session.

Alternatives

Adjunctive therapies include electrotherapy and low laser irradiation. However, at present, insufficient research has been completed to recommend their general use.

Not all wounds need debridement. Sometimes it is better to leave a hardened crust of dead tissue (eschar), than to remove it and create an open wound, particularly if the crust is stable and the wound is not inflamed. Before performing debridement, the physician will take a medical history with attention to factors that might complicate healing, such as medications being taken and smoking. The physician will also note the cause of the wound and the ways it has been treated. Some ulcers and other wounds occur in places where blood flow is impaired, for example, the foot ulcers that can accompany diabetes mellitus. In such cases, the physician or nurse may decide not to debride the wound because blood flow may be insufficient for proper healing.

Resources

BOOKS

Falanga, V., and K. G. Harding, eds. *The Clinical Relevance of Wound Bed Preparation*. New York: Springer Verlag, 2002.

Harper, Michael S. *Debridement*. Berkeley, CA: Paradigm Press, 2001.

Maklebust, JoAnn and Mary Y. Sieggreen. *Pressure Ulcers: Guidelines for Prevention and Nursing Management*. 2nd ed. Springhouse, PA: Springhouse Corporation, 1996.

PERIODICALS

Dervin, G. F., I. G. Stiell, K. Rody, and J. Grabowski. "Effect of Arthroscopic Debridement for Osteoarthritis of the Knee on Health-Related Quality of Life." *The Journal of Bone and Joint Surgery (American)* 85-A (January 2003): 10–19.

Friberg, T. R., M. Ohji, J. J. Scherer, and Y. Tano. "Frequency of Epithelial Debridement During Diabetic Vitrectomy." *American Journal of Ophthalmology* 135 (April 2003): 553–554.

Reynolds, N., N. Cawrse, T. Burge, and J. Kenealy. "Debridement of a Mixed Partial and Full Thickness Burn With an Erbium: YAG Laser." *Burns* 29 (March 2003): 183–188.

Schirmer, B. D., A. D. Miller, and M. S. Miller. "Single Operative Debridement for Pancreatic Abscess." *Journal of Gastrointestinal Surgery* 7 (February 2003): 289.

Terzi, C., A. Bacakoglu, T. Unek, and M. H. Ozkan. "Chemical Necrotizing Fasciitis Due to Household Insecticide Injection: Is Immediate Radical Surgical Debridement Necessary?" *Human & Experimental Toxicology* 21 (December 2002): 687–690.

Wolff, H., and C. Hansson. "Larval Therapy—an Effective Method of Ulcer Debridement." *Clinical and Experimental Dermatology* 28 (March 2003): 134–137.

ORGANIZATIONS

American Academy of Wound Management. 1255 23rd St., NW, Washington, DC 20037. (202) 521-0368. <http://www.aawm.org>.

Wound Care Institute. 1100 N.E. 163rd Street, Suite #101, North Miami Beach, FL 33162. (305) 919-9192. <http://woundcare.org>.

OTHER

Moses, Scott. "Wound Debridement." *Family Practice Notebook.* February 12, 2003 [cited May 15, 2003]. <http://www.fpnotebook.com/SUR12.htm>.

"Types of Wound Debridement." Wound Care Information Network: Types of Wound Debridement. 2002 [cited May 15, 2003]. <http://www.medicaledu.com/debridhp.htm>.

Richard H. Camer
Monique Laberge, Ph.D.

Decubitus ulcers *see* **Bedsores**

Deep brain stimulation

Definition

Deep brain stimulation (DBS) delivers a constant low electrical stimulation to a small region of the brain, through implanted electrodes connected to an implanted battery. It is used to partially restore normal movements in Parkinson's disease, essential tremor, and dystonia.

Purpose

Parkinson's disease is due to degeneration of a group of cells called the substantia nigra. These cells interact with other brain regions to help control movement. The normal signals from the substantia nigra inhibit these other regions, and so when it degenerates, these regions become overactive. The electrical signals from the DBS electrodes mimic the inhibitory function of the substantia nigra, helping to restore more normal movements.

The substantia nigra normally releases the chemical dopamine, which exerts its inhibitory action on the globus pallidus interna (GPi) and the subthalamic nucleus (STN). For Parkinson's disease, deep brain stimulation is performed on these two centers. The target for DBS in dystonia is the GPi as well. Treatment of essential tremor usually targets the thalamus.

Each of these brain regions has two halves, which control movement on the opposite side of the body: right controls left, and left controls right. Unilateral DBS may be used if the symptoms are much more severe on one side. Bilateral DBS is used to treat symptoms on both sides.

Demographics

Parkinson's disease affects approximately one million Americans. The peak incidence is approximately age 62, but young-onset PD can occur as early as age 40. Because young-onset patients live with their disease for so many more years, they are more likely to become candidates for surgery than older-onset patients. In addition, younger patients tend to do better and have fewer adverse effects of surgery. Approximately 5% of older PD patients receive one form or another of PD surgery. Many more develop the symptoms for which surgery may be effective, but either develop them at an advanced age, making surgery inadvisable, or decide the risks of surgery are not worth the potential benefit, or do not choose surgery for some other reason.

Essential tremor is more common than Parkinson's disease, but rarely becomes severe enough to require surgery. Dystonia is a very rare condition, and the number of patients who have received DBS as of 2003 is under 100.

Description

Deep brain stimulation relies on implanting a long thin electrode deep into the brain, through a hole in the top of the skull. In order to precisely locate the target area and to ensure the probe is precisely placed in the target, a "stereotactic frame" is used. This device is a rigid frame attached to the patient's head, providing an immobile three-dimensional coordinate system, which can be used to precisely track the location of the GPi or STN and the movement of the electrode.

For unilateral DBS, a single "burr hole" is made in the top of the skull. Bilateral DBS requires two holes. A strong topical anesthetic is used to numb the skin while this hole is drilled. Since there are no pain receptors in the brain, there is no need for deeper anesthetic. In addition, the patient must remain awake in order to report any sensory changes during the surgery. The electrode is placed very close to several important brain structures. Sensory changes during electrode placement may indicate the electrode is too close to one or more of these regions.

Once the burr hole is made, the surgeon inserts the electrode. Small electric currents from the electrode are used to more precisely locate the target. This is harmless, but may cause twitching, light flashes, or other sensations. A contrast dye may also be injected into the spinal fluid, which allows the surgeon to visualize the brain's structure using one or more imaging techniques. The patient will be asked to make various movements to assist in determining the location of the electrode.

The electrode is connected by a wire to an implanted pulse generator. This wire is placed under the scalp and skin. A small incision is made in the area of the collarbone, and the pulse generator is placed there. This portion of the procedure is performed under general anesthesia.

Diagnosis/Preparation

DBS for Parkinson's disease is considered as an option in a patient who is still responsive to levodopa (used to treat symptoms) but has developed motor complications. These include the rapid loss of benefit from a single dose (wearing off), unpredictable fluctuations in benefit (on-off), and uncontrolled abnormal movements (dyskinesias). Essential tremor patients who are candidates for surgery are those whose tremor is unsatisfacto-

rily controlled by medications and whose tremor significantly impairs activities of daily living. Similar criteria apply for dystonia patients.

The patient who is a candidate for DBS discusses all the surgical options with his neurologist before deciding on deep brain stimulation. A full understanding of the risks and potential benefits must be understood before consenting to the surgery.

The patient will undergo a variety of medical tests, and one or more types of neuroimaging procedures, including MRI, CT scanning, **angiography** (imaging the brain's blood vessels) and ventriculography (imaging the brain's ventricles). On the day of the surgery, the stereotactic frame is fixed to the patient's head. A local anesthetic is used at the four sites where the frame's pins contact the head; there may nonetheless be some initial discomfort. A final MRI is done with the frame in place, to set the coordinates of the targeted area of the brain in relation to the frame.

The patient will receive a mild sedative to ease the anxiety of the procedure. Once the electrodes are positioned, the patient receives general anesthetic to implant the pulse generator.

Aftercare

The procedure is lengthy, and the patient will require a short hospital stay afterward to recover from the surgery. Following the procedure itself, the patient meets several times with the neurologist to adjust the stimulation. The pulse generator is programmable, and can be fine-tuned to the patient's particular needs. This can provide a higher degree of symptom relief than lesioning surgeries, but requires repeated visits to the neurologist. Pulse generator batteries must be replaced every three to five years. This is done with a small incision as an outpatient procedure. Since the generator is in the chest area, no additional brain surgery is required.

The patient's medications are adjusted after surgery, with a reduction in levodopa likely in most patients who receive DBS of the subthalamic nucleus.

Risks

Deep brain stimulation entails several risks. There are acute surgical risks, including hemorrhage and infection, and the risks of general anesthesia. The electrodes can be placed too close to other brain regions, which can lead to visual defects, speech problems, and other complications. These may be partially avoided by adjusting the stimulation settings after the procedure. Because a device is left implanted under the skin, there is the risk of breakage or malfunction, which requires surgical removal.

A patient with implanted electrodes must not receive diathermy therapy. Diathermy is the passage of radiowaves through the tissue to heat it, and is used as a physical therapy for muscle pain and other applications. Diathermy poses a risk of death in a patient with DBS electrodes.

Patients who are cognitively impaired may become more so after surgery, and cognitive impairment usually prevents a patient from undergoing surgery.

Normal results

Deep brain stimulation improves the movement disorder symptoms of Parkinson's disease by 25–75%, depending on the care of the placement and the ability to find the optimum settings. These improvements are seen most while off levodopa; DBS does little to improve the best response to levodopa treatment. Levodopa dose will likely be reduced, leading to a significant reduction in dyskinesias.

Morbidity and mortality rates

The rate of complications depends highly on the skill and experience of the **surgical team** performing the procedure. Rates from one of the most experienced teams, in a study of over 200 patients, were as follows.

Post-operative complications:

• asymptomatic intracranial bleed (10% of procedures)

• symptomatic intracranial bleed (2%)

• seizures (3%)

• headache (25%)

• infection (6%)

Device-related complications:

• lead replacements (9%)

• lead repositionings (8%)

• extension wire replacements (6%)

• implantable pulse generator replacements (17%), approximately half of which were due to malfunction

The risk of death is less than 1%.

Alternatives

Patients who are candidates for deep brain stimulation have usually been judged to require surgery for effective treatment of their symptoms. Other surgical alternatives for Parkinson's disease include **pallidotomy** and thalamotomy, which destroy brain tissue to achieve the same effect as the stimulation. Pallidotomy is rarely performed for Parkinson's disease, unless tremor is the only debilitating symptom. It is common in essential tremor. DBS for dystonia is the only really promising neurosur-

gical treatment for this condition. Some peripheral surgeries may be appropriate for selected patients.

Resources

BOOKS

Jahanshahi, M., and C. D. Marsden. *Parkinson's Disease: A Self-Help Guide.* New York: Demos Medical Press, 2000.

ORGANIZATIONS

National Parkinson's Disease Foundation. Bob Hope Parkinson Research Center, 1501 N.W. 9th Avenue, Bob Hope Road, Miami, FL 33136-1494. (305) 547-6666. (800) 327-4545. Fax: (305) 243-4403. <http://www.parkinson.org>.

WE MOVE, Worldwide Education and Awareness for Movement Disorders. 204 West 84th Street, New York, NY 10024. (800) 437-MOV2, Fax: (212) 875-8389. <http://www.wemove.org>.

Richard Robinson

Deep vein thrombosis *see* **Venous thrombosis prevention**

Defibrillation

Definition

Defibrillation is a process in which an electrical device called a defibrillator sends an electric shock to the heart to stop an arrhythmia resulting in the return of a productive heart rhythm.

Purpose

Defibrillation is performed to correct life-threatening arrhythmias of the heart including ventricular fibrillation and cardiac arrest. In cardiac emergencies it should be performed immediately after identifying that the patient is experiencing an arrhythmia, indicated by lack of pulse and unresponsiveness. If an electrocardiogram is available, the arrhythmia can be displayed visually for additional confirmation. For medical treatment by a physician, in non-life threatening situations, atrial defibrillation can be used to treat atrial fibrillation or flutter.

Precautions

Defibrillation should not be performed on a patient who has a pulse or is alert, as this could cause a lethal heart rhythm disturbance or cardiac arrest. The paddles used in the procedure should not be placed on a woman's breasts or over an internal pacemaker.

A portable defibrillator is used in an attempt to revive a man who had a heart attack before he is transported to an emergency room. *(Photograph by Adam Hart-Davis. Science Source/Photo Researchers. Reproduced by permission.)*

Cardiac arrhythmias that prevent the heart from pumping blood to the body can cause irreversible damage to the major organs including the brain and heart. These arrhythmias include ventricular tachycardia, fibrillation, and cardiac arrest. About 10% of the ability to restart the heart is lost with every minute that the heart fibrillates. Death can occur in minutes unless a productive heart rhythm, able to generate a pulse, is restored through defibrillation. Because immediate defibrillation is crucial to the patient's survival, the American Heart Association has called for the integration of defibrillation into an effective emergency cardiac care system. The system should include early access, early **cardiopulmonary resuscitation**, early defibrillation, and early advanced cardiac care.

Defibrillators deliver a brief electric shock to the heart, which enables the heart's natural pacemaker to regain control and establish a productive heart rhythm. The defibrillator is an electronic device that includes defibrillator paddles and electrocardiogram monitoring.

During external defibrillation, the paddles are placed on the patient's chest with a conducting gel ensuring good contact with the skin. When the heart can be visualized directly, during **thoracic surgery**, sterile internal paddles are applied directly to the heart. Direct contact with the patient is discontinued by all caregivers. If additional defibrillation is required the paddles should be repositioned exactly to increase the likelihood of further

shocks being effective in stopping the arrhythmia. The patient's pulse and/or electrocardiogram are continually monitored when defibrillation is not in progress. Medications to treat possible causes of the abnormal heart rhythm may be administered. Defibrillation continues until the patient's condition stabilizes or the procedure is ordered to be discontinued.

Early defibrillators, about the size and weight of a car battery, were used primarily in ambulances and hospitals. The American Heart Association now advocates public access defibrillation; this calls for placing automated external defibrillators (AEDS) in police vehicles, airplanes, and at public events, etc. The AEDS are smaller, lighter, less expensive, and easier to use than the early defibrillators. They are computerized to provide simple, verbal instructions to the operator and to make it impossible to deliver a shock to a patient whose heart is not fibrillating. The placement of AEDs is likely to expand to many public locations.

Preparation

Once a patient is found in cardiac distress, without a pulse and non-responsive, and help is summoned, cardiopulmonary resuscitation (CPR) is begun and continued until the caregivers arrive and are able to provide defibrillation. Electrocardiogram leads are attached to the patient chest. Gel or paste is applied to the defibrillator paddles, or two gel pads are placed on the patient's chest. The caregivers verify lack of a pulse while visualizing the electrocardiogram, assure contact with the patient is discontinued, and deliver the electrical charge.

Atrial defibrillation is a treatment option that will be ordered for treatment of atrial fibrillation or flutter. The electrocardiogram will be monitored throughout the procedure. The paddles are placed on the patients chest with conducting gel to ensure good contact between the paddles and skin. If the heart can be visualized directly during thoracic surgery, the paddles will be applied directly to the heart. The defibrillator is programmed to recognize distinct components of the electrocardiogram and will only fire the electrical shock at the correct time. Again, all direct contact with the patient is discontinued prior to defibrillation.

Aftercare

After defibrillation, the patient's cardiac status, breathing, and **vital signs** are monitored with a **cardiac monitor**. Additional tests to measure cardiac damage will be performed, which can include a 12 lead electrocardiogram, a chest x-ray, and **cardiac catheterization**. Treatment options will be determined from the outcome of these procedures. The patient's skin is cleansed to remove gel and, if necessary, electrical burns are treated.

Risks

Skin burns from the defibrillator paddles are the most common complication of defibrillation. Other risks include injury to the heart muscle, abnormal heart rhythms, and blood clots.

Normal results

Defibrillation performed to treat life-threatening ventricular arrhythmias is most likely to be effective within the first five minutes, preventing brain injury and death by returning the heart to a productive rhythm able to produce a pulse. Patients will be transferred to a hospital critical care unit for additional monitoring, diagnosis, and treatment of the arrhythmia. Intubation may be required for respiratory distress. Medications to improve cardiac function and prevent additional arrhythmias, are frequently administered. Some cardiac function may be lost due to the actual defibrillation, but is also associated with the underlying disease.

Atrial defibrillation is successful at restoring cardiac output, alleviating shortness of breath, and decreasing the occurrence of clot formation in the atria.

Resources

BOOKS

Giuliani, E. R., et al., eds. "Arrhythmias." In *Mayo Clinic Practice of Cardiology.* 3rd ed. St. Louis: Mosby, 1996.

PERIODICALS

Bur, Andreas, et al. "Effects of Bystander First Aid, Defibrillation and Advanced Life Support on Neurological Outcome and Hospital Costs in Patients after Ventricular Fib-

rillation Cardiac Arrest." *Intensive Care Medicine* 27 (2001): 1474–1480.

Herlitz, J., et al. "Characteristics and Outcome Among Patients Suffering In-hospital Cardiac Arrest in Monitored and Non-monitored Areas." *Resuscitation* 48 (2001): 125–135.

Matarese, Leonard. "Police and AEDS: A Chance to Save Thousands of Lives Each Year." *Public Management* 79 (June 1997): 4.

"Medical Breakthroughs That Could Save Your Life." *Body Bulletin* (February 1998): 1.

"Upping the Odds of Survival." *Hospitals and Health Networks* 71 (June 5, 1997): 13.

ORGANIZATIONS

American Heart Association. 7320 Greenville Ave. Dallas, TX 75231. (214) 373-6300. <http://www.americanheart.org>

OTHER

"AARC Clinical Practice Guideline: Defibrillation During Resuscitation." *Respiratory Care* 40 (1995): 744–748. [cited May 2003]. <http://www.hsc.missouri.edu/~shrp/rtwww/rcweb/aarc/ddrcpg.html>

"Defibrillation." *American Heart Association.* [cited May 2003]. <http://www.americanheart.org>

Lori De Milto
Allison J. Spiwak, MSBME

Defibrillator, automatic *see* **Implantable cardioverter-defibrillator**

Dental implants

Definition

Dental implants are surgically fixed substitutes for roots of missing teeth. Embedded in the jawbone, they act as anchors for a replacement tooth, also known as a crown, or a full set of replacement teeth.

Purpose

The purpose of dental implant surgery is to fix metallic anchors in the jaw bone so that they can receive the replacement teeth and hold them in place. Dental implants should be considered as an option for replacing failing or missing teeth and often provide more predictable results than bridgework, resin bonded bridges, or endodontic treatment.

Demographics

In 2000, the estimated number of dental implants placed in the United States was 910,000 and this number

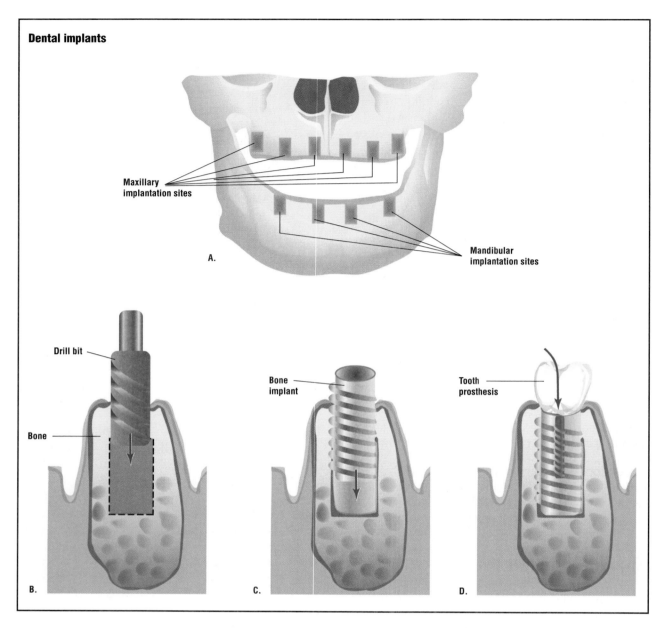

Dental implants

Maxillary implantation sites

Mandibular implantation sites

A.

Drill bit

Bone

B.

Bone implant

C.

Tooth prosthesis

D.

A dental drill is used to make a hole for the implant in the jawbone (B). The bone implant is secured into the drilled hole (C), and the tooth prosthesis is built onto the implant (D). *(Illustration by GGS Inc.)*

is expected to increase at a rate of about 18% per year through 2005.

Description

By replacing a lost tooth with a dental implant, the overall health and function of the surrounding teeth is maintained. The implant can prevent tooth migration and loss of structure and will help avoid loss of bone from the jaw in that area. Further, implants reduce the impact of the lost tooth on surrounding teeth, as traditional bridge structures often require reduction (filing down) of the two flanking teeth to hold the bridge in place with a crown. Implanting avoids such alterations to the surrounding teeth when replacing a lost tooth.

When replacing dentures, implants can provide even more benefits. Implants do not slip nor do they have the potential of limiting the diet to easily chewed foods as can happen with poorly fitting dentures. If appropriate, implants are the method most able to surgically restore one or more missing teeth to their original conditions.

The actual procedure occurs as follows. Under local anesthesia, the first step for many implant procedures is the exposure of the bone where the implant is to be made. This is followed by placement of the implant into the exposed jawbone. Implants that are placed in the bone are called endosteal implants and are made of titanium or a titanium alloy because this metal does not adversely interact with biological tissue. After placement of the implant a cover screw is put in and the wound is closed with stitches and allowed to heal. In general, placements in the lower jaw need to heal about three months, while placements in the upper jaw need to heal about six months.

After healing, in a second surgical procedure, the implant is uncovered, the cover screw is removed, and a healing abutment or a temporary crown is placed in the implant. Temporary crowns are generally used for esthetic reasons, when the implant is in a place that is visible. Both healing abutments and temporary crowns allow the tissue around the implant to be trained to grow around the final prosthetic tooth.

After about two months the soft tissue will be healed to receive the final prosthetic tooth. Impressions are used to make custom abutments that take into account the neck morphology of the implant. The prosthetic tooth is sometimes attached to a gold cylinder that can be screwed into the abutment or it can be directly cemented onto the abutment. This multi-stage process, where the two surgical procedures are separated by a lengthy healing time, has proven to provide excellent stability in the final implant. Single step surgical implants are available, but some stability of the final implant is often lost by eliminating the healing step.

Preparation/Diagnosis

At the first appointment, the dentist or oral surgeon performs a thorough examination to determine whether implants are appropriate to replace the missing teeth. Often, x rays are necessary to discover the state of the jawbone, particularly if the teeth have been lost for some time. This information is used to determine if implants

are appropriate and, if so, what particular type of implant would be best for the clinical situation.

There are two solutions commonly used if the initial examination indicates that the bone in the area where the implant is to occur is too resorbed to support the implant. The first is **bone grafting**. This involves undergoing a procedure that moves bone from one place in the body to another to enlarge the bone structure at the implant site. Often, bone can be moved from one place in the mouth to another. Sometimes a graft from a donor or an animal or artificial bone can be used if bone from the patient is not available. Grafting usually is done four to eight months before the implant procedure, to allow the graft a chance to heal before it is disturbed with the implant process.

A second solution is the use of subperiosteal implants that ride above the bone but beneath the gum. These types of implants are not placed in the bone. A **CT scan** is commonly used to obtain a model of the bone structure and then the implant fixture is molded to precisely fit the bone model.

Risks

The greatest risk following the surgical procedures is that the implant will fail. For implants placed within the bone, most failures occur within the first year and then occur at a rate of less than 1% per year thereafter. Recent research has indicated that tobacco use by the patient and use of a single-stage implant procedure are two risk factors that increase failure rate.

Normal results

Overall, the success rate for all implants runs from 90% to 95%. Most failed implants can be replaced with a second attempt.

Resources

BOOKS

Balshi, Tom, William Becker, Edmond Bedrossian, and Peter Wohrle. *A Patient's Guide to Dental Implants.* Omaha, NE: Addicus Books, 2003.

Wiland, Michael R., Michael Mastromarino, and Joseph N. Pipolo. *Smile: How Dental Implants can Transform Your Life.* Boca Raton, FL: CRC Press-Parthenon Publishers. 2001.

PERIODICALS

Vehemente, V. A., et al. "Risk Factors Affecting Dental Implant Survival." *Journal of Oral Implantology* 28 (2002): 74–81.

ORGANIZATIONS

American Academy of Implant Dentistry. 211 E. Chicago Avenue, Suite 750, Chicago, IL 60611. (312) 335-1550, Fax: (312) 335-9090. <http://www.aaid-implant. org>.

American Dental Association. 211 E. Chicago Ave. Chicago, IL 60611. (312) 440-2500, Fax: (312) 440-7494. <http://www.ada.org>.

Michelle Johnson, M.S., J.D.

Dermabrasion

Definition

Dermabrasion is a procedure to improve the look of the skin involving the mechanical removal of the damaged top layer using a high speed rotary wheel.

Purpose

Originally developed as a means of treating acne scars, dermabrasion can be used to treat many kinds of skin problems including scars from other types of wounds, wrinkles, skin coloration abnormalities, and other more serious conditions such as rhinophyma, a disfiguring form of rosacea that affects the nose. Although the treatment is not a cure, in that the scar or other abnormality cannot be entirely removed, dermabrasion does soften the edges of the scar or other abnormality and can radically improve its appearance.

Dermabrasion is often used in combination with other plastic surgery techniques, such as chemical peels, excisions, punch grafting, and CO_2 laser resurfacing to achieve an overall smoothing of various skin abnormalities, particularly of the face.

Demographics

Dermabrasion is a technique that has been used in dermatology for over 100 years. Although used much less often since the advent of laser resurfacing, dermabrasion continues to be a viable treatment that has been reported to have quicker healing times, similar rates of complications, and is more effective in eliminating some types of lesions, particularly surgical scars. According to the American Society for Aesthetic Plastic Surgery, there were about 60,000 dermabrasion procedures performed in 2001.

Description

Dermabrasion is commonly performed using a handheld engine that can reach rotational speeds of 18,000–35,000 rpm. Rapid planing of the skin is achieved through the combination of this rotational speed, the abrading attachment, and pressure applied by the operator. Because of the importance of the skill of the operator, patients should select doctors with significant experience with the procedure.

There are three types of abrading attachments in common use: diamond fraises, wire brushes, and serrated wheels. Diamond fraises are stainless steel wheels that have diamond chips of various coarseness bonded

Dermabrasion

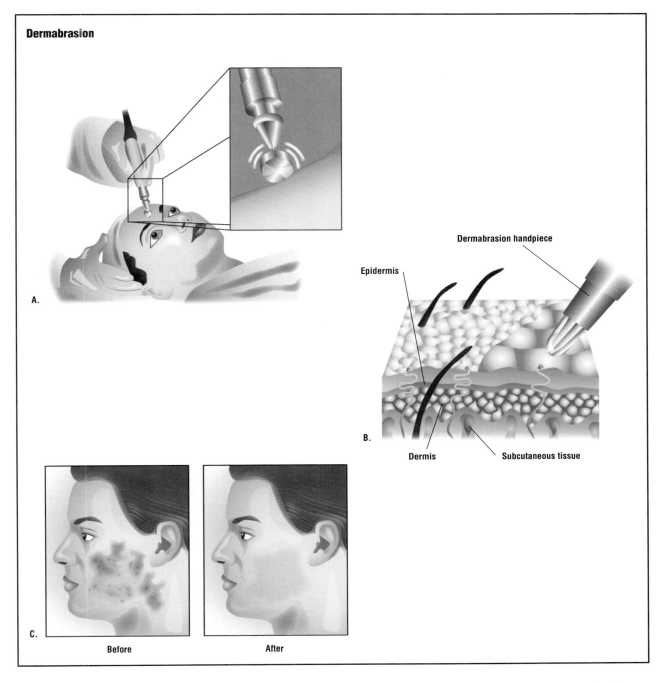

A.

Dermabrasion handpiece

Epidermis

B.

Dermis

Subcutaneous tissue

C.

Before

After

A doctor performs dermabrasion with a high-speed rotary wheel (A). The tool takes off the top layers of the skin (B) to improve the appearance of wrinkles or scars (C). *(Illustration by GGS Inc.)*

to its surface. Cylinder and pear-shaped diamond fraises are also used for work in various locations. The wire brush is a wheel with wires attached at various angles. In experienced hands, it is the most effective attachment for deep scars. The serrated wheel or diamond fraise is often used to soften the edges of skin removed with a wire brush.

Before the procedure begins, medication is often given to relax the patient and reduce pain. For small areas, local anaesthetic nerve blocks are often used to numb the area being treated. Alternatively, topical cryoanaesthesia (numbing the skin using cold) can be used. This is done by spraying a cold-inducing agent on the skin. Sometimes the skin is pre-chilled with ice to increase the anaesthetic effect.

During the procedure the patient lies on his back on the surgical table, eyes covered with disposable eye patches. The area being treated is parted with Gentaian violet, a stain that will help gauge how deep the treatment is going. A gloved and gowned assistant holds the skin taut while each section of the face is abraded using the hand-held engine. The surgeon works in sections to avoid obvious lines of demarcation in the final results. If the entire face is to be dermabraded, laser is commonly used for the lower eyelids and lip as less than satisfactory results often occur in these areas.

Diagnosis/Preparation

Because there are several different skin surfacing techniques now available, the initial meetings with the dermatological or plastic surgeon must ensure that dermabrasion is the technique of choice for the particular skin abnormality and location that is being treated. Although controversial, some studies have reported abnormal scarring in patients previously treated with 13 cis-retinoic acid (Accutane), so many surgeons will require a six month break from the medication before performing dermabrasion. A second contraindication for dermabrasion is HIV or hepatitis infection, as small droplets of blood becomes aerosolized (distributed within the air) during the treatment, creating a risk for the doctor and other staff.

Finally, even if there is no patient history of cold sores, it is important that anti-viral medicine is administered to anyone undergoing the procedure, as an outbreak after dermabrasion can be very severe and spread beyond the mouth to other areas of the face.

Aftercare

After the procedure, any treated areas are dressed for healing. For example, a dressing that is primarily water held on a mesh support, called Vigilon, can be used to cover the wound. It is changed daily for about five days, then the wound is left open to the air. This kind of treatment speeds the restoration of the epithelium, the cellular covering of the body. Using this technique, healing occurs in about five to seven days.

Generally, the patient is given pain medication, **antibiotics**, and anti-swelling medication during recovery. Antiviral drugs are also continued. Patients should avoid the sun during the healing process.

Risks

The most common complication of the procedure is the formation of keloid, a type of abnormal scar that results from excessive collagen production. Because this type of scarring tends to be associated with darker skin types, patients with this kind of skin should approach dermabrasion with caution. Other potential complications include abnormal pigmentation of the treated skin, persistent redness of the skin, and a localized dilation of small groups of blood vessels called telangiectasia. Finally, the formation of milia, bumps that form due to obstruction of the sweat glands, although this can be treated after healing with retinoic acid.

Normal results

Normal results include significant improvement in the appearance of the skin's surface after healing of the skin. It should be emphasized, however, that many scars will not be completely removed and the change in appearance is to due a softening of the edges of the abnormality, not elimination. If a patient cannot tolerate a residual presence of the scar or other abnormality, the treatment should not be used.

Morbidity and mortality rates

The morbidity and mortality rate of this cosmetic procedure is extremely low.

Alternatives

A variety of other skin resurfacing techniques are available and include chemical (phenol or trichloroacetic acid, TCA) peels and laser (CO_2 and Erbium) resurfacing.

See also Laser skin resurfacing.

Resources

BOOKS

Stuzin, James M., Thomas J. Baker, and Tracy M. Baker. "Treatment of Photoaging: Facial Chemical Peeling." In *Plastic Surgery: Indications, Operations, and Outcomes.* Vol. 5, edited by Craig A. Vander Kolk, et al. St. Louis: Mosby, 2000.

KEY TERMS

Chemical peel—A skin treatment that uses the application of chemicals, such as phenol or trichloroacetic acid (TCA), to remove the uppermost layer of skin.

Cryoanaesthesia—The use of the numbing effects of cold as a surgical anaesthetic. For dermabrasion, this involves the spraying of a cold-inducing chemical on the area being treated.

Epithelium—The cellular covering of the body. This covering is disturbed during dermabrasion and reheals.

Gentaian violet—An antibacterial, antifungal dye that is commonly applied to the skin during dermabrasion.

Keloid—An abnormal type of scarring that involves progressive enlargement, elevated edges, and irregular shapes because of excessive collagen formation during healing.

Laser skin resurfacing—The use of laser light to remove the uppermost layer of skin. Two types of lasers commonly used in this manner are CO_2 and Erbium.

Punch grafting—A method of treating a deep scar involving excision of the damaged area, followed by the suturing in of similarly shaped punch of skin that is often taken from behind the ear.

Rosacea—A disease of the skin marked by constant flushing and acne-like lesions.

PERIODICALS

Roenigk, Henry H. "Dermabrasion: State of the Art 2002." *Journal of Cosmetic Dermatology* 1 (2002): 72–87.

ORGANIZATIONS

American Society for Aesthetic Plastic Surgery, 11081 Winners Circle, Los Alamitos, CA 90720. (800) 364-2147 or (562) 799-2356. <http://www.surgery.org>

American Society of Plastic Surgeons. 444 E. Algonquin Rd. Arlington Heights, IL 60005. (800) 475-2784. <http://www.plasticsurgery.org>

Michelle Johnson, M.S., J.D.

Diabetes surgery *see* **Islet cell transplantation**

Dialysis, kidney *see* **Kidney dialysis**

Differential count *see* **White blood cell count and differential**

Dilatation and curettage

Definition

Dilatation and curettage (D & C) is a gynecological procedure in which the cervix is dilated (expanded) and the lining of the uterus (endometrium) is scraped away.

Purpose

D & C is used to diagnose and treat heavy or irregular bleeding from the uterus. Possible reasons for abnormal uterine bleeding include:

• Hormonal imbalance. Often women with abnormal bleeding are first treated with hormones in an attempt to normalize bleeding. D & C may be used to determine the cause of bleeding if hormone treatment is ineffective.

• Endometrial polyps. Polyps are benign growths that may protrude from the uterus by a stem or stalk, usually to the endometrium or cervix. D & C may be used to diagnose polyps or to remove them.

• Uterine fibroids. Also called leiomyomas, fibroids are benign growths in the smooth muscle of the uterus. Abnormal bleeding is often the only symptom of fibroids. D & C is often used to diagnose fibroids and may be used to scrape away small tumors; additional surgery may be needed to remove more extensive growths.

• Endometrial hyperplasia (EH). EH is a condition where the endometrium grows excessively, becoming too thick and causing abnormal bleeding. Tissue samples procured during D & C can be assessed for early signs of cancer.

• Cancer. D & C may be used to obtain tissue for microscopic evaluation to rule out cancer. Women over the age of 40 are at an increased risk of developing endometrial cancer.

• Miscarriage, incomplete abortion, or childbirth. Abnormal bleeding may result if some of the products of pregnancy remain in the uterus after a miscarriage or induced abortion, or if parts of the placenta are not expelled naturally after childbirth. These retained products can be scraped out by D & C.

Description

D & C is usually performed under general anesthesia, although local or epidural anesthesia can also be used.

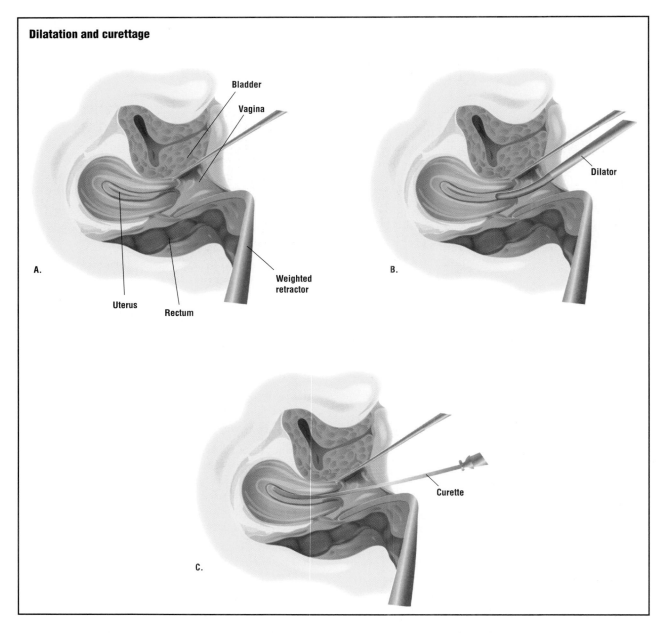

Dilatation and curettage

A.
- Bladder
- Vagina
- Uterus
- Rectum
- Weighted retractor

B.
- Dilator

C.
- Curette

For a D & C, the patient lies on her back, and a weighted retractor is placed in the vagina (A). A dilator is used to open the cervix (B), and a curette is used to scrape the inside of the uterus (C). *(Illustration by GGS Inc.)*

Local anesthesia lessens risk and costs, but the woman will feel cramping during the procedure. The type of anesthesia used often depends upon the reason for the D & C.

During the procedure (which takes only minutes to perform), the doctor inserts an instrument called a speculum to hold open the vaginal walls, and then stretches the opening of the uterus (the cervix) by inserting a series of tapering rods, each thicker than the previous one, or by using other specialized instruments. This process of opening the cervix is called dilation.

Once the cervix is dilated, the physician inserts a spoon-shaped surgical device called a curette into the uterus. The curette is used to scrape away the uterine lining. One or more small tissue samples from the lining of the uterus or the cervical canal are sent for analysis by microscope to check for abnormal cells.

Although simpler, less expensive techniques such as a vacuum aspiration are quickly replacing the D & C as a diagnostic method, it is still often used to diagnose and treat a number of conditions.

Diagnosis/Preparation

If general anesthesia will be used, the patient will be instructed to refrain from eating and drinking for at least eight hours before the procedure. The doctor may order blood and/or urine tests to scan for certain abnormalities. Because opening the cervix can be painful, sedatives may be given before the procedure begins. Deep breathing and other relaxation techniques may help ease cramping during cervical dilation.

Aftercare

A woman who has had a D & C performed in a hospital can usually go home the same day or the next day. Many women experience backache and mild cramps after the procedure, and may pass small blood clots for a day or so. Vaginal staining or bleeding may continue for several weeks.

Most women can resume normal activities almost immediately. Patients should avoid sexual intercourse, douching, and tampon use for at least two weeks to prevent infection while the cervix is closing and to allow the endometrium to heal completely.

Risks

The primary risk after the procedure is infection. If a woman experiences any of the following symptoms, she should report them immediately to her doctor, who can treat the infection with antibiotics:

• fever

• heavy bleeding

• severe cramps

• foul-smelling vaginal discharge

D & C is a surgical operation that has certain risks associated with general anesthesia such as pulmonary aspiration and failed intubation. Rare complications include perforation of the uterus (which usually heals on its own) or puncture of the bowel or bladder (which requires further surgery to repair).

Extensive scarring of the uterus may occur after over-aggressive scraping during D & C, leading to a condition called Asherman's syndrome. The major symptoms of Asherman's syndrome are light or absent menstrual periods, infertility, and recurrent miscarriages. Scar tissue can be removed with surgery in most women, although approximately 20–30% of women will remain infertile after treatment.

Normal results

Removal of the uterine lining will normally cause no side effects, and may be beneficial if the lining has

thickened so much that it causes heavy periods. The uterine lining soon grows again normally, as part of the menstrual cycle.

Morbidity and mortality rates

D & C has been associated with a 4–10% rate of postoperative complications.

Alternatives

There are a number of alternatives to D & C, depending on the reason for doing the procedure. The following are some examples of procedures that allow doctors alternative ways of evaluating, sampling, or treating disorders of the inner lining of the uterus:

• Expectant management of spontaneous abortion. D & C is the most commonly used method of treatment for incomplete abortion; one study showed that over 90% of women who visited hospital emergency rooms for incomplete spontaneous abortion were treated by D & C. Recent studies, however, have shown that expectant management (i.e., no active intervention) is a viable option for women who do not wish to undergo surgery and who are in otherwise good health. Up to 72% of women indicated that that expectant management of incomplete abortion was preferable to medical or surgical intervention.

• Endometrial biopsy. This procedure is similar to D & C in that a curette is used to obtain a sample of endometrial tissue. Little or no cervical dilation is necessary, however, because the curette used in endometrial biop-

KEY TERMS

Endometrial polyps—Growths in the lining of the uterus (endometrium) that may cause bleeding and can develop into cancer.

Epidural anesthesia—A type of anesthesia that is injected into the epidural space of the spinal cord to numb the nerves leading to the lower half of the body.

Uterine fibroid—A noncancerous tumor of the uterus that can range from the size of a pea to the size of a grapefruit. Small fibroids require no treatment, but those causing serious symptoms may need to be removed.

sy is narrower. The cervix is numbed with a local anesthetic but the patient will still experience cramping.

- Vacuum scraping. A thin plastic tube attached to a suction machine is passed through the cervix and scraped along the endometrium. Vacuum scraping has been shown to have similar success in diagnosing uterine cancer as D & C. Local anesthesia is also used for this procedure.

- Hysteroscopy. A thin telescope called a hysteroscope is inserted through the cervix and used to view the inside of the uterus after it has been expanded with a liquid or gas. The view afforded by the hysteroscope can help to diagnose abnormal growths, accumulation of scar tissue, or other conditions.

- **Hysterectomy**. A total hysterectomy permanently removes the uterus and cervix. This procedure is generally recommended only if a woman no longer desires to have children and no other forms of treatment have been successful. Most hysterectomies are done to treat uterine fibroids and endometriosis (a condition in which the endometrium grows outside of the uterus).

Resources

PERIODICALS

Geyman, John, Lynn Oliver, and Sean Sullivan. "Expectant, Medical, or Surgical Treatment of Spontaneous Abortion in First Trimester of Pregnancy?" *Journal of the American Board of Family Practice* 12, no. 1 (1999): 55–64.

Molnar, Alexandra, Lynn Oliver, and John Geyman. "Patient Preferences for Management of First-Trimester Incomplete Spontaneous Abortion." *Journal of the American Board of Family Practice* 13, no. 5 (2000): 333–337.

ORGANIZATIONS

American College of Obstetricians and Gynecologists. 409 12th St., SW, PO Box 96920, Washington, DC 20090-6920. <http://www.acog.org>

OTHER

"Asherman's Syndrome." *International Adhesions Society.* April 24, 2002 [cited February 24, 2003]. <http://www.adhesions.org/relatedconditions/asherman.htm>.

"Dilatation and Curettage." *eTenet.* 2001 [cited February 24, 2003]. <http://www.etenet.com/Apps/Library/Corporate.asp?ID=713>.

"Dilatation and Curettage." *Patient Education Institute.* December 21, 2001 [cited February 24, 2003]. <http://www.nlm.nih.gov/medlineplus/tutorials/dilationandcurettage/og059101.html>.

"Dysfunctional Uterine Bleeding." *WomenOne.org.* 2001 [cited February 24, 2003. <http://www.womenone.org/health04.htm>.

"Endometrial Hyperplasia." *American College of Obstetricians and Gynecologists.* 2001 [cited February 24, 2003]. <http://www.medem.com/MedLB/article_detaillb.cfm?article_ID=ZZZ7Z2GWQMC&sub_cat=9>.

"Hysterectomy." *American College of Obstetricians and Gynecologists.* 2001 [cited February 24, 2003]. <http://www.medem.com/search/article_display.cfm?path=n:&mstr=/ZZZMULQGSWC.html&soc=ACS&srch_typ=NAV_SERCH>.

"Hysteroscopy." *American College of Obstetricians and Gynecologists.* 2001 [cited February 24, 2003]. <http://www.medem.com/MedLB/article_detaillb.cfm?article_ID=ZZZAXX8MA7C&sub_cat=8>.

Williams, Carmine. "Dilation and Curettage." *eMedicine.* April 26, 2001 [cited February 24, 2003]. <http://www.emedicine.com/aaem/topic156.htm>.

Carol A. Turkington
Stephanie Dionne Sherk

Discharge from the hospital

Definition

Discharge from the hospital is the point at which the patient leaves the hospital and either returns home or is transferred to another facility such as one for rehabilitation or to a nursing home. Discharge involves the medical instructions that the patient will need to fully recover. Discharge planning is a service that considers the patient's needs after the hospital stay, and may involve several different services such as visiting nursing care, physical therapy, and home blood drawing.

Description

Hospitalization is often a short-term event, so planning for discharge may begin shortly after admission. The physicians, nurses, and case managers involved in a patient's care are part of an assessment team that keeps in mind the patient's pre-admission level of functioning, and whether the patient will be able to return home following the current hospital admission. Information that could affect the discharge plan should be noted in the patient's medical record so that it will be taken into account when discharge is being scheduled. The primary questions include:

• Can this patient return to his or her preadmission situation?

• Has there been a change in the patient's ability to care for him- or herself?

• Is the patient in need of services to be able to care for him- or herself?

• Which services will the patient need?

• Are there mental health needs that must be met?

• Does the patient agree with the discharge plan?

While a person has been in the hospital, physicians other than the primary care physician have been in charge of the patient's care. Good discharge planning involves clear communication between the hospital physician(s) and the primary care physician. This may be done by telephone and/or in writing. The information to be conveyed includes:

• a summary of the hospital stay

• a list of test and surgeries performed, with results

• a list of test results still pending

• a list of tests needed after discharge, such as a repeat chest x ray

• a list of medications the patient is being discharged with, including the dosage and frequency

• a copy of the patient's discharge instructions

• when the patient should see the primary care physician for a follow-up appointment

• the plan for outpatient treatment, such as home intravenous **antibiotics** or parenteral nutrition to ensure that

responsibility for this treatment has been clearly transferred and that the primary care physician accepts the treatment responsibility

• discharge instructions to the patient on activity level, diet, and **wound care**

Before leaving the hospital, the patient will receive discharge instructions that should include:

• an explanation of the care the patient received in the hospital

• a list of medications the patient will be taking (the dosage, times, and frequency)

• a list of potential side effects of any newly prescribed medications

• a prescription for any newly prescribed medications

• when to see the primary care physician for a follow-up appointment

• **home care** instructions such as activity level, diet, restrictions on bathing, wound care, as well as when the patient can return to work or school, or resume driving

• signs of infection or worsening condition, such as pain, fever, bleeding, difficulty breathing, or vomiting

• an explanation of any services the patient will now be receiving, such as for a visiting nurse, and to include contact information

The term discharge planning may be used to refer to the service provided to help patients arrange for services such as rehabilitation, physical therapy, occupational therapy, visiting nurses, or nursing home care. This service may be provided by a case manager or by the hospital's social service department. The patient may request this service, or the physician may make the request in the form of a referral to the department. The patient will need to be evaluated to see what services he or she requires, as well as what services he or she qualifies for (such as meals-on-wheels), or what services the patient's insurance will cover. The patient may be discharged home with a visit from a visiting nurse later the same day to assess the patient's need for these services and to make arrangements for him or her in the home. A person may be discharged home only when certain equipment such as a hospital-style bed and oxygen has been delivered to the home. If a patient feels he or she is being discharged before he or she is ready, the patient can file a complaint with the hospital's ombudsman.

A follow-up from the hospital staff, either physician, nurse, or case manager, should take place within two weeks of discharge to review the results of any tests that were done in the hospital that came in after the patient was discharged, to remind the patient of the follow-up appointment with the physician, to see if the patient has any questions about any new medications that were added in the hospital, and to be sure that no problems arose after discharge that have not been addressed. Such follow-up calls help to ensure a successful recovery.

A patient may experience a complication or an adverse effect as a result of care received in the hospital. The complication may be due to medication that was given, or from a test or surgery performed. In the February 2003 issue of *The Annals of Internal Medicine,* researchers reported how often these adverse effects arose, and how severe they were. Patients were interviewed by telephone a few weeks after discharge. About 20% had experienced an adverse effect such as a new or worsening symptom, medication-related problems, the need for an unexpected visit to the doctor, or death. Of the 20%, about one third had preventable adverse effects, and another third had problems that would have been less severe if they had received proper medical care. Three percent developed permanent disability.

See also Admission to the hospital.

Resources

BOOKS

Wachter, Robert M., Lee Goldman, and Harry Hollander, editors. *Hospital Medicine.* Baltimore: Lippincott Williams & Wilkins, 2000.

PERIODICALS

Forster, A. J., et al. "The Incidence and Severity of Adverse Events Affecting Patients after Discharge from the Hospital." *Annals of Internal Medicine,* 138 (February 2003): 161–167.

ORGANIZATIONS

The American Hospital Association. One North Franklin, Chicago, IL 60606.

National Center for Health Statistics. *National Hospital Discharge Survey,* Vital Health Stat. 153 (November 2002): 1–194.

National Institute on Aging. <http://www.nih.gov/nia>.

Esther Csapo Rastegari, RN, BSN, EdM

Disk removal

Definition

Disk removal is one of the most common types of back surgery. Diskectomy (also called discectomy) is the removal of an intervertebral disk, the flexible plate that connects any two adjacent vertebrae in the spine. Intervertebral disks act as shock absorbers, protecting the brain and spinal cord from the impact produced by the body's movements.

Purpose

Removing the invertebral disk is performed after completion of unsuccessful conservative treatment for back pain that has been present for at least six weeks. Surgery is also performed if there is pressure on the lumbosacral nerve roots that causes weakness, bowel dysfunction, or bladder dysfunction.

As a person ages, the disks between vertebrae degenerate and dry out, and tears form in the fibers holding them in place. Eventually, the disk can develop a blister-like bulge, compressing nerves in the spine and causing pain. This is called a "prolapsed" (or herniated) disk. If such a disk presses on a nerve root and causes muscle weakness, or problems with the bladder or bowel, immediate disk removal surgery may be needed.

The goal of the surgery is to relieve all pressure on nerve roots by removing the pulpy material from the disk, or the entire disk. If it is necessary to remove material from several nearby vertebrae, the spine may become unsteady. In this case, the surgeon will perform a **spinal fusion**, removing all disks between two or more vertebrae, and roughening the bones so that the vertebrae heal together. Bone strips taken from the patient's leg or hip may be used to help hold the vertebrae together. Spinal fusion decreases pain, but decreases spinal mobility.

Demographics

Approximately 150,000 Americans undergo disk removal each year in the United States.

Description

The surgery is performed under general anesthesia. The surgeon cuts an opening into the vertebral canal, and moves the dura and the bundle of nerves called the "cauda equina" (horse's tail) aside, which exposes the disk. If a portion of the disk has moved out from between the vertebrae and into the nerve canal, it is sim-

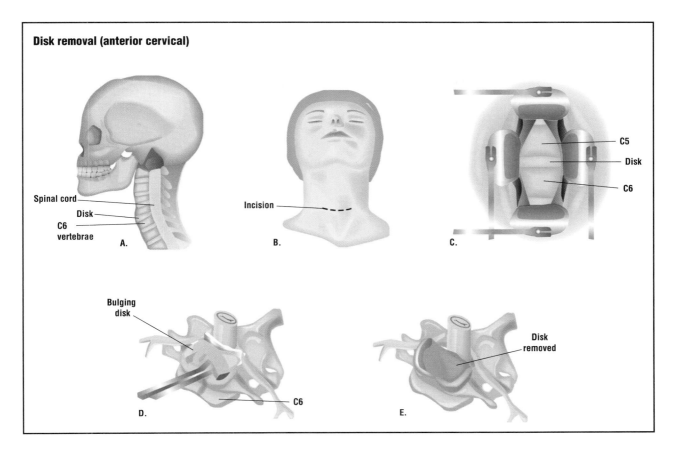

Disk removal (anterior cervical)

Spinal cord
Disk
C6 vertebrae
A.

Incision
B.

C5
Disk
C6
C.

Bulging disk
C6
D.

Disk removed
E.

In the anterior cervical disk removal, an incision is made into the patient's neck (B). The cervical disk, which may be herniated, is visualized (C). It is removed completely (D and E). *(Illustration by GGS Inc.)*

ply removed. If the disk itself has become fragmented and partially displaced, or is not fragmented but bulges extensively, the surgeon removes the damaged part of the disk and the part that lies in the space between the vertebrae.

There are minimally invasive surgical techniques for disk removal, including microdiskectomy. In this procedure, the surgeon uses a magnifying instrument or special microscope to view the disk. Magnification makes it possible to remove a herniated disk with a smaller incision, causing less damage to nearby tissue. Video-assisted arthroscopic microdiskectomy has exhibited good results with less use of narcotics and a shortened period of disability. Newer forms of diskectomy are still in the research stage, and are not yet widely available. These include laser diskectomy and automated percutaneous diskectomy.

Total disk replacement research in the United States is underway. Products under investigation include the ProDisc (made by Spine Solutions, Inc.), and the SB Charite III (made by Link Spine Group, Inc.). In these clinical studies, a significant number of patients who received artificial disk implants report a reduction in back and leg pain; 92.7% state they are satisfied or extremely satisfied with the procedure.

Diagnosis/Preparation

The physician will obtain x rays and neuroimaging studies, including a computed tomography (CT) scan, myelogram, and **magnetic resonance imaging** (MRI); and clinical exams to determine the precise location of the affected disk.

An hour before surgery, the patient is given an injection to dry up internal fluids and encourage drowsiness.

Aftercare

After the operation, the patient is lying flat and face down when he or she awakens. This position must be maintained for several days, except for occasional positional changes to avoid **bedsores**. There may be slight pain or stiffness in the back area.

Patients usually leave the hospital on the fourth or fifth day after surgery. They must:

- Avoid sitting for more than 15–20 minutes.

- Use a reclined chair.

- Avoid bending at the waist, twisting, or lifting heavy objects.

- Begin gentle walking (indoors or outdoors), and gradually increase **exercise**. Exercise should be continued for the next four weeks.

- Begin stationary biking or gentle swimming after two weeks.

- Sleep on a firm mattress.

- Slow down if they experience more than minor pain in the back or leg.

- Refrain from sitting in one place for an extended period of time (e.g., long car ride).

Patients should be able to resume normal activities in four to six weeks.

Risks

All surgery carries some risk due to heart and lung problems or the anesthesia itself, but this risk is generally very small. (The risk of death from general anesthesia for all types of surgery, for example, is only approximately one in 1,600 surgeries.)

The most common risk of the surgery is infection, which occurs in 1–2% of cases. Rarely, the surgery damages nerves in the lower back or major blood vessels in front of the disk. Occasionally, there may be some residual paralysis of a leg or bladder muscle after surgery, but this is the result of the disk problem that necessitated the surgery, not the operation itself.

Normal results

In properly evaluated patients, there is a very good chance that disk removal will be successful in easing pain. The surgery can relieve pain in 90% of cases; however, there are some people who do not achieve pain relief. This depends on a number of factors, including the length of time that they had the condition requiring surgery. Disk surgery has a "good to excellent" result in 87% of patients over age 60. The surgery can relieve both back and leg pain, especially the latter.

Alternatives

Prior to disk removal surgery, a patient usually undergoes treatment with medical or physical therapy. Disk removal surgery may be indicated if these treatments are ineffective, or if emergency symptoms (i.e., bladder and bowel dysfunction) develop.

See also Bone grafting; Spinal fusion.

Resources

BOOKS

Beauchamp, M.D., Daniel R., Mark B. Evers, M.D., Kenneth L. Mattox, M.D., Courtney M. Townsend, and David C. Sabiston (Editors). *Sabiston Textbook of Surgery: The Biological Basis of Modern Surgical Practice*. 16th edition. London: W B Saunders Co., 2001.

Bogduk, Nikolai, Brian McGuirk, and Boriana Dirk Van Der Deliiska. *Medical Management of Acute and Chronic Low Back Pain*. Philadelphia, PA: Elsevier Health Sciences, 2002.

Cailliet, Rene. *Low Back Disorders: A Medial Enigma*. Philadelphia, PA: Lippincott Williams & Wilkins, 2003.

Lawrence, Peter F., Richard M. Bell, and Merril T. Dayton, eds. *Essentials of General Surgery*. 3rd edition. Philadelphia, PA: Lippincott, Williams & Wilkins, 2000.

Resnick, Daniel K., ed. *Surgical Management of Low Back Pain (Neurosurgical Topics)*. 2nd edition. Rolling Meadows, IL: American Association of Neurological Surgeons, 2001.

Watkins, Robert G. *Surgical Approaches to the Spine*. 2nd edition. Berlin, Germany: Springer Verlag. 2003.

PERIODICALS

Alini, M., P. J. Roughley, J. Antoniou, T. Stoll, and M. Aebi. "A Biological Approach to Treating Disc Degeneration: Not for Today, But Maybe for Tomorrow." *European Spine Journal* 11, no. 2 (October 2002): S215-20.

Deyo, R., and J. Weinstein. "Low Back Pain." *New England Journal of Medicine* 344, no. 5 (2001): 363-70.

Oskouian, R .J., Jr., J. P. Johnson, and J. J. Regan. "Thoracoscopic Microdiscectomy." *Neurosurgery* 5, no.1 (January 2002): 103-9.

KEY TERMS

Cauda equina—A bundle of nerve roots in the lower back (lumbar region) of the spinal canal that controls the leg muscles and functioning of the bladder, intestines, and genitals.

Computed tomography (CT) scan—A special type of x ray that produces detailed images of structures inside the body.

Diskectomy (or discectomy)—The surgical removal of a portion of an invertebral disk.

Dura—The strongest and outermost of three membranes that protect the brain, spinal cord, and nerves of the cauda equina.

Fusion—A union, joining together; e.g., bone fusion.

Myelogram—The film produced by myelography; a graphic representation of the differential count of cells found in a stained representation of bone marrow.

Herniated disk—A blister-like bulging or protrusion of the contents of the disk out through the fibers that normally hold them in place. Also called ruptured disk, slipped disk, or displaced disk.

Intervertebral disk—Cylindrical elastic-like gel pads that separate and join each pair of vertebrae in the spine.

Laminectomy—An operation in which the surgeon cuts through the covering of a vertebra to reach a herniated disk in order to remove it.

Magnetic resonance imaging (MRI)—A test that provides pictures of organs and structures inside the body by using a magnetic field and pulses of radio wave energy to detect tumors, infection, and other types of tissue disease or damage, or conditions affecting blood flow. The area of the body being studied is positioned inside a strong magnetic field.

Percutaneous—Denoting the passage of substances through unbroken skin; also refers to passage through the skin by needle puncture, including introduction of wires and catheters by the Seldinger technique.

Vertebra—The bones that make up the back bone (spine).

Silber, J. S., D. G. Anderson, V. M. Hayes, and A. R. Vaccaro. "Advances in Surgical Management of Lumbar Degenerative Disease." *Orthopedics* 25, no.7 (July 2002): 767-71.

ORGANIZATIONS

North American Spine Society. 22 Calendar Court, 2nd Floor, LaGrange, IL 60525. (877) Spine-Dr. E-mail: info@spine.org. <http://www.spine.org>.

National Institutes of Health. 9000 Rockville Pike, Bethesda, MD 20892. (301) 496-4000. Email: NIHInfo@od.nih.gov. <http://www.nih.gov/>.

OTHER

Spine Health.com. *Total Disc Replacement.* 2003. <http://www.spine-health.com/research/discupdate/artificial/artificial04.html>. [cited March 19, 2003].

American Academy of Orthopaedic Surgery (AAOS) and American Association of Orthopaedic Surgery. *Low Back Surgery.* 2001. <http://orthoinfo.aaos.org/booklet/thr_report.cfm?thread_id=10&topcategory=sp>. [cited March 19, 2003].

Carol A. Turkington
Crystal H. Kaczkowski, MSc.

Diskectomy *see* **Disk removal**

Diuretics

Definition

Diuretics are medicines that help reduce the amount of water in the body.

Purpose

Diuretics are used to treat the buildup of excess fluid in the body that occurs with some medical conditions such as congestive heart failure, liver disease, and kidney disease. Some diuretics are also prescribed to treat high blood pressure. Most of these drugs act on the kidneys to increase urine output. This reduces the amount of fluid in the bloodstream, which in turn lowers blood pressure.

Diuretics may be used in surgery to reduce blood pressure and swelling. Mannitol, an osmotic diuretic, may be used to reduce swelling in the brain, which may be necessary for some neurosurgical procedures.

Description

There are several types of diuretics, also called water pills:

- Loop diuretics, such as bumetanide (Bumex) and furosemide (Lasix), get their name from the loop-shaped part of the kidneys where they have their effect.

- Thiazide diuretics include such commonly used diuretics as hydrochlorothiazide (HydroDIURIL, Esidrix), chlorothiazide (Diuril), and chlorthalidone (Hygroton).

- Potassium-sparing diuretics prevent the loss of potassium, which is a problem with other types of diuretics; examples of potassium-sparing diuretics are amiloride (Midamor) and triamterene (Dyrenium).

- Osmotic diuretics keep water from being reabsorbed in the kidney. Mannitol, which is given by intravenous drip, is commonly used to reduce cerebral edema (swelling of the brain).

- Carbonic anhydrase inhibitors are another form of diuretic. While they cause water loss through the kidneys by changing the acidity of urine, their most common use is in treatment of glaucoma, an eye disease caused by increased pressure inside the eyeball. Acetazolamide (Diamox) is the most commonly used carbonix anhydrase inhibitor. Acetazolamide is given by mouth, but other drugs may be given as eye drops.

In addition, some medicines contain combinations of two diuretics. The brands Dyazide and Maxzide, for example, contain the thiazide diuretic hydrochlorothiazide with the potassium-sparing diuretic triamterene.

Some nonprescription (over-the-counter) medicines contain diuretics. However, the medicines described here cannot be bought without a physician's prescription. They are available in tablet, capsule, liquid, and injectable forms.

Recommended dosage

Warnings and cautions apply to the thiazide and loop diuretics, which are given by mouth over a long period of time. They do not apply to a single dose of an osmotic diuretic, which may be given immediately before or during surgery.

The recommended dosage depends on the type of diuretic and may be different for different patients, but they should check with the physician who prescribed the drug or the pharmacist who filled the prescription for the correct dosage, and take the medicine exactly as directed.

Precautions

Seeing a physician regularly while taking a diuretic is important. The physician will check to make sure the medicine is working as it should and will watch for unwanted side effects.

Some people feel unusually tired when they first start taking diuretics. This effect usually becomes less noticeable over time, as the body adjusts to the medicine.

Because diuretics increase urine output, people who take this medicine may need to urinate more often, even during the night. Health care professionals can help patients schedule their doses to avoid interfering with their sleep or regular activities.

For patients taking the kinds of diuretics that rob potassium from the body, physicians may recommend adding potassium-rich foods or drinks such as citrus fruits and juices to the diet. Or, they may suggest taking a potassium supplement or taking another medicine that keeps the body from losing too much potassium. If the physician recommends any of these measures, the patient must make sure to closely follow the directions. The patient should not make other diet changes without checking with the physician. People who are taking potassium-sparing diuretics should not add potassium to their diets, as too much potassium may be harmful.

People who take diuretics may lose too much water or potassium when they get sick, especially if they have severe vomiting and diarrhea. They should check with their physicians if they become ill.

These medicines make some people feel lightheaded, dizzy, or faint when they get up after sitting or lying down. Older people are especially likely to have this problem. Drinking alcohol, exercising, standing for long periods, or being outdoors in hot weather may make the problem worse. To lessen the problem, a person should get up gradually and hold onto something for support if possible. The patient should avoid drinking too much alcohol and be careful in hot weather or when exercising or standing for a long time.

Anyone who is taking a diuretic should be sure to tell the health care professional in charge before having surgical or dental procedures, medical tests, or emergency treatment.

Some diuretics make the skin more sensitive to sunlight. Even brief exposure to sun can cause severe sunburn, itching, a rash, redness, or other changes in skin color. While being treated with this medicine, the person should avoid being in direct sunlight, especially between 10 A.M. and 3 P.M.; wear a hat and tightly woven clothing that covers the arms and legs; use a sunscreen with a skin protection factor (SPF) of at least 15; protect the lips with a sun-block lipstick; and not use tanning beds, tanning booths, or sunlamps. People with fair skin may need to use a sunscreen with a higher skin protection factor.

Special conditions

People who have certain medical conditions or who are taking certain other medicines may have problems if they take diuretics. Before taking these drugs, they should be sure to let the physician know about any of these conditions.

ALLERGIES. Anyone who has had unusual reactions to diuretics or **sulfonamides** (sulfa drugs) in the past should let the physician know. The physician should also be told about any allergies to foods, dyes, preservatives, or other substances.

PREGNANCY. Diuretics will not help the swelling of hands and feet that some women experience during pregnancy. In general, pregnant women should not use diuretics unless a physician recommends their use. Although studies have not been done on pregnant women, studies of laboratory animals show that some diuretics can cause harmful effects when taken during pregnancy.

BREASTFEEDING. Some diuretics pass into breast milk, but no reports exist of problems in nursing babies whose mothers use this medicine. However, thiazide diuretics may decrease the flow of breast milk. Women who are breastfeeding and need to use a diuretic should check with the physician.

OTHER MEDICAL CONDITIONS. Side effects of some diuretics may be more likely in people who have had a recent heart attack or who have liver disease or severe kidney disease. Other types of diuretics may not work properly in people with liver disease or severe kidney disease. Diuretics may worsen certain medical conditions such as gout, kidney stones, pancreatitis, lupus erythematosus, and hearing problems. In addition, people with diabetes should be aware that diuretics might increase blood sugar levels. People with heart or blood vessel disease should know that some diuretics increase cholesterol or triglyceride levels. The risk of an allergic reaction to certain diuretics is greater in people with bronchial asthma. Before using diuretics, people with any of these medical problems should make sure their physicians are aware of their conditions. Also, people who have trouble urinating or who have high potassium levels in their blood may not be able to take diuretics and should check with a physician before using them.

USE OF CERTAIN MEDICINES. Taking diuretics with certain other drugs may affect the way the drugs work or may increase the chance of side effects.

Side effects

Some side effects such as loss of appetite, nausea and vomiting, stomach cramps, diarrhea, and dizziness, usually lessen or go away as the body adjusts to the med-

icine. These problems do not need medical attention unless they continue or interfere with normal activities.

Patients taking potassium-sparing diuretics should know the signs of too much potassium and should check with a physician as soon as possible if any of these symptoms occur:

- irregular heartbeat
- breathing problems
- numbness or tingling in the hands, feet, or lips
- confusion or nervousness
- unusual tiredness or weakness
- weak or heavy feeling in the legs

Patients taking diuretics that cause potassium loss should know the signs of too little potassium and should check with a physician as soon as possible if they have any of these symptoms:

- fast or irregular heartbeat
- weak pulse
- nausea or vomiting
- dry mouth
- excessive thirst
- muscle cramps or pain
- unusual tiredness or weakness
- mental or mood changes

Interactions

Diuretics may interact with other medicines. When this happens, the effects of one or both of the drugs may change or the risk of side effects may be greater. Anyone who takes a diuretic should let the physician know all other medicines he or she is taking and should ask whether the possible interactions can interfere with drug therapy. Among the drugs that may interact with diuretics are:

- Angiotensin-converting enzyme (ACE) inhibitors such as benazepril (Lotensin), captopril (Capoten), and enalapril (Vasotec), which are used to treat high blood pressure. Taking these drugs with potassium-sparing diuretics may cause levels of potassium in the blood to be too high, increasing the chance of side effects.

- Cholesterol-lowering drugs such as cholestyramine (Questran) and colestipol (Colestid). Taking these drugs with combination diuretics such as Dyazide and Maxzide may keep the diuretic from working. The person should take the diuretic at least one hour before or four hours after the cholesterol-lowering drug.

- Cyclosporine (Sandimmune), a medicine that suppresses the immune system. Taking this medicine with

KEY TERMS

Inflammation—Pain, redness, swelling, and heat that usually develop in response to injury or illness.

Lupus erythematosus—A chronic disease that affects the skin, joints, and certain internal organs.

Pancreas—A gland located beneath the stomach. The pancreas produces juices that help breakdown food.

Potassium—A mineral found in whole gains, meat, legumes, and some fruits and vegetables. Potassium is important for many body processes, including proper functioning of the nerves and muscles.

Triglyceride—A substance formed in the body from fat in the diet; they are the main fatty materials in the blood. Triglyceride levels are important in the diagnosis and treatment of many diseases, including high blood pressure, diabetes, and heart disease.

potassium-sparing diuretics may increase the chance of side effects by causing levels of potassium in the blood to be too high.

• Potassium supplements, other medicines containing potassium, or salt substitutes that contain potassium. Taking these with potassium-sparing diuretics may lead to too much potassium in the blood, increasing the chance of side effects.

• Lithium, used to treat bipolar disorder (manic-depressive illness). Using this medicine with potassium-sparing diuretics may allow lithium to build up to poisonous levels in the body.

• Digitalis heart drugs such as digoxin (Lanoxin). Using this medicine with combination diuretics such as triamterene-hydrocholorthiazide (Dyazide, Maxzide) may cause blood levels of the heart to be too high, making side effects such as changes in heartbeat more likely.

The list above does not include every drug that may interact with diuretics. The patient is advised to check with a physician or pharmacist before combining diuretics with any other prescription or nonprescription (over-the-counter) medicine.

Resources

BOOKS

AHFS: Drug Information. Washington, DC: American Society Healthsystems Pharmaceuticals, 2002.

Drug Facts and Comparisons. St. Louis: Facts & Comparisons, 2003.

Reynolds, J. E. F., ed. *Martindale: The Extra Pharmacopeia*, 31st ed. London: The Pharmaceutical Press, 1993.

OTHER

"Carbonic Anhydrase Inhibitors (Systemic)." Medline Plus Drug Information. [cited June 2003]. <http://www.nlm.nih.gov/medlineplus/druginfo/uspdi/202114.html>.

"Diuretics, Loop (Systemic)." Medline Plus Drug Information. [cited June 2003]. <http://www.nlm.nih.gov/medlineplus/druginfo/uspdi/202205.html>.

"Diuretics, Potassium-Sparing (Systemic)." Medline Plus Drug Information. [cited June 2003]. <http://www.nlm.nih.gov/medlineplus/druginfo/uspdi/202206.html>.

"Diuretics, Thiazide (Systemic)." Medline Plus Drug Information. [cited June 2003]. <http://www.nlm.nih.gov/medlineplus/druginfo/uspdi/202208.html>.

Nancy Ross-Flanigan
Sam Uretsky, PharmD

Diverticulectomy *see* **Meckel's diverticulectomy**

DNR order *see* **Do not resuscitate (DNR) order**

Do not resuscitate (DNR) order

Definition

Do not resuscitate (DNR) order is a part of advanced medical directives allowed by federal law passed in 1991, expanding the notion of patient autonomy to situations in which they may not be able to make crucial medical decisions due to incapacitation. It instructs medical personnel not to perform life-saving **cardiopulmonary resuscitation** (CPR) or other procedures to restart the heart or breathing once they have ceased. By law, the DNR directive must be offered as an option to patients by health providers in, and in some states, out of a hospital setting. Once signed, the DNR directive must be placed in the in the patient's chart.

Purpose

With such advanced cardiopulmonary techniques as CPR, it is possible to keep almost any patient's heart and lungs functioning, independent of how terminal or hopeless their medical condition becomes. The DNR program is designed to help people in the final stages of a terminal illness or who have intractable pain the option for deciding against life-saving measures that may only prolong their pain and death. The option of deciding against life-saving measures is considered to be a formal part of patient autonomy and is respected as an ethical subset of medical **informed consent**.

Description

DNR orders affect a small group of patients and are designed to avoid the suffering of a terminal illness or other serious conditions that are medically irreversible. The order actually authorizes medical treatment to be withheld. It is included with the medical orders in the medical chart, and with it, hospital and pre-hospital personnel are restricted from using CPR techniques and other measures to revive the patient.

Some states allow DNR orders only in hospital settings. Other states allow DNR orders to be honored by emergency responders working outside the hospital setting. Over half of the states in the United States have pre-hospital DNR orders. A physician must sign the pre-hospital DNR directives. The state's Emergency Medical Service (EMS) department or state medical association administers the programs. In some states, the DNR may be called a pre-hospital medical care directive or a comfort care only document.

A DNR order can be revoked at any time in any way that effectively communicates the patient's desire. It can come from the patient in the form of a letter or document. It can come from the patient telling an emergency provider to disregard the order. The revocation can be invoked by removing any bracelet or medallion that indicates DNR status. It can be communicated by the designated health agent or patient representative who has the power to express the patient's wishes to health providers. Some states maintain a registry for individuals with DNR orders. It is important to find out about a state's service for DNR and its particular legal forms and requirements. Many patients who die in a hospital have had a DNR order.

Preparation

Do not resuscitate orders are a part of advanced medical directives. This a legal document that places limits on medical treatment, guides medical providers on the wishes and options of the patient and helps family members and providers make decisions in accordance with the wishes of patients. Advanced directives are prepared in advance and may include a **living will** that lays out all of the patient's wishes should they become incapacitated. A DNR order is a very specific order that medical treatment be withheld, especially CPR. Finally, a health agent or a person with a durable medical **power of attorney** is usually appointed to carry out all wishes of the patient and to make sure that specific wishes, like DNR, are honored.

KEY TERMS

Advanced medical directive—A legal document drafted by a patient in advance ordering specific medical procedures to be offered or withheld if they are incapacitated.

CPR—Cardiopulmonary resuscitation. A set of medical procedures used in an emergency to restart the heart and lungs.

Medical agent—A designated representative for the patient who, in advance, is legally empowered to carry out their wishes with respect to medial care.

Medical surrogate—Another name for a medical agent or person legally designated to represent the patient with medical providers.

An advanced directive for resuscitation being withheld can be prepared by requesting a form from the physician, by writing down that wish, by having a lawyer draft a living will or by using computer software for legal documents. States differ in the respect of whether the documents must be cosigned or notarized. Crucial to the effort is that the physician be told of the wishes of the patient and discuss what occurs when the DNR order is carried out.

Normal results

DNR law varies from state to state but the common features include:

- Formal documents that providers or responders can readily recognize in charts or on display in the home.

- DNR bracelets or medallions that the patient wears and providers are trained to recognize.

- DNR must be signed by a physician before responders or other providers may honor them.

- Once in effect, DNR orders include only certain life-preserving procedures, like CPR. Comfort treatment is not withheld and the alleviation of pain is still pursued by providers.

- Physicians or other providers who are unwilling to carry out the order (for moral or professional reasons) are required to transfer the care of the patient to another provider who will carry out the DNR order.

Resources

BOOKS

"Death and Dying." In *Merck Manual, Home Edition.* [cited May 5, 2003]. <http://www.merck.com/mrkshared/mmanual_home/sec1/4.jsp.>

PERIODICALS

Kish, S. K. "Advance Directives in Critically Ill Cancer Patients." In *Critical Care Nursing Clinics North America* 12 (September 1, 2000): 373–83.

Matousek, M. "Start the Conversation: The Modern Maturity Guide to End-of-Life Care." and "The Last Taboo." *Modern Maturity/AARP* (September-October 2000).

ORGANIZATIONS

Cancer Information Service. (800) 4-CANCER (800-422-6237). TTY: (800) 332-8615. < www.cancer.gov>.

Partnership for Caring. 1620 Eye St., NW, Suite 202, Washington, DC 20006. (202) 296-8071. Fax: (202) 296-8352. Toll-free hotline: (800) 989-9455 (option 3).

OTHER

"Advanced Directives and Do Not Resuscitate Orders." American Academy of Family Physicians. March 2002 [cited May 5, 2003]. <http://familydoctor.org/handouts/003.html>.

"Choosing a Health Care Agent." *Healthwise.* WebMD Health [cited May 5, 2003]. <http://www.WebMD.com.>

"Death and Dying." *Health Topics.* National Library of Medicine, NIH/MedlinePlus. [cited May 5, 2003]. <http://www.nlm.nih.gov/medlineplus/deathanddying.html.>

Nancy McKenzie, Ph.D.

Dopamine *see* **Adrenergic drugs**

Doppler echocardiography *see* **Echocardiography**

Doxycycline *see* **Tetracyclines**

Dressings *see* **Bandages and dressings**

Drugs used in labor *see* **Uterine stimulants**

Durable medical power of attorney *see* **Power of attorney**

E

Ear, nose, and throat surgery

Definition

Ear, nose, and throat surgery is the the surgical treatment of diseases, injuries, or deformations of the ears, nose, throat, head, and neck areas.

Purpose

The purpose of surgery to the ears, nose, throat, head, and neck is to treat an abnormality (defect or disease) in these anatomical areas. An anatomical deformity is a change that usually occurs during embryological development, leaving the affected person with the apparent defect. A disease in this area usually develops later in life, such as head and neck cancer. Additionally, the specialty known as otorhinolaryngology (ears [*oto*], nose [*rhino*], and throat [*laryn*], referring to the larynx or throat) also includes surgical intervention for diseases in the head and neck regions. Most ears, nose, and throat (ENT) surgeons in the United States are referred to as otolaryngologist and the specialty as otolaryngology. Ear surgery is usually performed to correct specific causes of hearing loss. Nose surgery can include different types of procedures necessary to treat sinus problems (sinus surgery). Throat surgery can include complicated procedures such as cancer of the larynx (**laryngectomy**), or more simple procedures such as surgical removal of the adenoids (**adenoidectomy**) or tonsils (**tonsillectomy**). Head and neck surgery may be necessary to remove a tumor or reconstruct an area after disfigurement from trauma or injury.

Demographics

Ears, nose, throat surgery comprises many different types of surgical procedures and spans over all age groups regardless of gender or ethnicity. A special subspecialty, pediatric otolaryngology, is the branch that treats ENT disease for infants and children.

Description

ENT surgery is the oldest surgical specialty in the United States, and it is one of the most elaborate fields of surgical specialty services, using advanced technology and a broad range of procedures that also includes major reconstructive surgery to correct deformity or injury. Cosmetic surgery can include surgical procedures to improve wrinkles in the face, contours of the nose and ears, chin augmentation, and **hair transplantation**.

Typically, ear surgery is utilized to correct defects causing hearing loss or impairment. Such procedures in-

QUESTIONS TO ASK THE DOCTOR

- What can I expect in the postoperative period?
- What are the specific aftercare recommendations for my specific surgical procedure?
- What are the expected normal results for my specific procedure?
- What medications will I be given to relieve any postoperative discomfort?
- Are there any side effects that I should expect in the postoperative period?

clude **stapedectomy** (removal of all or part of a bone in the middle ear called the stapes), **tympanoplasty** (reconstruction of the ear drum), and **cochlear implants** (implantation of a device to stimulate nerve ends within the inner portion of the ear to enable hearing). Surgery of the ear also includes myringotomy (insertion of ear tubes to drain fluid in persons with chronic ear infections).

Common surgical procedures of the throat include removal of tonsils (tonsillectomy) or adenoids (adenoidectomy). The tonsils (either side and in back of the throat) and adenoids (higher up the throat behind the nose) are masses of lymph tissue that play an active role in body defenses to fight infection. The tonsils and adenoids can get chronically infected, in which case surgical removal is usually indicated to relieve breathing problems and infection recurrence. Furthermore, chronic inflammation of the adenoids can cause repeated middle ear infections that can ultimately impair hearing.

Surgery of the nose can include procedures that treat sinus diseases (sinus surgery). Advanced endoscopic surgery for sinus and nasal disorders can eliminate the need for external incisions and greater surgical precision. Other common surgical procedures include correction of a deviated nasal septum (**septoplasty**) and for chronic nasal obstruction (congestion).

Surgery of the neck region can commonly include **tracheotomy** (a surgical procedure in which an opening is made in the trachea or window). Tracheotomy is indicated for a person who is unable to deliver enough air (oxygen) to the lungs. Additionally, ENT surgeons perform complicated surgical procedures for the treatment of malignant head and neck cancers. In addition to **tumor removal**, when indicated, ENT surgeons may perform an operation called **radical neck dissection**, during which the ENT will remove cancer that has spread via lymphat-

ic vessels to regional neck lymph nodes. Neck dissection is also useful since specimens can be removed for pathological examination, which can provide important information concerning metastasis (spread) and can direct the treatment plan (i.e., radiation therapy and/or chemotherapy may be recommended for aggressive cancers). ENT surgeons also treat sleep-related disorders such as sleep apnea and excessive snoring; a procedure called laser-assisted uvula palatoplasty (LAUP) will remove tissue to allow for unobstructed airflow.

Other ENT procedures include surgical reconstruction of ear deformities (otoplasties), special surgery for diseases in the inner ear, and skull-based surgeries (neuro-otology). As well, ENT surgeons can surgically treat abnormalities near the eye, perform oral surgery for treatment of dental and jaw injury, and remove skin cancer within the head and neck region. ENT surgeons also perform special surgical techniques that can preserve nerve and blood vessel function (**microsurgery**) and reconstruction of bone and soft tissue.

Diagnosis/Preparation

A careful history and **physical examination** of the ears, nose, throat, head, and neck is a standard approach during initial consultation. Different instruments with light sources (i.e., otoscope for ear examinations) enable ENT surgeons to quickly visualize the ears, nose, and throat. Visualization of these areas can reveal the severity of the disease or deformity. The head and neck area is inspected and the neck and throat area is typically felt with the surgeon's hands (palpation). Special technological advancements have enabled ENT surgeons to further visualize deep internal anatomical structures. Nasal endoscopy allows visualization of the upper airway to detect anatomical problems related to sinuses. Videostroboscopy can be used to visualize the vocal cords, and triple endoscopy (laryngoscopy, esophagoscopy, and **bronchoscopy**) can diagnose and stage head and neck cancers. Preparation before surgery is fairly standardized and includes blood work-up and instructions to have nothing to eat or drink after midnight of the night before the procedure.

Aftercare

The aftercare for ENT surgery depends on the procedure and state of the health of the patient. The aftercare for a patient who is 60 years old with head/neck cancer is more extensive than a tonsillectomy performed in a young adolescent or child. Generally, aftercare should be directed toward **wound care** and knowledge gained from the surgeon specifically detailing the expected length of average convalescence. Wound care (cleansing, dressing changes, etc.) and postoperative follow-up with the ENT surgeon is essential. Medications for pain may be prescribed. Patients stay in the hospital for eight to 10 hours (for the effects of anesthesia to subside) for same-day surgical procedures (i.e., tonsillectomy), or they may be admitted for a few days for more complicated procedures (i.e., cancer). Aftercare and convalescence may take longer for complicated procedures such as advanced cancer and temporal-bone (two bones on both sides of the skull near the ear) surgery for nerve disorders (that can affect balance) or for tumors.

Risks

The risk of ENT surgery depends on the procedure and the health status of the patient. Some procedures do not have much risk, while complications for other procedures can carry considerable risk. For example, the risk of a complicated operation such as neck dissection could result in loss of ear sensation, since the nerve that provides the feeling of sensation is commonly severed during the procedure.

Normal results

There will be a cure (i.e., tonsillectomy) or an improvement (i.e., cancer of the head and neck) of the primary disease. Ear surgery should help individuals hear well. Throat surgery can help remove chronically inflamed tonsils, or adenoids, polyps, or cancer. Nose surgery for deviated septums or nasal congestion will improve breathing problems and help a person breath more easily and effectively through the nose. Neck surgery can help remove diseased tissue and prevent further spread of cancer. Surgery for sleep apnea will remove redundant tissue that blocks airways and obstructs normal airflow.

Morbidity and mortality rates

Outcome and disease progression vary for each disease state. There are no general statistics for all ENT procedures. Some procedures are generally correlated with excellent morbidity (over 90% success rates for all cases receiving tympanoplasty) and no mortality, while others may be associated with poor outcome and much illness (i.e., advanced head/neck cancer).

Alternatives

Usually, surgery is indicated when benefit from surgery is a clear-cut primary intervention or when medical (also referred to as conservative) treatment has failed to provide sustained symptomatic improvement. A person diagnosed with cancer may not have an alternative conservative treatment, depending on the stage (progression of cancer). However, a person with sinus problems may be treated conservatively (with **antibiotics**, saline nasal spray wash, steroid nasal spray, and/or antihista-

mine spray) before indication or necessity for surgery. There are many other services that the ENT surgeon uses to treat specific diseases, including audiology services for diagnostic and therapeutic (hearing aids) purposes, and services to treat disorders of speech and voice.

Resources

BOOKS

McPhee, Stephen, et al. "Ears, Nose, and Throat." In *Current Medical Diagnosis and Treatment*. 35th ed. Stamford: Appleton & Lange, 1995.

ORGANIZATIONS

American Academy of Otolaryngology-Head and Neck Surgery, Inc. One Prince Street, Alexandria, VA 22314-3357. (703) 836-4444. <http://www.entnet.org>.

American Hearing Research Foundation. 55 E. Washington St., Suite 2022, Chicago, Il 60602. (312) 726-9670. <http://www.american-hearing.org/>.

American Speech-Language-Hearing Association. 10801 Rockville Pike, Rockville, MD 20852. (800) 638-8255. <http://www.asha.org>.

Laith Farid Gulli, MD,MS
Robert Ramirez, BS

Ear surgery *see* **Otoplasty**
Ear tubes *see* **Myringotomy and ear tubes**
Eardrum repair *see* **Tympanoplasty**
ECCE *see* **Extracapsular cataract extraction**
ECG *see* **Electrocardiography**

Echocardiography

Definition

Echocardiography is a diagnostic test that uses ultrasound waves to produce an image of the heart muscle and the heart's valves.

Purpose

Echocardiography is used to diagnose certain cardiovascular diseases, and is one of the most widely used diagnostic tests for heart disease. Ultrasound waves that rebound or echo off the heart can show the size, shape, and movement of the heart's valves and chambers, as well as the flow of blood through the heart. Echocardiography may show abnormalities such as a poorly functioning heart valve or damage to the heart tissue from a heart attack. Echocardiography is especially useful for assessing disorders of the heart valves. It not only allows doctors to evaluate the heart valves, but can also detect abnormalities in the pattern of blood flow. For example, echocardiography can show the backward flow of blood through heart valves that are partially open (that should be fully closed). This backward flow of blood through a valve is known as regurgitation. By assessing the motion of the heart wall, echocardiography can help detect the presence, and assess the severity, of coronary artery disease, as well as help determine whether chest pain is related to heart disease. Additionally, echocardiography can help detect hypertrophic cardiomyopathy, in which the walls of the heart thicken in an attempt to compensate for heart muscle weakness.

Echocardiography is also used to evaluate heart murmurs (abnormal heart sounds), determine the causes of congestive heart failure, assess enlarged hearts or hearts with septal defects (holes between pumping chambers), and monitor the heart in patients with diseases that may affect heart function (e.g., lupus, lung diseases). The biggest advantage to echocardiography is that it is noninvasive (it does not involve breaking the skin or entering body cavities) and has no known risks or side effects. Echocardiography is often used in conjunction with other diagnostic tests for the heart such as **electrocardiography**.

Echocardiography is usually performed in the cardiology department at a hospital, but may also be performed in a cardiologist's office or an outpatient imaging center. Because the ultrasound scanners used to perform echocardiography are portable (handheld) or mobile, echocardiography can be performed in the hospital's emergency department or at the bedside of patients who cannot be transported to the cardiology department.

Description

Echocardiography creates an image of the heart using ultra-high-frequency sound waves—sound waves that are too high in frequency to be heard by the human ear. The technique is very similar to ultrasound scanning commonly used to visualize the fetus during pregnancy.

An echocardiography examination generally lasts between 15–30 minutes. The patient lies bare-chested on an examination table. A special gel is spread over the chest to help the transducer make good contact and slide smoothly over the skin. The transducer, also called a probe, is a small handheld device at the end of a flexible cable. The transducer, essentially a modified microphone, is placed against the chest and directs ultrasound waves into the chest. Some of the waves get echoed (or reflected) back to the transducer. Since different tissues and blood reflect ultrasound waves differently, these sound waves can be translated into a meaningful image of the heart that can be displayed on a monitor or recorded on paper or tape. The patient does not feel the sound waves, and the entire procedure is painless.

Occasionally, variations of the echocardiography test are used. For example, Doppler echocardiography employs a special microphone that allows technicians to measure and analyze the direction and speed of blood flow through blood vessels and heart valves. This makes it especially useful for detecting and evaluating regurgitation through the heart valves. By assessing the speed of blood flow at different locations around an obstruction, it can also help to precisely locate the obstruction.

An **exercise** echocardiogram, or stress echo, is an echocardiogram performed during exercise, when the heart muscle must work harder to supply blood to the body. This allows doctors to detect heart problems that might not be evident when the body is at rest and needs less blood. For patients who are unable to exercise, certain drugs can be used to mimic the effects of exercise by dilating the blood vessels and making the heart beat faster.

During the examination the sonographer can take measurements and, using the ultrasound scanner's computer, make calculations, including measuring blood flow speed. Most ultrasound scanners are equipped with videotape recorders or digital imaging/archiving devices to record the real-time examination, and with medical image printers to print out hard copies of still images.

Preparation

The patient removes any clothing and jewelry above the chest.

Aftercare

No special measures need to be taken following echocardiography.

Risks

There are no known complications associated with the use of echocardiography. There is a slight risk of having a heart attack during an exercise echocardiogram, due to the stress put on the heart during the test, mostly for patients with a history of heart attack or other risk factors.

Normal results

A normal echocardiogram shows a normal heart structure and the normal flow of blood through the heart chambers and heart valves. However, a normal echocardiogram does not rule out the possibility of heart disease.

An echocardiogram may show a number of abnormalities in the structure and function of the heart, including:

- thickening of the wall of the heart muscle (especially the left ventricle)
- abnormal motion of the heart muscle
- blood leaking backward through the heart valves (regurgitation)
- decreased blood flow through a heart valve (stenosis)

Resources

BOOKS

The Patient's Book of Medical Tests. Boston, New York City: Houghton Mifflin Company, 1997.

PERIODICALS

Kosoff, George. "Basic Physics and Imaging Characteristics of Ultrasound." *World Journal of Surgery* 24 (February 2000): 134–142.

Lee, Thomas H., and Charles A. Boucher. "Noninvasive Tests in Patients with Stable Coronary Artery Disease." *New England Journal of Medicine* 344, no. 24 (June 14, 2001): 1840–6.

ORGANIZATIONS

American College of Cardiology. Heart House. 9111 Old Georgetown Road, Bethesda, MD 20814-1699. (800) 253-4636. <http://www.acc.org>.

American Heart Association National Center. 7272 Greenville Avenue, Dallas, TX 75231. (800) AHA-USA1. <http://www.americanheart.org>.

American Institute of Ultrasound in Medicine. 14750 Sweitzer Lane, Suite 100, Laurel, MD 20707-5906. (301) 498-4100. <http://www.aium.org>.

American Registry of Diagnostic Medical Sonographers. 600 Jefferson Plaza, Suite 360, Rockville, MD 20852-1150. (800) 541-9754. <http://www.ardms.org>.

American Society of Echocardiography. 1500 Sunday Drive, Suite 102, Raleigh, NC 27607. (919) 787-5181. <http://asecho.org>.

OTHER

Barasch, Eddy. "Why Doctors Use Echocardiography." <http://www.thedoctorwillseeyounow.com/articles/heart/echocard_3/>.

Jennifer E. Sisk, MA
Lee Shratter, MD

Ectopic pregnancy treatment *see* **Salpingostomy**

EECP *see* **Enhanced external counterpulsation**

EEG *see* **Electroencephalography**

EKG *see* **Electrocardiography**

Elective abortion *see* **Abortion, induced**

Elective surgery

Definition

An elective surgery is a planned, non-emergency surgical procedure. It may be either medically required (e.g., cataract surgery), or optional (e.g., breast augmentation or implant) surgery.

Purpose

Elective surgeries may extend life or improve the quality of life physically and/or psychologically. Cosmetic and reconstructive procedures, such as a facelift (rhytidectomy), tummy tuck (**abdominoplasty**), or nose surgery (**rhinoplasty**) may not be medically indicated, but they may benefit the patient in terms of raising self-esteem. Other procedures, such as cataract surgery, improve functional quality of life even though they are technically an "optional" or elective procedure.

WHO PERFORMS THE PROCEDURE AND WHERE IS IT PERFORMED?

An elective surgical procedure is typically performed by a surgeon or qualified physician in either an inpatient, hospital environment or an outpatient, ambulatory center. Some simple, minimally invasive procedures may be performed in a doctor's office. The type of elective surgery will mandate the qualifications and background of the surgeon or physician who performs it. For example, the removal of a mole or a skin biopsy may be performed in a doctor's office by a dermatologist, while **gastric bypass** surgery would be performed in a hospital setting by a bariatric surgeon.

QUESTIONS TO ASK THE DOCTOR

- Is surgery my only option?
- What type of anesthesia will be used for this procedure?
- What will my recovery time be?
- What postoperative restrictions will I face after surgery?
- Can the surgery be done as an outpatient procedure?
- How long can I safely wait to have the surgery?
- How many procedures of this nature have you performed? What's your success rate?
- What are the costs involved with both the surgery and necessary postoperative care?

Some elective procedures are necessary to prolong life, such as an **angioplasty**. However, unlike **emergency surgery** (e.g., **appendectomy**), which must be performed immediately, a required elective procedure can be scheduled at the patient's and surgeon's convenience.

Demographics

According to the National Center for Health Statistics of the U.S. Centers for Disease Control (CDC), in 2000 over 40 million inpatient surgical procedures were performed in the United States. Ambulatory surgery accounted for 31.5 million procedures in 1996, the most recent year for which CDC data is available. Statistically, women were more likely to have surgery, accounting for 58% of ambulatory and inpatient procedures. This data includes both emergency and elective procedures.

Description

There are literally hundreds of elective surgeries spanning all the systems of the body in modern medical practice. Several major categories of common elective procedures include:

- Plastic surgery. Cosmetic or reconstructive surgery that improves appearance and in some cases, physical function.

- Refractive surgery. **Laser surgery** for vision correction.

- Gynecological surgery. Either medically necessary or optional surgery (e.g., **hysterectomy**, **tubal ligation**).

- Exploratory or diagnostic surgery. Surgery to determine the origin and extent of a medical problem, or to biopsy tissue samples.

- Cardiovascular surgery. Non-emergency procedures to improve blood flow or heart function, such as angioplasty or the implantation of a pacemaker.

- Musculoskeletal system surgery. Orthopedic surgical procedures, such as **hip replacement** and ACL reconstruction.

Diagnosis/Preparation

In some cases, insurance companies may require a **second opinion** before approving payment on elective surgical procedures. Anyone considering an elective surgery should review their coverage requirements with their health insurance carrier before scheduling the procedure.

Diagnostic and/or radiological testing may be performed to confirm the diagnosis or assist the surgeon in planning the surgical procedure. Typically, a complete medical history, **physical examination**, and laboratory tests (e.g., **urinalysis**, **chest x ray**, bloodwork, and electrocardiogram) are administered as part of the preoperative evaluation.

Other preoperative preparations will be dependent on the surgery itself. If a general anesthetic is to be used, dietary restrictions may be placed on the patient prior to the operation. If blood loss is expected during the procedure, advance banking of blood by the patient (known as autologous donation) may be recommended.

Aftercare

Recovery time and **postoperative care** will vary by the elective procedure performed. Patients should receive complete, written postoperative care instructions prior to returning home after surgery, and these instructions should be explained completely to them by the physician or nursing staff.

Risks

The risks for an elective surgery will vary by the type of procedure performed. In general, by their invasive nature most surgeries carry a risk of infection, hemorrhage, and circulatory problems such as shock or thrombosis (clotting within the circulatory system). The anesthesia used may also present certain risks for complications such as anaphylactic shock (an allergic reaction).

Normal results

Elective surgical results depend on the type of procedure performed. Optimal results for an elective procedure should be discussed with the patient prior to surgery. In some cases, the "normal" results from a surgery may only be temporary (i.e., follow-up surgery may be required at a later date), while other results are life-long. For example, a facelift may eventually require a second procedure as a patient ages whereas a tubal ligation offers permanent results.

Morbidity and mortality rates

Success, morbidity, and mortality rates are also dependent on the elective procedure itself. A physician and/or surgeon should be able to provide a patient with statistical information on success rates for a specific elective surgery.

Alternatives

The alternatives available for a particular surgery will depend on the purpose of the procedure. For example, other birth control options would be an alternative to any elective surgery for the purpose of sterilization (i.e., tubal ligation, **vasectomy**, hysterectomy). Other elective surgeries may not have a treatment alternative other than foregoing the surgery and living with the medical consequences. As part of **informed consent**, a patient's physician should review all possible treatment options, surgical and otherwise, before scheduling elective surgery.

Resources

BOOKS

Cottrell, James, and Stephanie Golden. *Under the Mask: A Guide to Feeling Secure and Comfortable During Anesthesia and Surgery.* Piscataway, NJ: Rutgers University Press, 2001.

Klippel, John. *All You Need to Know About Joint Surgery: Preparing for Surgery and an Active New Lifestyle.* Atlanta, GA: The Arthritis Foundation, 2002.

PERIODICALS

O'Conner-Von, Susan. "Preparing Children for Surgery: An Integrative Research Review." *AORN Journal* 71, no. 2 (February 2000): 334–43.

ORGANIZATIONS

American College of Surgeons. 63 N. St. Clair Drive, Chicago, IL 60611. 1-312-202-5000. postmaster@facs.org. <http://www.facs.org>.

Paula Ford-Martin

Electrocardiography

Definition

Electrocardiography is a commonly used, noninvasive procedure for recording electrical changes in the heart. The record, which is called an electrocardiogram (ECG or EKG), shows the series of waves that relate to the electrical impulses that occur during each beat of the heart. The results are printed on paper and/or displayed on a monitor to provide a visual representation of heart function. The waves in a normal record are named P, Q, R, S, and T, and follow in alphabetical

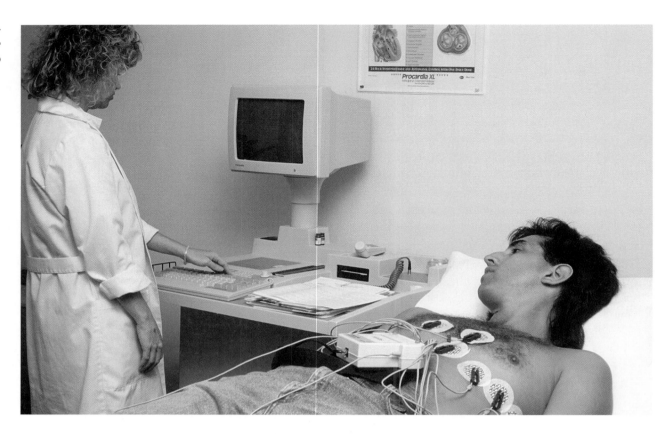

An electrocardiography unit uses electrodes to measure the electrical activity of the heart and translates it into a line on paper and a computer screen. Doctors, technicians, and others can use the line tracing to look for a number of cardiac problems. *(Custom Medical Stock Photo. Reproduced by permission.)*

order. The number of waves may vary, and other waves may be present.

Purpose

Electrocardiography is a starting point for detecting many cardiac problems, including angina pectoris, stable angina, ischemic heart disease, arrhythmias (irregular heartbeat), tachycardia (fast heartbeat), bradycardia (slow heartbeat), myocardial infarction (heart attack), and certain congenital heart conditions. It is used routinely in physical examinations and for monitoring a patient's condition during and after surgery, as well as in the intensive care setting. It is the basic measurement used in **exercise** tolerance tests (i.e., stress tests) and is also used to evaluate symptoms such as chest pain, shortness of breath, and palpitations.

Demographics

According to the U.S. Centers for Disease Control (CDC), nearly 23 million EKG procedures were performed in doctor's offices in the year 2000.

Men are more likely to experience heart attacks than women, although a woman's risk of heart attack rises after menopause. African-Americans, Hispanics, and Native Americans are all at greater risk for cardiovascular disease than Caucasians, in part because of the higher incidence of diabetes mellitus (a major risk factor for cardiovascular disease) in these populations.

Description

The patient disrobes from the waist up, and electrodes (tiny wires in adhesive pads) are applied to specific sites on the arms, legs, and chest. When attached, these electrodes are called leads; three to 12 leads may be employed for the procedure.

Muscle movement may interfere with the recording, which lasts for several beats of the heart. In cases where rhythm disturbances are suspected to be infrequent, the patient may wear a small Holter monitor in order to record continuously over a 24-hour period. This is known as ambulatory monitoring.

Special training is required for interpretation of the electrocardiogram. To summarize in the simplest manner the features used in interpretations, the P wave of the electrocardiogram is associated with the contraction of the atria—the two chambers of the heart that receive blood from the veins. The QRS series of waves, or QRS complex, is associated with ventricular contraction, with the T wave coming after the contraction. The ventricles are the two chambers of the heart that receive blood from the atria and that send the blood into the arteries. Finally, the P-Q or P-R interval gives a value for the time taken for the electrical impulse to travel from the atria to the ventricle (normally less than 0.2 seconds).

Diagnosis/Preparation

Patients are asked not to eat for several hours before a **stress test**. Before the leads are attached, the skin is cleaned to obtain good electrical contact at the electrode positions and, occasionally, shaving the chest may be necessary.

Heart problems are diagnosed by the pattern of electrical waves produced during the EKG, and an abnormal rhythm can be called dysrhythmia. The cause of dysrhythmia is ectopic beats. Ectopic beats are premature heartbeats that arise from a site other than the sinus node—commonly from the atria, atrioventricular node, or the ventricle. When these dysrhythmias are only occasional, they may produce no symptoms or simply a feeling that the heart is turning over or "flip-flopping." These occasional dysrhythmias are common in healthy people, but they also can be an indication of heart disease.

The varied sources of dysrhythmias provide a wide range of alterations in the form of the electrocardiogram. Ectopic beats display an abnormal QRS complex. This can indicate disease associated with insufficient blood supply to the heart muscle (myocardial ischemia). Multiple ectopic sites lead to rapid and uncoordinated contractions of the atria or ventricles. This condition is known as fibrillation. When the atrial impulse fails to reach the ventricle, a condition known as heart block results.

Aftercare

To avoid skin irritation from the salty gel used to obtain good electrical contact, the skin should be thoroughly cleaned after removal of the electrodes.

Risks

The EKG is a noninvasive procedure that is virtually risk-free for the patient. There is a slight risk of heart attack for individuals undergoing a stress test EKG, but patients are carefully screened for their suitability for this test before it is prescribed.

QUESTIONS TO ASK THE DOCTOR

- Why has an EKG been prescribed for me?
- When will I get the results of my EKG?
- Should I take my prescription and over-the-counter medications as normal before my EKG or stress test?
- Should I refrain from eating before my stress test?

Risk factors for heart disease include obesity, hypertension (high blood pressure), high triglycerides and total blood cholesterol, low HDL ("good") cholesterol, tobacco smoking, and increased age. People who have diabetes mellitus (either type 1 or type 2) are also at increased risk for cardiovascular disease.

Normal results

When the heart is operating normally, each part contracts in a specific order. Contraction of the muscle is triggered by an electrical impulse. These electrical impulses travel through specialized cells that form a conduction system. Following this pathway ensures that contractions will occur in a coordinated manner.

When the presence of all waves is observed in the electrocardiogram, and these waves follow the order defined alphabetically, the heart is said to show a normal sinus rhythm, and impulses may be assumed to be following the regular conduction pathway.

In the normal heart, electrical impulses—at a rate of 60–100 times per minute—originate in the sinus node. The sinus node is located in the first chamber of the heart, known as the right atrium, where blood reenters the heart after circulating through the body. After traveling down to the junction between the upper and lower chambers, the signal stimulates the atrioventricular node. From here, after a delay, it passes by specialized routes through the lower chambers or ventricles. In many disease states, the passage of the electrical impulse can be interrupted in a variety of ways, causing the heart to perform less efficiently.

The heart is described as showing arrhythmia or dysrhythmia when time intervals between waves, or the order or the number of waves do not fit the normal pattern described above. Other features that may be altered include the direction of wave deflection and wave widths.

KEY TERMS

Ambulatory monitoring—ECG recording over a prolonged period during which the patient can move around.

Arrhythmia or dysrhythmia—Abnormal rhythm in hearts that contract in an irregular way.

ECG or EKG—A record of the waves that relate to the electrical impulses produced at each beat of the heart.

Ectopic beat—Abnormal heart beat arising elsewhere than from the sinoatrial node.

Electrodes—Tiny wires in adhesive pads that are applied to the body for ECG measurement.

Fibrillation—Rapid, uncoordinated contractions of the upper or the lower chambers of the heart.

Lead—Name given the electrode when it is attached to the skin.

Reperfusion therapy—Restoration of blood flow to an organ or tissue; following a heart attack, quickly opening blocked arteries to reperfuse the heart muscles to minimize damage.

Morbidity and mortality rates

According to the American Heart Association, cardiovascular disease is the number one cause of death in the United States. It is also the leading cause of death among people with diabetes.

Alternatives

Electrocardiography is the gold standard for detecting heart conditions involving irregularities in electrical conduction and rhythm. Other tests that may be used in conjunction with an EKG include an echocardiogram (a sonogram of the heart's pumping action) and a stress test—an EKG that is done in conjunction with treadmill or other supervised exercise to observe the heart's function under stress—may also be performed.

Resources

BOOKS

Beasley, Brenda. *Understanding EKGs: A Practical Approach.* 2nd ed. Upper Saddle River, NJ: Prentice Hall, 2002.

PERIODICALS

Kadish, Alan, et al. "ACC/AHA Clinical Competence Statement on Electrocardiography and Ambulatory Electrocardiography." *Journal of The American College of Cardiology* 38, no. 7 (2001). <http://www.acc.org/clinical/competence/ECG/pdfs/ECG_pdf.pdf.>.

Fergusun, J. D., et al. "The Prehospital 12- Lead Electrocardiogram: Impact on Management of the Out-of-hospital Acute Coronary Syndrome Patient." *American Journal of Emergency Medicine* 21, no. 2 (March 2003): 136–42.

ORGANIZATIONS

The American College of Cardiology. Heart House, 9111 Old Georgetown Road, Bethesda, MD 20814-1699. (800) 253-4636. <http://www.acc.org>.

American Heart Association. 7272 Greenville Ave., Dallas, TX 75231. (800) 242-8721. <http://www.americanheart.org>.

Maggie Boleyn, R.N., B.S.N.
Paula Ford-Martin

Electroencephalography

Definition

Electroencephalography, or EEG, is a neurological test that involves attaching electrodes to the head of a person to measure and record electrical activity in the brain over time.

Purpose

The EEG, also known as a brain wave test, is a key tool in the diagnosis and management of epilepsy and other seizure disorders. It is also used to assist in the diagnosis of brain damage and diseases such as strokes, tumors, encephalitis, mental retardation, and sleep disorders. The results of the test can distinguish psychiatric conditions such as schizophrenia, paranoia, and depression from degenerative mental disorders such as Alzheimer's and Parkinson's diseases. An EEG may also be used to monitor brain activity during surgery to assess the effects of anesthesia. It is also used to determine brain status and brain death.

Demographics

The number of EEG tests performed each year can only be estimated. It is not a reportable event and is used in the diagnostic workup for a number of disorders. The number of EEG tests per year is estimated to be in the range of 10–25 million.

Description

Before an EEG begins, a nurse or technologist attaches approximately 16–21 electrodes to a person's scalp

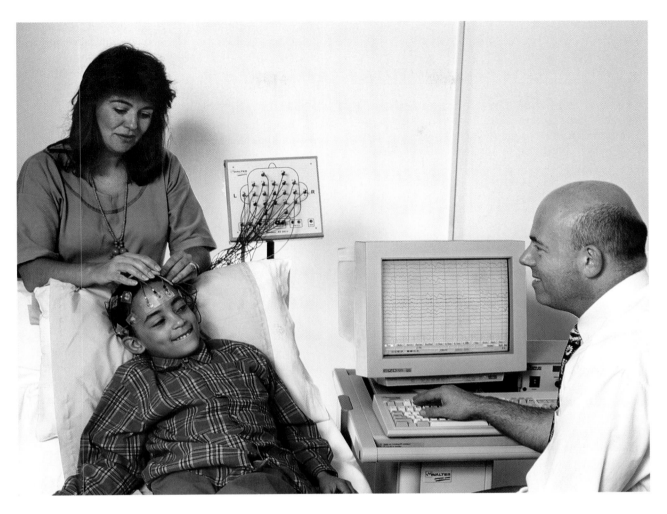

The electrodes taped to this boy's scalp monitor his brain activity (brain waves) by detecting the electric impulses generated by the brain's activity. *(Science Source/Photo Researchers. Reproduced by permission.)*

using an electrically conductive, washable paste. The electrodes are placed on the head in a standard pattern based on head circumference measurements. Depending on the purpose for the EEG, implantable, or invasive, electrodes are occasionally used. Implantable electrodes include sphenoidal electrodes, which are fine wires inserted under the zygomatic arch, or cheekbone. Depth electrodes, or subdural strip electrodes, are surgically implanted into the brain and are used to localize a seizure focus in preparation for epilepsy surgery. Once in place, even implantable electrodes do not cause pain. The electrodes are used to measure the electrical activity in various regions of the brain over the course of the test period.

For the test, a person lies on a bed, padded table, or comfortable chair and is asked to relax and remain still while measurements are being taken. An EEG usually takes no more than one hour, although long-term monitoring is often used for diagnosis of seizure disorders.

During the test procedure, a person may be asked to breathe slowly or quickly. Visual stimuli such as flashing lights or a patterned board may be used to stimulate certain types of brain activity. Throughout the procedure, the electroencephalography unit makes a continuous graphic record of the person's brain activity, or brain waves, on a long strip of recording paper or computer screen. This graphic record is called an electroencephalogram. If the display is computerized, the test may be called a digital EEG, or dEEG.

The sleep EEG uses the same equipment and procedures as a regular EEG. Persons undergoing a sleep EEG are encouraged to fall asleep completely rather than just relax. They are typically provided a bed and a quiet room conducive to sleep. A sleep EEG lasts up to three hours, or up to eight or nine hours if it is a night's sleep.

In an ambulatory EEG, individuals are hooked up to a portable cassette recorder. They then go about normal

WHO PERFORMS THE PROCEDURE AND WHERE IS IT PERFORMED?

Electroencephalography is often administered by specially trained technicians who are supervised by a neurologist or other physician with specialized training in administering and interpreting the test. Because of the equipment involved, an EEG is usually administered in a hospital setting. It may be conducted in a professional office.

activities and take normal rest and sleep for a period of up to 24 hours. During this period, individuals and their family members record any symptoms or abnormal behaviors, which can later be correlated with the EEG to see if they represent seizures.

An extension of the EEG technique, called quantitative EEG (qEEG), involves manipulating the EEG signals with a computer using the fast Fourier transform algorithm. The result is then best displayed using a colored gray scale transposed onto a schematic map of the head to form a topographic image. The brain map produced in this technique is a vivid illustration of electrical activity in the brain. This technique also has the ability to compare the similarity of the signals between different electrodes, a measurement known as spectral coherence. Studies have shown the value of this measurement in diagnosis of Alzheimer's disease and mild closed head injuries. The technique can also identify areas of the brain having abnormally slow activity when the data are both mapped and compared to known normal values. The result is then known as a statistical or significance probability map (SPM). This allows differentiation between early dementia (increased slowing) or otherwise uncomplicated depression (no slowing).

Diagnosis/Preparation

An EEG is generally performed as one test in a series of neurological evaluations. Rarely does the EEG form the sole basis for a particular diagnosis.

Full instructions should be given to individuals receiving an EEG when they schedule their test. Typically, individuals taking medications that affect the central nervous system, such as anticonvulsants, stimulants, or antidepressants, are told to discontinue their prescription for a short time prior to the test (usually one to two days). However, such requests should be cleared with the treating physician. EEG test candidates may be asked to avoid food and beverages that contain caffeine, a central nervous system stimulant. They may also be asked to arrive for the test with clean hair that is free of styling products to make attachment of the electrodes easier.

Individuals undergoing a sleep EEG may be asked to remain awake the night before their test. They may be given a sedative prior to the test to induce sleep.

Aftercare

If an individual has suspended regular medication for the test, the EEG nurse or technician should advise as to when to begin taking it again.

Risks

Being off certain medications for one to two days may trigger seizures. Certain procedures used during EEG may trigger seizures in persons with epilepsy. Those procedures include flashing lights and deep breathing. If the EEG is being used as a diagnostic for epilepsy (i.e., to determine the type of seizures an individual is experiencing) this may be a desired effect, although the person needs to be monitored closely so that the seizure can be aborted if necessary. This type of test is known as an ictal EEG.

Normal results

In reading and interpreting brain wave patterns, a neurologist or other physician will evaluate the type of brain waves and the symmetry, location, and consistency of brain wave patterns. Brain wave response to certain stimuli presented during the EEG test (such as flashing lights or noise) will also be evaluated.

The four basic types of brain waves are alpha, beta, theta, and delta, with the type distinguished by frequency. Alpha waves fall between 8 and 13 Hertz (Hz), beta are above 13 Hz, theta between 4 and 7 Hz, and delta are less than 4 Hz. Alpha waves are usually the dominant rhythm seen in the posterior region of the brain in older children and adults, when awake and relaxed. Beta waves are normal in sleep, particularly for infants and young children. Theta waves are normally found during drowsiness and sleep and are normal in wakefulness in children, while delta waves are the most prominent feature of the sleeping EEG. Spikes and sharp waves are generally abnormal; however, they are common in the EEG of normal newborns.

Different types of brain waves are seen as abnormal only in the context of the location of the waves, a person's age, and one's conscious state. In general, disease typically increases slow activity, such as theta or delta waves, but decreases fast activity, such as alpha and beta waves.

Not all decreases in wave activity are abnormal. The normal alpha waves seen in the posterior region of the brain are suppressed merely if a person is tense. Sometimes the addition of a wave is abnormal. For example, alpha rhythms seen in a newborn can signify seizure activity. Finally, the area where the rhythm is seen can be telling. The alpha coma is characterized by alpha rhythms produced diffusely, or, in other words, by all regions of the brain.

Some abnormal beta rhythms include frontal beta waves that are induced by sedative drugs. Marked asymmetry in beta rhythms suggests a structural lesion on the side lacking the beta waves. Beta waves are also commonly measured over skull lesions, such as fractures or burr holes, in activity known as a breach rhythm.

Usually seen only during sleep in adults, the presence of theta waves in the temporal region of awake, older adults has been tentatively correlated with vascular disease. Another rhythm normal in sleep, delta rhythms, may be recorded in the awake state over localized regions of cerebral damage. Intermittent delta rhythms are also an indication of damage of the relays between the deep gray matter and the cortex of the brain. In adults, this intermittent activity is found in the frontal region whereas in children, it is in the occipital region.

The EEG readings of persons with epilepsy or other seizure disorders display bursts, or spikes, of electrical activity. In focal epilepsy, spikes are restricted to one hemisphere of the brain. If spikes are generalized to both hemispheres of the brain, multifocal epilepsy may be present. The EEG can be used to localize the region of the brain where the abnormal electrical activity is occurring. This is most easily accomplished using a recording method, or montage, called an average reference montage. With this type of recording, the signal from each electrode is compared to the average signal from all the electrodes. The negative amplitude (upward movement, by convention) of the spike is observed for the different channels, or inputs, from the various electrodes. The negative deflection will be greatest as recorded by the electrode that is closest in location to the origin of the abnormal activity. The spike will be present but of reduced amplitude as the electrodes move farther away from the site producing the spike. Electrodes distant from the site will not record the spike occurrence.

A final variety of abnormal result is the presence of slower-than-normal wave activity, which can either be a slow background rhythm or slow waves superimposed on a normal background. A posterior dominant rhythm

QUESTIONS TO ASK THE DOCTOR

- How many EEG procedures has the technician performed?
- What preparations are being made to treat an induced seizure?
- Is the supervising physician appropriately certified to interpret an EEG?

of 7 Hz or less in an adult is abnormal and consistent with encephalopathy (brain disease). In contrast, localized theta or delta rhythms found in conjunction with normal background rhythms suggest a structural lesion.

Morbidity and mortality rates

There are few adverse conditions associated with an EEG test. Persons with seizure disorders may induce seizures during the test in reaction to flashing lights or by deep breathing. Mortality from an EEG has not been reported.

Alternatives

There are no equivalent tests that provide the same information as an EEG.

Resources

BOOKS

Chin, W. C., and T. C. Head. *Essentials of Clinical Neurophysiology,* 3rd ed. London: Butterworth-Heinemann, 2002.

Daube, J. R. *Clinical Neurophysiology,* 2nd edition. New York: Oxford University Press, 2002.

Ebersole, J. S., and T. A. Pedley. *Current Practice of Clinical Electroencephalography,* 3rd ed. Philadelphia: Lippincott Williams & Wilkins, 2002.

Rowan, A. J., and E. Tolunsky. *Primer of EEG.* London: Butterworth-Heinemann, 2003.

PERIODICALS

De Clercq, W., P. Lemmerling, S. Van Huffel, and W. Van Paesschen. "Anticipation of Epileptic Seizures from Standard EEG Recordings." *Lancet* 361, no. 9361 (2003): 971–972.

Harden, C. L., F. T. Burgut, and A. M. Kanner. "The Diagnostic Significance of Video-EEG Monitoring Findings on Pseudoseizure Patients Differs Between Neurologists and Psychiatrists." *Epilepsia* 44, no. 3 (2003): 453–456.

Stepien, R. A. "Testing for Non-linearity in EEG Signal of Healthy Subjects." *Acta Experimental Neurobiology* 62, no. 4 (2002): 277–281.

KEY TERMS

Encephalitis—Inflammation of the brain.

Fast Fourier transfer—A digital processing of the recorded signal resulting in a decomposition of its frequency components.

Ictal EEG—An EEG done to determine the type of seizure characteristic of a person's disorder. During this EEG, seizure medicine may be discontinued in an attempt to induce as seizure during the testing period.

Sphenoidal electrodes—Fine wire electrodes that are implanted under the cheek bones, used to measure temporal seizures.

Subdural electrodes—Strip electrodes that are placed under dura mater (the outermost, toughest, and most fibrous of the three membranes [meninges] covering the brain and spinal cord). They are used to locate foci of epileptic seizures prior to epilepsy surgery.

Zygomatic arch—Cheekbone. A quadrilateral bone forming the prominence of the cheek. It articulates (touches or moves) with the frontal, sphenoid, and maxillary, and temporal bones.

Vanhatalo, S., M. D. Holmes, P. Tallgren, J. Voipio, K. Kaila, and J. W. Miller. "Very Slow EEG Responses Lateralize Temporal Lobe Seizures: An Evaluation of Non-invasive DC-EEG." *Neurology* 60, no. 7 (2003): 1098–1104.

ORGANIZATIONS

American Association of Electrodiagnostic Medicine. 421 First Avenue SW, Suite 300 East, Rochester, MN 55902. (507) 288–0100, Fax: (507) 288–1225. aaem@aaem.net. <http://www.aaem.net/>.

American Board of Registration for Electroencephalographic Technologists. P.O. Box 916633, Longwood, FL 32791-6633 .

American Board of Registration of EEG and EP Technologists. PO Box 891663, Longwood, FL 32791. (407) 788–6308. <http://www.abret.org/index.htm>.

American Society of Electroneurodiagnostic Technologists Inc. 204 W. 7th Carroll, IA 51401. (712) 792–2978. <http://www.aset.org/>.

Epilepsy Foundation. 4351 Garden City Drive, Landover, MD 20785-7223. (800) 332–1000 or (301) 459–3700. <http://www.efa.org>.

Joint Review Committee on Electroneurodiagnostic Technology. 3350 South 198th Rd., Goodson, MO 65659-9110. (417) 253–5810. <http://www.caahep. org/about/coas.htm>.

OTHER

Hofstra University. "Electroencephalography." [cited April 27, 2003]. <http://people.hofstra.edu/faculty/sina_y_rabbany/engg181/EEG.html>.

Bergey, Gregory K., and Piotr J. Franaszczuk. "Epileptic Seizures are Characterized by Changing Signal Complexity." [cited April 17, 2003]. <http://erl.neuro.jhmi.edu/pfranasz/CN00/cn00.pdf>.

Rutherford, Kim, M.D. "EEG (Electroencephalography)." *Kid's Health For Parents.* June 2001 [cited April 27, 2003]. <http://kidshealth.org/parent/system/medical/eeg.html>.

National Society for Epilepsy. "Epilepsy Information: Electroencephalography." September 2002 [cited April 27, 2003]. <http://www.epilepsynse.org.uk/pages/info/leaflets/eeg.cfm>.

L. Fleming Fallon, Jr., MD, DrPH

Electrolyte tests

Definition

Electrolytes are positively and negatively charged molecules called ions, that are found within the body's cells and extracellular fluids, including blood plasma. A test for electrolytes includes the measurement of sodium, potassium, chloride, and bicarbonate. These ions are measured to assess renal (kidney), endocrine (glandular), and acid-base function, and are components of both renal function and comprehensive metabolic biochemistry profiles. Other important electrolytes routinely measured in serum or plasma include calcium and phosphorus. These are measured together because they are both affected by bone and parathyroid diseases, and often move in opposing directions. Magnesium is another electrolyte that is routinely measured. Like calcium, it will cause tetany (uncontrolled muscle contractions) when levels are too low in the extracellular fluids.

Purpose

Tests that measure the concentration of electrolytes are needed for both the diagnosis and management of renal, endocrine, acid-base, water balance, and many other conditions. Their importance lies in part with the serious consequences that follow from the relatively small changes that diseases or abnormal conditions may cause. For example, the reference range for potassium is 3.6-5.0 mmol/l. Potassium is often a STAT (needed immediately) test because values below 3.0 mmol/l are associated with arrhythmia (irregular heartbeat), tachycardia (rapid heartbeat), and cardiac arrest, and values above 6.0 mmol/L are associated with bradycardia (slow heartbeat) and heart failure. Abnormal potassium cannot be treated without reference to bicarbonate, which is a measure of the buffering capacity of the plasma. Sodium bicarbonate and dissolved carbon dioxide act together to resist changes in blood pH. For example, an increased plasma bicarbonate indicates a condition called metabolic alkalosis, which results in blood pH that is too high. This may cause hydrogen ions to shift from the cells into the extracellular fluid in exchange for potassium. As potassium moves into the cells, the plasma concentration falls. The low plasma potassium, called hypokalemia, should not be treated by administration of potassium, but by identifying and eliminating the cause of the alkalosis. Administration of potassium would result in hyperkalemia when the acid-base disturbance is corrected. Sodium measurements are very useful in differentiating the cause of an abnormal potassium result. Conditions such as the overuse of **diuretics** (drugs that promote lower blood pressure) often result in low levels of both sodium and potassium. On the other hand, Cushing's disease (adrenocortical over-activity) and Addison's disease (adrenocortical under-activity) drive the sodium and potassium in opposing directions. Chloride levels will follow sodium levels except in the case of acid-base imbalances, in which chloride may move in the opposing direction of bicarbonate. In short, diagnosis and management of a patient with an electrolyte disturbance is best served by measuring all four electrolytes.

Description

Sodium is the principal extracellular cation and potassium the principal intracellular cation. A cation is an ion with a positive charge. An anion is an ion with a negative charge. Sodium levels are directly related to the osmotic pressure of the plasma. In fact, since an anion is always associated with sodium (usually chloride or bicarbonate), the plasma osmolality (total dissolved solute concentration) can be estimated. Since water will often follow sodium by diffusion, loss of sodium leads to dehydration and retention of sodium leads to edema. Conditions that promote increased sodium, called hypernatremia, do so without promoting an equivalent gain in water. Such conditions include diabetes insipidus (water loss by the kidneys), Cushing's disease, and hyperaldosteronism (increased sodium reabsorption). Many other conditions, such as congestive heart failure, cirrhosis of the liver, and renal disease result in renal retention of sodium, but an equivalent amount of water is retained as well. This results in a condition called total body sodium excess, which causes hypertension and edema, but not an elevated serum sodium concentration. Low serum sodium, called hyponatremia, may result from Addison's disease,

excessive diuretic therapy, the syndrome of inappropriate secretion of antidiuretic hormone (SIADH), burns, diarrhea, vomiting, and cystic fibrosis. In fact, the diagnosis of cystic fibrosis is made by demonstrating an elevated chloride concentration (greater than 60 mmol/l) in sweat.

Potassium is the electrolyte used as a hallmark sign of renal failure. Like sodium, potassium is freely filtered by the kidney. However, in the distal tubule sodium is reabsorbed and potassium is secreted. In renal failure, the combination of decreased filtration and decreased secretion combine to cause increased plasma potassium. Hyperkalemia is the most significant and life-threatening complication of renal failure. Hyperkalemia is also commonly caused by hemolytic anemia (release from hemolysed red blood cells), diabetes insipidus, Addison's disease, and digitalis toxicity. Frequent causes of low serum potassium include alkalosis, diarrhea and vomiting, excessive use of thiazide diuretics, Cushing's disease, intravenous fluid administration, and SIADH.

Calcium and phosphorus are measured together because they are both likely to be abnormal in bone and parathyroid disease states. Parathyroid hormone causes resorption of these minerals from bone. However, it promotes intestinal absorption and renal reabsorption of calcium and renal excretion of phosphorus. In hyperparathyroidism, serum calcium will be increased and phosphorus will be decreased. In hypoparathyroidism and renal disease, serum calcium will be low but phosphorus will be high. In vitamin D dependent rickets (VDDR), both calcium and phosphorus will be low; however, calcium is normal while phosphorus is low in vitamin D resistant rickets (VDRR). Differential diagnosis of an abnormal serum calcium is aided by the measurement of ionized calcium (i.e., calcium not bound by protein). Approximately 45% of the calcium in blood is bound to protein, 45% is ionized, and 10% is complexed to anions in the form of undissociated salts. Only the ionized calcium is physiologically active, and the level of ionized calcium is regulated by parathyroid hormone (PTH) via negative feedback (high ionized calcium inhibits secretion of PTH). While hypoparathyroidism, VDDR, renal failure, hypoalbuminemia, hypovitaminosis D, and other conditions may cause low total calcium, only hypoparathyroidism (and alkalosis) will result in low ionized calcium. Conversely, while hyperparathyroidism, malignancies (those that secrete parathyroid hormone-related protein), multiple myeloma, antacids, hyperproteinemia, dehydration, and hypervitaminosis D cause an elevated total calcium, only hyperparathyroidism, malignancy, and acidosis cause an elevated ionized calcium.

Serum magnesium levels may be increased by hemolytic anemia, renal failure, Addison's disease, hyperparathyroidism, and magnesium-based antacids. Chronic alcoholism is the most common cause of a low serum magnesium owing to poor nutrition. Serum magnesium is also decreased in diarrhea, hypoparathyroidism, pancreatitis, Cushing's disease, and with excessive diuretic use. Low magnesium can be caused by a number of **antibiotics** and other drugs and by administration of intravenous solutions. Magnesium is needed for secretion of parathyroid hormone, and therefore, a low serum magnesium can induce hypocalcemia. Magnesium deficiency is very common in regions where the water supply does not contain sufficient magnesium salts. Magnesium acts as a calcium channel blocker, and when cellular magnesium is low, high intracellular calcium results. This leads to hypertension, tachycardia, and tetany. Unfortunately serum total magnesium levels do not correlate well with intracellular magnesium levels, and serum measurement is not very sensitive for detecting chronic deficiency because of compensatory contributions from bone. Ionized magnesium levels are better correlated with intracellular levels because the ionized form can move freely between the cells and extracellular fluids.

Measurement of electrolytes

Electrolytes are measured by a process known as potentiometry. This method measures the voltage that develops between the inner and outer surfaces of an ion selective electrode. The electrode (membrane) is made of a material that is selectively permeable to the ion being measured. This potential is measured by comparing it to the potential of a reference electrode. Since the potential of the reference electrode is held constant, the difference in voltage between the two electrodes is attributed to the concentration of ion in the sample.

Precautions

Electrolyte tests are performed on whole blood, plasma, or serum, usually collected from a vein or capillary.

Special procedures are followed when collecting a sweat sample for electrolyte analysis. This procedure, called pilocarpine iontophoresis, uses electric current applied to the arm of the patient (usually an infant) in order to convey the pilocarpine to the sweat glands where it will stimulate sweating. Care must be taken to ensure that the collection device (macroduct tubing or gauze) does not become contaminated and that the patient's parent or guardian understands the need for the electrical equipment employed.

Preparation

Usually no special preparation is necessary by the patient. Samples for calcium and phosphorus and for magnesium should be collected following an eight-hour fast.

Aftercare

Discomfort or bruising may occur at the puncture site, or the person may feel dizzy or faint. Pressure to the puncture site until the bleeding stops reduces bruising. Applying warm packs to the puncture site relieves discomfort.

Risks

Minor temporary discomfort may occur with any blood test, but there are no complications specific to electrolyte testing.

Normal results

Electrolyte concentrations are similar whether measured in serum or plasma. Values are expressed as mmol/L for sodium, potassium, chloride, and bicarbonate. Magnesium results are often reported as milliequivalents per liter (meq/L) or in mg/dL. Total calcium is usually reported in mg/dL and ionized calcium in mmol/L. Since severe electrolyte disturbances can be associated with life-threatening consequences such as heart failure, shock, coma, or tetany, alert values are used to warn physicians of impending crisis. Typical reference ranges and alert values are cited below:

- serum or plasma sodium: 135–145 mmol/l; alert levels: less than 120 mmol/l and greater than 160 mmol/l
- serum potassium: 3.6–5.4 mmol/l (plasma, 3.6–5.0 mmol/l); alert levels: less than 3.0 mmol/l and greater than 6.0 mmol/l
- serum or plasma chloride: 98–108 mmol/l
- sweat chloride: 4–60 mmol/l
- serum or plasma bicarbonate: 18–24 mmol/l (as total carbon dioxide, 22–26 mmol/l); alert levels: less than 10 mmol/l and greater than 40 mmol/l
- serum calcium: 8.5–10.5 mg/dl (2.0–2.5 mmol/l); alert levels: less than 6.0 mg/dl and greater than 13.0 mg/dl
- ionized calcium: 1.0–1.3 mmol/l
- serum inorganic phosphorus: 2.3–4.7 mg/dl (children, 4.0–7.0 mg/dl); alert level: less than 1.0 mg/dl
- serum magnesium: 1.8–3.0 mg/dl (1.2–2.0 meq/l or 0.5–1.0 mmol/l)
- ionized magnesium: 0.53–0.67 mmol/l
- osmolality (calculated) 280–300 mosm/kg

Resources

BOOKS

Henry, J. B. *Clinical Diagnosis and Management of Laboratory Methods.* 20th ed. Philadelphia: W. B. Saunders Company, 2001.

KEY TERMS

Anion—An ion with a negative charge.

Arrhythmia—Abnormal rhythm of the heart beat.

Bradycardia—Slow heart beat, usually under 50 beats per minute.

Cation—An ion with a positive charge.

Hypokalemia—An abnormally small concentration of potassium in the blood. This occurs in periodic paralysis and in potassium depletion due to excessive loss from the kidneys or gastrointestinal tract.

Tachycardia—Rapid heart beat, generally over 90 beats per minute.

Tetany—Inappropriately sustained muscle spasms.

Tierney, Lawrence M., Stephen J. McPhee, and Maxine A. Papadakis. *Current Medical Diagnosis and Treatment 2001.* 40th ed. New York: Lange Medical Books/McGraw-Hill, 2001.

Wallach, Jacques. *Interpretation of Diagnostic Tests.* 7th ed. Philadelphia: Lippincott Williams & Wilkins, 2000.

OTHER

MedLine Plus. "Electrolytes." October 18, 2001 [cited April 4, 2003]. <http://www.nlm.nih.gov/medlineplus/ency/article/002350.htm>.

National Institutes of Health. [cited April 5, 2003]. <http://www.nlm.nih.gov/medlineplus/encyclopedia.html>.

Erika J. Norris
Mark A. Best, M.D.

Electrophysiology study of the heart

Definition

An electrophysiology study (EPS) of the heart is a test performed to analyze the electrical activity of the heart. The test uses cardiac catheters and sophisticated computers to generate electrocardiogram (EKG) tracings and electrical measurements with exquisite precision from within the heart chambers.

Purpose

Heart disease is the leading killer in the United States, accounting for more than 50% of all annual deaths. The normal function of the heart depends on its electrical activity, and the effect of this activity on each of its cells. When a heart is diseased, impaired electical activity is often the factor that leads to sudden death, thus the need for EPS tests.

An EPS can be performed solely for diagnostic purposes or to pinpoint the exact location of electrical signals (cardiac mapping) in conjunction with a therapeutic procedure called catheter ablation (tissue removal). A cardiologist may recommend an EPS when the standard EKG, Holter monitor, event recorder, **stress test**, echocardiogram, or angiogram cannot provide enough information to evaluate an abnormal heart rhythm (arrhythmia).

An EPS offers more detailed information about the heart's electrical activity than many other noninvasive tests because electrodes are placed directly *on* heart tissue. This placement allows the electrophysiologist to determine the specific location of an arrhythmia and, often, to correct it during the same procedure. This corrective treatment is considered a permanent cure; in many cases, the patient may not need to take heart medications.

EPS may be helpful in assessing:

• certain tachycardias (fast hearbeats) or bradycardias (slow heartbeats) of unknown cause

• patients who have been resuscitated after experiencing sudden cardiac arrest

• various symptoms of unknown cause, such as chest pain, shortness of breath, fatigue, or syncope (dizziness/fainting)

• response to anti-arrhythmic therapy

Precautions

Pregnant patients should not undergo EPS because the study requires exposure to radiation, which may harm the growing baby. Patients who have coronary artery disease may need to be treated prior to EPS. EPS is contraindicated in patients with an acute myocardial infarction, as the infarct may be extended with rapid pacing. The test is also contraindicated for patients who are uncooperative.

Description

The rhythmic pumping action of the heart, which is essentially a muscle, is the result of electrical impulses traveling throughout the walls of the four heart chambers. These impulses originate in the sinoatrial (SA) node (specialized cells situated in the right atrium, or top right chamber of the heart). Normally, the SA node, acting like a spark plug, spontaneously generates the impulses, which travel through specific pathways through-

WHO PERFORMS THE PROCEDURE AND WHERE IS IT PERFORMED?

The relatively simple EPS is performed in a special laboratory under controlled clinical circumstances by cardiologists, nurses, and technicians with special training in electrophysiology.

QUESTIONS TO ASK THE DOCTOR

- What is the purpose of the EPS test?
- How do I prepare for cardiac electrophysiology?
- Will it hurt?
- How is the test performed?
- How long will it take?
- Are there any risks involved?

out the atria to the atrioventricular (AV) node. The AV node is a relay station sending the impulses to more specialized muscle fibers throughout the ventricles (the lower chambers of the heart). If these pathways become damaged or blocked or if extra (abnormal) pathways exist, the heart's rhythm may be altered (too slow, too fast, or irregular), which can seriously affect the heart's pumping ability.

To undergo EPS, the patient is placed on a table in the EPS lab and connected to various monitors. Sterile technique is maintained. A minimum of two catheters are inserted into the right femoral (thigh) vein in the groin area. Depending on the type of arrhythmia, the number of catheters used and their route to the heart may vary. For certain tachycardias, two additional catheters may be inserted in the left groin and one in the internal jugular (neck) vein or in the subclavian (below the clavicle) vein. The catheters are about 0.08 in (2 mm) in diameter, about the size of a spaghetti noodle. The catheters used in catheter ablation are slightly larger.

With the help of fluoroscopy (x rays on a television screen), all catheters are guided to several specific locations in the heart. Typically, four to 10 electrodes are located on the end of the catheters, which have the ability to send electrical signals to stimulate the heart (called pacing) and to receive electrical signals from the heart, but not at the same time (just as a walkie-talkie cannot send and receive messages at the same time).

First, the electrodes are positioned to receive signals from inside the heart chambers, which allows the doctor to measure how fast the electrical impulses travel in the patient's heart at that time. These measurements are called the patient's baseline measurements. Next, the electrodes are positioned to pace. That is, the EPS team tries to induce (sometimes in combination with various heart drugs) the arrhythmia that the patient has previously experienced so the team can observe it in a controlled environment, compare it to the patient's clinical or spontaneous arrhythmia, and decide how to treat it.

Once the arrhythmia is induced and the team determines that it can be treated with catheter ablation, cardiac mapping is performed to locate the precise origin and route of the abnormal pathway. When this is accomplished, the ablating electrode catheter is positioned directly against the abnormal pathway, and high radio-frequency energy is delivered through the electrode to destroy (burn) the tissue in this area.

Pediatric patients present challenges for EPS. In 2001, an analysis of 45 children who underwent EPS was conducted. The researchers concluded that success rates and the prevention of complications in children may be increased by using ultrasound guidance for access to the internal jugular vein for coronary sinus cannulation (insertion of a tube for the transport of fluid) during EPS. Access was successfully obtained in all 45 of the patients without major complications using this technique.

Diagnosis/Preparation

The following preparations are made for an EPS:

- Blood tests usually are ordered one week prior to the test.

- The patient may be advised to stop taking certain medications, especially cardiac medications, that may interfere with the test results.

- The patient fasts for six to eight hours prior to the procedure. Fluids may be permitted until three hours before the test.

- The patient undergoes conscious sedation (awake but relaxed) during the test.

- A local anesthetic is injected at the site of catheter insertion.

- Peripheral pulses are marked with a pen prior to catheterization. This permits rapid assessment of pulses after the procedure.

KEY TERMS

Ablation—Removal or destruction of tissue, such as by burning or cutting.

Angiogram—X ray of a blood vessel after special x-ray dye has been injected into it.

Bradycardia—Relatively slow heart action, usually considered as a rate under 60 beats per minute.

Cardiac catheter—Long, thin, flexible tube, which is threaded into the heart through a blood vessel.

Cardiologist—Doctor who specializes in diagnosing and treating heart diseases.

Echocardiogram—Ultrasound image of the heart.

Electrocardiogram—Tracing of the electrical activity of the heart.

Electrode—A medium, such as platinum wires, for conducting an electrical current.

Electrophysiology—Study of how electrical signals in the body relate to physiologic function.

Event recorder—A small machine, worn by a patient usually for several days or weeks, that is activated by the patient to record his or her EKG when a symptom is detected.

Fibrillation—Rapid, random contraction (quivering).

Holter monitor—A small machine, worn by a patient usually for 24 hours, that continuously records the patient's EKG during usual daily activity.

Stress test—Recording a patient's EKG during exercise.

Supraventricular tachycardia—A fast heart beat that originates above the ventricles.

Tachycardia—Fast heartbeat.

Thrombophlebitis—Venous inflammation with the formation of thrombus (a clot in the cardiovascular system).

Aftercare

The patient needs to rest flat in bed for several hours after the procedure to allow healing at the catheter insertion sites. The patient often returns home either the same day or the next day. Someone should drive the patient home. To minimize bleeding and pain, the patient is advised to keep the extremity in which the catheter was placed immobilized and straight for several hours after the test.

Risks

EPS and catheter ablation are considered low-risk procedures. There is a risk of bleeding and/or infection at the site of catheter insertion. Blood clot formation may occur and is minimized with anticoagulant medications administered during the procedure. Vascular injuries causing hemorrhage or thrombophlebitis are possible. Cardiac perforations are also possible. If the right internal jugular vein is accessed, the potential for puncturing the lung with the catheter exists and could lead to a collapsed lung.

Because ventricular tachycardia or fibrillation (lethal arrhythmias) may be induced in the patient, the EPS lab personnel must be prepared to defibrillate the patient as necessary.

Patients should notify their health care provider if they develop any of these symptoms:

- numbness or tingling in the extremities
- heavy bleeding
- change in color and/or temperature of extremities
- loss of function in extremities

Normal results

Normal EPS results show that the heart initiates and conducts electrical impulses within normal limits.

Abnormal results include confirmation of arrhythmias, such as:

- supraventricular tachycardias
- ventricular arrhythmias
- accessory pathways
- bradycardias

Resources

BOOKS

Grubb, Blair P., and Brian Olshansky. *Syncope: Mechanisms and Management.* Armonk, NY: Futura Publishing, 1997.

Hummel, J. D., S. J. Kalbfleisch, and J. M. Dillon. *Pocket Guide for Cardiac Electrophysiology.* Philadelphia: W. B. Saunders Co., 1999.

Josephson, M. E. *Clinical Cardiac Electrophysiology: Techniques and Interpretations.* Philadelphia: Lippincott Williams & Wilkins Publishers, 2001.

Pagana, Kathleen D., and Timothy J. Pagana. *Diagnostic Testing and Nursing Implications*. 5th ed. St. Louis: Mosby, 1999.

Singer, Igor. *Interventional Electrophysiology*. Baltimore: Williams & Wilkins, 1997.

PERIODICALS

Asirvatham, S. J., C. J. Bruce, and P. A. Friedman. "Advances in Imaging for Cardiac Electrophysiology." *Coronary Artery Disease* 14 (February 2003): 3–13.

Binah, O. "Cytotoxic Lymphocytes and Cardiac Electrophysiology." *Journal of Molecular and Cellular Cardiology* 34 (September 2002): 1147–1161.

Kocic, I. "Sudden Cardiac Death: From Molecular Biology and Cellular Electrophysiology to Therapy." *Current Opinions in Investigative Drugs* 3 (July 2002): 1045–1050.

Liberman, L., A. J. Hordof, D. T. Hsu, and R. H. Pass. "Ultrasound-Assisted Cannulation of the Right Internal Jugular Vein during Electrophysiologic Studies in Children." *Journal of Interventional Cardiology and Electrophysiology* 5, no. 2 (June 2001): 177–179.

ORGANIZATIONS

American Association of Critical-Care Nurses. 101 Columbia, Aliso Viejo, CA 92656-4109. (800) 899–2226. <www.aacn.org/>.

The American College of Cardiology Heart House, 9111 Old Georgetown Road, Bethesda, MD 20814-1699. (800) 253–4636 <www.acc.org>.

American Heart Association. 7272 Greenville Ave., Dallas TX 75231-4596. (800) 242–1793. <www.amhrt.org>.

Cardiac Arrhythmia Research and Education Foundation (C.A.R.E.). 2082 Michelson Dr. #301, Irvine, CA 92612. (800) 404–9500. <www.longqt.com/>.

Cardiac Electrophysiology Society. <www. Cardiaceps.org>.

Maggie Boleyn, R.N., B.S.N.
Monique Laberge, Ph. D.

Electrosurgery *see* **Curettage and electrosurgery**

Emergency airway puncture *see* **Cricothyroidotomy**

Emergency surgery

Definition

Emergency surgery is non-elective surgery performed when the patient's life or well-being is in direct jeopardy. Largely performed by surgeons specializing in emergency medicine, this surgery can be conducted for many reasons but occurs most often in urgent or critical cases in response to trauma, cardiac events, poison episodes, brain injuries, and pediatric medicine.

Purpose

Most surgery is elective and is performed after a diagnosis based upon a history and physical of the patient, with differential test results and the development of strategies for management of the condition. With emergency surgery, the team, as well as the surgeon, may have less information about the patient than would ordinarily be required and work under very time-dependent conditions to save a patient's life, help avoid critical injury or systemic deterioration of the patient, or to alleviate severe pain. Because of the unique conditions for urgent acute surgery, operations are usually performed by a **surgical team** specially trained for management of a critical, or life threatening event.

Acute surgical emergencies include:

- invasive types of resuscitation for acute respiratory failure, pulmonary embolism and pulmonary obstructions
- blunt and penetrating head, chest, abdomen injuries, largely from automobile accidents and gun shot wounds
- burns
- cardiac events, including heart attacks, cardiac shock and cardiac arrhythmia
- aneurysms
- brain injuries and other neurological conditions
- perforated ulcer and appendix, and peritonitis

Description

Emergency surgery can take place in any hospital setting. However, trauma centers or trauma sections of hospitals handle most emergency surgeries. Forty-four states have designated trauma centers, some states with better systems than others. A level 1 trauma center, the most advanced of the trauma center system, is equipped to get the patient to surgery beginning with trained first responders. The system relies on available operating rooms, readily available laboratory personnel, anesthesiologists, x-ray and blood bank access, intensive care nurses, and ward nurses—all trained to take the patient to the **operating room** within 60 minutes of the incident. If patients are in surgery within an hour they have a 25% chance of survival.

Diagnosis/Preparation

Emergency surgery follows a path from resuscitation and stabilization of the patient with a patient management team, to preparation of the patient for surgery, to post-operative and recovery procedures—all designed to deal quickly with the life-threatening situation. There is often little time or possibility for extensive diagnosis or the gathering of a patient history. Decisions are made quickly about surgery, often without family members present. The possibility of emergency surgery due to trauma, injury, emergency medical conditions and cardiac events make it wise for all patients to have a **living will** detailing their medical care wishes and to carry it with them at all times.

Normal results

Mortality rates are high for emergency surgeries. For instance, rupture of abdominal aneurysm results in death in about 50% of cases due to kidney failure from shock or disrupted blood supply. An untreated aneurysm is always fatal. Certain gastrointestinal disorders require emergency surgery, including bleeding in the digestive tract, obstructions, appendicitis and inflammation of the lining of the abdomen. Pediatric emergency surgery includes birth defects of the heart. One in 120 infants is born with a heart defect requiring surgery to unblock the flow of blood or to treat a malformed aortic valve. Heart attacks are very effectively treated with emergency surgery depending upon the part of the heart affected, whether there is arterial blockage and overall health. Arrhythmia can develop, as well as stroke. The first 48 hours are the most crucial with cardiac events and whether there is immediate medical and surgical attention. Many cardiac surgeries result in bypass procedures, with a higher death rate associated with bypass surgery done on an emergency basis. Women have more emergency heart bypass operations than men, probably due to lack of earlier cardiac care.

See also Elective surgery.

Resources

BOOKS

Marx: Rosen's Emergency Medicine: Concepts and Clinical Practice 5th ed. St. Louis: Mosby, Inc., 2002.

PERIODICALS

Thacker, C.V., et al. "ARF After Open-heart Surgery: Influence of Gender and Race." *American Journal of Kidney Diseases* 41, no. 4, (April 2003).

ORGANIZATIONS

American College of Emergency Physicians. <http://www.acep.org>.

OTHER

DeNoon, D. "Trauma Centers: Life-or-Death Difference." *WebMD Medical News.* October 23, 2002 [cited June 17, 2003]. <http://www.webmd.com>.

Smith, I. M. "U.S. Trauma Centers." *Virtual Hospital.* April 2003 [cited June 17, 2003]. <http://www.vh.org/adult/patient/internalmedicine/aba30/2003/traumacenter.html> .

Nancy Mckenzie, PhD

Endarterectomy, carotid *see* **Carotid endarterectomy**

Endarterectomy, peripheral *see* **Peripheral endarterectomy**

Endocardial resection *see* **Myocardial resection**

Endolymphatic shunt

Definition

An endolymphatic shunt is a surgical procedure in which a very small silicone tube is placed in the membranous labyrinth of the inner ear to drain excess fluid.

Purpose

An endolymphatic shunt is placed as part of the treatment of Ménière's disease, a disorder of the inner ear whose causes are still unknown. Ménière's disease is characterized by the following symptoms:

- a rise in the level of endolymphatic fluid in the labyrinth of the inner ear
- hearing loss that comes and goes
- a sensation that the environment or oneself is revolving or spinning (vertigo)
- ringing, buzzing, or hissing noises in the ears (tinnitus)
- a feeling that the ears are blocked or plugged

Endolymphatic shunt surgery is one of the surgical procedures available to treat Ménière's disease, which is also known as endolymphatic hydrops. The surgery is based on the theory that the disorder causes the inner ear to become overloaded with fluid and that draining this fluid will relieve the symptoms. The fluid is drained by opening the endolymphatic sac, a pouch located next to the mastoid bone at the end of the endolymphatic duct. The endolymphatic duct is a canal that leads to the inner ear.

Demographics

According to the National Institute on Deafness and Other Communication Disorders (NIDCD), there were an estimated three to five million cases of Ménière's disease in the United States in 1998, with nearly 100,000 new cases diagnosed annually. In most cases only one ear is affected, but as many as 15–40% of patients are affected in both ears. The onset of Ménière's disease occurs most often in adults between the ages of 20 and 50. Men and women are affected in equal numbers.

Description

An endolymphatic shunt is placed with the patient under general anesthesia. The operation takes about two hours to perform. The patient is usually positioned lying on the back with the head turned to one side and the affected ear lying uppermost. The head is immobilized and supported with a pad or brace. The operation itself begins with opening the mastoid bone and identifying the endolymphatic sac. To find the sac, the surgeon removes the bony cover of the sigmoid sinus, which is an S-shaped cavity behind the mastoid bone. The surgeon leaves intact a small rectangle of thin bone called Bill's Island (named for Dr. William House). The sigmoid sinus is then collapsed with gentle pressure. The surgeon exposes the endolymphatic sac and makes an incision in it in order to insert the shunt.

Diagnosis/Preparation

The diagnosis of Ménière's disease is based on the patient's medical history, a **physical examination**, and the results of hearing tests, balance tests, an electronystagmogram, and imaging studies. An MRI or CT scan is performed to rule out a tumor as the cause of the patient's symptoms. A hearing test (audiogram) identifies the hearing loss that is typical of Ménière's disease. Balance function tests are administered to assess the patient's vertigo.

The patient is prepared for surgery by having the hair removed and the skin shaved over an area of at least 1.5 in (3.8 cm) around the site of the incision. A mild solution of soap and water is commonly used to cleanse the outer ear and surrounding skin.

Aftercare

The operated ear is covered with a Glassock dressing, which is a special dressing applied to keep pressure on the site to reduce swelling. There is usually some tenderness and discomfort in the operated ear and the throat (from the breathing tube inserted during surgery), which can be controlled by such analgesic medications as meperidine (Demerol) or oxycodone (Percocet).

Risks

There are few risks associated with endolymphatic shunt surgery. The operation is considered the first-line surgical treatment for Ménière's disease precisely because it is very safe. The chance of hearing loss from the procedure is about 0.5%.

Normal results

Endolymphatic shunt surgery relieves the vertigo associated with Ménière's disease, with restoration of hearing dependent on the severity of the disease. The patient's ear may protrude slightly shortly after surgery but usually returns to its original position within two to three

KEY TERMS

Bony labyrinth—A series of cavities contained in a capsule inside the temporal bone of the skull. The endolymph-filled membranous labyrinth is suspended in a fluid inside the bony labyrinth.

Electronystagmogram—A test that involves the graphic recording of eye movements.

Endolymph—The watery fluid contained in the membranous labyrinth of the inner ear.

Endolymphatic sac—The pouch at the end of the endolymphatic duct that connects to the membranous labyrinth of the inner ear.

Mastoid—A large bony process at the base of the skull behind the ear. It contains air spaces that connect with the cavity of the middle ear.

Membranous labyrinth—A complex arrangement of communicating membranous canals and sacs, filled with endolymph and suspended within the cavity of the bony labyrinth.

Ménière's disease—Also known as idiopathic endolymphatic hydrops, Ménière's disease is a disorder of the inner ear. It is named for Prosper Ménière (1799–1862), a French physician.

Shunt—A channel through which blood or another body fluid is diverted from its normal path by surgical reconstruction or the insertion of a synthetic tube.

Sigmoid sinus—An S-shaped cavity on the inner side of the skull behind the mastoid process.

Tinnitus—A sensation of ringing, buzzing, roaring, or clicking noises in the ear.

Vertigo—An illusory feeling that either one's self or the environment is revolving. It is usually caused either by diseases of the inner ear or disturbances of the central nervous system.

---

weeks after the operation. Numbness around the ear is a common complication that may last for several months.

Morbidity and mortality rates

Endolymphatic shunt surgery is considered a low-morbidity procedure. It has been reported to achieve complete or substantial control of vertigo in 81% of patients, with significant improvement in hearing in about 20%. Overall, there is a 60% chance of curing the vertigo, a 20% chance that the attacks will remain at the same level of severity, and a 20% chance that the attacks will get worse. The patient's vertigo usually improves even if hearing does not improve.

Alternatives

Nonsurgical alternatives

There are several nonsurgical treatments recommended for patients with Ménière's disease:

• Vestibular suppressants. These are drugs designed to control vertigo attacks; they include mechzine (Antivert), diazepam (Valium), and dimenhydrinate (Dramamine).

• Diuretics. Medications that increase the body's output of urine can also help reduce the frequency of vertigo attacks in some patients by lowering the amount of fluid in the body.

• Dietary changes. Although the benefits of a low salt diet have not been confirmed by formal scientific research, many patients with Ménière's disease have noted that their symptoms improve when they restrict their salt intake.

• Steroids. Prednisone and other steroids have been used to treat patients in the early stages of Ménière's disease. Their use in this disorder, however, is still considered experimental as of 2003.

Surgical

Surgical alternatives to the placement of an endolymphatic shunt include:

• Selective vestibular neurectomy. In this procedure, the surgeon cuts the vestibular nerve, which relays balance, position and movement signals from the inner ear to the brain. Vestibular neurectomy prevents the transmission of faulty information from the affected ear and eliminates attacks of vertigo in many patients.

• Labyrinthectomy. In this procedure, the membranous labyrinth of the inner ear is removed. Labyrinthectomy is more successful than other surgeries in eliminating vertigo, but the patient suffers complete and permanent loss of hearing in the operated ear.

Resources

BOOKS

Graham, M. D. *Treatment Options for Ménière's Disease: Endolymphatic Sac Surgery: Do It or Don't Do It and Why?* San Diego: Singular Publishing, 1998.

Haybach, P. J., and J. Underwood. *Ménière's Disease: What You Need to Know*. Portland, OR: Vestibular Disorders Association, 1998.

"Ménière's Disease." In *The Merck Manual of Diagnosis and Therapy*, edited by Mark H. Beers, MD, and Robert Berkow, MD. Whitehouse Station, NJ: Merck Research Laboratories, 1999.

PERIODICALS

Brookler, K. H. "A Patient with Endolymphatic Hydrops Refractory to Shunt Surgery." *Ear Nose Throat Journal* 79 (July 2000): 493.

Goksu, N., Y. A. Bayazit, A. Abdulhalik, and Y. K. Kemaloglu. "Vestibular Neurectomy with Simultaneous Endolymphatic Subarachnoid Shunt." *European Archives of Otorhinolaryngology* 259 (May 2002): 243-246.

Mason, T. P. "What is Ménière's Disease, and How is it Treated?" *Health News* 9 (April 2003): 12.

Ostrowski, V. B., and J. M. Kartush. " Endolymphatic Sac-Vein Decompression for Intractable Ménière's Disease: Long Term Treatment Results." *Otolaryngology Head and Neck Surgery* 128 (April 2003): 550-559.

Welling, D. B., and H. N. Nagaraja. "Endolymphatic Mastoid Shunt: a Reevaluation of Efficacy." *Otolaryngology Head and Neck Surgery* 122 (March 2000): 340-345.

ORGANIZATIONS

American Academy of Otolaryngology—Head and Neck Surgery. One Prince Street, Alexandria, VA 22314. (703) 806-4444. <www.entnet.org>.

National Institute on Deafness and Other Communication Disorders (NIDCD). 31 Center Drive, MSC 2320, Bethesda, MD 20892-2320. (800) 241-1044. <www.nidcd.nih.gov/>.

Vestibular Disorders Association (VEDA). PO Box 4467, Portland, OR 97208-4467. (800) 837-8428. <www.vestibular. org>.

OTHER

"Ménière's Disease–Surgical Therapy." *UPennHealth*. <www.uphs.upenn.edu/balance/patient%20education%20brochures/Meniere's-Surgical%20Treatment.htm>.

Monique Laberge, PhD

Endometriosis surgery *see* **Laparoscopy for endometriosis**

Endoscopic retrograde cholangiopancreatography

Definition

Endoscopic retrograde cholangiopancreatography (ERCP) is an imaging technique used to diagnose dis-

eases of the pancreas, liver, gallbladder, and bile ducts. It combines endoscopy and x-ray imaging.

Purpose

ERCP is used in the management of diseases that affect the gastrointestinal tract, specifically the pancreas, liver, gall bladder, and bile ducts. The pancreas is an organ that secretes pancreatic juice into the upper part of the intestine. Pancreatic juice is composed of specialized proteins that help to digest fats, proteins, and carbohydrates. Bile is a substance that helps to digest fats; it is produced by the liver, secreted through the bile ducts, and stored in the gallbladder. Bile is released into the small intestine after a person has eaten a meal containing fat.

A doctor may recommend ERCP if a patient is experiencing abdominal pain of unknown origin, weight loss, or jaundice. These may be symptoms of biliary disease. For instance, gallstones that form in the gallbladder or bile ducts may become stuck there, causing cramping or dull pain in the upper right area of the abdomen, fever, and/or jaundice. Other causes of biliary obstruction include tumors, injury from gallbladder surgery, or inflammation. The bile ducts may also become narrowed (called a biliary stricture) as a result of cancer, blunt trauma to the abdomen, pancreatitis (inflammation of the pancreas), or primary biliary cirrhosis (PBC). PBC may be caused by a condition called primary sclerosing cholangitis, an inflammation of the bile ducts that may cause pain, jaundice, itching, or other symptoms. These symptoms may also be experienced by a patient with cholangitis, or with infection of the bile ducts caused by bacteria or parasites.

ERCP can also be used to diagnose a number of pancreatic disorders. Pancreatitis is an inflammation of the pancreas, caused by chronic alcohol abuse, injury, obstruction of the pancreatic ducts (e.g., by gallstones), or other factors. The condition may be either acute (having a severe but short course) or chronic (persistent). Symptoms of pan-

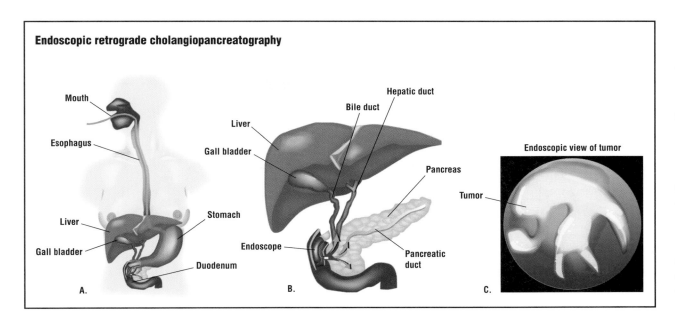

Endoscopic retrograde cholangiopancreatography

In endoscopic retrograde cholangiopancreatography, an endoscope is introduced into the patient's mouth and fed through the esophagus, stomach, and duodenum (small intestine) (A). A dye is released into the ducts (B). A series of x rays is taken, and a tumor may be visible with the endoscope (C). *(Illustration by GGS Inc.)*

creatitis include abdominal pain, weight loss, nausea, and vomiting. ERCP may be used to diagnose cancer of the pancreas; pancreatic pseudocysts (collections of pancreatic fluid); or strictures of the pancreatic ducts. Certain congenital disorders may also be identified by ERCP, such as pancreas divisum, a condition in which parts of the pancreas fail to fuse together during fetal development.

Demographics

Diseases of the pancreas and biliary tract affect millions of Americans each year. According to the National Health and Nutrition Survey, gallbladder disease affects approximately 6.3 million men and 14.2 million women in the United States between the ages of 24 and 74. Approximately one million new cases of gallstones are diagnosed each year. The incidence of gallstones is higher among women; adults over the age of 40; and people who are overweight. Primary sclerosing cholangitis occurs at a rate of two to seven cases per 100,000 persons. The rate of gallbladder cancer is approximately 2.5 out of 100,000 persons. In addition, approximately 87,000 cases of pancreatitis and 30,000 cases of pancreatic cancer are diagnosed each year in the United States.

Description

ERCP is performed with the patient given either a sedative or general anesthesia. The physician then sprays the back of the patient's throat with a local anesthetic. The endoscope (a thin, hollow tube attached to a viewing screen) is then inserted into the mouth. It is threaded down the esophagus, through the stomach, and into the duodenum (upper part of the small intestine) until it reaches the spot where the bile and pancreatic ducts empty into the duodenum. At this point a small tube called a cannula is inserted through the endoscope and used to inject a contrast dye into the ducts. The term "retrograde" in the name of the procedure refers to the backward direction of the dye as it is injected through the ducts. A series of x rays are then taken as the dye moves through the ducts.

If the x rays show that a problem exists, ERCP may be used as a therapeutic tool. Special instruments can be inserted into the endoscope to remove gallstones, take samples of tissue for further examination (e.g., in the case of suspected cancer), or place a special tube called a stent into a duct to relieve an obstruction.

Diagnosis/Preparation

ERCP is generally not performed unless other less invasive diagnostic tests have first been used to determine the cause of a patient's symptoms. Such tests include:

• complete medical history and physical examination

• blood tests (certain diseases can be diagnosed by abnormal levels of blood components)

• ultrasound imaging (a procedure that uses high-frequency sound waves to visualize structures in the human body)

- computed tomography (CT) scan (an imaging device that uses x rays to produce two-dimensional cross-sections on a viewing screen)

Before undergoing ERCP, the patient will be instructed to refrain from eating or drinking for at least six hours to ensure that the stomach and upper part of the intestine are empty. Arrangements should be made for someone to take the patient home after the procedure, as he or she will not be able to drive. The physician should also be given a complete list of all prescription, over-the-counter, and alternative medications or preparations that the patient is taking. The patient should also notify the doctor if he or she is allergic to iodine because the contrast dye contains it.

Aftercare

After the procedure, the patient will remain at the hospital or outpatient facility until the effects of the sedative wear off and no signs of any complications have appeared. A longer stay may be warranted if the patient experiences complications or if other procedures were performed.

Risks

Complications that have been reported with ERCP include pancreatitis, cholangitis (inflammation of the bile ducts), cholecystitis (inflammation of the gallbladder), injury to the duodenum, pain, bleeding, infection, and formation of blood clots. Factors that increase the risk of complications include liver damage, bleeding disorders, a history of post-ERCP complications, and a less experienced endoscopist.

Normal results

Following ERCP, the patient's biliary and pancreatic ducts should be free of stones and show no strictures, obstructions, or evidence of infection or inflammation.

Morbidity and mortality rates

The overall complication rate associated with ERCP is approximately 11%. Pancreatitis may occur in up to 7% of patients. Cholangitis and cholecystitis occur in less than 1% of patients. Infection, injury, bleeding, and blot clot formation also occur in less than 1%. The mortality rate for ERCP is approximately 0.1%.

Alternatives

Although less invasive techniques exist (such as computed tomography and ultrasonography) to help to diagnose gastrointestinal diseases, these imaging studies are often not precise enough to allow for definite diagnosis of certain conditions. Percutaneous transhepatic cholangiography (PTCA) is an alternative to ERCP that involves the insertion of a long, flexible needle through the skin to the bile ducts; contrast dye is then injected into the ducts so that they may be visualized by x ray. PTCA may be recommended if ERCP fails or cannot be performed. Magnetic resonance cholangiopancreatography (MRCP) is an imaging technology that allows for noninvasive examination of the biliary and pancreatic ducts. Its disadvantage, however, is that unlike ERCP, it cannot be used for therapeutic procedures as well as imaging.

Resources

BOOKS

Feldman, Mark, et al. *Sleisenger & Fordtran's Gastrointestinal and Liver Disease*, 7th ed. Philadelphia: Elsevier Science, 2002.

PERIODICALS

Ahmed, Aijaz, and Emmet B. Keeffe. "Gallstones and Biliary Tract Disease." *WebMD Scientific American Medicine* February 28, 2003 [cited April 7, 2003]. <www.medscape.com/viewarticle/449563_1>.

Aronson, Naomi, Carole Flamm, Rhonda L. Bohn, et al. "Evidence-Based Assessment: Patient, Procedure, or Operator Factors Associated with ERCP Complications." *Gastrointestinal Endoscopy* 56, no. 6 (December 2002)(6 Suppl): S294-S302.

Freeman, Martin L. "Adverse Outcomes of ERCP." *Gastrointestinal Endoscopy* 56, no. 6 (December 2002) (6 Suppl): S273-S282.

Vandervoort, Jo, et al. "Risk Factors for Complications After Performance of ERCP." *Gastrointestinal Endoscopy* 56, no. 5 (November 2002): 652-656.

Yakshe, Paul. "Biliary Disease." *eMedicine*, March 29, 2002 [cited April 7, 2003]. <www.emedicine.com/MED/topic 225.htm>.

Yakshe, Paul. "Pancreatitis, Chronic." *eMedicine*, January 8, 2003 [cited April 7, 2003]. <www.emedicine.com/med/topic1721.htm>.

KEY TERMS

Bile—A bitter yellowish-brown fluid secreted by the liver that contains bile salts, bile pigments, cholesterol, and other substances. It helps the body to digest and absorb fats.

Congenital—Present at birth.

Endoscope—An instrument with a light source attached that allows the doctor to examine the inside of the digestive tract or other hollow organ.

Gastrointestinal tract—A group of organs and related structures that includes the esophagus, stomach, liver, gallbladder, pancreas, small intestine, large intestine, rectum, and anus.

Jaundice—A condition characterized by deposits of bile pigments in the skin, mucous membranes, and the whites of the eyes. It is also known as icterus.

Magnetic resonance imaging—A technique that uses a strong magnetic field and pulses of radio waves to produce cross-sectional images of the body.

Stent—A thin rod-like or tube-like device made of wire mesh, inserted into a blood vessel or duct to keep it open.

Stricture—An abnormal narrowing of a duct or canal.

ORGANIZATIONS

American College of Gastroenterology. 4900 B South 31st St., Arlington, VA 22206. (703) 820-7400. <www.acg.gi.org>.

American Gastroenterological Association. 7910 Woodmont Ave., 7th Floor, Bethesda, MD 20814. (301) 654-2055. <www.gastro.org>.

American Society for Gastrointestinal Endoscopy. 1520 Kensington Rd., Suite 202, Oak Brook, IL 60523. (630) 573-0600. <www.asge.org>.

OTHER

National Digestive Diseases Information Clearinghouse. *Endoscopic Retrograde Cholangiopancreatography.* Bethesda, MD: NDDIC, 2002. [cited April 7, 2003]. <www.niddk.nih.gov/health/digest/pubs/diagtest/ercp.htm>.

Stephanie Dionne Sherk

Endoscopic sclerotherapy *see* **Sclerotherapy for esophageal varices**

Endoscopic sinus surgery

Definition

Functional endoscopic sinus surgery (FESS) is a minimally invasive surgical procedure that opens up sinus air cells and sinus ostia (openings) with an endoscope.

The use of FESS as a sinus surgical method has now become widely accepted; and the term "functional" is meant to distinguish this type of endoscopic surgery from nonendoscopic, more conventional sinus surgery procedures.

Purpose

The purpose of FESS is to restore normal drainage of the sinuses. Normal function of the sinuses requires ventilation through the ostia (mouth-like opening) and is facilitated by a mucociliary transport process that maintains a constant flow of mucus out of the sinuses. All sinuses need ventilation to prevent infection and inflammation, a condition known as sinusitis. In healthy individuals, sinus ventilation occurs through the ostia into the nose. The sinuses open into the middle meatus (curved passage in each nasal cavity) under the middle turbinate (thin, bony process that is the lower portion of the ethmoid bone in each nasal cavity), which together are known as the osteomeatal complex, the key area of the nose. The hair-like cilia direct the flow of mucus toward the ostia.

Sinusitis develops when there is a problem in the area where the maxillary and frontal sinuses meet near the nose or, occasionally, by dental infection. When sinusitis occurs, the cilia work less efficiently, preventing the flow of mucus. The mucous membranes of the sinuses become engorged, resulting in ostia closure. Poor ventilation and accumulation of mucus then produce the conditions required for bacterial infection.

WHO PERFORMS THE PROCEDURE AND WHERE IS IT PERFORMED?

This procedure is usually performed on an outpatient basis by an ear, nose, and throat (ENT) specialist, such as an otolaryngologist or an ophthalmic surgeon. ENT physicians are graduates of a school of medicine and typically undergo an otolaryngology residency with further specialization in sinus disease and endoscopic sinus surgery.

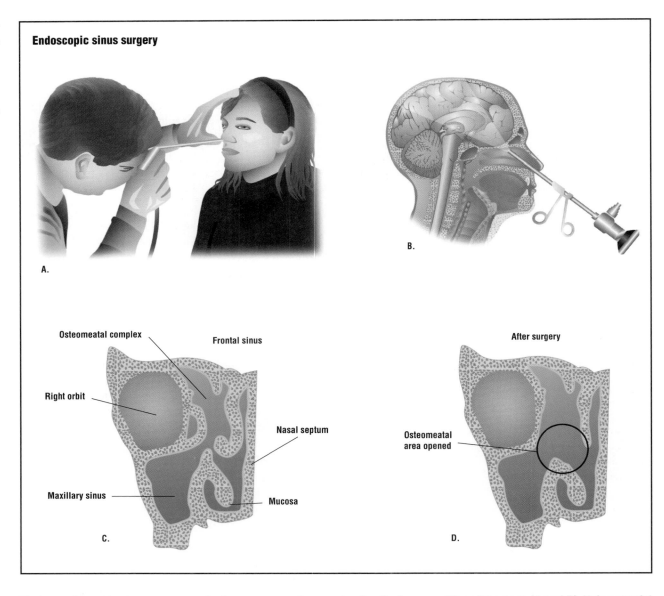

Endoscopic sinus surgery

Osteomeatal complex

Frontal sinus

Right orbit

Nasal septum

Maxillary sinus

Mucosa

C.

After surgery

Osteomeatal area opened

D.

A.

B.

During endoscopic sinus surgery, a doctor uses an endoscope to view the inner cavities of the nose (A and B). Using special instruments, the doctor opens the sinuses to alleviate problems with sinusitis (C and D). *(Illustration by GGS Inc.)*

Demographics

Sinusitis is a very common condition, affecting 31 million Americans each year; 30% of the United States population have sinusitis at some point in their lives. The average adult has three to four upper respiratory infections a year; 1% of these infections are complicated by sinusitis, accounting for 16 million visits to the doctor each year.

Description

After inducing adequate vasoconstriction with co-caine or ephedrine, the surgeon locates the middle turbinate, the most important landmark for the FESS procedure. On the side of the nose at the level of the middle turbinate lies the uncinate process, which the surgeon removes. The surgeon opens the back ethmoid air cells, to allow better ventilation, but leaves the bone covered with the mucous membrane. Following this step, the ostium located near the jaw is checked for obstruction and, if necessary, opened with a middle meatal antrostomy. This surgical procedure often greatly improves the function of the osteomeatal complex and provides better ventilation of the sinuses.

FESS offers several advantages:

- It is a minimally invasive procedure.
- It does not disturb healthy tissue.
- It is performed in less time with better results.
- It minimizes bleeding and scarring.

Diagnosis/Preparation

As with many diseases, the history of a patient with sinusitis represents a key part of the preoperative evaluation. Before considering FESS, the ear, nose and throat (ENT) specialist will proceed with a thorough diagnostic examination. The development of such diagnostic tools as the fiberoptic endoscope and CT scanning has greatly improved the treatment of sinus disease. The fiberoptic endoscope is used to examine the nose and all its recesses thoroughly. The specific features the physician must examine and evaluate are the middle turbinate and the middle meatus, any anatomic obstruction, and the presence of pus and nasal polyps.

CT scanning can also be used to identify the diseased areas, a process that is required for planning the surgery. It shows the extent of the affected sinuses, as well as any abnormalities that may make a patient more susceptible to sinusitis.

FESS is usually performed under local anesthesia with intravenous sedation on an outpatient basis with patients going home one to two hours after surgery. It usually does not cause facial swelling or bruising, and does not generally require nasal packing.

Aftercare

FESS usually does not cause severe postoperative sinus pain. After the procedure, it is important to keep the nose as free from crust build-up as possible. To achieve this, the surgeon may perform a lengthy cleaning two to three times per week or the patient may perform a simple nasal douching several times a day. Normal function usually reappears after one or two months. In patients with severe sinusitis or polyps, a short course of systemic steroids combined with **antibiotics** may quicken recovery.

Risks

The most serious risk associated with FESS is blindness resulting from damage to the optic nerve. The chances of this complication occurring, however, are extremely low. Cerebrospinal fluid leak represents the most common major complication of FESS, but it occurs in only about 0.2% of cases in the Unites States. The leak is usually recognized at the time of surgery and can easily be repaired. Other less serious and rare complications in-

clude orbital hematoma and nasolacrimal duct stenosis. All of these complications are also associated with conventional sinus surgery and not only with FESS.

Normal results

The FESS procedure is considered successful if the patient's sinusitis is resolved. Nasal obstruction and facial pain are usually relieved. The outcome has been compared with that of the Caldwell-Luc procedure and, although both methods are considered effective, there is a strong patient preference for FESS. The extent of the disease before surgery dictates the outcome, with the best results obtained in patients with limited nasal sinusitis.

Morbidity and mortality rates

According to the American Academy of Family Physicians (AAFP), FESS usually has a good outcome, with most studies reporting an 80–90% rate of success. Good results have also been obtained in patients who have had previous sinus surgery.

Alternatives

- Image-guided endoscopic surgery. This method uses image guidance techniques that feature a three-dimensional mapping system combining CT scanning and real-time data acquisition concerning the location of the **surgical instruments** during the procedure. It allows surgeons to navigate more precisely in the affected area. The surgeon can monitor the exact location of such vital organs as the brain and eyes as well as positively identifying the affected areas.
- Caldwell-Luc procedure. This procedure is directed at improving drainage in the maxillary sinus region located below the eye. The surgeon reaches the region

KEY TERMS

Antrostomy—The operation of opening an antrum for drainage.

Antrum—The cavity of a sinus.

Caldwell-Luc procedure—A surgical procedure in which the surgeon enters the maxillary sinus by making an opening under the upper lip above the teeth.

Cilia—Short hair-like processes that make a lashing movement.

CT scan—A sectional imaging of the body constructed by computed tomography.

Endoscope—An instrument for visualizing the interior of a hollow organ.

Ethmoid sinuses—Paired labyrinth of air cells between the nose and eyes.

Maxillary sinuses—Sinuses located in the cheek under the eye next to the ethmoid sinus.

Meatus—A general term for an opening or passageway in the body.

Middle meatus—A curved passage in each nasal cavity located below the middle nasal concha and extending along the entire superior border of the inferior nasal concha.

Middle turbinate—The lower of two thin bony processes on the ethmoid bone on the lateral wall of each nasal fossa that separates the superior and middle meatus of the nose.

Mucociliary—Involving cilia of the mucous membranes of the respiratory system.

Mucous membrane—A membrane rich in mucous glands that lines body passages and cavities communicating directly or indirectly with the exterior of the body (as for example, the alimentary, respiratory, and genitourinary tracts). Mucous membranes function in protection, support, nutrient absorption, and secretion of mucus, enzymes, and salts.

Mucus—A viscous, slippery secretion that is produced by mucous membranes which it moistens and protects.

Nasal concha—Any of three thin bony plates on the lateral wall of the nasal fossa on each side with or without their covering of mucous membrane.

Ostia—A mouth-like opening in a bodily part.

Polyp—A projecting mass of swollen and hypertrophied or tumorous tissue.

Sinus—A cavity in a bone of the skull that usually communicates with the nostrils and contains air.

Sinusitis—Inflammation of a sinus.

Stenosis—Narrowing of a duct or canal.

Turbinate—Relating to a nasal concha.

Uncinate process—A downwardly and backwardly directed process of each lateral mass of the ethmoid bone that joins with the inferior nasal conchae.

Vasoconstriction—Narrowing of blood vessels, especially as a result of vasomotor action.

---

through the upper jaw above one of the second molars. He or she creates a passage to connect the maxillary sinus to the nose in order to improve drainage.

Resources

BOOKS

Bhatt, N. J. *Endoscopic Sinus Surgery: New Horizons.* Independence, KY: Singular Publishing Group, 1997.

Bhatt, N. J. *The Frontal Sinus: Advanced Surgical Techniques.* Independence, KY: Singular Publishing Group, 2002.

Marks, S. C., and W. A. Loechel. *Nasal and Sinus Surgery.* Philadelphia: W. B. Saunders Co., 2000.

PERIODICALS

Engelke, W., W. Schwarzwaller, A. Behnsen, and H. G. Jacobs. "Subantroscopic laterobasal sinus floor augmentation (SALSA): an up-to-5-year clinical study." *International Journal of Oral and Maxillofacial Implants* 18 (January-February 2003): 135–143.

Graham, S. M., and K. D. Carter. "Major complications of endoscopic sinus surgery: a comment." *British Journal of Ophthalmology* 87 (March 2003): 374–377.

Larsen, A. S., C. Buchwald, and S. Vesterhauge. "Sinus barotrauma—late diagnosis and treatment with computer-aided endoscopic surgery." *Aviation & Space Environmental Mediciine* 74 (February 2003): 180–183.

Ramadan, H. H. "Relation of age to outcome after endoscopic sinus surgery in children." *Archives of Otolaryngology & Head and Neck Surgery* 129 (February 2003): 175–177.

Wormald, P. J. "Salvage frontal sinus surgery: the endoscopic modified Lothrop procedure." *Laryngoscope* 113 (February 2003): 276–283.

ORGANIZATIONS

American Academy of Otolaryngology-Head and Neck Surgery. One Prince St., Alexandria, VA 22314-3357. (703) 836-4444. <http://www.entnet.org/>.

Association for Research in Otolaryngology. 19 Mantua Rd., Mt. Royal, NJ 08061. (856) 423-0041. (301) 733-3640. <http://www.aro.org/index.html>.

North American Society for Head and Neck Pathology. Department of Pathology, H179, P.O. Box 850, Milton S. Hershey Medical Center, Penn State University School of Medicine, Hershey, PA 17033. (717) 531-8246. <http://www.headandneckpathology.com/>.

OTHER

"Factsheet: Sinus Surgery." American Academy of Otolaryngology—Head and Neck Surgery [cited May 5, 2003]. <http://www.entlink.org/healthinfo/sinus/sinus_surgery.cfm>.

Slack, R. and G. Bates. "Sinus Surgery." *American Family Physician*. 1 September 1998 [cited May 5, 2003]. <http://www.aafp.org/afp/980901ap/slack.html>.

Monique Laberge, Ph.D.

Endotracheal intubation

Definition

Endotracheal intubation is the placement of a tube into the trachea (windpipe) in order to maintain an open airway in patients who are unconscious or unable to breathe on their own. Oxygen, anesthetics, or other gaseous medications can be delivered through the tube.

Purpose

Specifically, endotracheal intubation is used for the following conditions:

• respiratory arrest

• respiratory failure

• airway obstruction

• need for prolonged ventilatory support

• Class III or IV hemorrhage with poor perfusion

• severe flail chest or pulmonary contusion

• multiple trauma, head injury and abnormal mental status

• inhalation injury with erythema/edema of the vocal cords

• protection from aspiration

Description

To begin the procedure, an anesthesiologist opens the patient's mouth by separating the lips and pulling on the upper jaw with the index finger. Holding a laryngoscope in the left hand, he or she inserts it into the mouth of the patient with the blade directed to the right tonsil. Once the right tonsil is reached, the laryngoscope is swept to the midline, keeping the tongue on the left to bring the epiglottis into view. The laryngoscope blade is then advanced until it reaches the angle between the base of the tongue and the epiglottis. Next, the laryngoscope is lifted upwards towards the chest and away from the nose to bring the vocal cords into view. Often an assistant has to press on the trachea to provide a direct view of the larynx. The anesthesiologist then takes the endotracheal tube, made of flexible plastic, in the right hand and starts inserting it through the mouth opening. The tube is inserted through the cords to the point that the cuff rests just below the cords. Finally, the cuff is inflated to provide a minimal leak when the bag is squeezed. Using a **stethoscope**, the anesthesiologist listens for breathing sounds to ensure correct placement of the tube.

Preparation

For endotracheal intubation, the patient is placed on the operating table lying on the back with a pillow under the head. The anesthesiologist wears gloves, a gown and goggles. General anesthesia is administered to the patient before starting intubation.

Risks

The anesthesiologist should evaluate and follow the patient for potential complications that may include edema; bleeding; tracheal and esophageal perforation; pneumothorax (collapsed lung); and aspiration. The patient should be advised of the potential signs and symptoms associated with life-threatening complications of airway problems. These signs and symptoms include but are not limited to sore throat, pain or swelling of the face and neck, chest pain, subcutaneous emphysema, and difficulty swallowing.

Normal results

The endotracheal tube inserted during the procedure maintains an open passage through the upper airway and allows air to pass freely to and from the lungs in order to ventilate them.

Alternatives

Alternatives to endotracheal intubation include:

• Esophageal tracheal combitube (ETC). The ETC is a double-lumen tube, combining the function of an esophageal obturator airway and a conventional endotracheal airway. The esophageal lumen has an open upper end, perforations at the pharyngeal level, and a closed distal end. The tracheal lumen has open ends. The lumens are separated by a wall and each is linked via a short tube with a connector. An oropharyngeal balloon serves to seal the oral and nasal cavities after

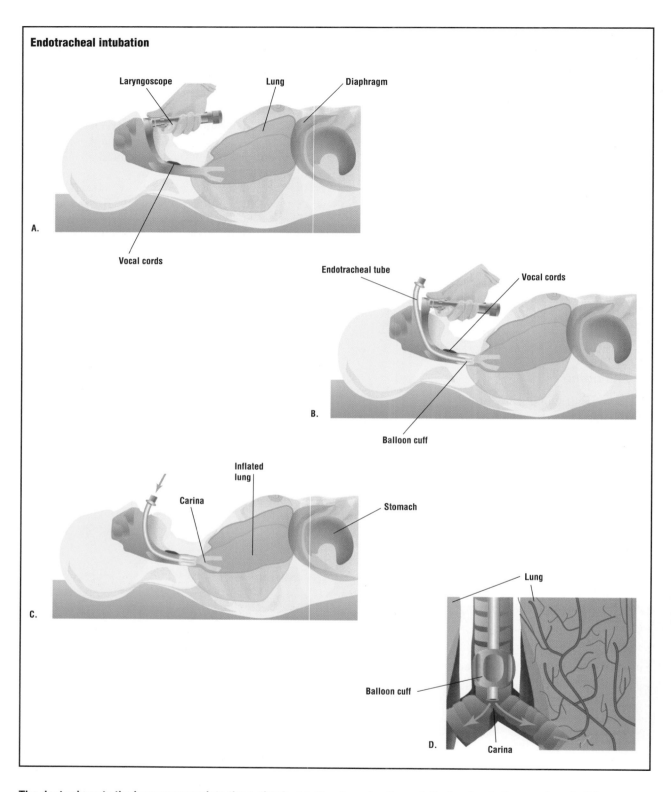

Endotracheal intubation

A.

Laryngoscope

Lung

Diaphragm

Vocal cords

B.

Endotracheal tube

Vocal cords

Balloon cuff

C.

Inflated lung

Carina

Stomach

D.

Lung

Balloon cuff

Carina

The doctor inserts the laryngoscope into the patient's mouth, advancing through the trachea to the vocal cords (A). An endotracheal tube is inserted into the airway (B). The balloon cuff is inflated, and the laryngoscope is removed (C). *(Illustration by GGS Inc.)*

insertion. At the lower end, a second cuff serves to seal either the trachea or esophagus.

- Laryngeal mask airway (LMA). The LMA consists of an inflatable silicone ring attached diagonally to a flexible tube. The ring forms an oval cushion that fills the space around and behind the larynx. It achieves a low-pressure seal between the tube and the trachea without insertion into the larynx.

- Tracheostomy. A tracheostomy is a surgically created opening in the neck that allows direct access to the trachea. It is kept open with a tracheostomy tube. A tracheostomy is performed when it is not possible to intubate the patient.

See also Anesthesia evaluation.

Resources

BOOKS

Finucane, B. T., and A. H. Santora. *Principles of Airway Management*. New York: Springer Verlag, 2003.

Roberts, J. T. *Fundamentals of Tracheal Intubation*. New York: Grune & Stratton, 1983.

Stewart, C. E. *Advanced Airway Management*. St. Louis: Quality Medical Publishing, 2002.

PERIODICALS

Bochicchio, G. V., et al. "Endotracheal intubation in the field does not improve outcome in trauma patients who present without an acutely lethal traumatic brain injury." *Journal of Trauma Injury, Infections and Critical Care* 54 (February 2003): 307–311.

Erhan, E., et al. "Tracheal intubation without muscle relaxants: Remifentanil or alfentanil in combination with propofol." *European Journal of Anaesthesiology* 20 (January 2003): 37–43.

Udobi, K. F., E. Childs, and K. Touijer. "Acute respiratory distress syndrome." *American Family Physician* 67 (January 2003): 315–322.

Van de Leur, J. P., J. H. Zwaveling, B. G. Loef, and C. P. Van der Schans. "Endotracheal suctioning versus minimally invasive airway suctioning in intubated patients: A prospective randomized controlled trial." *Intensive Care Medicine* 186 (February 8, 2003).

ORGANIZATIONS

American Society of Anesthesiologists. 520 N. Northwest Highway, Park Ridge, IL 60068-2573. (847) 825-5586. <http://www.asahq.org/>.

OTHER

"Endotracheal intubation." Health_encyclopedia. <http://www.austin360.com/search/healthfd/shared/health/adam/ency/article/003449.html>.

"Endotracheal intubation." PennHealth. <http://www.pennhealth.com/ency/article/003449.htm>.

"Intubation." Discovery_Health. <http://health.discovery.com/diseasesandcond/encyclopedia/1219.htmlgt;.

Monique Laberge, Ph.D.

KEY TERMS

Anesthesia—Loss of feeling or sensation. Anesthesia is administered during surgery by an anesthesiologist.

Edema—The presence of abnormally large amounts of fluid in the intercellular tissue spaces of the body.

Emphysema—A pathological accumulation of air in tissues or organs, especially in the lungs.

Endotracheal—Located inside the trachea.

Epiglottis—A cartilaginous lidlike appendage that closes the glottis while food or drink is passing through the pharynx.

Glottis—The vocal part of the larynx, consisting of the vocal cords and the opening between them.

Laryngoscope—An instrument used to examine the larynx.

Larynx—The voice box.

Pharynx—The cavity at the back of the mouth.

Pneumothorax—A collapse of the lung due to an abrupt change in the intrapleural pressure within the chest cavity.

Trachea—The windpipe; a tough, fibrocartilaginous tube passing from the larynx to the bronchi before the lungs.

Stethoscope—A rubber Y-shaped device used to listen to sounds produced by the human body.

Endovascular stent surgery

Definition

Endovascular stent surgery is a minimally invasive surgical procedure that uses advanced technology and instrumentation to treat such disorders of the circulatory system as blockage or damage to blood vessels caused by the build up of plaque (fatty deposits, calcium deposits, and scar tissue) in the arteries, a condition called atherosclerosis (hardening of the arteries). The surgeon may recommend the placement of an endovascular stent, a small wire-mesh tube that surgeons call a scaffold, in an affected artery. The procedure may be done in conjunction with cleaning or repairing the artery. The twofold procedure opens, enlarges, and supports artery walls for a long-lasting improvement in blood flow and a decrease in the risk of heart attack or stroke. In endovascular stent surgery (*endo*, within, and *vascular*, blood vessel), all of the work done by the surgeon is within the blood vessels themselves. Nearly all of the medium-sized and large blood vessels in the body's vascular system can be accessed from within the vessels. This fact has contributed to a rapid increase in the performance of endovascular stent surgery.

Purpose

The purpose of endovascular stent surgery is to improve or restore the flow of blood and oxygen throughout the body, a process called coronary revascularization. Endovascular stent surgery is used most often to correct the narrowing in medium-sized and large arteries blocked by plaque. Stents have been used in coronary arteries, the carotid arteries in the neck, and renal (kidney) or biliary (gall bladder) arteries. They are rarely used for smaller arteries in the legs, for example, or other smaller vessels in the body.

Endovascular stenting is also the newest treatment for such emergency vascular events, as abdominal or thoracic (related to chest and lung area) aortic aneurysms. Aortic aneurysms are life-threatening bulges in the walls of the aorta, the largest artery in the body, usually the result of progressive atherosclerosis.

Demographics

Candidates for endovascular stent surgery are patients with atheroslerosis who are at high risk for heart attack and stroke. Heart disease and stroke are the leading causes of death and disability in the United States for both men and women. People at greatest risk have high blood pressure and high cholesterol, and sometimes diabetes. Typically these people may also smoke, be overweight, and have close relatives with heart disease or coronary artery disease or who have had a stroke. More than 700,000 people per year have stent surgeries to clear obstructions in the coronary arteries. Abdominal aortic aneurysms are the 13th leading cause of death in the United States, occurring primarily in people over age 67. More than 190,000 aortic aneurysms are diagnosed each year; of these, 45,000 people have surgery. Although the use of stent grafting is increasing, most aneurysms are treated with conventional open surgery procedures.

Description

The conditions most often treated by endovascular stent surgery are: coronary artery disease; narrowing (stenosis) of the carotid artery in the neck, a risk factor for stroke; and aortic aneurysm.

• Coronary artery disease is a circulatory disorder resulting from plaque blockages in the arteries of the heart. The heart is a muscle that requires a constant flow of

blood and oxygen through its blood vessels so that it can perform the critical function of supplying the whole body with blood. When fatty deposits form in the heart's two main arteries, the arteries become narrowed and the flow of blood and oxygen is blocked. Blockages can cause pain in the chest (angina) and eventually, when the blood vessels are occluded (closed up), a heart attack.

• The carotid arteries in the neck carry blood and oxygen to the brain. When these major arteries are blocked by plaque, the narrowing can interrupt the flow of blood to the brain and cause a disabling stroke. A **carotid endarterectomy** is a surgical procedure performed on people with significant stenosis (50 to 70% narrowing); in this procedure, a surgeon removes the fatty deposits to correct the narrowing and allow blood and oxygen to flow freely to the brain. Although an effective surgical measure, it is a surgery that presents high risks to patients who are already greatly compromised. Endovascular stent surgery is a less invasive procedure, with fewer risks, and is sometimes the surgeon's choice to prevent stroke in certain high-risk patients.

• An aortic aneurysm, which is a life-threatening bulging of the aorta, can occur anywhere along this major artery, either in the abdomen (abdominal aortic aneurysm or AAA) or in the chest area (thoracic aneurysm). When the aorta is blocked by significant amounts of plaque, pressure may cause it to bulge like a balloon directly above or below the blockage, causing a weakening of the vessel wall. The aorta may eventually rupture, causing massive bleeding and death. Sometimes the aneurysm is diagnosed when the victim complains of pain; but there may also be no obvious symptoms. Sometimes the vessel ruptures, causing massive internal bleeding and eventual loss of consciousness, requiring **emergency surgery**. Endovascular stent surgery is the least invasive method of surgical intervention to repair an aneurysm.

Coronary artery disease and carotid stenosis can be treated in three ways: medically, which is the use of therapeutic drugs in combination with changes in diet and **exercise**; by such open surgery as the highly invasive coronary artery bypass surgery (CABG); or by such minimally invasive procedures as stent implantation, balloon **angioplasty**, and atherectomy or endarterectomy (the cutting of plaque from the inside of vessel walls). Sometimes combinations of these methods are used. The goal of all these procedures is to improve the flow of blood and oxygen throughout the body, reduce symptoms, and reduce the risk of heart attack or stroke.

Endovascular stent surgery was introduced in the 1980s to treat occlusive (blocking) coronary artery disease, without using open surgery. More recently, endovascular stent grafting, a variation of the procedure, is

466

also being used to repair life-threatening aortic aneurysms, which formerly could be treated only with open surgery. Because the incision for endovascular procedures is just large enough to allow passage of a small tube (catheter) into a blood vessel, the procedure does not disturb the patient's body processes as much as conventional **vascular surgery**. This advance in technique helps reduce the patient's stay in the hospital and makes recovery faster. At the same time, it satisfies a common goal of surgeons to use less invasive methods that offer patients the best result with the fewest risks.

An endovascular stent is a tiny wire mesh tube that can look like a cage or a coiled spring, depending on the manufacturer's design. The implantation of stents is performed through a tiny incision, using a catheter to deliver it to the site of treatment in a vessel. The stent provides a mechanical way to hold a blood vessel open and improve blood flow over the long term. Stents are sometimes implanted through the same incision after balloon angioplasty has been performed. Balloon angioplasty is another catheter-guided procedure that uses a balloon device to stretch the waxy plaque formation and open the vessel walls. Before stents were used, some patients undergoing angioplasty (in 5–10% of angioplasty procedures) suffered acute closure, which is the complete closing down of the treated artery either during or after the procedure. Stents reduce the likelihood of this medical emergency and the need for immediate cardiac surgery to correct it. Stents are implanted both to treat new blockages and to treat the repeat build-up of plaque after prior surgical treatment, a process called restenosis. Endovascular stent implantation has been shown to reduce the likelihood of restenosis. Some stents can deliver anti-plaque drugs to the area of blockage. These are called drug-eluting stents; they are aimed at preventing restenosis and eliminating the need for further surgeries.

Endovascular stent surgery is performed in a **cardiac catheterization** laboratory equipped with a fluoroscope, a special x-ray machine and an x-ray monitor that looks like a regular television screen. The patient will be placed on an x-ray table and covered with a sterile sheet. An area on the inside of the upper leg will be washed and treated with an antibacterial solution to prepare for the insertion of a catheter. The patient is given local anesthesia to numb the insertion site and will usually remain awake during the procedure. To implant stents in arteries, the stent is threaded through an incision in the groin up into the affected blood vessel on a catheter with a deflated balloon at its tip and inside the stent. The surgeon views the entire procedure with a fluoroscope. The surgeon guides the balloon catheter to the blocked area and inflates the balloon, causing the stent to expand and press against the vessel walls. The balloon is then deflat-

WHO PERFORMS THE PROCEDURE AND WHERE IS IT PERFORMED?

Endovascular stent surgery is performed by a vascular surgeon in a hospital or medical center cardiac catheterization laboratory.

ed and taken out of the vessel. The entire procedure takes from an hour to 90 minutes to complete. The stent remains in the vessel permanently to hold the vessel walls open and allow blood to pass freely as in a normally functioning healthy artery. Cells and tissue will begin to grow over the stent until its inner surface is covered. It then becomes a permanent part of the functioning artery.

Stent surgery for emergency treatment of aortic aneurysm is called endovascular stent grafting or endovascular repair. Candidates for this treatment have either aortic aneurysms or other abnormal conditions of the aorta, such as an **arteriovenous fistula** (abnormal communication between an artery and a vein) or other kinds of aortic blockage. Formerly these conditions were treated by highly invasive surgical procedures, with incisions that reached from the breastbone to the navel, to access the aorta, open it, and insert and attach a slender fabric-covered tube called a graft. During the less invasive endovascular stent surgery, a collapsed metal stent-graft (also called an endograft) is threaded through an artery beginning from a small incision in the groin and ending in the aorta. Threading is done through a tube-like delivery system lying in the vessel, which allows catheters and stents to move up and down during the procedure. A stent graft is similar to the stents used in coronary artery procedures, but has a ring of tiny hooks and barbs at each end that allow it to connect to the inner wall of the artery, replacing and repairing (grafting) the weakened area. The surgeon guides the stentgraft into the aneurysm by using fluoroscopic x-ray imaging. When the stent graft is in place, its outer sheath is withdrawn and the stent graft is expanded. It will anchor itself to the inside of the artery wall with the hooks and barbs on each end. Some stent-graft systems also use balloons to push the hooks into the vessel wall. Because the procedure is minimally invasive, patients recover quickly and are usually able to eat the same day, walk on the second day, and go home in two to three days after the surgery.

Diagnosis/Preparation

Often the first test done to diagnose coronary artery disease is an electrocardiogram, to show the heart's

QUESTIONS TO ASK
THE DOCTOR

- Why do I need this procedure?
- What kind of anesthesia will I have?
- Will I be uncomfortable during or after the procedure?
- Will I be able to resume all my normal activities when I go home?
- Will I need any follow-up care or tests after the surgery?
- How often do you perform this procedure?
- Is there any chance I would need this type of surgery again?
- What can I do after surgery to reduce my chances of having this condition again?

rhythm. A **stress test**, or exercise electrocardiogram, may be performed as well, though this test can be too strenuous for some patients. Cardiac catheterization is considered the most definitive test. It requires the injection of a special dye into the coronary arteries at the same time that a catheter is threaded up into the heart's arteries and x rays are displayed on a monitor to show any narrowing or blockage. To diagnose clogged arteries in other areas of the body, such imaging techniques, as computed tomography (CT) or **magnetic resonance imaging** (MRI) may be used to visualize the presence and extent of narrowing in the blood vessels. Diagnostic procedures for aneurysm may include these same imaging tests; but often, because of the emergency nature of aneurysm, there is little time to conduct extensive testing beyond immediate confirmation of the presence of the aneurysm.

For up to twelve hours before a stent procedure or combined angioplasty and stent surgery, the patient will have to avoid eating or drinking. An intravenous line will be inserted so that medications (anticoagulants to prevent clot formation and radioactive dye for x rays) can be administered during the surgery. The patient's groin area will be shaved and cleaned with an antiseptic to prepare for the incision. About an hour before the procedure, the patient may be given a mild sedative to ensure that he or she will relax sufficiently for the procedure.

Aftercare

After stent surgery, the patient will spend several hours in the **recovery room** to be monitored for **vital signs** (temperature, heart rate, and breathing) and heart sounds. Pressure will be applied to the catheter insertion site in the groin to prevent bleeding; a weight may be applied to the leg to restrict movement. For the first 24 hours, the patient will have to lie flat and limit activities. Drinking fluids will be especially important to help flush out the dye that was used for x rays during the procedure. Stent recipients are usually placed on **aspirin** therapy or anti-clotting (anticoagulant) medication immediately after surgery. They will remain on it indefinitely to prevent clots from occurring in the stent. There are no other postoperative precautions, although dietary and lifestyle changes may be recommended to reduce such risk factors as high cholesterol and smoking that could lead to new blockages from ongoing buildup of plaque in the body's blood vessels. Patients are advised not to have magnetic resonance imaging (MRI) procedures after the surgery because of the effect of magnetism on the metal stents. Stents are not affected by metal detectors.

Risks

The greatest risk with stent implantation is the formation of clots within the stent. Aspirin and oral anti-clotting medications are usually given after stent placement to minimize this risk, which has been reported to occur in about 1–1.5% of patients undergoing endovascular stent surgeries. There has been no evidence of long-term complications from stent implantation, according to the American Heart Association.

A variety of complications can occur with stent grafting for emergency aneurysm repair. Movement of the stent within the vessel can occur in up to 10% of cases, requiring repeat surgery. Clots can occur in the vessel and migrate to other areas of the body, causing heart attack or stroke. About 2% of patients will require an additional open surgical procedure to correct the aneurysm or complications that occur after emergency endovascular repair.

Normal results

People undergoing endovascular stent surgeries usually recover within a week or so, compared to months of recovery from conventional open surgery. They can quickly resume normal activities with a reduction of symptoms and little chance of repeat stenosis, depending upon their general health. The American Heart Association reports that 70–90% of procedures for coronary artery disease are endovascular stenting procedures. Stents have been shown to reduce the risk of restenosis after angioplasty or other catheter-based procedures have been performed.

Morbidity and mortality rates

Deaths have not been reported either during or immediately following endovascular stent surgeries that are linked to the surgical procedure. Stent procedures have been shown to increase survival (by reducing restenosis) among people with coronary artery disease.

The mortality rate for surgically treated abdominal aortic aneurysm is about 5% and increases to 50% for aneurysms that rupture. Thoracic aneurysms also have a mortality rate of about 5%, rising to 67% if ruptured. Stent grafting has been shown overall to have lower rates of morbidity and mortality than conventional open procedures.

Prevention

Preventive measures are the same to prevent heart attack and stroke. Any adult can reduce the likelihood of plaque formation by making such dietary and lifestyle changes, as:

• Eating healthy diet rich in fruits, vegetables, and whole grains, with limited meat and dairy products. Especially avoid trans-fatty-acids found in such chemical- or heat-extracted oils as margarine, some vegetable oils, and butter substitutes.

• Keeping blood pressure down by reducing the use of table salt and avoiding such salty foods, as chips, processed meats, pickles and sauerkraut, as well as prepared and packaged foods.

• Losing weight, if necessary, which helps to reduce blood pressure. Excess weight strains the whole circulatory system.

• Engaging in moderate exercise several times a week. Exercise that works up a sweat and increases heart rate is recommended. A brisk walk for 20 minutes on three days a week is thought to be sufficient for people who are less physically active.

• Controlling cholesterol through diet and certain medications.

• Having a heart examination at least once a year with an electrocardiogram. The patient should also consult the doctor about taking aspirin for clot prevention.

• Quitting smoking. Smoking encourages the build-up of plaque. Nicotine raises blood pressure, and carbon monoxide in smoke reduces the amount of oxygen circulating in the blood. Strong links have been made between smoking and heart attack or stroke.

• Keeping alcohol use moderate. Moderate alcohol use, one or two drinks a day, has been shown to help increase the levels of "good" cholesterol, improve circulation, and reduce the risk of clots forming in the blood.

Alternatives

Stent implantation helps to clear blocked arteries and keep them open mechanically. There are no mechanical

---

KEY TERMS

Aorta—The largest artery in the body, which passes through the abdomen and chest, supplying blood to the stomach and legs.

Aneurysm—A life-threatening enlargement or bulge in an artery caused by a weakening of the artery wall above or below an area of blockage.

Balloon angioplasty—X-ray-guided insertion of a balloon catheter into a blocked blood vessel to remove plaque and open the vessel for better blood flow.

Endovascular—Within the walls of a blood vessel.

Graft—Replacement of a diseased or damaged part of the body with a compatible substitute that can be artificial (metal or other substance) or taken from the body itself, such as a piece of skin, healthy tissue, or bone.

Revascularization—Restoring the body's blood flow after an interruption or blockage has disrupted normal circulation.

Rupture—The bursting of a blood vessel or organ that has suffered enlargement, bulging, and weakening from unusual pressure.

Stent—A specially designed wire-mesh device that is placed inside a blood vessel to open or support it.

Thoracic—Pertaining to the chest cavity, including the lungs and the area around the lungs.

Vascular—Pertaining to the blood vessels of the body that make up the circulatory system; veins and arteries.

---

alternatives however, to reduce plaque formation. Nutritional supplements and alternative therapies that have been recommended to help reduce risks and promote good vascular health include:

• Vitamins B_6 and B_{12} help to lower homocysteine, an amino acid that is believed to contribute to atherosclerosis. B_6 is also a mild diuretic and helps to balance fluids in the body.

• Folic acid helps lower homocysteine levels and increases the oxygen-carrying capacity of red blood cells.

• Antioxidant vitamins C and E work together to promote healthy blood vessels and improve circulation.

• Angelica, an herb that contains coumadin, a recognized anticoagulant, may help to prevent the formation of blood clots.

- Garlic has been shown in studies to reduce cholesterol and help prevent atherosclerosis.

- Essential fatty acids help reduce blood pressure and cholesterol, and maintain elasticity of blood vessels.

- Chelation therapy can be used to break up plaque and improve circulation.

- Citrin is an herbal extract that inhibits the synthesis of dangerous fats in the body.

- Certain herbs have been shown to improve circulation and help prevent plaque formation, including cayenne, chickweed, ginkgo biloba, and hawthorn berries.

- A vegetarian diet, with plenty of whole grains (brown rice, oats, spelt, whole wheat) showed a reversal of coronary artery disease in an American study called the Lifestyle Heart Trial.

Resources

BOOKS

Heart and Stroke Facts, and Stent Procedure. American Heart Association, 2002.

ORGANIZATIONS

American Heart Association. 7320 Greenville Ave. Dallas, TX 75231. (214) 373-6300. <http://www.americanheart.org>.

OTHER

"Angioplasty and Coronary Stent Implantation." Health Topics. Atlanta Health Pages [cited May 5, 2003]. <http://www.healthpages.org/AHP/LIBRARY/HLTHTOP/index.htm>.

Bellozo, J. "Endovascular Stent-Grafting Alternative to Traditional Abdominal Surgery." Scripps Health. Scripps Research Institute. August 12, 2002. [May 5, 2003]. <http://www.scripps.org>.

"Performing Endovascular Surgery:New Minimally Invasive Approach to Treating Vascular Disease." Patient Care. Department of Surgery, State University of New York, Stony Brook [cited May 5, 2003]. <http://galactica.informatics.sunysb.edu/surgery/endovasc-1.html>.

L. Lee Culvert

Enhanced external counterpulsation

Definition

Enhanced external counterpulsation (EECP) is a non-invasive procedure in which a set of inflatable cuffs (much like blood pressure cuffs) mechanically compress the blood vessels in the patient's lower limbs to increase blood flow in the coronary arteries of the heart. The blood pressure cuffs are wrapped around the patient's calves, thighs, and buttocks. Computer technology, **electrocardiography**, and blood pressure monitors enable the accurate timing of gentle but firm inflation and deflation of the pressure cuffs with the patient's heartbeat and blood pressure.

Purpose

EECP is performed to restore blood flow to the heart and to relieve chest pain (angina) and ischemia. The goals of the procedure are to relieve symptoms of coronary artery disease, enable the patient to resume a normal lifestyle, and lower the risk of a heart attack or other heart problems. EECP may encourage blood vessels to open small channels (called collaterals) to eventually bypass blocked vessels and improve blood flow to the heart.

Demographics

The concept of counterpulsation is not new (it was first introduced in the late 1950s at Harvard), but the computerized technology currently available with EECP makes it a relatively new procedure, introduced less than 10 years ago. As of 2003 it is available in only about 200 centers across the United States.

EECP is used to treat patients with chronic stable angina, coronary artery disease, or high blood pressure. Most recently, the Food and Drug Administration (FDA) has approved EECP for the treatment of congestive heart failure. The treatment may be appropriate for patients who are not eligible for such non-surgical interventional procedures as balloon **angioplasty**, stent placement, rotoblation, atherectomy, or brachytherapy. It may also be used for patients who do not qualify for such surgical treatment as **coronary artery bypass graft surgery**.

EECP is not the first-line treatment for angina. Rather, it is reserved for patients who have not achieved good results from medication or interventional management of their symptoms.

EECP may benefit patients with such other medical conditions as erectile dysfunction, kidney disease, eye disease, diabetic neuropathy, and other circulatory disorders. More research is needed to evaluate the outcomes of EECP for these patients.

Many insurance providers and **Medicare** have approved EECP treatment for reimbursement.

Contraindications

EECP is not recommended for patients who have certain types of valve disease; uncontrolled arrhythmias (irregular heart rhythms); severe hypertension; uncontrolled congestive heart failure; significant blockages or blood clots in the leg arteries; or those who have had a recent **cardiac catheterization**, angioplasty, or bypass surgery.

Description

While the patient lies on a bed, the leg cuffs are deflated and inflated with each heartbeat. A computer synchronizes the compression of the cuffs with the heartbeat. The electrocardiogram indicates when each heartbeat begins, triggering the cuffs to be mechanically deflated. As each heartbeat ends, the cuffs are mechanically inflated in sequential order, starting with the cuffs on the calves and working upward. The pressure produced by the inflation of the cuffs when the heart is at rest pushes the blood in the legs upward toward the heart. The deflating action that occurs just when the heart begins to beat reduces the work of the heart as it pumps blood to other parts of the body.

EECP treatments are performed on an outpatient basis and generally last one to two hours. Treatments must be repeated about five times a week for up to seven weeks to achieve improved circulation.

Diagnosis/Preparation

Preparation

The patient is usually instructed to wear tight-fitting, seamless cycling pants or athletic tights to prevent chafing, one of the main adverse side effects.

Before the procedure, the patient's weight, blood pressure, pulse, and breathing rate are measured and recorded. The patient's legs are examined for areas of redness and signs of potential vascular problems.

The patient is asked to record his or her symptoms during the course of treatment to determine if and how symptoms improve over time. The patient should record the severity and duration of troublesome symptoms, the time the symptoms occurred, and any activities that may have triggered the symptoms. This patient record is reviewed before each treatment session.

PATIENT EDUCATION. The health care team will ensure that the patient understands the potential benefits and risks of the procedure. Informative and instructional handouts are usually provided to explain the procedure. Because the procedure requires multiple outpatient visits (generally 35 visits over a seven-week period), the patient must be able to meet the treatment schedule.

INFORMED CONSENT. Informed consent is an educational process between health care providers and patients. Before any procedure is performed, the patient is asked to sign a consent form. Before signing the form, the patient should understand the nature and purpose of the diagnostic procedure or treatment; the risks and benefits of the procedure; and alternatives, including the option of not proceeding with the test or treatment. During the discussion about the procedure, the health

---

WHO PERFORMS THE PROCEDURE AND WHERE IS IT PERFORMED?

EECP is performed by health care providers trained in the procedure. Interventional cardiologists, registered nurses, and other health care professionals may perform the procedure. Currently, EECP credentialing is being investigated by the International EECP Therapists Association (IETA). EECP is generally performed in an outpatient clinic or hospital.

---

care providers are available to answer all of the patient's questions.

SMOKING CESSATION. Patients who will undergo any procedure to treat cardiovascular disease are encouraged to stop smoking and using any tobacco products before the procedure, and to make a commitment to be a nonsmoker after the procedure. There are several **smoking cessation** programs available in the community. The patient should ask a health care provider for more information if he or she needs help quitting smoking.

Aftercare

Discomfort

Patients report little or no discomfort during the procedure. Some people may feel tired after the first few treatments, but this loss of energy improves over time.

Lifestyle changes

To manage heart disease, the patient needs to make several lifestyle changes before and after the procedure, including:

- Quitting smoking. Smoking causes damage to blood vessels, increases the patient's blood pressure and heart rate, and decreases the amount of oxygen available in the blood.
- Managing weight. Maintaining a healthy weight, by watching portion sizes and exercising, is important. Being overweight increases the work of the heart.
- Participating in an **exercise** program. The cardiac rehabilitation exercise program is usually tailored for the patient, who will be supervised by professionals.
- Making dietary changes. Patients should eat a lot of fruits, vegetables, grains, and non-fat or low-fat dairy products, and reduce fats to less than 30% of all calories. Alcoholic beverages should be limited or avoided.

- Taking medications as prescribed. **Aspirin** and other heart medications may be prescribed, and the patient may need to take these medications for life.

- Following up with health care providers. The patient needs to visit the physician regularly to control risk factors.

Risks

EECP is a relatively safe and effective treatment, and few adverse side effects have been reported. The main adverse side effect is chafing (skin irritation from the compression of the cuffs). To reduce or prevent this side effect, patients are instructed to wear tight-fitting cycling pants or athletic tights. Leg pain is another adverse side effect.

Normal results

The benefits of EECP are comparable to the results of angioplasty and coronary artery bypass graft surgery: 80% of patients experience significant improvement after EECP treatment. The largest research study on EECP indicates that after receiving treatment, patients used less medication, had fewer angina attacks with less severe symptoms, and increased their capacity to exercise without experiencing symptoms. EECP improves the patient's sense of well-being and overall quality of life; and in some cases, prolongs the patient's life. Benefits five years after EECP treatment are comparable to surgical outcomes.

The effects of EECP treatment last from three to five years and sometimes longer.

EECP does not prevent coronary artery disease from recurring; therefore, lifestyle changes are strongly recommended and medications are prescribed to reduce the risk of recurrent disease.

Morbidity and mortality rates

Morbidity and mortality have not been reported with this procedure.

Alternatives

All patients with coronary artery disease can help improve their condition by making such lifestyle changes as quitting smoking, losing weight if they are overweight, eating healthful foods, reducing blood cholesterol, exercising regularly, and controlling diabetes and high blood pressure.

All patients with coronary artery disease should be prescribed medications to treat their condition. Such Antiplatelet medications as aspirin or clopidogrel (Plavix) are usually recommended. Other medications used to treat angina may include beta blockers, nitrates, and angiotensin-converting enzyme (ACE) inhibitors. Medications may also be prescribed to lower lipoprotein levels, since elevated lipoprotein levels have been associated with an increased risk of cardiovascular problems.

Treatment with vitamin E is not recommended because it does not lower the rate of cardiovascular events in people with coronary artery disease. Although such antioxidants as vitamin C, beta-carotene, and probucol show promising results, they are not recommended for routine use. Treatment with folic acid and vitamins B_6 and B_{12} lowers homocysteine levels (reducing the risk for cardiovascular problems), but more studies are needed to determine if lowered homocysteine levels correlate with a reduced rate of cardiovascular problems in treated patients.

KEY TERMS

Angina—Also called angina pectoris; chest pain or discomfort that occurs when diseased blood vessels restrict blood flow to the heart.

Aorta—The main artery that carries blood from the heart to the rest of the body; the largest artery in the body.

Artery—A vessel that carries oxygen-rich blood to the body.

Atherectomy—A nonsurgical technique for treating diseased arteries with a rotating device that cuts or shaves away obstructing material inside the artery.

Atria—The right and left upper chambers of the heart.

Balloon angioplasty—A nonsurgical technique for treating diseased arteries by temporarily inflating a tiny balloon inside an artery.

Beta blocker—An antihypertensive drug that limits the activity of epinephrine, a hormone that increases blood pressure.

Brachytherapy—The use of radiation during angioplasty to prevent the artery from narrowing again (a process called restenosis).

Calcium channel blocker—A drug that lowers blood pressure by regulating calcium-related electrical activity in the heart.

Cardiac catheterization—An invasive procedure used to create x rays of the coronary arteries, heart chambers and valves.

Coronary artery disease—Also called atherosclerosis, it is a buildup of fatty matter and debris in the coronary artery wall that causes narrowing of the artery.

Echocardiogram—An imaging procedure used to create a picture of the heart's movement, valves and chambers.

Electrocardiogram (ECG, EKG)—A test that records the electrical activity of the heart, using small electrode patches attached to the skin on the chest.

Ischemia—Decreased blood flow to an organ, usually caused by constriction or obstruction of an artery.

Rotoblation—A nonsurgical technique for treating diseased arteries in which a special catheter with a diamond-coated tip is guided to the point of narrowing in the artery. The catheter tip spins at high speeds and grinds away the blockage or plaque on the artery walls.

Stent—A device made of expandable metal mesh that is placed (by using a balloon catheter) at the site of a narrowing artery. The stent remains in place to keep the artery open.

Stress test—A test that determines how the heart responds to stress.

Vein—A blood vessel that returns oxygen-depleted blood from various parts of the body to the heart.

Ventricles—The lower pumping chambers of the heart that propel blood to the lungs and the rest of the body.

Such nonsurgical interventional procedures as balloon angioplasty, stent placement, rotoblation, atherectomy, or brachytherapy can be performed to open a blocked artery.

Coronary artery bypass graft surgery is a surgical procedure in which one or more blocked coronary arteries are bypassed by a blood vessel graft to restore normal blood flow to the heart. These grafts usually come from the patient's own arteries and veins located in the leg, arm, or chest.

Resources

BOOKS

McGoon, Michael D., ed., and Bernard J. Gersh. *Mayo Clinic Heart Book: The Ultimate Guide to Heart Health,* Second Edition. New York: William Morrow and Co., Inc., 2000.

Topol, Eric J. *Cleveland Clinic Heart Book: The Definitive Guide for the Entire Family from the Nation's Leading Heart Center.* New York: Hyperion, 2000.

Trout, Darrell, and Ellen Welch. "Enhanced External Counterpulsation (EECP)." In *Surviving with Heart: Taking Charge of Your Heart Care.* Golden, CO: Fulcrum Publishing, 2002.

PERIODICALS

Arora, R. R., et al. "The Multicenter Study of Enhanced External Counterpulsation (MUST-EECP): Effect of EECP on Exercise-Induced Myocardial Ischemia and Anginal Episodes." *The Journal of the American College of Cardiology* 33(7) 1999: 1833–1840.

Lawson, W. E., J. C. Hui, and P. F. Cohn. "Long-Term Prognosis of Patients with Angina Treated with Enhanced External Counterpulsation: Five-year Follow-Up Study." *Clinical Cardiology* 23(4) 2000: 254–258.

Soran, O. Z., et al. "Enhanced External Counterpulsation in the Management of Patients with Cardiovascular Disease." *Clinical Cardiology* 22 (1999): 173–178.

Urano, H., et al. "Enhanced External Counterpulsation Improves Exercise Tolerance, Reduces Exercise-Induced Myocardial Ischemia and Improves Left Ventricular Diastolic Filling in Patients with Coronary Artery Disease." *Journal of the American College of Cardiology* 37, no. 1 (2001): 93–99.

ORGANIZATIONS

American College of Cardiology. Heart House. 9111 Old Georgetown Rd., Bethesda, MD 20814-1699. (800) 253-4636, ext. 694, or (301) 897-5400. <http://www.acc.org>.

American Heart Association. 7272 Greenville Ave., Dallas, TX 75231. (800) 242-8721 or (214) 373-6300. <http://www.americanheart.org>.

Cleveland Clinic Heart Center. The Cleveland Clinic Foundation. 9500 Euclid Avenue, F25, Cleveland, Ohio, 44195. (800) 223-2273, ext. 46697, or (216) 444-6697. <http://www.clevelandclinic.org/heartcenter>.

International EECP Therapists Association. P.O. Box 650005, Vero Beach, FL 32965-0005. (800) 376-3321, ext. 140. <http://www.ietaonline.com>.

National Heart, Lung and Blood Institute. National Institutes of Health. Building 1. 1 Center Dr., Bethesda, MD 20892. E-mail: <NHLBIinfo@rover.nhlbi.>. <http://www.nhlbi.nih.gov>.

Texas Heart Institute. Heart Information Service. P.O. Box 20345, Houston, TX 77225-0345. <http://www.tmc.edu/thi>.

OTHER

Cardiac Renewal Centers of America. (800) LONG-LIFE. <http://www.cardiacrenewal.com/>.

HeartCenterOnline. <http://www.heartcenteronline.com>.

The Heart: An Online Exploration. Franklin Institute Science Museum. 222 North 20th Street, Philadelphia, PA, 19103. (215) 448-1200. <http://sln2.fi.edu/biosci/heart.html>.

Heart Information Network. <http://www.heartinfo.org>.

EECP.Com. Sponsored by Vasomedical, Inc.

VIDEOS

Straight to the Heart: The EECP Treatment Option for Angina. Featuring Larry King. Spotlight Health, Inc., 2001. <http://www.eecp.com/tr/larry.htm>.

Angela M. Costello

Enucleation, eye

Definition

Enucleation is the surgical removal of the eyeball that leaves the eye muscles and remaining orbital contents intact.

Purpose

Enucleation is performed to remove large-sized eye tumors or as a result of traumatic injury when the eye cannot be preserved. In the case of tumors, the amount of radiation required to destroy a tumor of the eye may be too intense for the eye to bear. Within months to years, many patients who are treated with radiation for large ocular melanomas lose vision, develop glaucoma, and eventually have to undergo enucleation.

The two types of eye tumors that may require enucleation are:

• Intraocular eye melanoma. This is a rare form of cancer in which malignant cells are found in the part of the eye called the uvea, which contains cells called melanocytes that house pigments. When the melanocytes become cancerous, the cancer is called a melanoma. If the tumor reaches the iris and begins to grow, or if there are symptoms, enucleation may be indicated.

• Retinoblastoma. Retinoblastoma is a malignant tumor of the retina. The retina is the thin layer of tissue that lines the back of the eye; it senses light and forms images. If the cancer occurs in one eye, treatment may consist of enucleation for large tumors when there is no expectation that useful vision can be preserved. If there is cancer in both eyes, treatment may involve enucleation of the eye with the larger tumor, and radiation therapy for the other eye.

WHO PERFORMS THE PROCEDURE AND WHERE IS IT PERFORMED?

Eye enucleation is usually performed by an ophthalmic surgeon or an ophthalmologist in a hospital setting. Young and healthy patients may undergo the surgery on an outpatient basis but most stay in the hospital for at least one night after surgery. Ophthalmic surgeons are members of the American College of Eye Surgeons, and are certified by the American Board of Eye Surgery after submitting to an extensive written application. Before ABES certification, they must be certified by the American Board of Ophthalmology (ABO). This certification indicates successful completion of an approved residency program and acquisition of sufficient knowledge in the areas of medical and surgical ophthalmology.

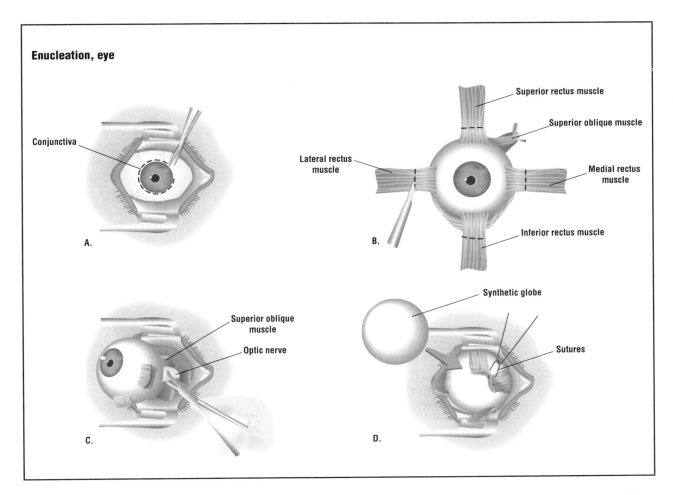

Enucleation, eye

Conjunctiva

A.

Superior rectus muscle

Superior oblique muscle

Lateral rectus muscle

Medial rectus muscle

Inferior rectus muscle

B.

Superior oblique muscle

Optic nerve

C.

Synthetic globe

Sutures

D.

The conjunctiva (outer covering of eye) is removed with blunt scissors (A). The four rectus muscles are removed from their attachments to the eyeball (B). The optic nerve is severed (C), and the eyeball is removed. A synthetic globe replaces the eyeball in the socket, and the rectus muscles are sutured around it (D). *(Illustration by GGS Inc.)*

Demographics

Data from the U.S. National Center for Health Statistics estimate that nearly 2.4 million eye injuries occur in the United States annually. This report calculated that nearly one million Americans have permanent significant visual impairment due to injury, with more than 75% of these individuals being blind in one eye. Eye injury is a leading cause of monocular blindness in the United States, and is second only to cataract as the most common cause of visual impairment. While no segment of the population escapes the risk of eye injury, the victims are more likely to be young. The majority of all eye injuries occur in persons under thirty years of age. Trauma is considered the most common cause of enucleation in children over three years of age.

For the year 2000, Texas demographics for cancer of the eye and orbit were fewer than five per 100,000.

According to the Nilt, there are about 2,200 cases of eye cancer diagnosed in the United States each year.

Description

Following anesthesia, the surgeon measures the dimensions of the eye globe, length of the optic nerve, and horizontal dimensions of the cornea. The surgeon then illuminates the globe of the eye before opening it. A dissecting microscope is used to detect major features and possible minute lesions. The eye is opened with a sharp razor blade by holding the globe with the left hand, cornea down against the cutting block, and holding the blade between the thumb and middle finger of the right hand. Enucleation proceeds with a sawing motion from back to front. The plane of section begins adjacent to the optic nerve and ends at the periphery of the cornea. The plane of section is dependent on whether a lesion has been detected. If not, the globe is cut along a horizontal plane, using as surface landmarks the superior and inferior oblique insertions and the long postciliary vein. If a lesion has been found, the plane of section is modified so that the lesion is included in the slab.

Diagnosis/Preparation

Enucleation may be performed under general or local anesthesia. In either case, the injection is given in the retrobulbar space. An antibiotic and an anti-inflammatory medication such as dexamethasone are also given intravenously.

Aftercare

Because the eye is surrounded by bones, it is much easier for patients to tolerate enucleation than the loss of a lung or kidney. When surgery is performed under general anesthesia, patients do not feel or see anything until they regain consciousness. Additional local anesthesia is often given at the end of the surgery so that the patient will have the least pain possible when waking up in the **recovery room**. Most patients have a headache for 24–36 hours after surgery that is relieved with two regular headache medication pills, such as Tylenol, every four hours. A firm pressure dressing is maintained for four to six days, such oral **antibiotics** are given for one week; and steroids, as prednisone, adjusted according to patient status, are given three times daily for four days. The socket is evaluated after removal of the pressure dressing. If the edema has disappeared, the sutures are removed. Topical antibiotics are applied four times daily for four weeks.

Risks

Enucleation surgery is very safe; only rarely do patients experience major complications. Complications include the following: bleeding, infection, scarring, persistent swelling, pain, wound separation, and the need for additional surgery. Complications may also occur with the orbital implants routinely used with patients who have undergone enucleation. Among these is the risk of infection.

Normal results

Within two to six weeks of enucleation surgery, patients are sent for a temporary ocular prosthesis (plastic eye). Besides the swelling and the black eye, patient features look normal. After a final prosthetic fitting, 90% of patients are usually quite happy with the way they look; 80% say others cannot even tell that they have only one eye.

Morbidity and mortality rates

In a study performed by the National Eye Institute on melanoma patients, at five-year follow-up, 82% of the patients who underwent enucleation remained alive. At a 10-year follow-up, 31% remained alive. As of 2003, the study is still ongoing and will follow all patients for up to 15 years.

Alternatives

There are no alternatives to enucleation because it is a procedure of last resort performed when other treatments have failed.

Resources

BOOKS

Linberg, J. W. *Oculoplastic and Orbital Emergencies.* New York: McGraw-Hill Professional, 1992.

Shields, J. A., and C. L. Shields. *Atlas of Orbital Tumors.* Philadelphia: Lippincott Williams & Wilkins, 1999.

Tasman, W., et al. *The Wills Eye Hospital Atlas of Clinical Ophthalmology.* Philadelphia: Lippincott Williams & Wilkins, 2001.

Vafidis, G. et al. *Perioperative Care of the Eye Patient.* Annapolis Junction, MD: BMJ Books, 2000.

PERIODICALS

Adenis, J. P., P. Y. Robert, and M. P. Boncoeur-Martel. "Abnormalities of orbital volume." *European Journal of Ophthalmology* 12 (September-October 2002): 345–350.

Burroughs, J. R., C. N. Soparkar, J. R. Patrinely, et al. "Monitored anesthesia care for enucleations and eviscerations." *Ophthalmology* 110 (February 2003): 311–313.

Chantada, G., A. Fandino, S. Casak, et al. "Treatment of overt extraocular retinoblastoma." *Medical Pediatric Oncology* 40 (March 2003): 158–161.

Gragoudas, E., W. Li, M. Goitein, et al. "Evidence-based estimates of outcome in patients irradiated for intraocular melanoma." *Archives of Ophthalmology* 120 (December 2002): 1665–1671.

KEY TERMS

Cornea—The transparent structure forming the anterior part of the fibrous tunic of the eye. It consists of five layers.

Glaucoma—A group of eye diseases characterized by an increase in intraocular pressure that causes changes in the optic disk and defects in the field of vision.

Intraocular melanoma—A rare form of cancer in which malignant cells are found in the part of the eye called the uvea.

Iris—The contractile eye membrane perforated by the pupil, and forming the colored portion of the eye.

Melanocytes—Color-containing cells in the uvea.

Melanoma—A malignant tumor arising from the melanocytic system of the skin and other organs.

Optic nerve—The nerve carrying impulses for the sense of sight.

Orbit—The cavity or socket of the skull in which the eye and its appendages are situated.

Retina—Thin nerve tissue that lines the back of the eye that senses light and forms images.

Retinoblastoma—Malignant (cancerous) tumor of the retina.

Jordan, D. R., S. R. Klapper, and S. M. Gilberg. "The use of vicryl mesh in 200 porous orbital implants: a technique with few exposures." *Ophthalmologic and Plastic Reconstruction Surgery* 19 (January 2003): 53–61.

ORGANIZATIONS

American Academy of Ophthalmology. P.O. Box 7424, San Francisco, CA 94120-7424. (415) 561-8500. <http://www.aao.org/index.html>.

American College of Eye Surgeons. 2665 Oak Ridge Court, Suite A, Fort Myers, FL 33901. (239) 275-8881. <http://www.aces-abes.org/>.

National Cancer Institute. Suite 3036A, 6116 Executive Boulevard, MSC8322, Bethesda, MD 20892-8322.(800) 422-6237. <http://cancer.gov/>.

OTHER

Finger, Paul T., MD, FACS. "Enucleation." Eye Cancer Network. [cited May 5, 2003]. <http://www.eyecancer.com/Enucleation/enuc.html>.

Monique Laberge, Ph.D.

Enzyme immmunoassay *see* **Immunoassay tests**

Epidural therapy

Definition

An epidural is a local (regional) anesthetic delivered through a catheter (small tube) into a vacant space outside the spinal cord called the epidural space.

The drugs commonly used in epidural anesthesia are bupivicaine (Marcaine, Sensorcaine); chloroprocaine (Nesacaine); and lidocaine (Xylocaine). The solutions of anesthetic should be preservative-free.

Purpose

The anesthetic agents that are infused through the small catheter block spinal nerve roots in the epidural space and the sympathetic nerve fibers adjacent to them. Epidural anesthesia can block most of the pain of labor and birth for vaginal and surgical deliveries. Epidural analgesia is also used after cesarean sections to help control postoperative pain.

Precautions

The primary problem associated with receiving epidural anesthesia is low blood pressure, otherwise known as hypotension, because of the blocking of sympathetic fibers in the epidural space. The decreased peripheral resistance that results in the circulatory system causes dilation of peripheral blood vessels. Fluid collects in the peripheral vasculature (vessels), simulating a condition that the body interprets as low fluid volume. A simple measure that prevents most hypotension is the infusion of 500–1000 cc of fluid intravenously into the patient prior to the procedure. Ringer's lactate is preferable to a solution containing dextrose, because the elevated maternal glucose that accompanies the rapid infusion of solutions containing dextrose can result in hyperglycemia in the newborn with rebound hypoglycemia.

It is important not to place a woman flat on her back after she has an epidural because the supine position can bring on hypotension. If a woman's blood pressure does drop, then the proper treatment is to turn her on her side, administer oxygen, increase the flow of intravenous fluids, and possibly administer ephedrine if the hypotension is severe. Very rarely, convulsions can result from severe

Epidural anesthesia may be administered to a woman in labor to ease the pain of labor and birth. *(M. English, MD/Custom Medical Stock Photo. Reproduced by permission.)*

reactions. Seizure activity would be treated with short-acting **barbiturates** or diazepam (Valium).

Description

Epidural anesthesia, because it virtually blocks all pain of labor and birth, is particularly helpful to women with such underlying medical problems as pregnancy-induced hypertension, heart disease, and pulmonary disease. Epidural anesthesia for labor is usually initiated at the woman's request, provided that the labor is progressing well, or if the mother feels severe pain during early labor.

Diagnosis/Preparation

To prepare for the administration of epidural anesthesia, the woman should have the procedure explained fully and sign consent forms if required. An intravenous line is inserted, if not already in place. She is positioned on her side or in a sitting position and connected to a blood pressure monitoring device. The nurse/assistant has the following equipment available: oxygen, epidural insertion equipment, fetal monitor, and additional intravenous fluid.

The health-care provider cleans the area with an antiseptic solution, injects a local anesthetic to create a small wheal at the L 3–4 area (between the third and fourth lumbar vertebrae), and inserts a needle into the epidural space. Once it is ascertained that the needle is in

the correct place, a polyethylene catheter is threaded through the needle. The needle is removed and a test dose of the anesthetic agent is administered. The catheter is taped in place along the patient's back with the end over her shoulder for easy retrieval when further doses are required.

If the patient responds well to the test dose, a complete dose is administered. Pain relief should come up to the level of the umbilicus. The epidural anesthesia lasts approximately 40 minutes to two hours, or longer as required. If necessary, additional doses of anesthetic, or top-up, are injected through the catheter or by continuous infusion on a special pump.

Epidural anesthesia can be given in labor in a "segmented" manner. In this instance, the laboring woman receives a small dose of anesthesia so that the perineal muscles do not fully relax. The baby's head is more apt to undergo internal rotation when the perineal muscles are not too loose, thus facilitating delivery. At the time of delivery, an additional dose can be administered for perineal relief.

Women who have cesarean deliveries may have additional medication injected into the epidural space to control intra-operative pain. Medications generally used are such narcotics as fentanyl or morphine (Duramorph). Side effects include severe itching, nausea, and vomiting. Treatment of these side effects with the appropriate medication can be helpful. Despite these problems, epidural analgesia is an effective method to relieve pain after cesarean delivery, allowing the woman to move easily and speed recovery.

Local anesthetics are generally safe when administered by the epidural route. There is a low frequency of allergic reaction to the drug. Most often the drug causes a mild skin reaction, but in more severe cases can cause breathing difficulty and an asthma-like reaction. A burning sensation at the site of injection may occur, sometimes with swelling and skin irritation. Other adverse reactions may occur if the epidural anesthetic is not properly administered.

Aftercare

It is important to carefully monitor **vital signs** after the administration of epidural anesthesia. Hypotension can result in fetal death and can also have grave consequences for the mother. The nurse should monitor the patient constantly and use a continuous blood pressure machine to obtain regular blood pressure readings for 20–30 minutes after each administration of anesthesia. The systolic blood pressure should not fall below 100 mm Hg or be 20 mm Hg less than a baseline systolic blood pressure for a hypertensive patient.

It is important to remind the woman to empty her bladder at least every two hours. With epidural anesthesia, there is loss of sensation of the need to void. Sometimes, an overfull bladder can block the descent of the baby's head. A catheter can be inserted into the bladder to drain the urine. The nurse needs to closely monitor intake and output and assess the bladder for signs of distension.

Risks

Side effects and complications are rare, but sometimes the patient will experience a "spinal headache" due to leakage of cerebrospinal fluid (CSF).

When a woman receives epidural anesthesia for labor pains, at times the labor can be prolonged because of excessive relaxation of the muscles. Also, the baby's head may not rotate—especially if it is in the occiput-posterior position (the back of the head is facing toward the woman's back). The woman may not have the sensation that results in the desire to push during contractions when she is fully dilated. These complications may result in an increased incidence of births with the use of vacuum extraction, forceps, or even cesarean deliveries. Administering a Pitocin (oxytocin) drip intravenously can counter this problem. Pitocin is a medication that causes the uterus to contract. Allowing the epidural to wear off in the second stage of labor when the woman is pushing may avoid this problem, but the return of the labor pains may be overwhelming to the woman.

Occasionally, slow absorption of the medication from the epidural space into the circulation can result in toxic reactions evident by decreased level of consciousness, slurred speech, loss of coordination, drowsiness, nervousness, and anxiety. The health-care provider should look out for these signs, and also report any elevation in temperature before a top-up dose is administered.

Normal results

Epidural anesthesia is a safe and effective method of giving pain relief to women during labor and delivery. It also can be used for cesarean births. It is believed that very little of the anesthetic is absorbed throughout the body (systemically), therefore epidural anesthesia is ideal because it does not pass the medication into the baby's circulation.

Resources

BOOKS

Pillitteri, Adele. *Maternal & Child Health Nursing,* 3rd edition. Philadelphia: Lippincott, 1999.

KEY TERMS

Analgesia—A medication that decreases the awareness of pain.

Anesthesia—Loss of sensation through the administration of substances that block the transmission of nerve impulses related to sensations of pain and pressure.

Regional anesthesia—Blocking of specific nerve pathways through the injection of an anesthetic agent into a specific area of the body.

ORGANIZATIONS

American Association of Nurse Anesthetists (AANA). 222 S. Prospect Avenue, Park Ridge, IL 60068. (847) 692-7050. <http://www.aana.com>.

OTHER

Anesthesia Options for Labor and Delivery: What Every Expectant Mother Should Know. AANA, 2001. <http://www.aana.com/patients/options.asp>.

Nadine M. Jacobson, RN
Samuel D. Uretsky, PharmD

Epilepsy surgery *see* **Anterior temporal lobectomy; Corpus callosotomy; Hemispherectomy**
Epinephrine *see* **Adrenergic drugs**

Episiotomy

Definition

An episiotomy is a surgical incision made in the perineum, the area between the vagina and anus. Episiotomies are done during the second stage of labor to expand the opening of the vagina to prevent tearing of the area during the delivery of the baby.

Purpose

An episiotomy is usually done during the birthing process in order to deliver a baby without tearing the perineum and surrounding tissue. Reasons for an episiotomy include:

- Evidence of maternal or fetal distress (i.e. no time to allow perineum to stretch).

- The baby is premature or in breech position, and his/her head could be damaged by a tight perineum.

- The baby is too large to be delivered without causing extensive tearing.

- The delivery is being assisted by forceps.

- The mother is too tired or unable to push.

- Existing trauma to the perineum.

Some experts believe that an episiotomy speeds up the birthing process, making it easier for the baby to be delivered. Speed can be important if there is any sign of distress that may harm the mother or baby. Because tissues in this area may tear during the delivery, another reason for performing an episiotomy is that a clean incision is easier to repair than a jagged tear and may heal faster. Although episiotomies are sometimes described as protecting the pelvic muscles and possibly preventing future problems with urinary incontinence, it is not clear that the procedure actually helps.

Demographics

In 2000, one study calculated the percentage of episiotomies performed in the United States out of all vaginal deliveries to be 19.4%. This was a dramatic reduction from the 1983 rate of 69.4%. Episiotomy rates were higher among white women (32.1%) than African American women (11.2%). Similar differences have been reported in other obstetric procedures (e.g. **cesarean section** and epidural use).

Episiotomy rates differ according to care provider—patients of midwives have lower rates than patients of medical doctors. One study comparing perineal outcomes for women being cared for by midwives or medical doctors found the episiotomy rate among midwives at 25% and 40% among medical doctors. Younger doctors are also less likely to perform an episiotomy than older doctors; one study found the rate of episiotomies performed by residents to be 17%, while the rate among doctors in private practice was 66%.

Description

An episiotomy is a surgical incision, usually made with sterile scissors, in the perineum as the baby's head is being delivered. This procedure may be used if the tissue around the vaginal opening begins to tear or does not seem to be stretching enough to allow the baby to be delivered.

In most cases, the physician makes a midline incision along a straight line from the lowest edge of the vaginal opening toward the anus. In other cases, the episiotomy is performed by making a diagonal incision across the midline between the vagina and anus (called a mediolateral incision). This method is used much less often, may be more painful, and may require more healing time than the midline incision. After the baby is delivered through the extended vaginal opening, the incision is closed with stitches. A local anesthetic may be applied or injected to numb the area before it is sewn up (sutured).

Episiotomies are classified according to the depth of the incision:

- A first-degree episiotomy cuts through skin only (vaginal/perineal).

- A second-degree episiotomy involves skin and muscle and extends midway between the vagina and the anus.

- A third-degree episiotomy cuts through skin, muscle, and the rectal sphincter.

Episiotomy

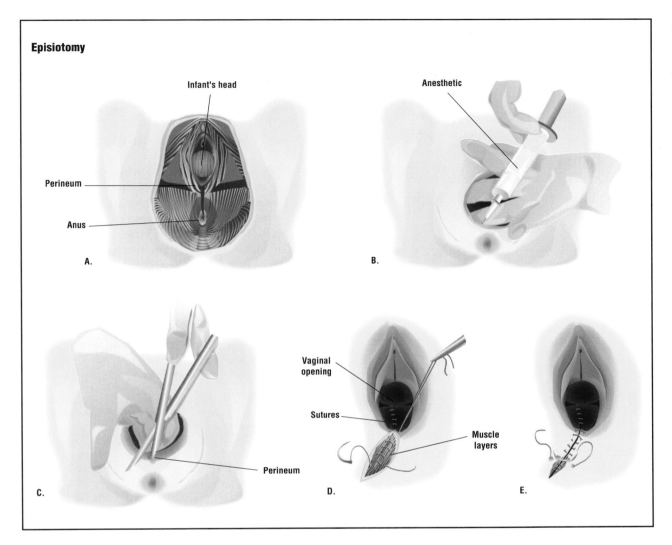

A. — Infant's head — Perineum — Anus

B. — Anesthetic

C. — Perineum

D. — Vaginal opening — Sutures — Muscle layers

E.

During childbirth, the area called the perineum is often cut to facilitate delivery (A). First, a local anesthetic may be given (B). The perineum is cut on an angle with scissors (C). After delivery, the layers of muscle and skin are repaired (D and E). *(Illustration by GGS Inc.)*

• A fourth-degree episiotomy extends through the rectum and cuts through skin, muscle, the rectal sphincter, and anal wall.

Diagnosis/Preparation

Although there are some reasons for anticipating an episiotomy before labor has begun (e.g. breech presentation of the baby), the decision to perform an episiotomy is generally not made until the second stage of labor, when delivery of the baby is imminent.

Aftercare

The area of the episiotomy may be uncomfortable or even painful for several days. Several practices can re-

lieve some of the pain. Cold packs can be applied to the perineal area to reduce swelling and discomfort. Use of a sitz bath can ease the discomfort. This unit circulates warm water over the area. A squirt bottle with water can be used to clean the area after urination or defecation rather than wiping with tissue. Also, the area should be patted dry rather than wiped. Cleansing pads soaked in witch hazel (such as the brand Tucks) are very effective for soothing and cleaning the perineum.

Risks

Several side effects of episiotomy have been reported, including infection (in 0.3% of cases), increased pain, increased bleeding, prolonged healing time, and in-

KEY TERMS

Kegel exercises—A series of contractions and relaxations of the muscles in the perineal area. These exercises are thought to strengthen the pelvic floor and may help prevent urinary incontinence in women.

Perineum—The area between the opening of the vagina and the anus in a woman, or the area between the scrotum and the anus in a man.

Sitz bath—A shallow tub or bowl, sometimes mounted above a toilet, that allows the perineum and buttocks to be immersed in circulating water.

Urinary incontinence—Inability to prevent the leakage or discharge of urine. It becomes more common as people age, and is more common in women who have given birth to more than one child.

creased discomfort once sexual intercourse is resumed. There is also the risk that the incision will be deeper or longer than is necessary to permit the birth of the infant. An incision that is too long or deep may extend into the rectum, causing more bleeding and an increased risk of infection. Additional tearing or tissue damage may occur beyond the episiotomy itself.

Normal results

In a normal and well-managed delivery, an episiotomy may be avoided altogether. If an episiotomy is considered necessary, a simple midline incision will be made to extend the vaginal opening without additional tearing or extensive trauma to the perineal area. Although there may be some pain associated with the healing of the incision, relief can usually be provided with mild pain relievers and supportive measures, such as the application of cold packs.

Morbidity and mortality rates

Studies have found that the rates of urinary/fecal incontinence, postpartum perineal pain, and sexual dysfunction are generally the same between women who have had an episiotomy and those who had a spontaneous tear of the perineum. There does appear to be a higher risk of more extensive perineal trauma when an episiotomy is performed (20.9% experienced third- or fourth-degree lacerations) then when it is not (3.1% experienced major perineal damage).

Alternatives

It may be possible to avoid the need for an episiotomy. Pregnant women may want to talk with their care providers about the use of episiotomy during the delivery. Kegel exercises are often recommended during the pregnancy to help strengthen the pelvic floor muscles. Prenatal perineal massage may help to stretch and relax the tissue around the vaginal opening. During the delivery process, warm compresses can be applied to the area along with the use of perineal massage. Coaching and support are also important during the delivery process. Slowed, spontaneous pushing during the second stage of labor (when the mother gets the urge to push) may allow the tissues to stretch rather than tear. Also, an upright birthing position (rather than one where the mother is lying down) may decrease the need for an episiotomy.

Resources

BOOKS

Enkin, Murray, Marc Keirse, James Neilson, et al. *A guide to effective care in pregnancy and childbirth.* Third edition. Oxford: Oxford University Press, 2000.

PERIODICALS

Carroli, G., and J. Belizan. "Episiotomy for vaginal birth." *The Cochrane Library* (2000).

Goldberg, Jay, David Holtz, Terry Hyslop, and Jorge Tolosa. "Has the Use of Routine Episiotomy Decreased? Examination of Episiotomy Rates From 1983 to 2000." *Obstetrics and Gynecology* 99 (March 2002): 395–400.

Kane-Low, Lisa, Julia Seng, Terri Murtland, and Deborah Oakley. "Clinician-specific episiotomy rates: Impact on perineal outcomes." *Journal of Midwifery and Women's Health* 45 (March 2000): 87–93.

Klein, M. C., R. J. Gauthier, J. Kaczorowski, et al. "Relationship of Episiotomy to Perineal Trauma and Morbidity, Sexual Dysfunction, and Pelvic Floor Relaxation." *American Journal of Obstetrics and Gynecology* 171 (1994): 591–8.

McCandlish, Rona. "Perineal Trauma: Prevention and Treatment." *Journal of Midwifery and Women's Health* 46 (November 2001): 396–401.

Roberts, Joyce E. "The 'Push' for Evidence: Management of the Second Stage." *Journal of Midwifery and Women's Health* 47 (January 2002): 2–15.

Yokoe, Deborah, Cindy Christiansen, Ruth Johnson, et al. "Epidemiology of and Surveillance for Postpartum Infections." *Emerging Infectious Diseases* 7 (2001).

ORGANIZATIONS

American College of Nurse-Midwives. 818 Connecticut Ave., NW, Suite 900, Washington, DC 20006. (202) 728-9860. <http://www.midwife.org>.

American College of Obstetricians and Gynecologists. 409 12th St., SW, PO Box 96920, Washington, DC 20090-6920. <http://www.acog.org>.

Midwives Alliance of North America. 4805 Lawrenceville Highway, Suite 116-279, Lilburn, GA 30047. (888) 923-MANA. <http://www.mana.org>.

OTHER

"Episiotomy FAQ Sheet." Perinatal Education Associates, Inc. 2002 [cited February 25, 2003]. <http://www.birthsource.com/proarticlefile/proarticle98.html>.

Marcus, Adam. "Episiotomy Rates Dropping in U.S." Healthfinder. May 7, 2002 [cited February 25, 2003]. <http://www.healthfinder.gov/news/newsstory.asp?docID=507067>.

Altha Roberts Edgren
Stephanie Dionne Sherk

EPS *see* **Electrophysiology study of the heart**
ERCP *see* **Endoscopic retrograde cholangiopancreatography**

Erythromycins

Definition

Erythromycins are medicines that kill bacteria or prevent their growth.

Purpose

Erythromycins are **antibiotics**, medicines used to treat infections caused by microorganisms. Physicians prescribe these drugs for many types of infections caused by bacteria, including strep throat, sinus infections, pneumonia, ear infections, tonsillitis, bronchitis, gonorrhea, pelvic inflammatory disease (PID), and urinary tract infections. Some medicines in this group are also used to treat Legionnaires' disease and ulcers caused by bacteria. These drugs will not work for colds, flu, and other infections caused by viruses.

Drugs in the erythromycin group may be used to eliminate such areas of infection as abscesses prior to surgery. For this purpose, they have been used in dentistry, eye surgery, and intestinal surgery. In some cases, erythromycin has been used to treat brain abscesses.

Description

The drugs described here include erythromycins (Erythrocin, Ery-C, E-Mycin, and other brands) and such medicines that are chemically related to erythromycins as azithromycin (Zithromax) and clarithromycin (Biax-

in). They are available only with a physician's prescription and are sold in capsule, tablet (regular and chewable), liquid, and injectable forms.

Recommended dosage

The recommended dosage depends on the type of erythromycin, the strength of the medicine, and the medical problem for which it is being taken. The person should check with the physician who prescribed the drug or the pharmacist who filled the prescription for the correct dosage.

The patient must always take erythromycins exactly as directed. The patient should never take larger, smaller, more frequent, or less frequent doses. To make sure the infection clears up completely, it is very important to take the medicine for as long as it has been prescribed. Patients must not stop taking the drug just because symptoms begin to improve. This is important with all types of infections, but it is especially important in streptococcal infections, which can lead to serious heart problems if they are not cleared up completely.

Erythromycins work best when they are at constant levels in the blood. To help keep levels constant, the medicine should be taken in doses spaced evenly through the day and night. The patient must not miss any doses. Some of these medicines are most effective when taken with a full glass of water on an empty stomach, but they may be taken with food if stomach upset is a problem. Others work equally well when taken with or without food. Patients should check package directions or ask the physician or pharmacist for instructions on how to take the medicine.

Precautions

There are warnings and cautions that apply to erythromycin and its related drugs when they are taken by mouth over a period of several days. These warnings may not apply when erythromycin is given intravenously (by vein), or as a single dose prior to or immediately after surgery.

Symptoms should begin to improve within a few days of beginning to take this medicine. If they do not, or if they get worse, the patient should check with the physician who prescribed the medicine.

Erythromycins may cause mild diarrhea, which usually goes away during treatment. Severe diarrhea, however, could be a sign of a very serious side effect. Anyone who develops severe diarrhea while taking erythromycin or related drugs should stop taking the medicine and call a physician immediately.

KEY TERMS

Abscess—A collection of pus, appearing in a localized infection, and associated with tissue destruction and frequently with swelling.

Bronchitis—Inflammation of the air passages in the lungs.

Gonorrhea—A sexually transmitted disease (STD) that causes infection in the genital organs and may cause disease in other parts of the body.

Inflammation—Pain, redness, swelling, and heat that usually develop in response to injury or illness.

Legionnaire's disease—A lung disease caused by a bacterium.

Microorganism—An organism that is too small to be seen with the naked eye.

Pelvic inflammatory disease (PID)—Inflammation of the female reproductive tract, caused by any of

several microorganisms. Symptoms include severe abdominal pain, high fever, and vaginal discharge. Severe cases can result in sterility.

Pneumonia—A disease in which the lungs become inflamed. Pneumonia may be caused by bacteria, viruses, or other organisms, or by physical or chemical irritants.

Sinus—Any of several air-filled cavities in the bones of the skull.

Strep throat—A sore throat caused by infection with *Streptococcus* bacteria. Symptoms include sore throat, chills, fever, and swollen lymph nodes in the neck.

Tonsillitis—Inflammation of a tonsil, a small mass of tissue in the throat.

Urinary tract—The passage through which urine flows from the kidneys out of the body.

Special conditions

Taking erythromycins may cause problems for people with certain medical conditions or people who are taking certain other medicines. Before taking these drugs, the patient should tell the physician about any of these conditions.

ALLERGIES. Anyone who has had unusual reactions to erythromycins, azithromycin, or clarithromycin in the past should let the physician know before taking the drugs again. The physician should also be told about any allergies to foods, dyes, preservatives, or other substances.

PREGNANCY. Some medicines in this group may cause problems in pregnant women and have the potential to cause birth defects. Women who are pregnant or who may become pregnant should check with their physicians before taking these drugs.

BREASTFEEDING. Erythromycins pass into breast milk. Mothers who are breastfeeding and who need to take this medicine should check with their physicians.

OTHER MEDICAL CONDITIONS. Before using erythromycins, people with any of these medical problems should make sure their physicians are aware of their conditions:

• heart disease

• liver disease

• hearing loss

USE OF CERTAIN MEDICINES. Taking erythromycins with certain other drugs may affect the way the drugs work or may increase the chance of side effects.

Side effects

The most common side effects are mild diarrhea, nausea, vomiting, and stomach or abdominal cramps. These problems usually go away as the body adjusts to the drug and do not require medical treatment. Less common side effects, such as sore mouth or tongue and vaginal itching and discharge also may occur. They do not need medical attention unless they persist or are bothersome.

More serious side effects are not common, but may occur. If any of the following side effects occur, the patient is advised to check with a physician immediately:

• severe stomach pain, nausea, vomiting, or diarrhea

• fever

• skin rash, redness, or itching

• unusual tiredness or weakness

Although rare, very serious reactions to azithromycin (Zithromax) are possible, including extreme swelling of the lips, face, and neck; and anaphylaxis (a violent allergic reaction). Anyone who develops these symptoms after taking azithromycin should stop taking the medicine and get immediate medical help.

Other rare side effects may occur with erythromycins and related drugs. Anyone who has unusual symptoms

---

after taking these medicines should get in touch with the physician.

Interactions

Erythromycins may interact with many other medicines. When an interaction occurs, the effects of one or both of the drugs may change or the risk of side effects may be greater. Anyone who takes erythromycins should let the physician know all other medicines he or she is taking. The drugs that may interact with erythromycins include:

- acetaminophen (Tylenol)
- medicine for overactive thyroid
- male hormones (androgens)
- female hormones (estrogens)
- other antibiotics
- blood thinners
- disulfiram (Antabuse), used to treat alcohol abuse
- such anti-seizure medicines as valproic acid (Depakote, Depakene)
- caffeine
- the antihistamines astemizole (Hismanal)
- such antiviral drugs as zidovudine (Retrovir)

The list above does not include every drug that may interact with erythromycins. A physician or pharmacist should be consulted before combining erythromycins with any other prescription or nonprescription (over-the-counter) medicine.

Resources

BOOKS

AHFS: Drug Information. Washington, DC: American Society of Healthsystems Pharmaceuticals, 2002.

Brody, T.M., J. Larner, K.P. Minneman, and H.C. Neu. *Human Pharmacology Molecular to Clinical,* 2nd ed. St. Louis: Mosby Year-Book, 1998.

Karch, A.M. *Lippincott's Nursing Drug Guide.* Springhouse, PA: Lippincott Williams & Wilkins, 2003.

Reynolds, J.E.F., ed. *Martindale The Extra Pharmacopoeia,* 31st ed. London: The Pharmaceutical Press, 1993.

PERIODICALS

Steps to keep antibiotics working effectively. Tufts University Health & Nutrition Letter. Medford, MA: Tufts University, May 2003.

OTHER

"Erythromycin." Medline Plus Drug Information. [cited May 2003] <http://www.nlm.nih.gov/medlineplus/druginfo/medmaster/a682381.html>.

"Erythromycins (Systemic)." Medline Plus Drug Information. [cited May 2003] <http://www.nlm.nih.gov/medlineplus/druginfo/uspdi/202223.html>.

Nancy Ross-Flanigan
Sam Uretsky

Esophageal atresia repair

Definition

Esophageal atresia repair, also known as tracheoesophageal fistula or TEF repair, is a surgical procedure performed to correct congenital defects of the esophagus (the muscular tube that connects the mouth to the stomach) and the trachea (the windpipe that carries air into the lungs). Esophageal atresia (EA) and tracheoesophageal fistula (TEF) are commonly found together (EA/TEF), but may also occur separately. As of 2003, there is no known cause for these congenital defects.

Purpose

In children born with EA, the esophagus has not developed as a continuous passage into the stomach but ends in a blind pouch. In the majority of cases (86%) it is also abnormally connected to the trachea by a small channel called a fistula. EA/TEF repair is performed to correct these defects, ensuring the survival of affected infants and their proper breathing and digestion.

Demographics

EA/TEF is reported to occur in about 1: 4500 births. It occurs equally among male and female infants and has been associated with prematurity. There are no other notable associations.

Description

The human esophagus and trachea are normally formed as two separate but parallel passageways early in fetal development. The esophagus leads from the throat to the stomach and digestive tract, and the trachea leads from the larynx to the lungs and respiratory system. Esophageal atresia occurs when the esophagus is incompletely formed; most typically, its upper portion ends in a pouch, failing to connect with the lower portion that leads to the stomach. Esophageal atresia with tracheoesophageal fistula, commonly known as EA/TEF, occurs when the membrane that divides the trachea from the esophagus (tracheoesophageal septum) is incompletely

Esophageal atresia repair

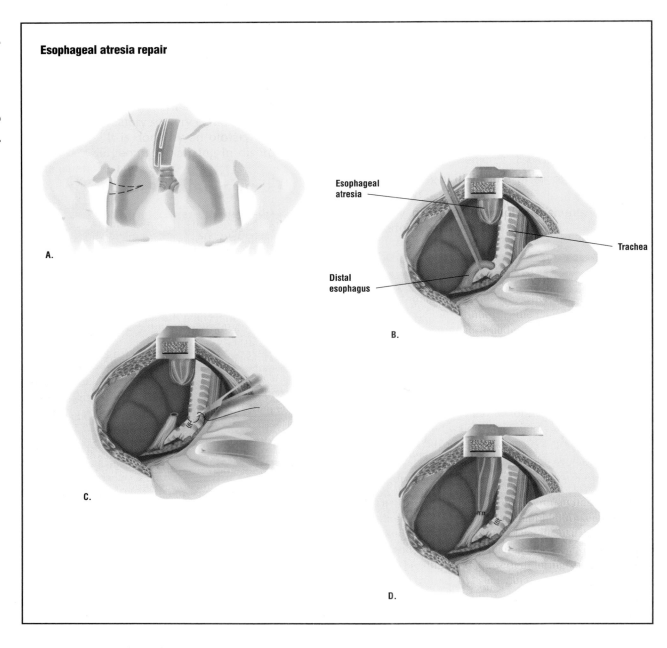

To repair esophageal atresia, an opening is cut into the chest (A). The two parts of the existing esophagus are identified (B). The lower esophagus is detached from the trachea (C) and connected to the upper part of the esophagus (D). The wound in the trachea is closed, and the chest incision is repaired. *(Illustration by GGS Inc.)*

formed, leaving a fistula between the two normally separate organs. The combined defect is found in 86% of children who need esophageal atresia repair. Isolated esophageal atresia, or esophageal atresia without TEF, is a much less common congenital defect thought to occur later in fetal development and requiring a more complicated operation. The presence of TEF without EA occurs also, but with fewer noticeable symptoms in the infant, making it more difficult to diagnose. It may not be diagnosed until months or even years later when digestive disturbances occur. Surgery is required to correct all of these congenital defects.

A classification system is commonly used to describe five types of esophageal atresia, with and without TEF:

• Type A: Esophageal atresia (7.7% of cases). EA alone is a condition in which both segments of the esophagus, upper and lower, end in blind pouches with neither segment attached to the trachea.

- Type B: Esophageal atresia with tracheoesophageal fistula (86.5%). This is the most common type of EA/TEF, in which the upper portion of the esophagus ends in a blind pouch and the lower segment of the esophagus is attached to the trachea by a fistula.

- Type C: Esophageal atresia with tracheoesophageal fistula (0.8%). Type C is a rare form of EA/TEF in which the upper segment of the esophagus forms a channel to the trachea (TEF) and the lower segment of the esophagus ends in a blind pouch (EA).

- Type D: Esophageal atresia with tracheoesophageal fistula (0.7%). Type D is the rarest form of EA/TEF, in which both segments of the esophagus are attached to the trachea.

- Type H: Tracheoesophageal fistula (4.2%). TEF alone is a condition in which a fistula is present between the esophagus and the trachea, while the esophagus has a normal connection to the stomach.

The incomplete esophagus in EA/TEF will not allow swallowed saliva, food, or liquids to pass into the stomach for normal digestion and nutrition. Because of the defect, normal eating or drinking can be dangerous because food and fluids have a direct route through the fistula into the lungs. Swallowed material in the dead-end esophagus as well as stomach fluids may be aspirated into the lungs through the fistula, compromising the child's breathing and potentially causing pneumonia or infection. The impossibility of normal eating, breathing, and digestion creates a life-threatening condition that requires immediate surgery.

The first signs of EA/TEF in a newborn infant may be tiny white frothy bubbles of mucus in the infant's mouth and sometimes in the nose as well. These bubbles reappear when they are suctioned away. Although the infant can swallow normally, the parents can often hear a rattling sound in the chest along with coughing and choking, especially when the baby is trying to nurse. Depending on the severity of the defect, some infants may develop a bluish complexion (cyanosis), caused by a lack of sufficient oxygen in the circulatory system. The infant's abdomen may be distended (swollen and firm) because the abnormally formed trachea will allow air to build up in the stomach and fill the space surrounding the abdominal organs. Saliva and stomach fluids may be aspirated into the lungs through the abnormal opening in the infant's trachea. Aspiration can lead to infection or even asphyxiation (impaired breathing or loss of consciousness due to lack of oxygen).

Other congenital defects are found in at least 50% of infants with EA/TEF. Typically more than one type of malformation will be found. These may include:

WHO PERFORMS THE PROCEDURE AND WHERE IS IT PERFORMED?

EA/TEF repair is performed in a hospital **operating room** by a pediatric or general surgeon.

- Heart defects (about 25% of affected infants)
- Gastrointestinal (digestive) anomalies, including malformed anus (rectum) or twisting of the small intestine (about 16%)
- Urinary tract and kidney defects (10%)
- Musculoskeletal (muscle and bone) defects, especially of the ribs and limbs

The multiple anomalies that can occur with EA/TEF have been described by an acronym, VATER or VACTRRL. This acronym stands for *v*ertebral defect, *a*norectal malformation, *c*ardiac defect, *t*racheoesophageal fistula, *r*enal anomaly, *r*adial dysplasia, and *l*imb defects. About 10% of children with EA have what is called the VATER syndrome. More infants with Type A esophageal atresia have multiple anomalies than those with Type B, the combined EA/TEF.

Healthy infants who have no complications, such as heart or lung problems or other types of intestinal malformations, can usually have esophageal surgery within the first 24 hours of life. The operation will be delayed for low birth weight infants or those with complicated malformations, usually until their nutritional status can be improved and other problems resolved sufficiently to reduce the risks of surgery. H-type TEF, which has fewer symptoms and is typically diagnosed when the child is at least four months old, is also easier to repair when the child's size and weight have increased. The esophagus can be dilated periodically during the growth period and a stomach tube used to decompress the stomach until the surgical repair is performed. All infants with some type of esophageal atresia will require surgery; many will have the repair performed in separate stages over a period of years. The procedures used to treat the five types of EA/TEF defects are similar.

Surgery is conducted while the infant is under general anesthesia, unconscious and free of pain. The surgeon makes an incision in the right chest wall between the ribs. If the gap between the two portions of the esophagus is short, the surgeon may join both ends of the esophagus together. This is called an anastomosis. If the upper portion of the esophagus is short and a long gap exists between the upper and lower portions, reconstructive surgery cannot be performed and the infant will have to be fed in another way to allow several months of growth. In this case, a **gastrostomy** (stomach tube) may be surgically placed directly into the stomach for feeding. In the most typical EA/TEF repair, the fistula will first be closed off, creating a separate airway. Then the blind esophageal pouch will be opened and connected to the other portion of the esophagus, creating a normal pathway directly into the stomach.

Diagnosis/Preparation

Diagnosis

A tentative diagnosis of EA/TEF may be made before the child is born. One of the first signs of esophageal atresia may be seen during the mother's prenatal ultrasound examination. Polyhydramnios, which is an excessive amount of amniotic fluid surrounding the fetus, is not always diagnostic but offers a warning sign. Fluid is normally exchanged between the fetus and the amniotic fluid through swallowing, urination, and discharges from the nose and mouth. In EA/TEF, the fetus may drool excessively because of a collection of fluid in the abnormal esophageal pouch, thus increasing the amount of amniotic fluid.

A newborn infant suspected of EA/TEF will be given an x-ray examination. The imaging study may reveal a dilated esophageal pouch that is larger than expected because it has collected a pool of amniotic fluid. During fetal development, the enlarged esophagus may also have pressed on and narrowed the trachea, a condition that may contribute to fistula development. Air in the stomach may confirm the presence of a fistula while gas in the large intestine will rule out duodenal atresia. The physician will also perform a comprehensive **physical examination**, looking for other congenital anomalies that are known to accompany EA/TEF. Chest x-rays may be taken to look for skeletal and cardiac abnormalities. Abdominal X-rays may be taken as well to look for intestinal obstruction and abnormalities. An echocardiogram (ECG) may be performed to evaluate heart function and an ultrasound of the kidneys performed to evaluate kidney function. A nasogastric (NG) tube may be placed in the infant; it may help to confirm a diagnosis of EA/TEF if it stops short of the usual distance (17 cm or about 6.7 in) to the stomach.

Preparation

When an infant is suspected of having EA/TEF, he or she will be transferred from the regular nursery to the neonatal (newborn) or pediatric intensive care department of the medical facility. Corrective surgery must be scheduled immediately to help ensure survival and promote proper swallowing, digestion, nutrition, and breathing. In patients with pneumonia or other lung problems, the doctor may clean out the baby's stomach and esophageal pouch with a suction tube to prevent the baby's stomach contents from being drawn through the fistula and into the trachea. A tube will be placed through the baby's mouth to continuously suction the esophageal pouch during surgery. The baby will be given fluids intravenously during surgery. **Oxygen therapy** will be administered if needed. An airway will be placed in the trachea if the baby has lung problems. **Antibiotics** may be given to treat or to prevent infection in the lungs, especially if the stomach contents have been drawn into the lungs. Preoperative blood and urine tests will also be performed.

Aftercare

Immediately after surgery, the patient will be cared for in the neonatal ICU with monitoring of breathing, body temperature, and heart and kidney function. Oxygen may be administered, and a mechanical respirator may also be necessary. Pain medication will be given if needed. Blood and urine tests may be performed to evaluate the infant's overall condition. Scans may be performed to evaluate esophageal functioning. The infant will be fed intravenously or will have a gastrostomy tube placed directly into the stomach until oral feedings can be swallowed and digested. Secretions may be suctioned from the throat and a nasogastric tube may be placed in the infant's nose to clear the stomach as needed. Hospitalization may be required for two weeks or longer, depending on the presence of complications or other underlying conditions. An x-ray procedure known as esophagography is usually performed at two months, six months, and one year of age to monitor the digestive function as the child grows. Long-term follow-up of patients who have had EA/TEF repair is essential.

Risks

There is some risk of postoperative breathing difficulties or respiratory complications, particularly infection or pneumonia due to aspiration of stomach contents. Pretreatment with antibiotics helps to prevent infection to some degree. Other risks of esophageal atresia repair include those that may occur with any surgery: reactions to anesthesia or medications; bleeding or clot formation; narrowing of the repaired organs; nerve injury; fluid imbalances; and collapsed lung (pneumothorax).

Complications that can occur in infants who have had EA/TEF repair include the following:

- Esophageal dysmotility. Dysmotility refers to weakness of the muscular walls of the esophagus. Some degree of dysmotility is expected to occur in all infants undergoing esophageal repair. This complication requires special precautions when the child is eating or drinking.

- About 50% of patients will develop gastroesophageal reflux disease (GERD) later in childhood or adult life. GERD is a condition in which the acid contents of the stomach flow back into the esophagus. The condition requires medical or surgical treatment.

- Recurrence of TEF. Recurrence is treated with repeat surgery.

- Swallowing difficulties (dysphagia). Dysphagia can cause food or pills to become stuck in the esophagus at the site of the surgical repair. Medications should be taken with water to prevent ulcers from developing.

- Breathing difficulties and choking. These complications are related to the slow passage of food, food stuck in the esophagus, or aspiration of food into the trachea.

- Chronic cough. The cough is characteristic of TEF repair; it is caused by weakness in the trachea and does not indicate a cold or illness.

- Increased susceptibility to colds, respiratory infections, and pneumonia. Precautions should be taken to avoid contact with other sick children. Parents and caregivers can seek advice about strengthening the child's immune system through appropriate nutrition and supplements.

KEY TERMS

Anastomosis—The connection of separate parts of a body organ or an organ system.

Anomaly (anomalies)—Abnormal development of a body organ or a defect in part of an organ system.

Aspiration—To take into the lungs by breathing.

Atresia—Absence of a normal opening.

Congenital—Present at birth.

Dysmotility—A lack of normal muscle movement (motility), especially in the esophagus, stomach, or intestines.

Dysplasia—The abnormal form or abnormal development of a body organ or organ system.

Esophagus—The upper portion of the digestive system, a tube leading from the mouth to the stomach.

Fistula—An abnormal tube-like passage between body organs or from a body organ to the body surface.

Trachea—The medical term for the windpipe.

Normal results

EA/TEF can usually be corrected with surgery, allowing the child to eat, breathe, and digest food in a normal fashion. Although almost 100% of children who have corrective surgery for EA/TEF survive the procedure, they may continue to have complications, some of which can be chronic. Ongoing medical care and additional surgery may be necessary.

Morbidity and mortality rates

The post-operative mortality rate in healthy infants is essentially zero. Prior to the development of a more advanced EA/TEF repair technique in 1939, the condition was often fatal. Pre- and postoperative neonatal care has also significantly improved the surgical outcome. Infants with multiple anomalies or cardiac or pulmonary problems are more subject to complications than otherwise healthy infants.

Alternatives

Esophageal atresia and tracheoesophageal fistula are congenital defects for which there are no recommended alternatives. These defects are commonly corrected surgically. There are no known measures to prevent these congenital defects.

Resources

BOOKS

Allan, W., MD, et al. *Pediatric Gastrointestinal Disease: Pathophysiology, Diagnosis, Management*, 3rd ed. Boston, MA: B.C. Decker, 2000.

ORGANIZATIONS

American Academy of Family Physicians. PO Box 11210, Shawnee Mission, KS 66207. (800) 274-2237. <www.aafp.org>.

EA/TEF Child and Family Support Connection. 111 West Jackson Blvd., Suite 1145, Chicago, IL 60604. (312) 987-9085. <www.eatef.org>.

OTHER

Allesandro, M. P., MD. *Esophageal Atresia and Tracheoesophageal Fistula (EA/TEF)*. Gastrointestinal Diseases, Virtual Children's Hospital Library. <www.vh.org/ pediatric/ provider/ radiology/PAP/GIDiseases/ EATEF.html>.

TEF/VATER International. *What is esophageal atresia?* <www.tefvater.org>.

L. Lee Culvert

Esophageal function tests

Definition

The esophagus is the muscular tube through which food passes on its way from the mouth to the stomach. The main function of the esophagus is to propel food into the stomach. To ensure that food does not move backward—a condition known as reflux—sphincters (constricting ring-shaped muscles) at either end of the esophagus close when the food is not passing through them in a forward direction. Esophageal function tests are used to determine whether the sphincters are working properly.

Purpose

The esophagus has two sets of sphincters at its upper and lower ends. Each of these muscular rings must contract in an exact sequence for swallowing to proceed normally. The upper esophageal sphincter normally stops the contents of the stomach from moving backward into the pharynx and larynx (voice box). The lower esophageal sphincter guards against stomach acid moving upward into the esophagus. The lower sphincter should be tightly closed except to allow food and fluids to enter the stomach.

The three major symptoms occurring with abnormal esophageal function are difficulty with swallowing (dysphagia); heartburn; and chest pain. Doctors perform a va-

riety of tests to evaluate these symptoms. Endoscopy, which is not a test of esophageal function, is often used to determine if the lining of the esophagus has any ulcers, tumors, or areas of narrowing (strictures). Many times, however, endoscopy only shows the doctor if there is an injury to the esophageal lining; it does not always provide information about the cause of the problem. Tests that measure the functioning of the esophagus are sometimes needed in addition to endoscopy. There are three basic types of tests used to assess esophageal function:

- Manometry. Manometry is used to study the way the muscles of the esophagus contract, and is most useful for investigating dysphagia.

- Esophageal pH monitoring. This test measures changes in the acidity of the esophagus, and is valuable for evaluating patients with heartburn or gastroesophageal reflux disease (GERD).

- X-ray studies. This type of imaging study is used to investigate dysphagia, either by using a fluoroscope to follow the progress of a barium mixture during the process of swallowing, or by using radioactive scanning techniques.

Description

Manometry

This study is designed to measure the pressure changes produced by contraction of the muscular portions of the esophagus. An abnormality in the function of any one of the segments of the esophagus can cause difficulty in swallowing (dysphagia). A manometric examination is most useful in evaluating patients when an endoscopy yields normal results.

During manometry, the patient swallows a thin tube carrying a device that senses changes in pressures in the esophagus. Readings are taken at rest and during the process of swallowing. Medications are sometimes given during the study to aid in the diagnosis. The results are then transmitted to recording equipment. Manometry is most useful in identifying diseases that produce disturbances of motility or contractions of the esophagus. In 2003, a solution containing five drops of peppermint oil in 10 mL of water was found to improve the manometric features of diffuse esophageal spasm (DES). The peppermint oil solution eliminated simultaneous esophageal contractions in all patients in the study.

Esophageal pH monitoring

This procedure measures the esophagus' exposure to acid reflux from the stomach. The test is ideal for evaluating recurrent heartburn or gastroesophageal reflux disease (GERD). Excessive acid reflux may produce ulcers, or strictures resulting from healed ulcers, in addition to the symptom of heartburn.

Normally, acid from the stomach washes backward into the esophagus in small amounts for short periods of time. The lower esophageal sphincter usually prevents excessive reflux in patients without disease. Spontaneous contractions that increase esophageal emptying and production of saliva also act to prevent damage to the esophagus.

Researchers have shown that in the esophagus, the presence of acid is damaging only if it lasts over long periods of time. Therefore, esophageal pH monitoring has been designed to monitor the level of acidity over a 24-hour period, usually in the patient's home. In this way, patients are able to maintain their daily routine, document their symptoms, and correlate symptoms with specific activities. During this period, a thin tube with a pH monitor remains in the esophagus to record changes in acidity. After the study, a computer is used to compare the changes with symptoms reported by the patient.

In addition to esophageal pH monitoring, the doctor may perform a Bernstein test (also known as the acid perfusion test) and an acid clearing test. In the Bernstein test, a small quantity of hydrochloric acid (HCl) is directed into the patient's esophagus. If the patient feels pain from the acid, the test is positive for reflux esophagitis. If there is no discomfort, another explanation must be sought for the patient's symptoms. In the acid clearing test, HCl is also directed into the esophagus. This test, however, measures the patient's ability to quickly swallow the acid. If the patient has to swallow more than 10 times to move the acid down the esophagus, he or she has a problem with esophageal motility.

pH monitoring is usually performed before surgery to confirm the diagnosis and to judge the effects of drug therapy. In 2003, studies showed that integrated esophageal and gastric acidity provided better quantitative measures of esophageal dysfunction in GERD than conventional measurements of pH. This finding may suggest better ways to evaluate the effectiveness of different treatments for GERD.

X-ray tests

X-ray tests of esophageal function fall into two categories: (1) tests performed with barium and a fluoroscope; and (2) those performed with radioactive materials. Studies performed with fluoroscopy are especially useful in identifying structural abnormalities of the esophagus. Sometimes the patient is given a sandwich or marshmallow coated with barium in order to identify the site of an obstruction. Fluoroscopy can diagnose or provide important information about a number of disorders involving esophageal function, however, including cricopharyngeal achalasia (a swallowing disorder of the throat); decreased or reverse peristalsis; and hiatal hernia.

During fluoroscopy, the radiologist can observe the passage of material through the esophagus in real time, and also make video recordings. These observations are particularly useful when the swallowing symptoms appear to occur mostly in the upper region of the esophagus. The most common cause of difficulty swallowing is a previous stroke, although other diseases of the neuromuscular system (like myasthenia gravis) can produce similar symptoms.

Scans using low-dose radioactive materials are useful because they may demonstrate that food passes more slowly than usual through the esophagus. They can also measure the speed of the bolus' passage. These studies involve swallowing food coated with radioactive material, followed by a nuclear medicine scan. Scans are often used when other methods have failed to make a diagnosis, or if it is necessary to determine the degree of the abnormality.

Preparation

Patients should not eat or drink anything after midnight before an esophageal function test. Many medications affect the esophagus; doses may need to be adjusted or even discontinued prior to testing. Patients must inform their physician of any and all medications they take, including over-the-counter medications and herbal preparations. They must also tell the doctor about any known allergies.

Aftercare

No special care is needed after most esophageal function tests. Patients can usually return to their normal daily activities following almost all of these tests.

Risks

Exposure to x rays, especially in the first three months of a woman's pregnancy, can be harmful to the fetus. Barium swallows may also cause impaction (hardening) of fecal matter. Additionally, although the tubes passed through the esophagus during some of the esophageal function tests are small, and most patients adjust to them quite well, some patients may gag and aspirate (breathe into the lungs rather than passing through the esophagus) some gastric juices.

Normal results

Normal findings include:

- lower esophageal sphincter pressure ranging from 10–20 mm Hg

KEY TERMS

Achalasia—Failure to relax. The term is often applied to sphincter muscles.

Barium—A metallic element used in its sulfate form as a contrast medium for x-ray studies of the digestive tract.

Bolus—A mass of food ready to be swallowed, or a preparation of medicine to be given by mouth or IV all at once rather than gradually.

Cathartic—A medication or other agent that causes the bowels to empty.

Craniopharyngeal achalasia—A swallowing disorder of the throat.

Diffuse esophageal spasm (DES)—An uncommon condition characterized by abnormal simultaneous contractions of the esophagus.

Dysphagia—Difficulty or discomfort in swallowing.

Esophagus—The muscular passageway between the throat and the stomach.

Heartburn—A sensation of warmth or burning behind the breastbone, rising upward toward the neck. It is often caused by stomach acid flowing upward from the stomach into the esophagus.

Hiatal hernia—A condition in which part of the stomach pushes up through the same opening in the diaphragm that the esophagus passes through.

Motility—Ability to move freely or spontaneously. Esophageal motility refers to the ability of the muscle fibers in the tissue of the esophagus to contract in order to push food or other material toward the stomach.

Peristalsis—The wavelike contraction of the muscle fibers in the esophagus and other parts of the digestive tract that pushes food through the system.

Sphincter—A circular band of muscle fibers that constricts or closes a passageway in the body. The esophagus has sphincters at its upper and lower ends.

- normal peristaltic waves

- normal size, shape, position, patency and filling of the esophagus

- negative acid reflux

- acid clearing in fewer than 10 swallows

- negative Bernstein test

Manometry is used to diagnose abnormalities related to contraction or relaxation of the various muscular regions of the esophagus. These studies cannot distinguish whether injury to either the muscle or nerves of the esophagus is producing the abnormal results—only the final effect on esophageal muscle is identified. The results of this test should be interpreted in light of the patient's entire medical history. For example, there are many diseases that affect the relaxation of the lower esophageal sphincter; one such condition is called achalasia. Achalasia is a frequent finding in individuals with Down's syndrome.

Abnormal results of pH tests can confirm symptoms of heartburn or indicate a cause of chest pain (or rarely, swallowing difficulties). The patient's doctor may want to prescribe or change medications based on these results, or even repeat the test using different doses of medication. As noted above, these studies should be done before surgical treatment of GERD.

X-ray tests can serve to document an abnormality in the esophagus. If the results are negative, other studies may be needed.

Resources

BOOKS

Castell, June A., and R. Matthew Gideon. "Esophageal Manometry," in Donald O. Castell and Joel E. Richter, eds., *The Esophagus*, 3rd ed. Philadelphia, PA: Lippincott, 1999.

Pagana, Kathleen D., and Timothy J. Pagana. *Diagnostic Testing and Nursing Implications*, 5th ed. St. Louis, MO: Mosby, 1999.

Smout, Andre. "Ambulatory Monitoring of Esophageal pH and Pressure." in Donald O. Castell and Joel E. Richter, eds., *The Esophagus*, 3rd ed. Philadelphia, PA: Lippincott, 1999.

PERIODICALS

Gardner, J.D., S. Rodriguez-Stanley, and M. Robinson. "Integrated Acidity and the Pathophysiology of Gastroesophageal Reflux Disease." *American Journal of Gastroenterology* 96, no. 5 (May 2001): 1363-70.

Mujica, V.R., R. S. Mudipalli, and S. S. Rao. "Pathophysiology of Chest Pain in Patients with Nutcracker Esophagus." *American Journal of Gastroenterology* 96, no.5 (May 2001): 1371-7.

Pimentel, M., G. G. Bonorris, E. J. Chow, and H. C. Lin. "Peppermint Oil Improves the Manometric Findings in Diffuse

Esophageal Spasm." *Journal of Clinical Gastroenterology* 33, no.1 (July 2001): 27-31.

Zarate, N., F. Mearin, A. Hidalgo, and J. R. Malagelada. "Prospective Evaluation of Esophageal Motor Dysfunction in Down's Syndrome." *American Journal of Gastroenterology* 96, no. 6 (June 2001): 1718-24.

ORGANIZATIONS

American Society for Gastrointestinal Endoscopy (ASGE). Thirteen Elm Street, Manchester, MA 01944-1314. (978) 526-8330. <http://www.asge.org>.

Illinois Nurses Association—Advanced Practices Registered Nurses (APRNs) Statistics. 105 W. Adams, Suite 2101, Chicago, IL 60603. <www.illinoisnurses.org/aprn.html>.

Society for Gastroenterology Nurses and Associates (SGNA). 401 North Michigan Avenue, Chicago, IL 60611-4267. (800) 245-7462. <www.sgna.org>.

Maggie Boleyn, RN, BSN
Lee Shratter, MD

Esophageal radiography *see* **Upper GI exam**

Esophageal resection

Definition

An esophageal resection is the surgical removal of the esophagus, nearby lymph nodes, and sometimes a portion of the stomach. The esophagus is a hollow muscular tube that passes through the chest from the mouth to the stomach—a "foodpipe" that carries food and liquids to the stomach for digestion and nutrition. Removal of the esophagus requires reconnecting the remaining part of the esophagus to the stomach to allow swallowing and the continuing passage of food. Part of the stomach or intestine may be used to make this connection. Several surgical techniques and approaches (ways to enter the body) are used, depending on how much or which part of the esophagus needs to be removed; whether or not part of the stomach will be removed; the patient's overall condition; and the surgeon's preference.

There are two basic esophageal resection surgeries. Esophagectomy is the surgical removal of the esophagus or a cancerous (malignant) portion of the esophagus and nearby lymph nodes. Esophagogastrectomy is the surgical removal of the lower esophagus and the upper part of the stomach that connects to the esophagus, performed when cancer has been found in both organs. Lymph nodes in the surrounding area are also removed.

An esophageal resection may be performed in combination with pre- and postoperative radiation and chemotherapy (chemoradiation).

Purpose

An esophagectomy is most often performed to treat early-stage cancer of the esophagus before the cancer has spread (metastasized) to the stomach or other organs. Esophagectomy is also a treatment for esophageal dysplasia (Barrett's esophagus), which is a precancerous condition of the cells in the lining of the esophagus. Lymph nodes are removed to be tested for the presence of cancer cells, which helps to determine if the cancer is spreading. Esophagectomy is also recommended when irreversible damage has occurred as a result of traumatic injury to the esophagus; swallowing of caustic (cell-damaging) agents; chronic inflammation; and complex motility (muscle movement) disorders that interfere with the passage of food to the stomach.

An esophagogastrectomy is performed when cancer of the esophagus has been shown to be spreading to nearby lymph nodes and to the stomach, creating new tumors. When cancer invades other tissues in this way, it is said to be metastatic. The goal of esophagogastrectomy is to relieve difficult or painful swallowing (dysphagia) in patients with advanced esophageal cancer, and to prevent or slow the spread of metastases to more distant organs such as the liver or the brain.

Demographics

The candidates for esophageal resection parallel those at high risk for esophageal cancer. Esophageal cancer is found among middle-aged and older adults, with the average age at diagnosis between 55 and 60. Esophageal cancer and esophageal dysplasia occur far more often in men than in women. One type of esophageal cancer (squamous cell carcinoma) occurs more frequently in African Americans; another type (adenocarcinoma) is more common in Caucasian males. Caucasian and Hispanic men with a history of gastroesophageal reflux disease (GERD) are also at increased risk, because GERD has been shown to cause changes in the cells of the esophagus that may lead to cancer. Higher risks are also associated with smoking (45%), alcohol abuse (20%), and lung disorders (23%).

Description

Esophageal cancer is diagnosed in about 13,000 people annually in the United States; it is responsible for approximately 1.5–5% of cancer deaths each year. Although it is not as prevalent as breast and colon cancer, its rate of occurrence is increasing. This rise is thought to be related to an increase in gastroesophageal reflux disease, or GERD.

The esophagus has a muscular opening, or sphincter, at the entrance to the stomach, which usually keeps acid from passing upward. In people with GERD, the esophageal sphincter allows partially digested food and excess stomach acid to flow back into the esophagus. This occurrence is known as regurgitation. Regurgitation continually exposes the lining of the esophagus to large amounts of acid, causing repetitive damage to the cells of the esophageal lining. The result is Barrett's esophagus, a condition in which the normal cells (squamous cells) of the esophageal lining are replaced by the glandular type of cells that normally line the stomach. Glandular cells are more resistant to acid damage but at the same time, they can more readily develop into cancer cells. Studies at New York's Memorial Sloan-Kettering Hospital have shown that only 30% of people diagnosed with Barrett's esophagus will later be diagnosed with cancer; the other 70% will not develop dysplasia, the precancerous condition. Effective medical treatment of acid reflux is thought to be a factor in the low incidence of cancer in people with Barrett's esophagus. Other types of cancer can also occur in the esophagus, including melanoma, sarcoma, and lymphoma.

The risk factors for esophageal cancer include:

• Use of tobacco. The highest risk for esophageal cancer is the combination of smoking and heavy alcohol use.

• Abuse of alcohol.

• Barrett's esophagus as a result of long-term acid reflux disease.

• A low-fiber diet; that is, a diet that is low in fruits and vegetables, and whole grains that retain their outer bran layer. Other dietary risk factors include such vitamin and mineral deficiencies, as low levels of zinc and riboflavin.

• Accidental swallowing of cleaning liquids or other caustic substances in childhood.

• Achalasia. Achalasia is an impaired functioning of the sphincter muscle between the esophagus and the stomach.

• Esophageal webs. These are bands of abnormal tissue in the esophagus that make it difficult to swallow.

• A rare inherited disease called tylosis, in which excess layers of skin grow on the hands and the soles of the feet. People with this condition are almost certain to develop esophageal cancer.

Cancer of the esophagus begins in the inner layers of the tissue that lines the passageway and grows outward. Cancer of the top layer of the esophageal lining is called squamous cell carcinoma; it can occur anywhere along the esophagus, but appears most often in the middle and upper portions. It can spread extensively within the esophagus, requiring the surgical removal of large parts of the esophagus. Adenocarcinoma is the type of cancer that develops in the lower end of the esophagus near the stomach. Both types of cancer may develop in people with Barrett's esophagus. Prior to 1985, squamous cell carcinoma was the most common type of esophageal cancer, but adenocarcinoma of the esophagus and the upper part of the stomach is increasing more rapidly than any other type of cancer in the United States. Up to 83% of patients undergoing esophagectomy have been shown to have adenocarcinoma. This development may be related to such changes in risk factors as decreased smoking and alcohol use as well as increased reflux disease. People at high risk for esophageal cancer should be examined and tested regularly for changes in cell types.

Esophageal cancer is classified in six stages determined by laboratory examination of tissue cells from the esophagus, nearby lymph nodes, and stomach. The six stages are:

• Stage 0. This is the earliest stage of esophageal cancer, in which cancer cells are present only in the innermost lining of the esophagus.

• Stage I. The cancer has spread to deeper layers of cells but has not spread into nearby lymph nodes or organs.

• Stage IIA. The cancer has invaded the muscular layer of the esophageal walls, sometimes as far as the outer wall.

• Stage IIB. The cancer has invaded the lymph nodes near the esophagus and has probably spread into deeper layers of tissue.

• Stage III. Cancer is present in the tissues or lymph nodes near the esophagus, especially in the trachea (windpipe) or stomach.

• Stage IV. The cancer has spread to more distant organs, such as the liver or brain.

Unfortunately, the symptoms of esophageal cancer usually don't appear until the disease has progressed beyond the early stages and is already metastatic. Without early diagnostic screening, patients may wait to consult a doctor only when there is little opportunity for cure. The symptoms of esophageal cancer may include difficulty swallowing or painful swallowing; unexplained weight loss; hiccups; pressure or burning in the chest; hoarseness; lung disorders; or pneumonia.

The decision to perform an esophageal resection will be made when staging tests have confirmed the presence of cancer and its stage. Two-thirds of people who undergo endoscopy, a close examination of the inside lining of the esophagus, and biopsies (testing esophageal tissue cells) will already have cancer, which can progress rapidly. Some will be treated with surgery and others with medical therapy, depending on the stage of the cancer, the patient's general health status, and the degree of risk. Removing the esophagus or the affected portion is the most common treatment for esophageal cancer; it can cure the disease if the cancer is in the early stages and the patient is healthy enough to undergo the stressful surgery. Esophagectomy will be recommended if early-stage cancer or a precancerous condition has been confirmed through extensive diagnostic testing and staging. Esophagectomy is not an option if the cancer has already spread to the stomach. In this case an esophagogastrectomy will usually be performed to remove the cancerous part of the esophagus and the upper part of the stomach.

Esophagectomy

An esophagectomy takes about 6 hours to perform. The patient will be given general anesthesia, keeping him or her unconscious and free of pain during surgery. One of several approaches or incisional strategies will be used, chosen by the surgeon to gain adequate access to the upper abdomen and remove the esophagus or the tumor and the nearby lymph nodes. The four common incisional approaches are: transthoracic, which involves a chest incision; Ivor-Lewis, a side entry through the fifth rib; three-hole esophagectomy, which uses small incisions in the chest and abdomen to accommodate the use of instruments; and transhiatal, which involves a mid-abdominal incision. The approach chosen depends on the extent of the cancer, the location of the tumor or obstruction, and the overall condition of the patient.

In a minimum-access laparoscopic and thorascopic procedure, the surgeon makes several small incisions on the chest and abdomen through which he or she can insert thin telescopic instruments with light sources. The abdomen will be inflated with gas to enlarge the abdominal cavity and give the surgeon a better view of the procedure. First, the camera-tipped laparoscope will be inserted through one small incision, allowing images of the organs in the abdominal area to be displayed on a video monitor in the **operating room**. If the surgeon is going to use a portion of the stomach to replace the resected esophagus, he or she will first locate the fundus, or upper portion of the stomach. The fundus will be manipulated, stapled off, and removed laparoscopically, to be sutured in place (gastroplasty) as a replacement esophagus.

Next, the surgeon will pass thorascopic instruments into the chest through another incision. The esophagus or cancerous portion of the esophagus will be visualized, manipulated, cut and removed. Lymph nodes in the area

will also be removed. Then the surgeon will either pull up a portion of the stomach and connect it to the remaining portion of the esophagus (anastomosis), or use a piece of the stomach or intestine, usually the colon, to reconstruct the esophagus. Either procedure will allow the patient to swallow and pass food and liquid to the stomach after recovery. As discussed above, other approaches may be used to gain access to the affected portion of the esophagus.

There are several variations of an esophagectomy, including:

- Standard open esophagectomy. This technique requires larger incisions to be made in the chest (**thoracotomy**) and in the abdomen so that the surgeon can dissect the esophagus or cancerous portion and remove it along with the nearby lymph nodes. The esophagus can then be reconnected to the stomach using a portion of either the stomach or the colon.

- Laparoscopic esophagectomy. This is a less invasive technique performed through several small incisions on the chest and abdomen with the camera-tipped laparoscope and a video monitor to guide removal of the esophagus or tumor along with nearby lymph glands.

- Vagal-sparing esophagectomy. This procedure preserves the branches of the vagus nerve that supply the stomach, with only minimal alteration of the size of the stomach and the nerves that control acid production and digestive functions.

Esophagogastrectomy

An esophagogastrectomy is also major surgery performed with the patient under general anesthesia. The surgeon will choose the incisional approach that allows the best possible access for resecting the lower portion of the esophagus and the upper portion of the stomach. The surgeon's decision will depend on the extent of the cancer, the amount of the esophagus that must be removed, and the patient's overall health status. An esophagogastrectomy can be performed as an open procedure through large incisions, or as a laparoscopic procedure through small incisions.

In a minimum-access laparoscopic procedure, several small incisions are made in the patient's abdomen. A laparoscope will be inserted through one small incision, allowing images of the abdominal organs to be displayed on a video monitor. As in an esophagectomy, gas may be used to inflate the abdominal cavity for better viewing and space for the surgeon to maneuver. The cancerous upper portion of the stomach will first be stapled off and resected. The cancerous portion of the esophagus will then be cut and removed along with nearby lymph nodes. Finally, a portion of the stomach will be pulled upward and connected to the remaining portion of the esophagus (anastomosis); or, if most of the esophagus has been removed, a piece of the colon will be used to construct a new esophagus. Sometimes the surgeon must make an incision in the neck in order to gain access to and resect the upper portion of the esophagus, followed by making an anastomosis between the esophagus and a portion of the stomach.

Diagnosis/Preparation

Diagnosis

The diagnosis of esophageal cancer begins with a careful history and a review of symptoms, and involves a number of different diagnostic examinations. An esophagoscopy may be performed in the doctor's office, allowing the doctor to examine the inside of the esophagus with a lighted telescopic tube (esophagoscope). A barium swallow is another common screening test, performed in the radiology (x ray) department of the hospital or in a private radiology office. In a barium swallow, the patient drinks a small amount of radiopaque (visible on x-ray) barium that will highlight any raised areas on the wall of the esophagus when chest x-rays are taken. The x-ray studies will reveal irregular patches that may be early cancer or larger irregular areas that may narrow the esophagus and could represent a more advanced stage of cancer. If either of these conditions is present, the doctors will want to confirm the diagnosis of esophageal cancer; determine how far it has invaded the walls of the esophagus; and whether it has spread to nearby lymph nodes or organs. This staging process is essential in order to determine the best treatment for the patient.

One staging technique is a diagnostic procedure called endoscopic ultrasound. The doctor will thread an endoscope, which is a tiny lighted tube with a small ultrasound probe at its tip, into the patient's mouth and down into the esophagus. This procedure allows the inside of the esophagus to be viewed on a monitor to show how far a tumor has invaded the walls of the esophagus. At the same time, the doctor can perform biopsies of esophageal tissue by cutting and removing small pieces for microscopic examination of the cells for cancer stag-

ing. Staging tests may also include computed tomography (**CT scans**); thorascopic and laparoscopic examinations of the chest and abdomen; and **positron emission tomography (PET)**.

Preparation

The patient will be admitted to the hospital on the day of the operation or the day before, and will be taken to a pre-operative nursing unit. The surgeon and anesthesiologist will visit the patient to describe the resection procedure and answer any questions that the patient may have. The standard preoperative blood and urine tests will be performed. Intravenous lines (IV) will be inserted in the patient's vein for the administration of fluids and pain medications during and after the surgery. Sedatives may be given before the patient is taken to the operating room.

Aftercare

Immediately after surgery the patient will be taken to a recovery area where the pulse, body temperature, and heart, lung, and kidney function will be monitored. Several hours later, the patient will be transferred to a concentrated care area. Surgical wound dressings will be kept clean and dry. Pain medication will be given as needed. A chest tube inserted during surgery will be checked for drainage and removed when the drainage stops. A nasogastric (nose to stomach) tube, also placed during surgery, will be used to drain stomach secretions. Nurses will check it regularly and rinse it out. It will eventually be removed by the surgeon. Until the patient is able to swallow soft foods, he or she will be fed intravenously or through a feeding tube that was placed in the small intestine during surgery. Patients will be encouraged to cough and to breathe deeply after surgery to fully expand the lungs and help prevent infection and collapse of the lungs. Walking and movement will also be encouraged to promote a quicker recovery.

About 10–14 days after the surgery, the patient will be given another barium swallow so that the doctor can examine the esophagus for any areas of leaking fluid. If none are seen, the nasogastric tube can be removed. The patient can then begin to sip clear liquids, followed gradually by small amounts of soft foods. Patients being treated for esophageal cancer may begin chemotherapy (cytotoxic or cell-killing medications), radiation therapy, or both, before or soon after **discharge from the hospital**. Patients typically remain in the hospital as long as two weeks after surgery if no complications have occurred.

When the patient goes home, any remaining bandages must be kept clean and dry. Frequent walking and gentle **exercise** are encouraged. Because laparoscopic and thorascopic surgery is less invasive and uses only small incisions, there is less trauma to the body, and activity can be resumed more quickly than with open procedures that require larger incisions. The patient should report any fever or chills, persistent pain, or incision drainage to the surgeon. The patient's diet will typically be restricted for a while to soft foods and small portions; a normal diet can be resumed in about a month, but with smaller quantities. Patients are advised not to drive if they are still taking prescribed narcotic pain medications. Daily care and assistance at home is recommended during the recuperation period. Regular medical care and periodic diagnostic testing, such as endoscopic ultrasound, is essential to monitor the condition of the esophagus and to detect recurrence of the cancer or the development of new tumors.

Risks

One of the primary risks associated with esophageal resection surgeries is leakage at the site of the anastomosis, where a new feeding tube was sutured (stitched) to the remaining esophagus. As many as 9% of all patients have been reported to develop leaks, most occurring when a portion of the stomach rather than the colon was used to construct the new section of the esophagus.

Other risks include:

- formation of blood clots that can travel to the heart, lungs, or brain
- nerve injury, which can cause defective emptying of the stomach
- infection
- breathing difficulties and pneumonia
- adverse reactions to anesthesia
- narrowing of the remaining esophagus (strictures), which may cause swallowing problems
- increased acid reflux and heartburn as a result of injury to or removal of the esophageal sphincter

Normal results

Esophageal resection, especially esophagectomy, can be curative if cancer has not spread beyond the esophagus. About 75% of patients undergoing esophagectomy will be found to have metastatic disease that has already spread to other organs. Esophagectomy will reduce symptoms in most patients, especially swallowing difficulties, which will improve the patient's nutritional status as well. Patients whose esophagectomy is preceded and followed by a combination of chemotherapy and radiation treatments have longer periods of survival.

The typical result of an esophagogastrectomy is palliation, which is the relief of symptoms without a cure.

QUESTIONS TO ASK THE DOCTOR

- Why do I need this surgery?
- How will the surgery be performed? How long will it take?
- How many times have you performed this procedure? How often is it performed in this hospital?
- How much discomfort can I expect in the short term? Over the long term?
- Will this surgery cure my cancer? Will it allow me to live longer?
- What are the chances that the cancer will come back?
- What are my options if I don't have the surgery?
- What are the risks involved in having this surgery?
- What kind of care will I need at home afterward?
- How quickly will I recover?

Because esophagogastrecomy is always performed when metastases have already been found elsewhere in the body, the procedure may relieve pain and difficulty in swallowing, and may delay the spread of the cancer to the liver and brain. Cure of the disease, however, is not an expectation.

Patients having less invasive laparoscopic and thorascopic resection procedures will experience less pain and fewer complications than patients undergoing open procedures.

Morbidity and mortality rates

Because 75% of all esophagectomy patients and 100% of all esophagogastrectomy patients will have metastatic disease, morbidity and mortality rates for these procedures are high. Thirty-day mortality for esophagectomy ranges from 6–12%; it is 10% or higher for esophagogastrectomy. Survival of early-stage cancer patients after esophagectomy ranges from 17 to 34 months if surgery alone is the treatment. The mortality rate for early-stage cancer patients having esophagectomy alone is higher than when surgery is combined with pre- and post-operative chemoradiation. The three-year survival rate for early-stage cancer patients who received pre- and post-esophagectomy chemoradiation is about 63%. Better

KEY TERMS

Achalasia—Failure to relax. The term is often applied to sphincter muscles.

Adenocarcinoma—A type of cancer that develops in the esophagus near the opening into the stomach.

Anastomosis—A surgically created joining or opening between two organs or body spaces that are normally separate.

Barrett's esophagus—A potentially precancerous change in the type of cells that line the esophagus, caused by acid reflux disease.

Carcinoma—The common medical term for cancer.

Dysphagia—Difficulty and pain in swallowing.

Dysplasia—The presence of precancerous cells in body tissue.

Endoscopic ultrasound—An imaging procedure that uses high-frequency sound waves to visualize the esophagus via a lighted telescopic instrument (endoscope) and a monitor.

Esophagus—The upper portion of the digestive system, a tube that carries food and liquids from the mouth to the stomach.

Gastroesophageal reflux disease (GERD)—A condition of excess stomach acidity in which stomach acid and partially digested food flow back into the esophagus during or after eating.

Malignancy—The presence of tumor-causing cancer cells in organ tissue.

Metastasis (plural, metastases)—The spread of cancer cells from a cancerous growth or tumor into other organs of the body.

Resection—The surgical cutting and removing of a body organ, portion of an organ, or other body part.

Sphincter—A circular band of muscle fibers that constricts or closes a passageway in the body. The esophagus has sphincters at its upper and lower ends.

Squamous cell carcinoma—A type of cancer that develops in the cells in the top layer of tissue.

Thoracotomy—An open surgical procedure performed through an incision in the chest.

Thorascopy—Examination of the chest through a tiny incision using a thin lighted tube-like instrument (thorascope).

staging techniques, more careful selection of patients, and improved surgical techniques are also believed to be responsible for the increase in postoperative survival rates. Recurrence of cancer in esophagectomy patients has been shown to be about 43%. A higher percentage of patients undergoing esophageal resections survive beyond the 30-day postoperative period in hospitals where the surgeons perform these procedures on a regular basis.

Alternatives

People with Barrett's esophagus can be treated with medicine and dietary changes to reduce acid reflux disease. These nonsurgical approaches are effective in relieving heartburn, calming inflamed tissues, and preventing further cell changes.

Fundoplication, or anti-reflux surgery, can strengthen the barrier to acid regurgitation when the lower esophageal sphincter does not work properly, curing GERD and reducing the exposure of the esophagus to excessive amounts of acid.

Photodynamic therapy (PDT) is the injection of a cytotoxic (cell killing) drug in conjunction with laser

treatments, delivering benefits comparable to more established treatments. Endoscopic laser treatments that deliver short, powerful laser beams to the tumor through an endoscope can improve swallowing difficulties; however, multiple treatments are required and the benefits are neither long-lasting nor shown to prevent cancer.

Resources

BOOKS

American Cancer Society. *The American Cancer Society's Complementary and Alternative Cancer Methods Handbook*. Atlanta, GA: American Cancer Society, 2002.

Harpham, Wendy S., MD. *Diagnosis Cancer: Your Guide Through the First Few Months*. New York: W. W. Norton, Inc., 1998.

Heitmiller, R. F., et al. "Esophagus," in Martin D. Abeloff, ed., *Clinical Oncology*, 2nd ed. New York: Churchill Livingstone, 2000.

ORGANIZATIONS

American Cancer Society. 1599 Clifton Road NE, Atlanta, GA 30329. (800)ACS-2345. <www.cancer.org>.

American Gastroenterological Association. 4930 Del Ray Avenue, Bethesda, MD 20814. (301) 654-2055. <www.gastro.org>.

OTHER

Ferguson, Mark, MD. *Esophageal Cancer*. Society of Thoracic Surgeons. <www.sts.org/doc4121>.

National Cancer Institute (NCI). *General Information About Esophageal Cancer*. Bethesda, MD: NCI, 2003.

L. Lee Culvert

Esophagogastroduodenoscopy

Definition

An esophagogastroduodenoscopy (EGD), which is also known as an upper endoscopy or upper gastrointestinal endoscopy, is a diagnostic procedure that is performed to view the esophagus, stomach, and duodenum (part of the small intestine). In an EGD, the doctor uses an endoscope, a flexible, tube-like, telescopic instrument with a tiny camera mounted at its tip, to examine images of the upper digestive tract displayed on a monitor in the examination room. Small instruments may also be passed through the tube to treat certain disorders or to perform biopsies (remove small samples of tissue).

Purpose

An EGD is performed to evaluate, and sometimes to treat, such symptoms relating to the upper gastrointestinal tract as:

- pain in the chest or upper abdomen
- nausea or vomiting
- gastroesophageal reflux disease (GERD)
- difficulty swallowing (dysphagia)
- bleeding from the upper intestinal tract and related anemias

In addition, an EGD may be performed to confirm abnormalities indicated by such other diagnostic procedures as an upper gastrointestinal (upper GI) x-ray series or a CT scan. It may be used to treat certain conditions, such as an area of narrowing (stricture) or bleeding in the upper gastrointestinal tract.

Description

Upper endoscopy is considered to be more accurate than x-ray studies for detecting inflammation, ulcers, or tumors. It is used to diagnose early-stage cancer and can frequently help determine whether a growth is benign or malignant. The doctor can obtain biopsies of inflamed or suspicious tissue for examination in the laboratory by a pathologist or cytologist. Cell scrapings can also be taken by introducing a small brush through the endoscope; this technique is especially helpful in diagnosing cancer or an infection.

Besides its function as an examining tool, an endoscope has channels that permit the passage of instruments. This feature gives the physician an opportunity to treat on the spot many conditions that may be seen in the esophagus, stomach, or duodenum. These treatments may include:

- removal of polyps and other noncancerous (benign) tissue growths
- stretching narrowed areas (strictures) in the esophagus
- stopping bleeding from ulcers or blood vessels
- removing foreign objects that have been swallowed, such as coins, pins, buttons, small nails, and similar items

Some of the diseases and conditions that are investigated, identified, or treated using EGD include:

- abdominal pain
- achalasia, a defect in the muscular opening between the esophagus and the stomach
- Barrett's esophagus, a precancerous condition of the cells lining the esophagus
- Crohn's disease and inflammatory disease of the small intestine
- esophageal cancer
- gastroesophageal reflux disease (GERD), a condition caused by excess stomach acid
- hiatal hernia
- irritable bowel syndrome
- rectal bleeding
- stomach cancer
- stomach ulcers
- swallowing problems

An EGD procedure is usually performed by a gastroenterologist, who is a physician specializing in the diagnosis and treatment of disorders of the digestive tract. GI (gastrointestinal) assistants, **operating room** nurses, or technicians may be involved in the collection of samples and care of the patient. Patients will be asked to either gargle using a local anesthetic or will have an anesthetic sprayed into their mouths onto the back of the throat to numb the gag reflex. Then the endoscopist will guide the endoscope through the mouth into the upper gastrointestinal tract while the patient is lying on his or her left side. The lens or camera at the end of the instru-

KEY TERMS

Cytologist (cytology)—A medical technologist who specializes in preparing and examining biopsy specimens and cell specimens for changes that may indicate precancerous conditions or a specific stage of cancer.

Diverticulum (plural, diverticula)—A blind tubular sac or pouch created when the mucous tissue lining the esophagus or colon herniates through its muscular wall.

Duodenum—The first portion of the small intestine below the stomach.

Endoscope—A tube-like telescopic tool used to view areas of the body that cannot be directly observed, such as the esophagus, stomach, or colon, and to allow treatment of these areas.

Endoscopist—A physician or other medical professional highly trained in the use of the endoscope and related diagnostic and therapeutic procedures.

Esophagus—The hollow muscular tube that passes from the mouth to the stomach, carrying food and liquids to the stomach to be digested and absorbed.

Gastroenterologist—A physician who specializes in digestive disorders and diseases of the organs of the digestive tract, including the esophagus, stomach, and intestines.

Gastroesophageal reflux disease (GERD)—A condition of excess stomach acidity in which stomach acid and partially digested food flow back into the esophagus during or after meals.

Pathologist (pathology)—A doctor who specializes in the anatomic (structural) and pathologic (disease-causing) chemical changes in the body and the related results of diagnostic testing.

Stricture—An abnormal narrowing of the esophagus or other duct or canal in the body.

---

ment allows the endoscopist to examine each portion of the upper gastrointestinal tract by observing images on a monitor. Photographs are usually taken for reference. During the procedure, air is pumped in through the instrument to expand the structure that is being studied and allow better viewing. Biopsies and other procedures will be performed as needed. The patient's breathing will not be disturbed and there will be little if any discomfort. Many patients fall asleep during all or part of the procedure.

Some patients should not have an EGD. This examination is contraindicated in patients who have:

- severe upper gastrointestinal (UGI) bleeding

- a history of such bleeding disorders as platelet dysfunction or hemophilia

- esophageal diverticula, which are small pouches in the esophagus that can trap food or pills and become infected

- a suspected perforation (puncture or rupture) of the esophagus or stomach

- recent surgery of the upper gastrointestinal tract (throat, esophagus, stomach, pyloric valve, duodenum)

An EGD is also contraindicated for those patients who are unable to cooperate fully with the procedure or whose overall condition includes a severe underlying illness that increases the risk of complications.

Diagnosis/Preparation

Certain medications (such as **aspirin** and the anti-inflammatory drugs called NSAIDs) should be discontinued at least seven days before an EGD to reduce the risk of bleeding. Patients will be asked not to eat or drink anything for at least six to 12 hours before the procedure to ensure that the upper intestinal tract will be empty. Before the procedure, patients may be given a sedative and/or pain medication, usually by intravenous injection.

Aftercare

After the procedure, the patient will be observed in the endoscopy suite or in a separate recovery area for an hour, or until the sedative or pain medication has worn off. Someone should be available to take the patient home and stay with them for a while. Eating and drinking should be avoided until the local anesthetic has worn off in the throat and the gag reflex has returned, which may take two to four hours. To test if the gag reflex has returned, a spoon can be placed on the back of the tongue for a few seconds with light pressure to see if the patient gags. Hoarseness and a mild sore throat are normal after the procedure; the patient can drink cool fluids or gargle to relieve the soreness.

The patient may experience some bloating, belching, and flatulence after an EGD because air is introduced into the digestive tract during the procedure. To prevent any injury to the esophagus from taking medications by mouth, patients should drink at least 4 or more ounces of liquid with any pill, and remain sitting upright for 30 minutes after taking pills that are likely to cause injury. The doctor should be notified if the patient develops a fever; difficult or painful swallowing (dysphagia); breathing difficulties; or pain in the throat, chest, or abdomen.

Risks

Endoscopy is considered a safe procedure when performed by a gastroenterologist or other medical professional with special training and experience in endoscopy. The overall complication rate of EGD performance is less than 2%; many of these complications are minor, such as inflammation of the vein through which medication is given. Serious complications can and do occur, however, with almost half being related to the heart or lungs. Bleeding or perforations are also reported, especially when tumors or strictures have been treated or biopsied. Infections have been reported, though rarely; careful attention to cleaning the instrument should prevent this complication. Perforation, which is the puncture of an organ, is very rare and can be surgically repaired if it occurs during an EGD.

Normal results

The results of the procedure or probable findings are often available to the patient prior to discharge from the endoscopy suite or the recovery area. The results of tissue biopsies or cell tests (cytology) will take from 72–96 hours. Normal results will show that the esophagus, stomach and duodenum are free of strictures, ulcers or erosions, diverticula, tumors, or bleeding. Abnormal results include the presence of any of these problems, as well as esophageal infections, fissures, or tears. An increasingly common finding is medication-induced esophageal injury, caused by tablets and capsules that have lodged in the esophagus. These injuries are thought to be associated with damage to the esophageal tissue from gastrointestinal reflux disease (GERD) and the related exposure of the esophagus to large amounts of stomach acid.

Resources

BOOKS

Edmundowicz, Steven. "Endoscopy." In *The Esophagus*, 3rd ed., edited by Donald O. Castell and Joel E. Richter. Philadelphia, PA: Lippincott, 1999.
Pagana, Kathleen D., and Timothy J. Pagana. *Diagnostic Testing and Nursing Implications*, 5th ed. St. Louis, MO: Mosby, 1999.

ORGANIZATIONS

American Society for Gastrointestinal Endoscopy (ASGE). 13 Elm Street, Manchester, MA 01944-1314. (978) 526-8330. <www.asge.org>.

Society for Gastroenterology Nurses and Associates (SGNA). 401 North Michigan Avenue, Chicago, IL 60611-4267. (800) 245-7462. <www.sgna.org>.

OTHER

Johns Hopkins Consumer Guide to Medical Tests. *Upper Gastrointestinal Endoscopy*. <www.hopkinsafter50.com>.

Maggie Boleyn, RN, BSN
L. Lee Culvert

Essential surgery

Definition

Essential surgery is an operative procedure that is considered to be vitally necessary for treating a disease or injury. Postponing or deciding against an essential procedure may result in a patient's death or permanent impairment.

Description

Essential surgery may be performed on either an elective or emergency basis. **Elective surgery** is defined as surgery that can be scheduled in advance and is not considered an emergency. Some elective surgeries, however, may be considered essential. For example, an aortic aneurysm is a weak spot in the wall of the aorta, a major blood vessel. If an aortic aneurysm is found during a **physical examination** or imaging procedure, an aneurysmectomy (surgical repair of an aneurysm) may be scheduled as an elective procedure. In most cases, complications can be avoided if the aneurysm is repaired in a timely manner. If no repair is performed, however, the aneurysm may grow larger and eventually burst; this serious medical emergency is most often fatal.

In other cases, essential surgery arises out of a medical emergency, giving the patient and physician less time to prepare for surgery or seek alternatives. An example of such an emergency is appendicitis, or an infection of the appendix (a pouch-shaped organ in the abdomen). If left untreated, appendicitis may result in a ruptured appendix, which is a life-threatening condition. An **appendectomy** (surgical removal of the appendix) is usually considered essential in treating appendicitis and avoiding rupture. Another example is trauma surgery, or surgery to repair serious injuries to the body.

A surgical procedure may be optional under some circumstances and essential under others. An example is surgery for Crohn's disease, or chronic inflammation of the intestines. This condition is associated with such symp-

Townsend, Jr., ed., *Sabiston Textbook of Surgery*, 16th ed. Philadelphia, PA: W. B. Saunders Company, 2001.

KEY TERMS

Aorta—The largest artery in the body; carries oxygenated blood from the heart to the extremities and major organs.

Appendix—A pouch-shaped organ that is attached to the upper part of the large intestine.

Cosmetic surgery—Surgery that is intended to improve a patient's appearance or correct disfigurement. It is also called aesthetic surgery.

Elective surgery—Surgery that would be beneficial to the patient but is not urgent, and is therefore a matter of choice.

PERIODICALS

O'Connor, Robert. "Aneurysms, Abdominal." *eMedicine*, February 11, 2002 [cited May 18, 2003]. <www.emedicine.com/emerg/topic27.htm>.

ORGANIZATIONS

American College of Surgeons. 633 N. Saint Clair St., Chicago, IL 60611-3211. (312) 202-5000. <www.facs.org>.

American Society of Plastic Surgeons (ASPS). 444 East Algonquin Road, Arlington Heights, IL 60005. (847) 228-9900. <www.plasticsurgery.org>.

OTHER

Centers for Medicare and Medicaid Services. *The Women's Health and Cancer Rights Act*, January 20, 2003 [cited May 18, 2003]. <www.cms.hhs.gov/hipaa/hipaa1/content/whcra.asp>.

Crohn's and Colitis Foundation of America. *When is Surgery Necessary for Crohn's Disease?*, 2002 [cited May 18, 2003]. <www.ccfa.org/medcentral/library/surgery/surgcd.htm>.

Stephanie Dionne Sherk

toms as abdominal pain, fatigue, fever, loss of appetite, and weight loss. Patients who are not able to manage their symptoms with medication may choose surgical treatment (such as the removal of a segment of bowel) as a means of improving their quality of life. Without surgery, a patient's condition wouldn't necessarily deteriorate. In contrast, the presence of severe bleeding, a bowel obstruction, or a hole in the intestinal wall— all potential complications of Crohn's disease— would be considered a medical emergency. Surgery subsequently becomes necessary for preventing permanent damage or to save the patient's life.

Whether a surgical procedure is essential is important in determining whether it will be covered by health insurance. If a procedure is not considered "medically necessary" (i.e. is considered elective), most insurance companies will not pay for the procedure, or will provide only minimal coverage. A common example of an elective procedure that is not usually covered by insurance is cosmetic surgery. In some cases, however, an elective procedure is covered by health insurance because it is considered essential in improving the patient's quality of life. An example is **breast reconstruction** following mastectomy (surgical removal of the breast). While breast reconstruction is an elective procedure according to most definitions (i.e. it is not medically necessary nor considered an emergency), it is considered essential in restoring a woman's self-image following the removal of a breast for the treatment of cancer. A 1998 federal law (the Women's Health and Cancer Rights Act) states that insurance companies are required to cover breast reconstruction in patients who are covered for mastectomy.

Resources

BOOKS

Lally, Kevin P., Charles S. Cox Jr., and Richard J. Andrassy. "Appendix: Appendicitis" (Chapter 45), in Courtney M.

Excessive sweating surgery *see* **Sympathectomy**

Excimer laser photoreflective keratectomy *see* **Photorefractive keratectomy (PRK)**

Exenteration

Definition

Exenteration is a major operation during which all the contents of a body cavity are removed. Pelvic exenteration refers to the removal of the pelvic organs and adjacent structures; orbital exenteration refers to the removal of the entire eyeball, orbital soft tissues, and some or all of the eyelids.

Purpose

The pelvis is the basin-shaped cavity that contains the bladder, rectum, and reproductive organs. The internal reproductive organs include the ovaries, fallopian tubes, uterus, and cervix for women, and the prostate and various ducts and glands for men. Pelvic exenteration is performed to surgically remove cancer that involves these organs and that has not responded well to other types of treatment.

Exenteration

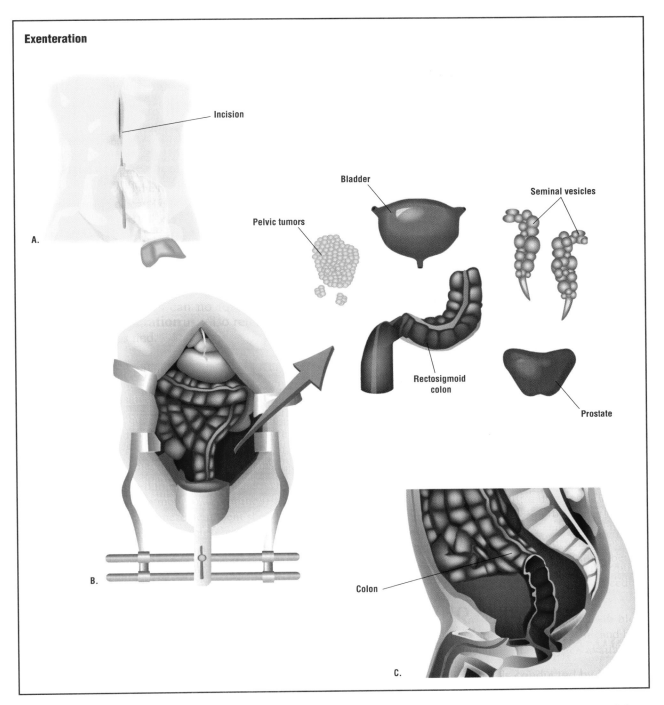

Incision

A.

Pelvic tumors

Bladder

Seminal vesicles

Rectosigmoid colon

Prostate

B.

Colon

C.

A large abdominal incision exposes abdominal and pelvic contents for pelvic exenteration (A). Contents of the lower abdominal cavity, including the rectosigmoid colon, prostate and seminal vesicles (if male), bladder, and any pelvic tumors are removed (B). *(Illustration by GGS Inc.)*

Pelvic exenteration is also indicated when cancer returns after an earlier treatment. In women, the operation is performed mostly for advanced and invasive cases of endometrial, ovarian, vaginal, and cervical cancer; for aggressive prostate cancer in men; and rectal cancer in either sex.

Orbital exenteration is performed to remove the eye and surrounding tissues when cancer of the orbital contents cannot be controlled by simple removal or irradiation. It is often the only course of treatment for advanced cancers of the eyelid, eyeball, optic nerve, or retina.

Exenteration is a major operation for both patient and surgeon; it is technically very challenging because it involves elaborate reconstructive surgery. Although it is a radical surgical procedure, exenteration often provides the only opportunity available for patients to eliminate the cancer and to prevent it from recurring.

Demographics

No data are available regarding the demographic nature of patients undergoing exenteration, given the numerous conditions that may warrant it. Cancer affects individuals of any age, sex, race, or ethnicity, although incidence may differ among these groups by cancer type.

Description

Both pelvic and orbital exenterations are considered to be major surgery and are performed under general anesthesia. The exact surgical procedure performed depends on the type of exenteration.

Pelvic exenteration

Pelvic exenterations start with an incision in the lower abdomen. Blood vessels are clamped and the organs specified by the procedure are removed. The site of incision is then stitched up. There are three types of pelvic exenteration: anterior, posterior, and total.

ANTERIOR EXENTERATION. This operation is called anterior exenteration because it removes organs toward the front of the pelvic cavity. It usually involves the removal of the female reproductive organs, bladder, and urethra. (In males, an operation that removes the bladder and prostate is called a cystoprostatectomy). Patients selected for this operation have cancers in areas that allow the rectum to be spared.

A new method for excreting urine must be created. One common approach, called an ileal conduit, diverts the ureters to a pouch made of small intestine, which is then connected to the abdominal wall. Urine exits the body through a small opening called a stoma, and collects in a small bag attached to the body. Vaginal reconstruction may also be performed during the exenteration, or in a later procedure.

POSTERIOR EXENTERATION. Posterior exenteration removes organs that are located in the back part of the pelvic cavity. These include the reproductive organs, plus the lower part of the bowel; the bladder and urethra are kept intact. A patient who has undergone posterior exenteration will require a **colostomy**, a procedure that connects the colon to the abdominal wall; waste exits the body through a stoma and is collected in a small bag.

TOTAL PELVIC EXENTERATION. This operation removes the bladder, urethra, rectum, anus, and supporting muscles and ligaments, together with the reproductive organs. Total pelvic exenteration is performed when there is no opportunity to perform a less extensive operation, because of the location and size of the cancer. A urinary stoma and a colostomy stoma will be created to collect waste.

Orbital exenteration

This operation removes the eyeball and surrounding tissues of the orbit. (Since the eye is surrounded by bone, orbital exenteration is often easier to tolerate than pelvic exenteration.) Orbital exenteration with partial preservation of eyelids and conjunctiva can sometimes be achieved. After the surgical site has healed, patients can be fitted with a temporary ocular prosthesis (plastic eye), although many patients prefer to wear an eye patch. Later, facial prostheses can be attached to the facial skeleton.

Diagnosis/Preparation

The evaluation of patients before pelvic exenteration includes a thorough physical examination with rectal and pelvic examination. Endorectal ultrasound and imaging studies such as computed tomography scans (**CT scans**) and **magnetic resonance imaging** (MRI) are routinely used to obtain pictures of the abdominal and pelvic areas and evaluate the spread of the cancer.

Ocular ultrasound examination, CT scan, and **angiography** evaluation (used to image blood vessels) are usually performed to prepare for orbital exenteration.

Some patients begin treatment with chemotherapy and/or radiation before the procedure. Surgery is typically performed approximately six weeks later.

In the case of pelvic exenteration, the patient will be given a bowel prep to cleanse the colon and prepare it for surgery. This procedure is required to lower the level of intestinal bacteria, thus helping to prevent post-surgical infections. **Antibiotics** are also typically given to help decrease bacteria levels in the bowel.

Aftercare

Pelvic exenteration

After a pelvic exenteration, a drainage tube is inserted at the site of the incision. There usually is some bleeding, discharge, and considerable tenderness and pain for a few days. At least a three- to five-day hospital stay is usually required. Side effects depend on the type of pelvic exenteration performed, but often include urination difficulty, especially if adjustment to a catheter is required; and a very painful lower abdomen.

Stitches are usually removed from the skin on the third day, or before the patient is sent home. A prescription for pain medication is usually given as well as instructions for follow-up care.

Ocular exenteration

After ocular exenteration, most patients have a headache for several days, which goes away with over-the-counter pain medications. An eye ointment is also prescribed that contains antibiotics and steroids to help the healing process.

Risks

As with any operation, there is a risk of complications due to anesthesia, wound infection, or injury to adjacent organs or structures.

In the case of pelvic exenteration, the following complications are also possible:

• hemorrhage that may require a blood transfusion
• injury to the bowel
• urinary tract infection
• urinary retention requiring permanent use of a catheter
• bowel obstruction

After removal of the reproductive organs, women will no longer have monthly periods nor will they be able to become pregnant. For men, surgery involving the prostate and the nerves around the rectum may also result in the inability to produce sperm or to have an erection.

In the case of orbital exenteration, the following complications have been known to occur:

• growth of an orbital cyst (rare)
• chronic throbbing orbital pain
• sinusitis (nasal stuffiness)

• ear problems
• reoccurrence of malignancy

Normal results

During and after recovery from exenteration, it is normal for a patient to undergo a period of psychological adjustment to the major change in lifestyle (e.g., learning to care for a urostomy or colostomy) or appearance (e.g., following orbital exenteration). It is important that all aspects of the procedure be discussed with the patient before undergoing surgery, and that any psychosocial distress that the patient experiences after exenteration be addressed.

Morbidity and mortality rates

There is a 30–44% chance of complications during pelvic exenteration, and the operative mortality rate ranges from 3–5%. About one-third of patients will experience such postoperative complications as bowel obstruction, fistula formation, inflammation or failure of the kidneys, narrowing of the ureters, or pulmonary embolism (a blood clot that travels to the lungs). The five-year survival rate after pelvic exenteration ranges from 23–61%. For patients who undergo pelvic or orbital exenteration, short- and long-term morbidity and mortality rates depend on the particular condition that required the procedure.

Alternatives

Exenteration is generally pursued only if no other less invasive options are available to the patient. Alternatives, however, include chemotherapy, radiation therapy, and more conservative surgery.

KEY TERMS

Anus—The terminal orifice of the gastrointestinal (GI) or digestive tract that includes all organs responsible for getting food in and out of the body.

Catheter—Long thin tubes that carry urine from the kidneys to the bladder.

Conjunctiva—A clear membrane that covers the inside of the eyelids and the outer surface of the eye.

General anesthesia—Method used to stop pain from being felt during an operation. General anesthesia is generally used only for such major operations as brain, neck, chest, abdomen, and pelvis surgery.

Ocular orbit—Bony cavity containing the eyeball.

Rectum—The last part of the large intestine (colon) that connects to the anus.

Resection—The complete or partial removal of an organ or tissue.

Resources

BOOKS

Yanoff, Myron, and Jay Duker. *Ophthalmology,* 1st ed. London: Mosby International Ltd., 1999.

PERIODICALS

Clarke, A., N. Rumsey, J. R. O. Collin, and M. Wyn-Williams. "Psychosocial Distress Associated with Disfiguring Eye Conditions." *Eye* 17, no. 1 (January 2003): 35–40.

Ramamoorthy, Sonia L., and James W. Fleshman. "Surgical Treatment of Rectal Cancer." *Hematology/Oncology Clinics of North America* 16, no. 4 (August 2002): 927.

Sevin, B. U., and O. R. Koechlie. "Pelvic Exenteration." *Surgical Clinics of North America* 81, no. 4 (August 1, 2001): 771–9.

Turns, D. "Psychosocial Issues: Pelvic Exenterative Surgery." *Journal of Surgical Oncology* 76 (March 2001): 224–36.

ORGANIZATIONS

American Academy of Ophthalmology. P.O. Box 7424, San Francisco, CA 94120-7424. (415) 561-8500. <http://www.aao.org>.

American Cancer Society. 1599 Clifton Road NE, Atlanta, GA 30329. (800) ACS-2345. <http://www.cancer.org>.

American College of Obstetricians and Gynecologists. 409 12th St., SW, P.O. Box 96920, Washington, DC 20090-6920. <http://www.acog.org>.

OTHER

Husain, Amreen, and Nelson Teng. "Pelvic Exenteration." *eMedicine,* January 31, 2003 [cited April 5, 2003]. <http://www.emedicine.com/med/topic3332.htm>.

Monique Laberge, PhD
Stephanie Dionne Sherk

Exercise

Definition

The Surgeon General of the United States defines exercise as physical activity that involves planned, structured, and repetitive bodily movements in order to improve or maintain physical fitness. As an element of health, exercise involves both strength training of the muscles and cardiovascular fitness, with stretching activities for flexibility. Most research on physical activity for fitness stresses the intensity and regularity of exercise as key elements. Typical exercise activities include fast walking, running, cycling, swimming, or aerobics classes. The latest Centers for Disease Control and Prevention report, in conjunction with the American Council on Sports Medicine, recommends that all adults perform 30 or more minutes a day of moderate-intensity activity for 5–7 days per week. The National Institutes of Health Consensus Development Conference Statement on Physical Activity and Cardiovascular Health identifies inactivity as a major public health problem in the United States. They have recommended exercise regimens 5–7 days a week for people who are already active, and such leisure activities as gardening, walking, using stairs instead of an elevator, cleaning house and recreational pursuits etc., for people who are largely sedentary.

Purpose

One important purpose of exercise is speeding recovery from surgery. Nowhere is being fit as important as when a person is facing surgery or recovering from surgery. Regular exercise leads to important health advantages, including weight loss; greater cardiovascular efficiency; lower cholesterol levels; increased musculoskeletal strength and flexibility; and better functioning of the metabolic, endocrine and immune systems. These effects diminish with lack of exercise within two weeks if physical activity is substantially reduced; the fitness effects disappear altogether within two to eight months if physical activity is not resumed.

With regard to **preparing for surgery**, the effects of regular exercise on all body systems create optimal responses both to the surgical procedures itself and during the postoperative recovery period.

Demographics

Most adults in North America would benefit from increasing their level of physical activity. The majority of adults in the United States (55%) are overweight, and two-thirds of those with weight problems are likely also to have diabetes, heart disease, high blood pressure, or

Exercise can be used to restore muscle strength after surgery. A computer monitors this man's performance and provides a visual display of his progress. *(Photograph by Geoff Tompkinson. Science Source/Photo Researchers. Reproduced by permission.)*

other obesity-related conditions. A sedentary lifestyle and unhealthy eating patterns are responsible for at least 300,000 deaths each year from chronic diseases. It is estimated that two-thirds of people over 65 have at least one chronic condition, with 36 million Americans suffering from some form of arthritis. More than 300,000 total joint replacement procedures are performed each year due to osteoarthritis. Lack of physical activity contributes substantially to conditions like osteoarthritis, low back pain, and osteoporosis.

Obesity reached epidemic proportions among adults in the United States in the years between 1987 and 2000. Over 45 million adults are obese; in addition, the percentage of young people who are overweight has more than doubled in the last 20 years. Despite the benefits of physical activity, more than 60% of American adults do not get enough physical activity to provide health benefits. More than 25% are not active in their leisure time. Insufficient activity increases with age; it is also more common in women than men and among those with lower levels of economic stability and educational achievement.

The direct consequences of obesity include:

• Heart disease and stroke, the leading causes of death and disability in the United States.

• Type 2 diabetes (also known as NIDDM, or non-insulin-dependent diabetes mellitus).

• Cancer. Obesity increases the risk of cancer of the uterus, gallbladder, cervix, ovary, breast, and colon in women; it increases the risk of cancer of the colon, rectum, and prostate in men.

• Osteoarthritis. Obesity adds to daily "wear and tear" on joints, primarily the knees, as well as the hips and lower back.

• Gallbladder disease. The risk of gallbladder disease and gallstones increases as a person's weight increases.

• Stress incontinence in women, especially those over 65 years old.

• Gastroesophageal reflux disease (GERD).

Diagnosis/Preparation

Over 25 million Americans will undergo surgery in 2003. Each patient's surgical risk, complications and outcomes will depend upon how fit they are; how well their cardiovascular and pulmonary systems withstand the stress of anesthesia; how quickly their bones and muscles recover after surgical procedures; and how well their metabolic and immune systems respond to surgery and the risk of infection. The general physical status of the patient is the most important factor in preparing for surgery. This status is determined by the physician, including his or her evaluation of the specific procedures to be performed. On the other hand, however, the patient's lifestyle may affect management of the surgery both before and after the actual procedures. A healthful diet, regular exercise, and quitting smoking are highly recommended before surgery. Each of these factors has an important role to play in optimal functioning of the circulatory and pulmonary systems. Smoking should cease two weeks before surgery to be beneficial.

Aftercare

After surgery, it is important to return to daily activities when the physician gives permission to do so. Most doctors encourage their patients to be as active as possible as soon as possible. While aftercare is individualized, and physicians may place certain limitations on physical activity for specific patients, walking as soon as the patient is able to walk is generally recommended. The patient should be as active as possible within the limits set by the physician for postoperative recovery, with the goal of returning to his or her normal daily activities and exercise routines. The patient should ask the physician for explicit guidelines about returning to an established exercise program or other physical or recreational activities.

Risks

The benefits of exercise before, after surgery and continuing as a daily life activity cannot be overemphasized. There are risks, however, for people who begin an exercise program without having had one in the past. Patients should always have a **physical examination** before taking up an exercise program for the first time or after a long period of inactivity.

Such high-intensity exercise regimens as high-impact aerobics and jogging are not recommended as often as they once were for helping patients attain a specific fitness level as measured by resting heart rate and muscle mass. Walking, swimming, and gardening can all contribute to aerobic fitness. Strength training with resistance exercises for the arms and legs using weights or bands is now an important aspect of physical fitness. These exercises can be done at a moderate rate, with the number of repetitions increased over time. Stretching is very important to both kinds of exercise activities.

Morbidity and mortality rates

Without exercise and a healthful diet, people burn fewer calories than they take in, resulting in increasing weight gain. While the formula is familiar, the outcomes are surprising. According to studies based on a newer index for obesity—the body mass index or BMI—people who are overweight or obese have dramatically shorter life spans. In fact, some studies are showing that individuals who are fat in middle age are as likely to lose years of life as those who smoke. Researchers have found obesity and overweight combined are the second leading cause of preventable death in the United States, behind tobacco use. Correlating the BMI—calculated from a person's weight in kilograms divided by height in meters squared—and the mortality of different cohorts of subjects in large longitudinal studies, researchers have found that the lowest mortality rates from all causes were found among those having a BMI between 23.5 and 24.9 for men and 22.0–23.4 for women. The strongest association between obesity and death from all causes are found among individuals with the highest BMI—people with a BMI of 40+. Clinical obesity is defined as a BMI of 30 or above. Morbid obesity is defined as a BMI of 40 or above.

With respect to health care, people who are obese have higher rates of complications in the hospital. Researchers in New York studied a group of patients who were in the **intensive care unit** (ICU) for a variety of causes, and found that those who were morbidly obese were far more likely to die of their illness than those who were closer to their desirable weight (23.3% vs. 6.1%). Patients who were morbidly obese had higher rates of transferrals to **nursing homes** from the ICU, rather than being discharged to their homes—over 16% for the obese patients compared to 3% for patients who were less overweight.

Resources

BOOKS

"Nutritional Disorders: Obesity." Section 1, Chapter 5 in *The Merck Manual of Diagnosis and Therapy*, edited by Mark

KEY TERMS

Aerobic exercise—Any type of exercise that is intended to increase the body's oxygen consumption and improve the functioning of the cardiovascular and respiratory systems.

Body mass index (BMI)—A measurement that has replaced weight as the preferred determinant of obesity. The BMI can be calculated (in English units) as 703.1 times a person's weight in pounds divided by the square of the person's height in inches.

Obesity—Excessive weight gain due to accumulation of fat in the body, sometimes defined as a BMI of 30 or higher, or body weight greater than 30% above one's desirable weight on standard height-weight tables.

Physical activity—Any activity that involves moving the body and results in the burning of calories.

Physical fitness—The combination of muscle strength and cardiovascular health usually attributed to regular exercise and good nutrition.

Sedentary—Characterized by inactivity and lack of exercise. A sedentary lifestyle is a major risk factor for becoming overweight or obese.

H. Beers, MD, and Robert Berkow, MD. Whitehouse Station, NJ: Merck Research Laboratories, 1999.

Report of the Surgeon General. *Physical Activity and Health.* Centers for Disease Control and Prevention, National Center for Chronic Disease Prevention and Health Promotion, The President's Council on Physical Fitness and Sports, 1996. <www.sgreports.nlm.nih.gov >

PERIODICALS

Bolliger, C. T. "Evaluation of Operability Before Lung Resection." *Current Opinion in Pulmonary Medicine* 9 (July 2003): 321-326.

Cummings, S., E. S. Parham, and G. W. Strain. "Position of the American Dietetic Association: Weight Management." *Journal of the American Dietetic Association* 102 (August 2002): 1145-1155.

Morey, M. C., and C. W. Zhu. "Improved Fitness Narrows the Symptom-Reporting Gap Between Older Men and Women." *Journal of Women's Health (Larchmont)* 12 (May 2003): 381-390.

Pollock, M. L., et al. "Resistance Exercise in Individuals With and Without Cardiovascular Disease: American Heart Association Advisory." *Circulation* 101 (February 22, 2000): 828-833.

Wallace, J. "Exercise in Hypertension: A Clinical Review." *Journal of Sports Medicine* 33 (2003): 585-598.

ORGANIZATIONS

Shape Up America! c/o WebFront Solutions Corporation, 15757 Crabbs Branch Way, Rockville, MD 20855. (301) 258-0540. <www.shapeup.org>.

Weight-control Information Network (WIN). 1 WIN Way, Bethesda, MD 20892-3665. (202) 828-1025 or (877) 946-4627.

OTHER

Agency for Health Care Practice and Research. *Assessing a Patient's Willingness to Adopt Dietary and Lifestyle Changes is the First Step Toward Sustained Weight Loss.* Research Archives, No. 237 (May 2000). <www.ahcpr.gov/research/may00/050.>

American Association of Orthopaedic Surgeons. *People With Chronic Conditions Benefit from Daily Exercise.* <www.aaos.org/wordhtml/home2.htm,>

National Center for Chronic Disease Prevention and Health Promotion, Centers for Disease Control and Prevention. *Nutrition and Physical Activity.* <www.cdc.gov/nccdphp/dnpa/physical/index.htm.>

Nancy McKenzie, PhD

Exercise electrocardiogram *see* **Stress test**

Exercise stress test *see* **Stress test**

Exploratory laparotomy *see* **Laparotomy, exploratory**

Extracapsular cataract extraction

Definition

Extracapsular cataract extraction (ECCE) is a category of eye surgery in which the lens of the eye is removed while the elastic capsule that covers the lens is left partially intact to allow implantation of an intraocular lens (IOL). This approach is contrasted with intracapsular cataract extraction (ICCE), an older procedure in which the surgeon removed the complete lens within its capsule and left the eye aphakic (without a lens). The patient's vision was corrected after intracapsular extraction by extremely thick eyeglasses or by contact lenses.

There are two major types of ECCE: manual expression, in which the lens is removed through an incision made in the cornea or the sclera of the eye; and phacoemulsification, in which the lens is broken into fragments inside the capsule by ultrasound energy and removed by aspiration.

Purpose

Historical background

The purpose of ECCE is to restore clear vision by removing a clouded or discolored lens and replacing it with an IOL. Cataract operations are among the oldest recorded surgical procedures; there are references to cataract surgery in the Code of Hammurabi in 1750 B.C. and in the treatises written around 600 B.C. by Susruta, a famous surgeon from India. In the ancient world, lenses damaged by cataracts were dislocated rather than removed in the strict sense; the surgeon used a lance to push the clouded lens backward into the vitreous body of the eye. This operation, known as couching, was standard practice until the mid-eighteenth century. Couching is still performed by some traditional healers in Africa and parts of Asia.

The first extracapsular extraction of a cataract was performed by a French surgeon named Jacques Daviel in 1753. Daviel removed the lens through a fairly long incision in the cornea of the eye. In 1865, the German ophthalmologist Albrecht von Graefe refined the operation by removing the lens through a much smaller linear incision in the sclera of the eye. After von Graefe, however, intracapsular extraction gradually became the favored method of cataract removal even though it left the patient without a lens inside the eye. The two inventions that made extracapsular extraction preferable again were the operating microscope and the intraocular lens. The first eye surgery performed with an operating microscope was done in Portland, Oregon, in 1948; in the same year, a British ophthalmologist named Harold Ridley implanted the first IOL in the eye of a cataract patient. Between 1948 and the 1980s, manual expression was the standard form of ECCE. Although phacoemulsification was first introduced in 1967, it was not widely accepted at first because it requires special techniques that take time for the surgeon to learn as well as expensive specialized equipment. As of 2003, phacoemulsification is now performed more often in the United States and Europe than "standard" ECCE. The manual expression technique, however, is still widely used in developing countries with large numbers of patients with eye disorders and limited hospital budgets.

The lens and cataract formation

To understand cataract surgery, it is helpful to have a basic description of the structure of the lens in the human eye. The lens, which is sometimes called the crystalline lens because it is transparent, is located immediately behind the iris. In humans, the lens is about 9 mm long and 4 mm wide. It consists of protein fibers and water, with the fibers arranged in a pattern that allows light to pass through the lens. There are three layers of cells in the lens: a central nucleus, which becomes denser and harder as a person ages; a cortex surrounding the nucleus, which contains cells that are metabolically active and continue to grow and divide; and a layer of cells between the cortex and the lens capsule known as the subcapsular epithelium.

Although a few people are born with cataracts or develop them in childhood, most cataracts are the result of the aging process. As people grow older, the protein fibers in the lens become denser, start to clump together, and form cloudy or opaque areas in the lens. Cataracts vary considerably in their speed of progression; they may develop in a few months or over a period of many years. Some people have cataracts that stop growing at an early stage of development and do not interfere with their vision. Although most people develop cataracts in both eyes, they do not usually progress at the same rate, so that the person has much better vision in one eye than in the other.

Ophthalmologists classify cataracts according to their location in the lens. It is possible for a person to have more than one type of cataract.

- Nuclear cataracts. Nuclear cataracts grow slowly over many years but can become very large and hard, which complicates their removal. They are sometimes called brunescent cataracts because they are characterized by deposits of brown pigment that give the lens an amber color. Nuclear cataracts are most commonly associated with age and with smoking as risk factors.

- Cortical cataracts. Cataracts in the cortex of the lens develop more rapidly than nuclear cataracts but remain softer and are easier to remove. They are thought to be caused by an increase in the water content of the lens. Risk factors for cortical cataracts include female sex and African or Caribbean heritage.

- Posterior subcapsular (PSC) cataracts. This type of cataract, which develops between the back of the lens and the lens capsule, is the softest and most rapidly growing type. PSC cataracts tend to scatter light at night and thus interfere with nighttime driving. Risk factors for PSC cataracts include diabetes and a history of treatment with steroid medications.

Demographics

Cataract extraction is one of the most frequently performed surgical procedures in industrialized countries. It is estimated that 300,000–400,000 cases of visually disabling cataracts occur each year in the United States alone, and that between 1 and 1.5 million cataract extractions are performed annually in the United States. This frequency reflects the importance of cataracts as a

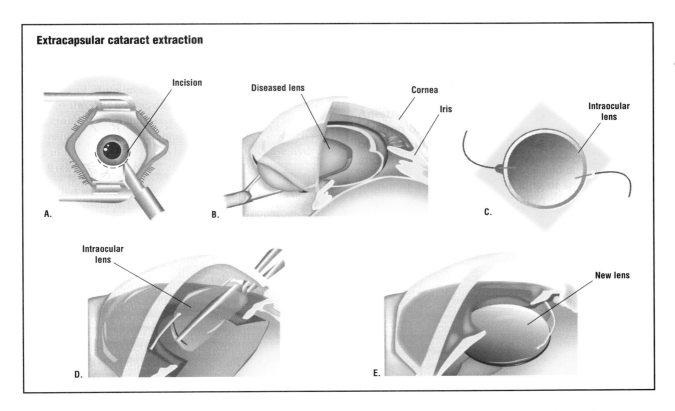

Extracapsular cataract extraction

In extracapsular cataract extraction, an incision is made in the eye just beneath the iris, or colored part (A). The diseased lens is pulled out (B). A prosthetic intraocular lens is placed through the incision (D), and is opened to replace the old lens (E). *(Illustration by GGS Inc.)*

major public health problem. The World Health Organization (WHO) estimated in 1997 that cataracts are responsible for 50% of cases of blindness around the world, or 19 million people. By 2020, that figure is expected to rise to 50 million. More recent publications estimate that 1.2% of the general population of Africa is blind, with cataracts responsible for 36% of these cases of blindness.

About one person in every 50 in the general American population will eventually have to have a cataract removed. It is difficult, however, to compare the rates of cataract formation among various subgroups because present published studies use a number of different grading systems for defining and detecting cataracts. In addition, the elderly are often under-represented in general population studies even though age is the greatest single risk factor for cataract development. Three recent research projects carried out in the United States, Australia, and England, respectively, reported that 50% of people over the age of 60 have some degree of cataract formation, with the figure rising to 100% for those over 80. As of 2003, little conclusive information is available regarding the incidence of cataracts in different racial and ethnic groups in the United States.

A variety of risk factors in addition to age have been associated with cataracts, but their precise significance is debated among researchers:

- Genetic factors. Twin studies show that the identical twin of a patient with a nuclear cataract has a 48% chance of developing one.

- Sex. Women are slightly more likely than men to develop cataracts. One American study found that 53.3% of women over 60 had nuclear cataracts compared to 49.7% of the men; 25.9% of the women had cortical cataracts versus 21.1% of the men.

- Exposure to ultraviolet radiation. Cortical cataracts are more likely to develop in people with frequent exposure to sunlight; however, nuclear cataracts are not related to sun exposure.

- Smoking. People who smoke more than 25 cigarettes per day are three times as likely as nonsmokers to develop nuclear or PSC cataracts. Smoking does not appear to be related to cortical cataracts.

- Alcohol consumption. Heavy drinking has been reported to increase the risk of developing all three types of cataracts.

- Diabetes. Patients with diabetes are at increased risk of developing all three types of cataracts.

- Use of steroid medications. PSC cataracts are known to be induced by steroids, even though they represent less than 10% of all cataracts.

- Socioeconomic status (SES). People with college or professional-school education have lower rates of cataract formation than people who did not finish high school, even attempting to correct for environmental and nutritional factors. There is, however, no obvious biochemical or medical explanation for this correlation, and some researchers treat it with caution.

- Chronic dehydration, diarrhea, and malnutrition. Studies carried out in India indicate that severe malnutrition or repeated episodes of diarrhea in childhood carry a three- to fourfold increase in risk of developing cataracts in later life. It is not yet known, however, whether this statistic would hold true for people in other countries.

Description

Conventional extracapsular cataract extraction

Although phacoemulsification has become the preferred method of extracapsular extraction for most cataracts in the United States since the 1990s, conventional or standard ECCE is considered less risky for patients with very hard cataracts or weak epithelial tissue in the cornea. The ultrasound vibrations that are used in phacoemulsification tend to stress the cornea.

A conventional extracapsular cataract extraction takes less than an hour to perform. After the area around the eye has been cleansed with antiseptic, sterile drapes are used to cover most of the patient's face. The patient is given either a local anesthetic to numb the tissues around the eye or a topical anesthetic to numb the eye itself. An eyelid holder is used to hold the eye open during the procedure. If the patient is very nervous, the doctor may administer a sedative intravenously.

After the anesthetic has taken effect, the surgeon makes an incision in the cornea at the point where the sclera and cornea meet. Although the typical length of a standard ECCE incision was 10–12 mm in the 1970s, the development of foldable acrylic IOLs has allowed many surgeons to work with incisions that are only 5–6 mm long. This variation is sometimes referred to as small-incision ECCE. After the incision is made, the surgeon makes a circular tear in the front of the lens capsule; this technique is known as capsulorrhexis. The surgeon then carefully opens the lens capsule and removes the hard nucleus of the lens by applying pressure with special instruments. After the nucleus has been expressed, the surgeon uses suction to remove the softer cortex of the lens. A special

viscoelastic material is injected into the empty lens capsule to help it keep its shape while the surgeon inserts the IOL. After the intraocular lens has been placed in the correct position, the viscoelastic substance is removed and the incision is closed with two or three stitches.

Phacoemulsification

In phacoemulsification, the surgeon uses an ultrasound probe inserted through the incision to break up the nucleus of the lens into smaller pieces. The newer technique offers the advantages of a smaller incision than standard ECCE, fewer or no stitches to close the incision, and a shorter recovery time for the patient. Its disadvantages are the need for specialized equipment and a steep learning curve for the surgeon. One study found that surgeons needed to perform about 150 cataract extractions using phacoemulsification before their complication rates fell to a baseline level.

Diagnosis/Preparation

Diagnosis

The diagnosis of cataract is usually made when the patient begins to notice changes in his or her vision and consults an eye specialist. In contrast to certain types of glaucoma, there is no pain associated with the development of cataracts. The specific changes in the patient's vision depend on the type and location of the cataract. Nuclear cataracts typically produce symptoms known as myopic shift (in nearsighted patients) and second sight (in farsighted patients). What these terms mean is that the nearsighted person becomes more nearsighted while the farsighted person's near vision improves to the point that there is less need for reading glasses. Cortical and posterior subcapsular cataracts typically reduce visual acuity; in addition, the patient may also complain of increased glare in bright daylight or glare from the headlights of oncoming cars at night.

Because visual disturbances may indicate glaucoma as well as cataracts, particularly in older adults, the examiner will first check the intraocular pressure (IOP) and the anterior chamber of the patient's eye. The examiner will also look closely at the patient's medical history and general present physical condition for indications of diabetes or other systemic disorders that affect cataract development. The next step in the diagnostic examination is a test of the patient's visual acuity for both near and far distances, commonly known as the Snellen test. If the patient has mentioned glare, the Snellen test will be conducted in a brightly lit room.

The examiner will then check the patient's eyes with a slit lamp in order to evaluate the location and size of the cataract. After the patient's eyes have been dilated with eye drops, the slit lamp can also be used to check the other structures of the eye for any indications of metabolic disorders or previous eye injury. Lastly, the examiner will use an ophthalmoscope to evaluate the condition of the optic nerve and retina at the back of the eye. The ophthalmoscope can also be used to detect the presence of very small cataracts.

Imaging studies of the eye (ultrasound, MRI, or CT scan) may be ordered if the doctor cannot see the back of the eye because of the size and density of the cataract.

Preparation

ECCE is almost always elective surgery—emergency removal of a cataract is performed only when the cataract is causing glaucoma or the eye is severely injured or infected. After the surgery has been scheduled, the patient will need to have special testing known as keratometry if an IOL is to be implanted. The testing, which is painless, is done to determine the strength of the IOL needed. The ophthalmologist measures the length of the patient's eyeball with ultrasound and the curvature of the cornea with a device called a keratometer. The measurements obtained by the keratometer are entered into a computer that calculates the correct power for the IOL.

The IOL is a substitute for the lens in the patient's eye, not for corrective lenses. If the patient was wearing eyeglasses or contact lenses before the cataract developed, he or she will continue to need them after the IOL is implanted. The lens prescription should be checked after surgery, however, as it is likely to need adjustment.

Aftercare

Patients can use their eyes after ECCE, although they should have a friend or relative drive them home after the procedure. The ophthalmologist will place some medications—usually steroids and antibiotics—in the operated eye before the patient leaves the office. Patients can go to work the next day, although the operated eye will take between three weeks and three months to heal completely. At the end of this period, they should have their regular eyeglasses checked to see if their lens prescription should be changed. Patients can carry out their normal activities within one to two days of surgery, with the exception of heavy lifting or extreme bending. Most ophthalmologists recommend that patients wear their eyeglasses during the day and tape an eye shield over the operated eye at night. They should wear sunglasses on bright days and avoid rubbing or bumping the operated eye. In addition, the ophthalmologist will prescribe eye drops for one to two weeks to prevent infection, manage

pain, and reduce swelling. It is important for patients to use these eye drops exactly as directed.

Patients recovering from cataract surgery will be scheduled for frequent checkups in the first few weeks following ECCE. In most cases, the ophthalmologist will check the patient's eye the day after surgery and about once a week for the next several weeks.

About 25% of patients who have had a cataract removed by either extracapsular method will eventually develop clouding in the lens capsule that was left in place to hold the new IOL. This clouding, which is known as posterior capsular opacification or PCO, is not a new cataract but may still interfere with vision. It is thought to be caused by the growth of epithelial cells left behind after the lens was removed. PCO is treated by capsulotomy, which is a procedure in which the surgeon uses a laser to cut through the clouded part of the capsule.

Risks

The risks of extracapsular cataract extraction include:

• Edema (swelling) of the cornea.

QUESTIONS TO ASK THE DOCTOR

- What type of cataract do I have and how fast is it developing?
- Would you recommend watchful waiting to see if surgery is necessary?
- How many cataract extractions do you perform each year, and what technique do you use?
- What is your success rate with cataract extractions?

- A rise in intraocular pressure (IOP).

- Uveitis. Uveitis refers to inflammation of the layer of eye tissue that includes the iris.

- Infection. Infection of the external eye may develop into endophthalmitis, or infection of the interior of the eye.

- Hyphema. Hyphema refers to the presence of blood inside the anterior chamber of the eye and is most common within the first two to three days after cataract surgery.

- Leaking or rupture of the incision.

- Retinal detachment or tear.

- Malpositioning of the IOL. This complication can be corrected by surgery.

- Cystoid macular edema (CME). The macula is a small yellowish depression on the retina that may be affected after cataract surgery by fluid collecting within the tissue layers. The patient typically experiences blurring or distortion of central vision. CME rarely causes loss of sight but may take between two and 15 months to resolve completely.

Normal results

Extracapsular cataract extraction is one of the safest and most successful procedures in contemporary eye surgery; about 95% of patients report that their vision is substantially improved after the operation. In the words of a British ophthalmologist, "The only obstacle lying between cataract sufferers and surgical cure is resource allocation."

Morbidity and mortality rates

Mortality as a direct result of cataract surgery is very rare. On the other hand, several studies have indicated that patients over the age of 50 who undergo cataract extraction have higher rates of mortality in the year follow-ing surgery than other patients in the same age group who have other types of **elective surgery**. Some researchers have interpreted these data to imply that cataracts related to the aging process reflect some kind of systemic weakness rather than a disorder limited to the eye.

About 23% of patients who have undergone cataract extraction have a postoperative complication. The majority of these, however, are not vision-threatening. The most common complication is swelling of the cornea (9.5%), followed by raised IOP (7.9%); uveitis (5.6%); leaking from the incision (1.2%); hyphema (1.1%); external eye infection (0.06%); endophthalmitis (0.03%); retinal detachment (0.03%); retinal tear (0.02%), and CME (0.017%). Of these complications, only endophthalmitis and retinal detachment or tear are considered potentially vision-threatening.

Standard ECCE and phacoemulsification have very similar success rates and complication rates when performed by surgeons of comparable skill and length of experience.

Alternatives

Medical treatment

As of 2003 there are no medications that can prevent or cure cataracts. Many ophthalmologists, however, recommend a well-balanced diet as beneficial to the eyes as well as the rest of the body, on the grounds that some studies suggest that poor nutritional status is a risk factor for cataract. While vitamin supplements do not prevent cataracts, there is some evidence that an adequate intake of vitamins A, C, and E helps to slow the rate of cataract progression. Elderly people who may be at risk of inadequate vitamin intake due to loss of appetite and other reasons may benefit from supplemental doses of these vitamins.

Watchful waiting

Not all cataracts need to be removed. A patient whose cataracts are not interfering with his or her normal activities and are progressing slowly may choose to postpone surgery indefinitely. It is important, however, to have periodic checkups to make sure that the cataract is not growing in size or density. In the recent past, surgeons often advised patients to put off surgical treatment until the cataract had "ripened," which meant that the patient had to wait until the cataract had caused significant vision loss and was interfering with reading, driving, and most daily activities. At present, ophthalmologists prefer to remove cataracts before they get to this stage because they are harder and consequently more difficult to remove. In addition, a rapidly growing cataract that is not

KEY TERMS

Acuity—Sharpness or clarity of vision.

Aphakic—Without a lens. An older form of cataract surgery known as intracapsular extraction left patients' eyes aphakic.

Aspiration—Removal by suction.

Brunescent—Developing a brownish or amber color over time. Nuclear cataracts are sometimes called brunescent.

Capsulorrhexis—The creation of a continuous circular tear in the front portion of the lens capsule during cataract surgery to allow for removal of the lens nucleus.

Capsulotomy—A procedure that is sometimes needed after ECCE to open a lens capsule that has become cloudy.

Cataract—A cloudy or opaque area on or in the lens of the eye.

Cornea—The transparent front portion of the exterior cover of the eye.

Couching—The oldest form of cataract surgery, in which the lens is dislocated and pushed backward into the vitreous body with a lance.

Endophthalmitis—An infection on the inside of the eye that may result in vision loss.

Hyphema—Bleeding inside the anterior chamber of the eye.

Keratometer—A device that measures the curva-

ture of the cornea. It is used to determine the correct power for an IOL prior to cataract surgery.

Lens capsule—A clear elastic membrane-like structure that covers the lens of the eye.

Macula—A small yellowish depression on the retina of the eye slightly below the optic disk that is the central point of sharpest vision. Its primary function is the absorption of shorter wavelengths of light.

Ophthalmology—The branch of medicine that deals with the diagnosis and treatment of eye disorders.

Phacoemulsification—A method of extracapsular cataract extraction in which the lens is broken apart by ultrasound energy and the fragments removed by suction.

Sclera—The tough white fibrous membrane that forms the outermost covering of the eyeball.

Uvea—The middle of the three coats of tissue surrounding the eye, comprising the choroid, iris, and ciliary body. The uvea is pigmented and well supplied with blood vessels.

Uveitis—Inflammation of any part of the uvea.

Vitreous body—The transparent gel that fills the inner portion of the eyeball between the lens and the retina. It is also called the vitreous humor or crystalline humor.

treated surgically may lead to swelling of the lens, secondary glaucoma, and eventual blindness. In most cases, however, it is up to the patient to decide when the cataract is troublesome enough to schedule surgery.

Surgical alternatives

The major surgical alternative to ECCE is intracapsular cataract extraction, or ICCE. It is rarely performed at present in Europe and North America, but is still done in countries where operating microscopes and high-technology equipment are not always available. In ICCE, the surgeon makes an incision about 150 degrees of arc, or about half the circumference of the cornea, in order to extract the lens and its capsule in one piece. The surgeon then inserts a cryoprobe, which is an instrument for applying extreme cold to eye tissue. The cryoprobe is placed on the lens capsule, where it freezes into place. It is then used to slowly pull the capsule and lens together

through the long incision around the cornea. Because of the length of the incision needed to perform ICCE and the pressure placed on the vitreous body, the procedure has a relatively high rate of complications. In addition, the recovery period is much longer than for standard ECCE or phacoemulsification.

See also Cryotherapy for cataracts; Phacoemulsification for cataracts.

Resources

BOOKS

"Cataract." Section 8, Chapter 97 in *The Merck Manual of Diagnosis and Therapy*, edited by Mark H. Beers, MD, and Robert Berkow, MD. Whitehouse Station, NJ: Merck Research Laboratories, 1999.

PERIODICALS

Basti, S., P. Garg, and M. K. Reddy. "Posterior Capsule Dehiscence During Phacoemulsification and Manual Extracap-

sular Cataract Extraction: Comparison of Outcomes."
Journal of Cataract and Refractive Surgery 29 (March
2003): 532-536.

Brown, Nicholas Phelps. "Medical Treatment of Cataract." *Optometry Today* (November 30, 2001): 28-32.

Grinbaum, A., M. Blumenthal, and E. Assia. "Comparison of
Intraocular Pressure Profiles During Cataract Surgery by
Phacoemulsification and Extracapsular Cataract Extrac-
tion." *Ophthalmic Surgery, Lasers and Imaging* 34 (May-
June 2003): 182-186.

Guzek, J. P., and A. Ching. "Small-Incision Manual Extracapsular Cataract Surgery in Ghana, West Africa." *Journal of
Cataract and Refractive Surgery* 29 (January 2003): 57-64.

Hammond, Chris. "The Epidemiology of Cataract." *Optometry
Today* (February 9, 2001): 24-28.

Kalpadakis, P., et al. "A Comparison of Endophthalmitis After
Phacoemulsification or Extracapsular Cataract Extraction
in a Socio-Economically Deprived Environment: A Retrospective Analysis of 2,446 Patients." *European Journal of
Ophthalmology* 12 (September-October 2002): 395-400.

Minassian, D. C., et al. "Extracapsular Cataract Extraction
Compared with Small Incision Surgery by Phacoemulsification: A Randomised Trial." *British Journal of Ophthalmology* 85 (July 2001): 822-829.

Pesudovs, Konrad, and David B. Elliott. "The Evolution of
Cataract Surgery." *Optometry Today* (October 19, 2001):
30-32.

Rowden, A., and R. Krishna. "Resident Cataract Surgical
Training in United States Residency Programs." *Journal
of Cataract and Refractive Surgery* 28 (December 2002):
2202-2205.

Thomas, R., T. Kuriakose, and R. George. "Towards Achieving
Small-Incision Cataract Surgery 99.8% of the Time." *Indi-
an Journal of Ophthalmology* 48 (June 2000): 145-151.

ORGANIZATIONS

American Academy of Ophthalmology. P. O. Box 7424, San
Francisco, CA 94120-7424. (415) 561-8500. <www.aao.
org>.

American Optometric Association. 243 North Lindbergh Blvd.,
St. Louis, MO 63141. (314) 991-4100.

American Society of Cataract and Refractive Surgery
(ASCRS). 4000 Legato Road, #850, Fairfax, VA 22033.
(888) 949-6753. <www.ascrs.org>.

Canadian Ophthalmological Society (COS). 610-1525 Carling
Avenue, Ottawa ON K1Z 8R9. <www.eyesite.ca>.

National Eye Institute. 2020 Vision Place, Bethesda, MD
20892-3655. (301) 496-5248. <www.nei.nih.gov>.

Prevent Blindness America. 500 East Remington Road,
Schaumburg, IL 60173. (800) 331-2020. <www.prevent-
blindness.org>.

Wills Eye Hospital. 840 Walnut Street, Philadelphia, PA 19107.
(215) 928-3000. <www.willseye.org>.

OTHER

D'Ocampo, Vicente Victor, and C. Stephen Foster. "Cataract,
Senile." *eMedicine* July 18, 2002 [May 25, 2003]. <www.
emedicine.com/oph/topic49.htm>.

National Eye Institute (NEI). *Are You at Risk for Cataract?*
Bethesda, MD: NEI, 2001. NIH Publication No. 94-3463.

National Eye Institute (NEI). *Facts About Cataract*. Bethesda,
MD: NEI, 2001. NIH Publication No. 99-201.

Royal College of Ophthalmologists. *Cataract Surgery Guidelines*. London, UK: Royal College of Ophthalmologists,
2001.

Thomas, Ravi, and Thomas Kuriakose. "Surgical Techniques
for a Good Outcome in Cataract Surgery: Personal Perspectives." *Journal of Community Eye Health* 13 (2000)
[May 24, 2003]. <www.jceh.co.uk/journal/35_4.asp>.

Rebecca Frey, Ph.D.

Extracorporeal shock-wave therapy *see*
Lithotripsy

Eye muscle surgery

Definition

Eye muscle surgery is performed to weaken,
strengthen, or reposition any of the extraocular muscles
(small muscles) located on the surface of the eye that
move the eyeball in all directions.

Purpose

The extraocular muscles attach via tendons to the
sclera (the white, opaque, outer protective covering of
the eyeball) at different places just behind an imaginary
equator circling the top, bottom, left, and right of the
eye. The other end of each of these muscles attaches to a
part of the orbit (the eye socket in the skull). These muscles enable the eyes to move up, down, to one side or the
other, or any angle in between.

Normally, both eyes move together, receiving the
same image on corresponding locations on both retinas.
The brain fuses these matching images into one three-dimensional image. The exception is in strabismus, which is
a disorder where one or both eyes deviate out of alignment, most often outwardly (exotropia) or toward the nose
(esotropia). In this case, the brain receives two different
images, and either suppresses one or allows the person to
see double (diplopia). By weakening or strengthening the
appropriate muscles to center the eyes, a person can correct this deviation. For example, if an eye turns upward,
the muscle at the bottom of the eye could be strengthened.

The main purpose of eye muscle surgery is thus to
restore straight eye alignment. The surgery is performed
to align both eyes so that they gaze in the same direction

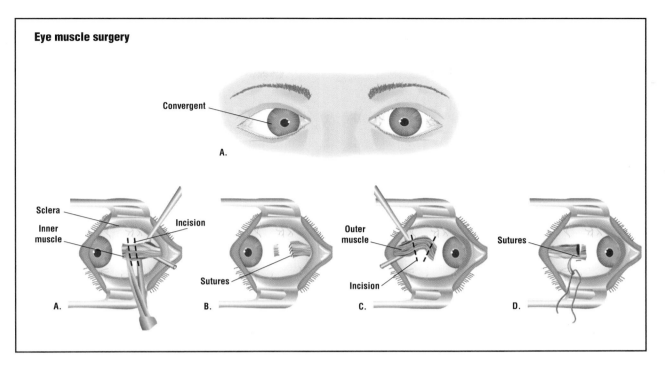

Eye muscle surgery

To repair a convergent gaze, the ophthalmogist cuts the muscles that move the eye from side to side (A). On one side, the muscles are attached further back on the eyeball (B). On the other, the muscle is shortened (C) and stitched (D). *(Illustration by GGS Inc.)*

and move together as a team; to improve appearance; and to promote the development of binocular vision in a young child. To achieve binocular vision, the eyes must align so that the location of the image on the retina of one eye corresponds to the location of the image on the retina of the other eye.

In addition to being used to correct strabismus, eye muscle surgery is also performed to treat such other eye disorders as nystagmus or such special types of congenital strabismus as Duane syndrome. Nystagmus is a condition in which one or both eyes move rapidly or oscillate; this condition can be improved by moving the eyes to the position of least oscillation. Duane syndrome is a disorder in which there is limited horizontal eye movement; it can sometimes be relieved by surgery that weakens an eye muscle.

Demographics

According to doctors at Wills Eye Hospital, Philadelphia, the most common divergent strabismus in childhood has a variable onset, often between six months and four years. The disorder occurs in 1.2% of children by seven years of age and occurs equally in males and females.

Duane syndrome commonly affects girls more often than boys, and the left eye more often than the right eye.

Congenital nystagmus is thought to be present at birth, but is usually not apparent until the child is a few months old. Acquired nystagmus occurs later than six months of age, and can be caused by stroke, such diseases as multiple sclerosis, or even a heavy blow to the head. It is not known how many people suffer from nystagmus, but it is thought to be one in 1,000 adults, and one in 640 children in the United States, according to the Nystagmus Network.

Description

The procedure used by the surgeon depends on the condition that needs correcting. During surgery, eye muscles can be:

- Weakened. This usually involves recessing the eye muscle or moving it posteriorly on the eye to elongate the muscle and allow the muscle tissue to relax.

- Tightened. Muscles are tightened by resection, which involves removing a piece of the muscle near its point of insertion and then reinserting the muscle into its original location. By removing a piece of muscle, the muscle is shortened and therefore strengthened.

- Repositioned. For some forms of strabismus, the eye muscles are neither weakened nor strengthened, but repositioned: i.e., the muscle's point of insertion is moved to a different location.

WHO PERFORMS THE PROCEDURE AND WHERE IS IT PERFORMED?

Eye muscle surgery is performed by surgeons with specialized training in eye surgery. These physicians are usually board-certified ophthalmologists and fellowship-trained pediatric and/or adult strabismus specialists.

The surgery is almost always performed as **outpatient surgery**; that is, the patient comes into the hospital or day surgery facility the morning of the surgery and goes home the same day.

There are two methods to alter extraocular muscles. Traditional surgery can be used to strengthen, weaken, or reposition an extraocular muscle. The surgeon first makes an incision in the conjunctiva (the clear membrane covering the sclera), then puts a suture into the muscle to hold it in place, and loosens the muscle from the eyeball with a surgical hook. During a resection, the muscle is detached from the sclera, a piece of muscle is removed so that the muscle is now shorter, and the muscle is reattached to the same place. This strengthens the muscle. In a recession, the muscle is made weaker by repositioning it. More than one extraocular eye muscle might be operated on at the same time.

Eye muscle surgery is performed with the eye in its normal position and usually takes an hour and a half. At no time during the operation is the eye removed from the socket. The surgeon determines where to reattach the muscles based on eye measurements taken before surgery. Most of the time, it can hardly be seen except with magnification.

Diagnosis/Preparation

Depth perception (stereopsis) in humans develops around the age of three months. For successful development of binocular vision and the ability to perceive three-dimensionally, eye muscle surgery should not be postponed past the age of four years. The earlier the surgery, the better the outcome, so an early diagnosis is important. Surgery may even be performed before the child is two years old.

Patients (or their caregivers) should make sure their doctors are aware of any medications that they are taking, even over-the-counter medications. Patients should not take **aspirin**, or any other blood-thinning medica-

tions for 10 days prior to surgery, and should not eat or drink after midnight the night before.

Aftercare

After surgery, the eyes feel scratchy, but not very painful. Postoperatively, the eyes are also a little red and watery. There may be some hemorrhage under the conjunctival membrane over the white of the eye that usually settles over a period of two to three weeks. It usually takes on a yellowish discoloration similar to a bruise as it clears. Sometimes there is some thickening of the membranes over the eye, which can take several more weeks to clear. Very fine dissolving sutures are used to reposition the conjunctival membrane at the end of surgery and, until these sutures dissolve, there may be some scratchiness in the eyes. This feeling usually disappears after two or three weeks.

There will also be some swelling and discharge after the surgery. The swelling is usually minor, and patients should be able to open their eyes within the next two days, as the swelling should gradually disappear.

Patients will need someone to drive them home after the operation. They should continue to avoid aspirin and other nonsteroidal anti-inflammatory agents for an additional three days, but they can take **acetaminophen** (e.g., Tylenol). Patients should discuss what medications they can or cannot take with the surgeon. Pain will subside after two or three days, and patients can resume most normal activities within a few days. Again, the period of recovery may vary with the patient and the patient can discuss with the surgeon when to return to normal activities. Patient's should not get their eyes wet for three to four days and should refrain from swimming for 10 days. Operated eyes will be red for about two weeks.

Adults and children over the age of six often experience double vision for a limited period of time after surgery. Children younger than six sometimes will have double vision for a short period of time. Double vision is rarely permanent.

Patients generally do not have to wear patches after surgery, although occasionally a temporary patch may be recommended. They are usually required to use eye drops for a week until the follow-up examination. If the eye is healing on schedule, then the eye drops are usually discontinued at that stage. A further postoperative appointment is usually made for six to eight weeks later, by which time the eye will have stabilized.

After surgery for strabismus, the patient usually needs corrective lenses and eye exercises (vision therapy) if binocular vision is to develop.

Risks

As with any surgery, there are risks involved. Eye muscle surgery is relatively safe, but very rarely a cut muscle cannot be retrieved. This, and other serious reactions, including those caused by anesthetics, can result in vision loss in the affected eye. Occasionally, retinal or nerve damage occurs. Permanent double vision is also a risk of eye muscle surgery. The success rate of this surgery varies from person to person and depends on each person's particular condition.

Some infrequent complications include, but are not limited to, allergy to the sutures, bleeding, and change in pupil size.

The major risk of eye muscle surgery is failure to achieve a satisfactory alignment of the eyes. This may be an undercorrection or an overcorrection, with the eyes turning the other way after the operation. Surgeons aim to achieve perfect alignment, but this is not always possible. If the alignment is still unsatisfactory at the final postoperative visit, then a second operation may be required.

Infection is an unusual postoperative complication and can be treated with antibiotic drops.

Because an incision is made through the conjunctiva and muscle, there is always some residual scarring. Usually, this is detectable only under a microscope, although it may be possible to see it on close examination.

As with any eye surgery, there is a potential risk of visual loss from strabismus operations, but this is a very rare complication.

Normal results

Normal results of eye muscle surgery are an improved alignment of the eyes and improved cosmetic appearance without complications. The surgery usually has a very good outcome.

Morbidity and mortality rates

Cosmetic improvement is likely with success rate estimates varying from about 65–85%. According to the latest statistics from 1998, binocular vision is improved in young children about 35% of the time, following eye muscle surgery. Between 15 and 35% of patients have either no improvement or a worsening of their condition. A second operation may rectify less than perfect outcomes.

Alternatives

Surgery is not the only treatment to correct eye muscle disorders. Options and outcomes vary considerably based on such factors as the presence of double vision.

QUESTIONS TO ASK THE DOCTOR

- What is the chance of needing a second operation?
- What are the possible risks and complications?
- Will I need eyeglasses?
- How much eye muscle surgery do you perform each year?
- Are there alternatives to surgery?
- Is a patch worn after surgery?
- Are there any scars after surgery?

Nonsurgical treatment is also available, such as orthoptics and vision therapy.

Orthoptics

Orthoptics is a medical term for the eye muscle training programs provided by orthoptists and optometrists. Vision therapy programs include orthoptics, but there are broad differences between vision therapy and orthoptics. Orthoptics dates back to the 1850s and is limited in scope to eye muscle training and the cosmetic straightening of eyes. Orthoptics treats muscle problems by considering only strength; it does not focus on neurological and visual-motor factors as vision therapy does. Treatment is home-based.

Vision therapy

Vision therapy is an individualized, supervised, non-surgical treatment program designed to correct eye movements and visual-motor deficiencies. Vision therapy sessions include procedures designed to enhance the brain's ability to control:

- eye alignment
- eye teaming
- eye focusing abilities
- eye movements
- visual processing

Visual-motor skills and endurance may be developed through the use of specialized computer and optical devices, including therapeutic lenses, prisms, and filters. During the final stages of therapy, the patient's newly acquired visual skills are reinforced and made automatic through repetition and by integration with motor and cognitive skills.

KEY TERMS

Conjunctiva—The mucous membrane that covers the eyes and lines the eyelids.

Duane syndrome—A hereditary congenital syndrome in which the affected eye shows a limited capacity to move, and is deficient in convergence with the other eye.

Extraocular muscles—The muscles (lateral rectus, medial rectus, inferior rectus, superior rectus, superior oblique, and inferior oblique) that move the eyeball.

Nystagmus—An involuntary rapid rhythmic movement of the eyeball, which may be horizontal, vertical, rotatory, or mixed.

Orbit—The cavity in the skull containing the eyeball; formed from seven bones: frontal, maxillary, sphenoid, lacrimal, zygomatic, ethmoid, and palatine.

Retina—The inner light-sensitive layer of the eye containing rods and cones. The retina transforms the image it receives into electrical messages sent to the brain via the optic nerve.

Sclera—The tough fibrous white outer protective covering of the eyeball.

Strabismus—A disorder in which the two eyes cannot be directed at the same object at the same time.

Resources

BOOKS

Dyer, J. A., and D. A. Lee. *Atlas of Extraocular Muscle Surgery.* Westport, CT: Praeger Publishers, 1984.

Good, William V., and Craig S. Hoyt. *Strabismus Management.* Boston: Butterworth-Hienemann, 1996.

Roth, A., and C. Speeg-Schatz, eds. *Eye Muscle Surgery.* Lisse, The Netherlands: Swets & Zeitlinger, 2001.

Salmans, Sandra. *Your Eyes: Questions You Have...Answers You Need.* Allentown, PA: People's Medical Society, 1996.

von Noorden, Gunter K. *Binocular Vision and Ocular Motility: Theory and Management of Strabismus,* 5th edition. St. Louis: Mosby-Year Book, 1996.

PERIODICALS

Bosman, J., M. P. ten Tusscher, I. de Jong, J. S. Vles, and H. Kingma. "The Influence of Eye Muscle Surgery on Shape and Relative Orientation of Displacement Planes: Indirect Evidence for Neural Control of 3D Eye Movements." *Strabismus* 10 (September 2002): 199–209.

Mayr, H. "Virtual Eye Muscle Surgery Based upon Biomechanical Models." *Studies in Health and Technology Information* 81 (2001): 305–311.

Murray, T. "Eye Muscle Surgery." *Current Opinion in Ophthalmology* 11 (October 2000): 336–341.

Rubsam, B., W. D. Schafer, B. Schulte, and N. Roewer. "Preliminary Report: Analgesia with Remifentanil for Complicated Eye Muscle Surgery." *Strabismus* 8 (December 2000): 287–289.

Watts, J. C. "Total Intravenous Anesthesia Without Muscle Relaxant for Eye Surgery in a Patient with Kugelberg-Welander Syndrome." *Anaesthesia* 58 (January 2003): 96.

ORGANIZATIONS

American Academy of Ophthalmology. 655 Beach Street, P.O. Box 7424, San Francisco, CA 94120-7424. <http://www.eyenet.org>.

American Academy of Pediatric Ophthalmology and Strabismus (AAPOS). <http://med-aapos.bu.edu>.

OTHER

Olitsky, Scott E., and Leonard B. Nelson. *Strabismus Web Book.* <www.members.aol.com/scottolitsky/webbook.htm>.

Kellogg Eye Center: Eye Muscle Surgery. <www.kellogg.umich.edu/patient/surg/eyemuscle.html>.

Pediatric Ophthalmic Consultants Webpage: Strabismus Surgery. <www.pedseye.com/StrabSurg.htm>.

Lorraine Lica, PhD
Monique Laberge, PhD

Eye surgery *see* **Ophthalmologic surgery**
Eyeball removal *see* **Enucleation, eye**
Eyelid plastic surgery *see* **Blepharoplasty**
Eyelid surgery *see* **Tarsorrhaphy**

Face lift

Definition

Face-lift surgery is a cosmetic procedure that involves removing sagging skin and tightening muscle tissue of the face and neck to counter signs of aging. The procedure is also called facialplasty, rhytidoplasty, and cervicofacial rhytidectomy.

Purpose

The purpose of face-lift surgery is to improve the appearance of the face by repositioning the skin and tightening some of the underlying muscle and tissue. The procedure is designed to counter sagging and looseness in skin and muscle tissue that becomes more pronounced as individuals age. Face-lift surgery will not eliminate all facial wrinkles. For example, wrinkles around the mouth and eyes may benefit little from face-lift surgery. Also, additional procedures including **blepharoplasty**, chemical peel, botox injections, or **dermabrasion** may be necessary to achieve desired results.

Demographics

The American Society for Aesthetic Plastic Surgery estimated that nearly 6.9 million cosmetic surgical and nonsurgical procedures were performed in the United States in 2002. The number of face-lift procedures increased by 6% from the previous year (2001). Among members of the American Academy of Cosmetic Surgery, 15,478 face-lift procedures were performed. The average fee for a face lift in 2002 was $7,000.

Description

A face lift takes about two hours and may be performed as an outpatient procedure or it may require hospitalization. General or local anesthetics will be used to sedate the patient. Typically, patients receiving local anesthesia will augment it with "twilight anesthesia," an intravenous sedative that helps to lower their awareness of the procedure being performed. An anesthesiologist will be present to administer the anesthetics and assist in monitoring and maintaining the patient's vital life functions.

The surgeon makes an incision within the hairline just above the ear. The incision continues down along the front edge of the ear, around the earlobe, and then up and behind the ear extending back into the hairline. The location of this incision is designed to hide any sign of the procedure later. The same procedure is repeated on the other side of the face. The surgeon separates the skin of the face from its underlying tissue, moving down to the cheek and into the neck area and below the chin. Fat deposits over the cheeks and in the neck may be removed surgically or with **liposuction** at this time. The surgeon tightens certain bands of muscle and tissue that extend up from the shoulder, below the chin, and up and behind the neck. If these muscles and tissue are not tightened, the looseness and sagging appearance of the skin will return. The surgeon trims excess skin from the edges of the original incision and the skin is pulled back into place. The incision is closed with sutures or staples.

Diagnosis/Preparation

Prior to the procedure, candidates meet with the surgeon to discuss the procedure, clarify the results that can be achieved, and the potential problems that can occur. Having realistic expectations is important in any cosmetic procedure. People will learn, for example, that although a face lift can improve the contour of the face and neck, other procedures will be necessary to reduce the appearance of many wrinkles. Candidates will be advised to stop taking **aspirin**, birth control pills or female hormones, and other medications affecting blood clotting two weeks before the procedure. Some physicians prescribe vitamin C and K to promote healing. Candidates are advised to stop smoking

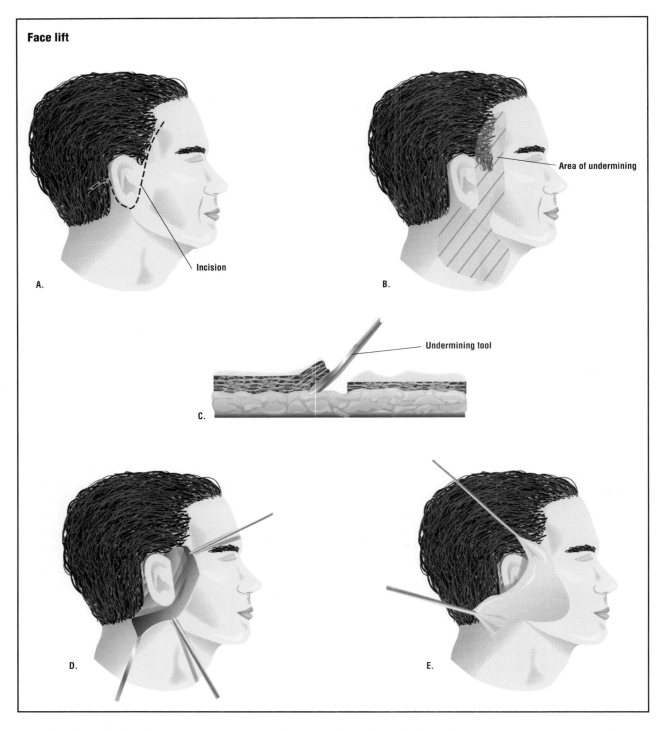

Face lift

A.

Incision

B.

Area of undermining

Undermining tool

C.

D.

E.

For a face lift, an incision is made around the ear at the base of the hairline (A). The skin is removed from underlying tissues in a procedure called undermining (B and C). The skin is pulled up to tighten it (D). The skin is stitched into place and excess is removed (E). *(Illustration by GGS Inc.)*

and to avoid exposure to passive smoke at least two weeks before and after the procedure. Some surgeons also recommend taking **antibiotics** prior to surgery to limit the risk of infection. Often a steroid injection is administered before or after the procedure to reduce swelling.

Aftercare

A pressure bandage is applied to the face to reduce the risk of hematoma, which is a pocket of blood below the skin. The person may spend a few hours resting in a **recovery room** to ensure that no bleeding has occurred. The individual then returns home. Some surgeons recommend that people stay in a reclining position for the 24 hours immediately following surgery, consuming a liquid diet, and avoiding flexing or bending the neck. Ice packs for the first few days can help to reduce swelling and lower the risk of hematoma. Individuals continue taking antibiotics until the first stitches come out about five days after the procedure. The remaining sutures are removed seven to ten days later. Many people return to work and limited activities within two weeks of the procedure.

Risks

Candidates with other medical conditions should consult with their primary care physician before undergoing a face lift. Lung problems, heart disease, and certain other conditions can lead to a higher risk of complications. Persons who use medications that affect blood clotting (including female hormones, aspirin, and some non-aspirin pain relievers) should stop taking these medications prior to surgery to lower the risk that a hematoma will form. A hematoma is the most frequent complication of face-lifts. Most hematomas form within 48 hours of surgery. The typical sign is pain or swelling affecting one side of the face but not the other.

Another risk is nerve damage. Sometimes it can affect a person's ability to raise an eyebrow, or distort the smile, or result in limited sensation in the earlobe. Most of these nerve injuries, however, repair themselves within two to six months.

Normal results

Some swelling and bruising is normal following a face lift. There should be a noticeable improvement in the contour of the face and neck. Some fine wrinkling of the skin may be improved, but deep wrinkles are likely to require another cosmetic procedure to improve their appearance.

Morbidity and mortality rates

In general, mortality and morbidity rates for forehead lifts and similar facial cosmetic procedures are very low. Almost all cases of mortality following facial cosmetic surgery involve patients who were treated for facial disfigurement because they had been severely

WHO PERFORMS THE PROCEDURE AND WHERE IS IT PERFORMED?

Face-lifts are performed by surgeons with specialized training in plastic and reconstructive surgery. They are most commonly performed in outpatient facilities or in private professional offices. The procedure may also be performed in a hospital.

burned or attacked by animals. Moreover, many plastic surgeons do not consider morbidity and mortality rates to be as significant as other factors in evaluating the success of facial cosmetic procedures. One group of researchers at the University of Washington maintains that "[t]he most important measures of outcome in facial cosmetic surgery are quality of life and patient satisfaction, in contrast to other, more objective measures such as complications or mortality rates."

Alternatives

Isometric exercises are recommended as non-surgical alternatives to face-lift procedures.

Injections of Botox (botulinum toxin) have been used to achieve the same results as a face lift. Botulinum toxin is a compound produced by the spores and growing cells of the organism that causes botulism, *Clostridium botulinum*. The toxin causes muscle paralysis. It was first used clinically in the 1960s to treat neurological disorders but also proved to be effective in paralyzing the facial muscles that cause "crow's feet" and frown wrinkles. Botulinum toxin, or Botox, was approved by the Food and Drug Administration (FDA) in April 2002 as a treatment for facial lines and wrinkles. Botox treatments must be repeated in approximately six months.

Coherent ultrapulse carbon dioxide laser treatment is a promising new treatment alternative to traditional face lift procedures. As of 2003, this equipment has been used by a few major institutions.

Some plastic surgeons have used a procedure called fat rebalancing to achieve outcomes similar to a traditional face lift procedure. Fat rebalancing involves relocation of fatty tissue from distant sites on the body to the face.

Resources

BOOKS

Engler, Alan M. *BodySculpture: Plastic Surgery of the Body for Men and Women,* 2nd edition. Hudson Publishing, 2000.

KEY TERMS

Hematoma—A complication of surgery in which a collection of blood forms below the skin.

Rhytidectomy—Wrinkle excision. It is an older alternative term for face lift.

Twilight anesthesia—An intravenous mixture of sedatives and other medications that decreases people's awareness of the procedure being performed.

Irwin, Brandith, and Mark McPherson. *Your Best Face: Looking Your Best Without Plastic Surgery.* Carlsbad, CA: Hay House, Inc, 2002.

Man, Daniel, and L. C. Faye. *New Art of Man: Faces of Plastic Surgery: Your Guide to the Latest Cosmetic Surgery Procedures*, New York: BeautyArt Press, 2003.

Papel, I. D., and S. S. Park. *Facial Plastic and Reconstructive Surgery*, 2nd edition. New York: Thieme Medical Publishers, 2000.

PERIODICALS

Bisson, M. A., R. Grover, and A. O. Grobbelaar. "Long-term results of facial rejuvenation by carbon dioxide laser resurfacing using a quantitative method of assessment." *British Journal of Plastic Surgery* 55 (2002): 652–656.

Byrd, H. S. and J. D. Burt. "Achieving aesthetic balance in the brow, eyelids, and midface." *Plastic and Reconstructive Surgery* 110 (2002): 926–939.

Donofrio, L. M. "Fat rebalancing: the new 'Facelift'" *Skin Therapy Letter* 7 (2002): 7–9.

Morgenstern, K. E. and J. A. Foster. "Advances in cosmetic oculoplastic surgery." *Current Opinions in Ophthalmology* 13 (2002): 324–330.

ORGANIZATIONS

American Board of Plastic Surgery. Seven Penn Center, Suite 400, 1635 Market Street, Philadelphia, PA 19103-2204, (215) 587-9322. <http://www.abplsurg.org/>

American College of Plastic and Reconstructive Surgery. <http://www.breast-implant.org>

American College of Surgeons. 633 North Saint Clair Street, Chicago, IL, 60611. (312) 202-5000. <http://www.facs.org/>

American Society for Aesthetic Plastic Surgery. 11081 Winners Circle, Los Alamitos, California 90720. (800) 364-2147 or (562)799-2356. <http://www.surgery.org/>

American Society for Dermatologic Surgery. 930 N. Meacham Road, P.O. Box 4014, Schaumburg, IL 60168-4014. (847) 330-9830. <http://www.asds-net.org>.

American Society of Plastic and Reconstructive Surgeons. 444 E. Algonquin Rd., Arlington Heights, IL 60005. (847) 228-9900. <http://www.plasticsurgery.org>.

American Society of Plastic Surgeons. 444 E. Algonquin Rd., Arlington Heights, IL 60005. (888) 475-2784. <http://www.plasticsurgery.org/>

OTHER

Mayo Clinic. [cited March 23, 2003]. <http://www.mayoclinic.org/facialcosmeticsurgery-jax/>.

National Library of Medicine. [cited March 23, 2003]. <http://www.nlm.nih.gov/medlineplus/plasticcosmeticsurgery.html>.

Online Surgery. [cited March 23, 2003]. <http://www.onlinesurgery.com/procedures/face_lift.php>.

L. Fleming Fallon, Jr., MD, DrPH

Fallopian tube ligation *see* **Tubal ligation**

Fallopian tube removal *see* **Salpingostomy**

Fasciotomy

Definition

Fasciotomy is a surgical procedure that cuts away the fascia to relieve tension or pressure.

Purpose

Fascia is thin connective tissue covering, or separating, the muscles and internal organs of the body. It varies in thickness, density, elasticity, and composition, and is different from ligaments and tendons.

The fascia can be injured either through constant strain or through trauma. Fasciitis is an inflammation of the fascia. The most common condition for which fasciotomy is performed is plantar fasciitis, an inflammation of the fascia on the bottom of the foot that is sometimes called a heel spur or stone bruise.

Plantar fasciitis is caused by long periods on one's feet, being overweight, or wearing shoes that do not support the foot well. Teachers, mail carriers, runners, and others who make heavy use of their feet are especially likely to suffer from plantar fasciitis.

Plantar fasciitis results in moderate to disabling heel pain. If nine to 12 months of conservative treatment (reducing time on feet, nonsteroid anti-inflammatory drugs, arch supports) under the supervision of a doctor does not result in pain relief, a fasciotomy may be performed. Fasciotomy removes a small portion of the fascia to relieve tension and pain. Connective tissue grows back into the space left by the incision, effectively lengthening the fascia.

When a fasciotomy is performed on other parts of the body, the usual goal is to relieve pressure from a compression injury to a limb. This type of injury often occurs during contact sports or after a snake bite. Blood vessels of the limb are damaged. They swell and leak, causing inflammation. Fluid builds up in the area contained by the fascia. A fasciotomy is performed to relieve this pressure and prevent tissue death. Similar injury occurs in high-voltage electrical burns that cause deep tissue damage.

Demographics

People who are likely to need a fascictomy include the following:

- athletes who have sustained one or more serious impact injuries
- people who spend long periods of time on their feet
- people with severe burns
- persons who are overweight
- snakebite victims

There is a slight male predominance among people undergoing a fasciotomy.

Description

Fasciotomy in the limbs is usually performed by a surgeon under general or regional anesthesia. An incision is made in the skin, and a small area of fascia is removed where it will best relieve pressure. Then the incision is closed.

Plantar fasciotomy is an endoscopic (performed with the use of an endoscope) procedure. The doctor makes two small incisions on either side of the heel. An endoscope is inserted in one incision to guide the doctor. A tiny knife is inserted in the other. A portion of the fascia near the heel is removed. The incisions are then closed.

Diagnosis/Preparation

In the case of injury, fasciotomy is performed on an emergency basis, and the outcome of the surgery depends

---

WHO PERFORMS THE PROCEDURE AND WHERE IS IT PERFORMED?

Fasciotomy in a limb is usually performed by a general surgeon. The typical location is an outpatient facility using regional anesthesia. For persons with burns or others who require extensive fasciotomy, the procedure is performed in a hospital **operating room** under general anesthesia.

Plantar fasciotomy is performed by a foot specialist in a professional office or outpatient surgical clinic under local anesthesia. The procedure requires 20 minutes to one hour.

---

largely on the general health of the injured person. Plantar fasciotomies are appropriate for most people whose foot problems cannot be resolved in any other way.

Little preparation is needed before a fasciotomy. When the fasciotomy is related to burn injuries, the fluid and electrolyte status of the affected person are constantly monitored.

Aftercare

Aftercare depends on the reason for the fasciotomy. People who have endoscopic plantar fasciotomy can walk without pain almost immediately, return to wearing their regular shoes within three to five days, and return to normal activities within three weeks. Most will need to wear arch supports in their shoes.

Persons who require fasciotomy as a result of an injury or snake bite are usually able to resume their normal activities in a few weeks.

Risks

The greatest risk with endoscopic plantar fasciotomy is that the arch will drop slightly as a result of this surgery, causing other foot problems. Risks involved with other types of fasciotomy are those associated with the administration of anesthesia and the development of blood clots or postsurgical infections.

Normal results

Fasciotomy in the limbs reduces pressure, thus reducing tissue death. Endoscopic plantar fasciotomy has a success rate in excess of 95%.

Morbidity and mortality rates

The most common morbidity in a fasciotomy is an incomplete response that requires a repeat fasciotomy procedure. Mortality is very rare and usually due to a problem related to the original condition.

Alternatives

Conservative nonoperative treatment for plantar fasciitis consists of nonsteroidal anti-inflammatory drugs for several weeks. For persons who spend excessive time on their feet, a change of occupation or the use of arch supports may be useful. Overweight individuals may consider weight reduction to reduce the stress placed on their feet. For persons bitten by a poisonous snake, there are no acceptable alternatives to a fasciotomy, and there are rarely acceptable alternatives to fasciotomy for a person who has been burned.

Resources

BOOKS

Bland, K. I., W. G. Cioffi, and M. G. Sarr. *Practice of General Surgery.* Philadelphia: Saunders, 2001.

Canale, S. T. *Campbell's Operative Orthopedics.* St. Louis, MO: Mosby, 2003.

Schwartz, S. I., J. E. Fischer, F. C. Spencer, G. T. Shires, and J. M. Daly. *Principles of Surgery.* 7th ed. New York: McGraw-Hill, 1998.

Townsend, C., K. L. Mattox, R. D. Beauchamp, B. M. Evers, and D. C. Sabiston. *Sabiston's Review of Surgery.* 3rd ed. Philadelphia: Saunders, 2001.

PERIODICALS

Cook, S., and G. Bruce. "Fasciotomy for Chronic Compartment Syndrome in the Lower Limb." *Australia New Zealand Journal of Surgery* 72, no. 10 (2002): 720–723.

Fulkerson, E., A. Razi, and N. Tejwani. "Review: Acute Compartment Syndrome of the Foot." *Foot and Ankle International* 24, no. 2 (2003): 180–187.

Lin, Y. M. "Will Fasciotomy Help in the Patients with Crush Syndrome?" *American Journal of Kidney Diseases* 41, no. 1 (2003): 265–266.

Watson, T. S., R. B. Anderson, W. H. Davis, and G. M. Kiebzak. "Distal Tarsal Tunnel Release with Partial Plantar Fasciotomy for Chronic Heel Pain: An Outcome Analysis." *Foot and Ankle International* 23, no. 6 (2002): 530–537.

ORGANIZATIONS

American Academy of Orthopaedic Surgeons. 6300 North River Road, Rosemont, IL 60018-4262. (847) 823-7186 or (800) 346-AAOS. Fax: (847) 823-8125. <http://www.aaos.org/wordhtml/home2.htm>.

American College of Foot and Ankle Surgeons. 515 Busse Highway, Park Ridge, IL 60068-3150. (888) 843-3338). mail@acfas.org. <http://www.acfas.org/index.html>.

American College of Surgeons. 633 North St. Clair Street, Chicago, IL 60611-32311. (312) 202-5000. Fax: (312) 202-5001. postmaster@facs.org. <http://www.facs.org>.

American Orthopaedic Foot and Ankle Society. 2517 Eastlake Avenue E., Seattle, WA 98102. (206) 223-1120. Fax: (206) 223-1178. aofas@aofas.org. <http://www.aofas.org>.

American Podiatric Medical Association. 9312 Old Georgetown Road, Bethesda, MD 20814. (301) 571-9200 or (800) 275-2762. Fax: (301) 530-2752. <http://www.apma.org>.

OTHER

Swain, R., and D. Ross. "Lower Extremity Compartment Syndrome." *Postgraduate Medicine* March 1999 [cited April 2, 2003]. <http://www.postgradmed.com/issues/1999/03_99/swain.htm>.

U. S. Department of Defense. "Postoperative Care." *Virtual Naval Hospital* (University of Iowa) [cited April 2, 2003]. <http://www.vnh.org/EWSurg/ch18/18PostoperativeCare.html>.

University of North Dakota School of Medicine. "Compartment Syndrome of the Foot." [cited April 2, 2003]. <http://www.med.und.nodak.edu/depts/fammed/Fractures/fracture.dir/oa2/76.htm>.

Yale University School of Medicine. "What Are the Signs of Compartment Syndrome?" [cited April 2, 2003]. <http://yalesurgery.med.yale.edu/surgery/sections/plastics/Core%20Curriculum%20Pages/Lower%20Extremity%20Page/LegAns2.html>.

L. Fleming Fallon, Jr., MD, DrPH

Femoral hernia repair

Definition

A femoral hernia repair, or herniorraphy is a surgical procedure performed to reposition tissue that has come out through a weak point in the abdominal wall near the groin. In general, a hernia is a protrusion of a loop or piece of tissue through a weak spot or opening in the abdominal wall. There are several different kinds of hernias; they are named according to their location. A femoral hernia is one that occurs in a person's groin near the thigh. In a child, a femoral hernia is usually the result of incomplete closing of this area during development in the womb.

Purpose

Femoral hernia repair is done to reduce the patient's risk of a future surgical emergency. A hernia may be congenital (present at birth) or may develop later in life because of a weakness in the abdominal wall. If the opening is very small, the amount of tissue that can push through it is small, and the person may barely be aware of the problem. One complication that may arise, however, is that the tissue that comes out through the opening can become incarcerated, or trapped. If the herniated tissue has its blood supply diminished because of pressure from other nearby organs or structures, it is referred to as strangulated. Strangulation may lead to gangrene, which means that the affected tissue can die and be invaded by bacteria. Femoral hernias are more likely than other hernias to become incarcerated or strangulated because the affected tissue pushes through a relatively small and closely confined space. Because of the increased risk of eventual strangulation and gangrene, the patient's doctor may recommend surgical repair of the hernia.

Demographics

Femoral hernias are a relatively uncommon type, accounting for only 3% of all hernias. While femoral hernias can occur in both males and females, almost all of them develop in women because of the wider bone structure of the female pelvis. Femoral hernias usually grow larger over time; any activity that involves straining, such as heavy lifting or a chronic cough, may cause the hernia to enlarge. Poor abdominal muscle tone, obesity, and pregnancy also increase a woman's risk of developing a femoral hernia. Most femoral hernias develop on only one side of the patient's abdomen, but about 15% of femoral hernias are bilateral. These bilateral hernias are more likely to become strangulated. An additional 20% of femoral hernias become incarcerated.

Femoral hernias are more common in adults than in children. Those that do occur in children are more likely

to be associated with a connective tissue disorder or with conditions that increase intra-abdominal pressure. Seventy percent of pediatric cases of femoral hernias occur in infants under the age of one.

Description

Femoral hernia repair may be performed under either general or local anesthesia. The repair of the hernia involves a cut, or incision, in the groin area (near the thigh), adjacent to the femoral artery. The surgeon locates the hernia, and reduces it by pushing the protruding tissue back inside the abdominal cavity. A hernia is referred to as reducible when the tissue that has come out through the opening can be pushed back and the opening closed. If incarceration or strangulation has occurred, the hernia is referred to as irreducible.

The procedure may be performed using the traditional open method, which requires a larger surgical incision, or by a laparoscopic approach. A laparoscopic procedure is performed through a few very small incisions. The hole in the abdominal wall may be closed with sutures, or by the use of a fine sterile surgical mesh. The mesh, which provides additional strength, is sewn into the abdominal wall with very small stitches. Some surgeons may choose to use the mesh when repairing a larger hernia. A hernia repair done with a mesh insert is called a tension-free procedure because the surgeon does not have to put tension on the layer of muscle tissue in order to bring the edges of the hole together. A laparoscopic hernia repair takes about 40 minutes to complete.

Diagnosis/Preparation

Diagnosis

A femoral hernia is usually diagnosed during a **physical examination**. In many cases, the patient will

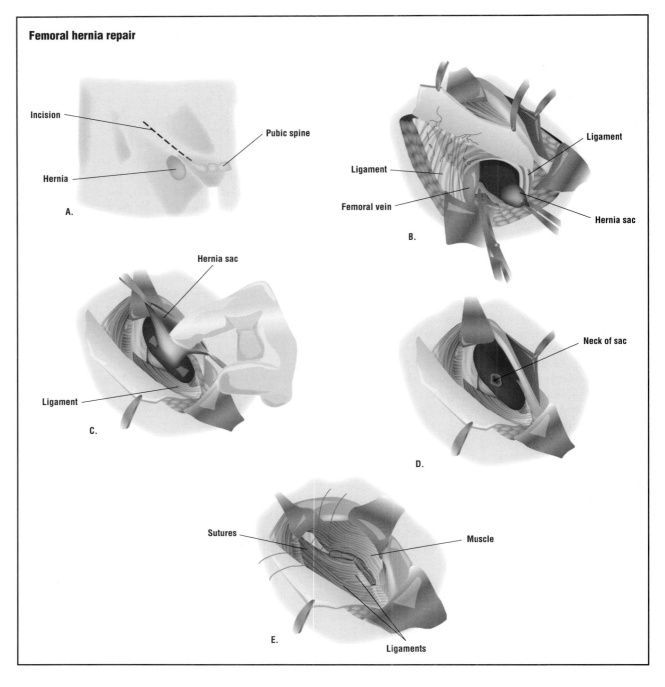

Femoral hernia repair

Incision

Pubic spine

Hernia

A.

Ligament

Ligament

Femoral vein

Hernia sac

B.

Hernia sac

Neck of sac

Ligament

C.

D.

Sutures

Muscle

Ligaments

E.

To repair a femoral hernia, an incision is made in the groin area near the hernia (A). Skin and ligaments are pulled aside to expose the hernia (B). The hernia sac is opened, and the contents are pushed back into the abdominal cavity (C). The neck of the sac is tied off, and excess tissue is removed (D). Layers of skin and tissues are repaired (E). *(Illustration by GGS Inc.)*

consult the doctor because of pain in the groin area or the inside of the upper thigh. The pain or discomfort of a femoral hernia may come and go, increasing when the person coughs or strains. If the pain is severe, the patient may go to an emergency room. In young children, symptoms of an incarcerated femoral hernia in-clude severe irritability, abdominal pain, cramping, and vomiting. Adult patients may have also felt a mass in the groin that may be tender when it is pressed. Pa-tients in severe pain may be given a sedative or pain-killing medication so that the doctor can examine the groin area and try to guide the herniated tissues back through the abdominal opening with gentle manual pressure.

In adult patients, the doctor will rule out the possibility that the pain is caused by an enlarged lymph node, a lipoma, or an inguinal hernia. Imaging studies are not generally used in diagnosing a hernia unless the doctor suspects that the hernia is incarcerated or strangulated. A strangulated hernia can be distinguished from an incarcerated hernia by the presence of fever; pain that persists after the doctor has reduced the hernia manually; and pain that is more severe than warranted by the examination findings.

Preparation

If the doctor suspects that the hernia is strangulated, he or she will give the patient a broad-spectrum antibiotic (usually cefoxitin) intravenously before the patient is taken to the **operating room**.

Adults scheduled for a nonemergency herniorraphy are given standard blood tests and a **urinalysis**. They should not eat breakfast on the morning of the procedure, and they should wear loose-fitting, comfortable clothing that they can easily pull on after the surgery without straining their abdomen.

Aftercare

Aftercare depends on several factors: the patient's age and general health status; the type of surgery (open or laparoscopic); and the type of anesthesia administered. Immediately after the procedure, the patient will be taken to the recovery area of the surgical center and monitored for signs of excessive bleeding, infection, uncontrolled pain, or shock. An uncomplicated femoral hernia repair is usually performed on an outpatient basis, which allows the patient to go home within a few hours of the surgery.

The patient will be given instructions about **incision care**, which will depend on the type of surgery and the way in which the incision was closed. Sometimes a transparent dressing is placed on the wound that the patient can remove about three days after the procedure. Very small incisions, such as those used for laparoscopic surgery, may be closed with Steri-strips® instead of sutures. The incision should be kept dry, so patients should take a sponge bath rather than a shower or tub bath for several days after surgery.

Adults should avoid heavy lifting for several weeks after a hernia repair. The surgeon can give the patient advice about specific weight limits on lifting. Contact sports and vigorous **exercise** should be avoided for about three weeks after a femoral hernia repair. Many patients will be able to return to most of their daily activities in a

few days, with complete recovery taking about a month in patients without other medical conditions.

Risks

All surgical procedures have associated risks, both surgical and anesthesia-related. Bleeding and infection are the two primary surgical risks. The risk of infection for an uncomplicated femoral hernia repair is about 1%. Anesthesia-related risks include reactions to the anesthetic agents, including interactions with over-the-counter and herbal preparations, as well as potential respiratory problems. There is a small risk of recurrence of a femoral hernia. In addition, female patients are at some risk of injury to the nerves and blood supply of their reproductive organs, because femoral hernias develop in a part of the abdominal wall that is close to the uterus and ovaries.

Normal results

Normal results with timely diagnosis and repair of a femoral hernia are a smooth recovery with no recurrence of the hernia.

Morbidity and mortality rates

The mortality rate following an uncomplicated femoral hernia repair is essentially zero. The mortality rate for repair of a strangulated hernia that has necessitated a **bowel resection** is higher, however, ranging from 5–19%. Morbidity following an uncomplicated herniorraphy is low; one Danish study reported that the most common complication, reported by 8% of patients, was pain during procedures performed under local anesthesia. A British study of laparoscopic hernia repairs found

---

QUESTIONS TO ASK THE DOCTOR

- How many femoral hernia repairs have you performed?
- Am I a candidate for laparoscopic surgery?
- How many femoral hernia repairs have you performed with a laparoscope?
- What kinds of complications have your patients experienced?
- How long is my recovery likely to take?
- What limitations will there be on my daily activities, such as returning to work, driving, or lifting a toddler?

KEY TERMS

Bilateral—Occurring on both the right and left sides of the body.

Femoral—Pertaining to the thigh region.

Gangrene—The death of a considerable mass of tissue, usually associated with loss of blood supply and followed by bacterial infection.

Hernia—The protrusion of a loop or piece of tissue through an incision or abnormal opening in other tissues. A femoral hernia is one that develops near the upper thigh in the groin area.

Herniorrhaphy—The medical term for a hernia repair.

Incarceration—The abnormal confinement of a section of the intestine or other body tissues. A femoral hernia may lead to incarceration of part of the intestine.

Intra-abdominal pressure—Pressure that occurs within the abdominal cavity. Pressure in this area builds up with coughing, crying, and the pressure exerted when bearing down with a bowel movement.

Reduction—The correction of a hernia, fracture, or dislocation.

Strangulation—A condition in which a vessel, section of the intestine, or other body part is compressed or constricted to the point that blood cannot circulate.

that only 22 out of 3017 patients reported recurrence of the hernia. The incidence of postoperative swelling and bruising was 8%.

Alternatives

There are no medical or surgical alternatives to a femoral hernia repair other than watchful waiting. There is some risk that the hernia will enlarge, however, which increases the risk of incarceration or strangulation. Moreover, the complications and risks of surgery increase with incarcerated or strangulated hernias. Once a hernia is suspected or diagnosed, it should be evaluated by a surgeon within a month to lower the risk of complications.

See also Incisional hernia repair; Inguinal hernia repair.

Resources

BOOKS

Ashcraft, Keith W. *Pediatric Surgery*. Philadelphia, PA: W. B. Saunders Company, 2000.

Delvin, David. *Coping with a Hernia*. London, UK: Sheldon Press, 1998.

PERIODICALS

Callesen, T., K. Bech, and H. Kehlet. "Feasibility of Local Infiltration Anaesthesia for Recurrent Groin Hernia Repair." *European Journal of Surgery* 167 (November 2001): 851-854.

Kapiris, S. A., W. A. Brough, C. M. Royston, et al. "Laparoscopic Transabdominal Preperitoneal (TAPP) Hernia Repair. A 7-Year Two-Center Experience in 3017 Patients." *Surgical Endoscopy* 15 (September 2001): 972-975.

Kulah, B., A. P. Duzgun, M. Moran, et al. "Emergency Hernia Repairs in Elderly Patients." *American Journal of Surgery* 182 (November 2001): 455-459.

Manthey, David, MD. "Hernias." *eMedicine*, June 22, 2001 [June 6, 2003]. <www.emedicine.com/EMERG/topic251.htm>.

ORGANIZATIONS

American Academy of Family Physicians. 11400 Tomahawk Creek Parkway, Leawood, KS 66211-2672. (913) 906-6000. E-mail: fp@aafp.org. <www.aafp.org>.

American Academy of Pediatrics. 141 Northwest Point Boulevard, Elk Grove Village, IL 60007-1098. (847) 434-4000. Fax: (847) 434-8000. E-mail: kidsdoc@aap.org. <www.aap.org>.

American College of Surgeons. 633 North St. Clair Street, Chicago, IL 60611-3231. (312) 202-5000. Fax: (312) 202-5001. <www.facs.org>.

OTHER

Hernia Resource Center. <www.herniainfo.com>.
National Library of Medicine. <www.nlm.nih.gov>.

Esther Csapo Rastegari, R.N., B.S.N., Ed.M.

Femoropopliteal bypass *see* **Peripheral vascular bypass surgery**

Fetal lung maturity test *see* **Lipid tests**

Fetal surgery

Definition

Fetal surgery allows doctors to treat certain abnormalities of the fetus that might otherwise be fatal or cause significant problems if permitted to progress.

Purpose

Approximately 3% of babies born in the United States each year have a complex birth defect. Parents are often left with the options of choosing to abort the fetus or treat the condition after birth. Certain birth defects, however, are complicated by the labor and delivery process; others may progress quickly after birth to cause significant disability or death. Fetal surgical techniques offer early intervention in order to treat such defects before they become more serious. The first open fetal surgery took place at the University of California at San Francisco (UCSF) in 1981.

Some of the fetal abnormalities that may be treated by fetal surgery are:

- Myelomeningocele. Also called spina bifida, myelomeningocele is a condition in which the spine fails to close properly during early fetal development. The spinal cord may protrude or be exposed through an opening in the lower back. Paralysis, neurological problems, bowel and bladder problems, and hydrocephalus (fluid buildup in the brain) may result. Myelomeningocele affects one out of every 1,000 babies born in the United States.

- Congenital diaphragmatic hernia (CDH). In babies with CDH, the diaphragm (the thin muscle that separates the chest from the abdomen) doesn't develop properly. The abdominal organs may enter the chest cavity through a hole (hernia) and cause pulmonary hyperplasia (underdeveloped lungs). CDH occurs in about one out of every 2,000 births.

- Urinary tract obstruction. The urethra (the tube that carries urine from the bladder to the outside of the body) may become obstructed *in utero* or fail to develop normally. When this happens, urine can back up into the kidneys and destroy tissue or cause the bladder to become enlarged. The amount of amniotic fluid also decreases because fetal urine is its major component. Pulmonary hypoplasia usually results because the lungs rely on amniotic fluid in their development.

- Congenital cystic adenomatoid malformation of the lung (CCAM). CCAM is a large mass of malformed lung tissue that does not function properly. As a result of its large size, it may put pressure on the heart and lead to heart failure. Lung development is also affected, and pulmonary hyperplasia may result.

- Twin/twin transfusion syndrome (TTTS). In some twin pregnancies, the two fetuses will share a placenta. TTTS occurs in approximately 15% of these twins when blood volume between the fetuses is unequal, causing abnormally low blood volume in the donor twin and abnormally high blood volume in the "recipient" twin. There is often a large difference in size between the twins. Approximately 70–80% of fetuses suffering from TTTS will die without intervention.

- Sacrococcygeal teratoma (SCT). This usually benign fetal tumor develops at the base of the spine (coccyx) and affects approximately one in 35,000 to 40,000 newborns in the United States. The tumor may become very large (sometimes as large as the fetus) and filled with blood vessels, causing stress on the heart.

Description

What fetal surgical technique is used depends on the specific condition of the fetus and its severity. The fetoscopic temporary tracheal occlusion procedure is used to treat CDH. The trachea is temporarily blocked (occluded) by a small balloon to trap fluid in the lungs (that normally escapes into the amniotic fluid); buildup of the fluid enlarges the lungs and stimulates their growth, pushing any abdominal organs that have moved into the chest cavity back into the abdomen. The occlusion is removed immediately after birth of the baby. The procedure is performed endoscopically. Rather than make a large incision into the abdomen and uterus, the surgeon inserts telescopic instruments through a tiny 1 in (2.5 cm) incision and uses them to perform the surgery. Other conditions that are treated with fetoscopic surgery are TTTS (to remove abnormal connections between blood vessels with a laser) and urinary tract obstruction (to insert a wire mesh tube called a stent into the bladder to allow urine to exit the body).

Open fetal surgery is used for conditions that cannot be treated endoscopically. An incision is made through the abdomen and the uterus is partially removed from the body. Amniotic fluid is drained from the uterus and kept in a warmer for replacement after completion of the surgery. An incision is made in the uterus (called a hysterotomy). In order to minimize bleeding of the uterus, an instrument called a uterine stapler is used to make an incision while simultaneously placing staples around the perimeter of the incision to prevent bleeding. Surgery is then performed on the fetus through the opening in the uterus to locate the abnormality and remove or fix it. Open fetal surgery is used for CCAM (to remove the cystic mass), myelomeningocele (to close the exposed spine), and SCT (to remove the tumor). Because of the nature of open fetal surgery, delivery for this child and all subsequent children of this mother will have to be performed by **cesarean section**.

Diagnosis/Preparation

Detection of many birth defects is possible through the use of sophisticated imaging and diagnostic techniques such as:

- Ultrasound. This imaging technique uses a machine that transmits high frequency sound waves to visualize structures in the human body, including the uterus and fetus.

Ultrasound is used to determine the size, position, and age of the fetus; to measure the amount of amniotic fluid; and to assess the fetus for any congenital abnormalities.

- Chorionic villus sampling (CVS). Cells are collected from the placenta with a thin plastic tube inserted through the cervix (opening to the uterus) or a needle inserted through the abdomen. The cells may then be analyzed for possible genetic disorders.
- Alpha-fetoprotein (AFP) testing. AFP is a protein made by the developing fetus. Large amounts of AFP in the mother's bloodstream may indicate certain fetal abnormalities.
- Amniocentesis. A needle is inserted through the woman's abdomen and into the uterus to procure a sample of amniotic fluid. Fetal cells in the fluid are then analyzed for possible genetic disorders.

Once a congenital abnormality has been diagnosed, the condition will be assessed to determine if the fetus is eligible for fetal surgery. Generally only the most severe conditions that are certain to cause fetal death or significant disability are treated with fetal surgery. If fetal surgery is indicated, the parents will meet with the team of health care providers that will be involved in the surgery.

To prepare for the surgery, the steroid betamethasone will be given in order to speed up the development of the fetus's lungs. A complete history and **physical examination** will be performed. A monitor will be used to track uterine contractions and fetal heart rate. The patient will be instructed to refrain from eating and drinking after midnight the day of surgery, and will sign a surgical consent. Blood samples may be taken for laboratory tests and to type match the patient's blood in case a blood transfusion is necessary. An intravenous (IV) catheter will be used to infuse fluids and/or medications to the patient.

Aftercare

Postoperative recovery generally takes from five to 10 days. The patient will be closely monitored to ensure that she does not go into premature labor. She may be put on bed rest to minimize this risk. Some signs of premature labor include contractions, cramping, lower back pain or abdominal pain or pressure, vaginal bleeding, and leaking of fluid from the vagina. Tocolytics are drugs given to delay or stop labor; some commonly administered tocolytics are terbutaline, indocin, and magnesium sulfate. **Antibiotics** will usually be administered to prevent postsurgical infection.

Risks

Some risks associated with fetal surgery include infection of the incision or lining of the uterus, premature

KEY TERMS

Cesarean section—A surgical procedure in which incisions are made through a woman's abdomen and uterus to deliver her baby.

Hernia—The protrusion of an organ or other structure through an opening in the wall that normally contains it.

Hydrocephalus—The buildup of cerebrospinal fluid in the brain.

Hysterotomy—Surgical incision of the uterus.

Oligohydramnios—Low levels of amniotic fluid during pregnancy.

Placenta—The organ that develops along with the fetus to connect the fetus to the mother.

Pulmonary hyperplasia.—Underdeveloped lungs.

Tocolytics—Drugs administered to stop or delay the onset of labor.

labor and delivery, bleeding, gestational diabetes, leakage of amniotic fluid, and infertility as well as those complications associated with anesthesia.

Normal results

The results of fetal surgery depend on the reason for the procedures. Successful results of fetal surgery generally include halting the progression of the congenital malformation and perhaps reversing some of the potential complications that would arise without intervention.

Morbidity and mortality rates

One study of open fetal surgery used to repair myelomeningocele indicated that the risk of going into premature labor was significantly increased among women who had had the procedure (50% compared to 9% of similar cases with no fetal surgery performed). There was also an increased risk of oligohydramnios or low amniotic fluid (48% compared to 4% of similar cases with no fetal surgery performed). Because of the high risk of premature labor associated with fetal surgery, some fetuses have died during premature birth.

Alternatives

There are some alternative procedures that are offered for treating specific birth defects, depending on their severity. Fetal surgery is generally recommended only for the most severe defects. For example, myelomeningocele may be treated by closing of the lesion soon after delivery.

SCTs and CCAMs may also be removed soon after the baby is born. Parents are often given the option of aborting the fetus (termed therapeutic abortion); or they may decide to refrain from medical intervention.

Resources

PERIODICALS

Bruner, Joseph, Noel Tulipan, Ray Paschall, Frank Boehm, William Walsh, Sandra Silva, Marta Hernanz-Schulman, Lisa Lowe, and George Reed. "Fetal Surgery for Myelomeningocele and Incidence of Shunt-Dependent Hydrocephalus." *Journal of the American Medical Association* 282, no. 19 (November 17, 1999): 1819–25.

ORGANIZATIONS

Center for Fetal Diagnosis and Treatment, Children's Hospital of Philadelphia. 34th Street and Civic Center Boulevard, Philadelphia, PA 19104-4399. (800) IN-UTERO. <http://fetalsurgery.chop.edu>.

Fetal Diagnosis & Therapy, Vanderbilt University Medical Center. B-1100 Medical Center North, Nashville, TN 37232. (615) 343-5227.

Fetal Treatment Center, University of California at San Francisco. 513 Parnassus Ave., HSW 1601, San Francisco, CA 94143-0570. (800) RX-FETUS. <http://www.fetus.ucsf.edu>.

Spina Bifida Association of America. 4590 MacArthur Blvd., SW, Washington, DC 20007. (800) 621-3141. <http://www.sbaa.org>.

OTHER

Danielpour, Moise, and Diana L. Farmer. "Fetal Surgery for Congenital CNS Abnormalities." *Cedars-Sinai Net Journal.* 2002 [cited February 28, 2003]. <http://www.cedars-sinai.edu/mdnsi/images/fetalsurg.pdf>.

"The Fetal Treatment Center: Our Treatments." *University of California* at *San Francisco.* 2001 [cited February 28, 2003]. <http://www.fetus.ucsf.edu/ourtreatments.htm>.

Iannelli, Vincent. "Surgery Before Birth?" *Pediatrics.* January 29, 2000 [cited February 28, 2003]. <http://pediatrics.about.com/library/weekly/aa012900.htm>.

Stephanie Dionne Sherk

Fetoscopy

Definition

Fetoscopy is a procedure that utilizes an instrument called a fetoscope to evaluate or treat the fetus during pregnancy.

Purpose

There are two different types of fetoscopy: external and endoscopic.

Health-care profesionals who may use the external fetoscope include a nurse practitioner, nurse midwife, and obstetrician. External fetoscopy may be performed in any setting with the pregnant woman lying supine or in a semi-sitting position. Endoscopic fetoscopy requires a high level of skill and experience by fetal surgeons and is performed in a hospital setting. During the procedures, a radiology technician may perform an ultrasound, and a laboratory technician may be involved in blood sampling. Nurses will participate in both outpatient and inpatient procedures.

External fetoscopy

An external fetoscope resembles a **stethoscope**, but with a headpiece. It is used externally on the mother's abdomen to auscultate (listen to) the fetal heart tones after about 18 weeks gestation. It also allows a birth attendant to monitor the fetus intermittently and ensure that the baby is tolerating labor without the mother having to be attached to a continuous fetal monitor.

Endoscopic fetoscopy

The second type of fetoscope is a fiber-optic endoscope. It is inserted into the uterus either transabdominally (through the abdomen) or transcervically (through the cervix) to visualize the fetus, to obtain fetal tissue samples, or to perform **fetal surgery**.

Approximately 3% of babies born in the United States each year have a complex birth defect. Certain birth defects are complicated by the labor and delivery process, while others may progress quickly after birth to cause significant disability or death. Fetal surgical techniques utilizing the endoscopic fetoscope offer early intervention in order to treat such defects before they become serious.

Some of the fetal abnormalities that may be treated by endoscopic fetoscopy are:

• Congenital diaphragmatic hernia (CDH). In babies with CDH, the diaphragm (the thin muscle that separates the chest from the abdomen) doesn't develop properly. The abdominal organs may enter the chest cavity through a hole (hernia) and cause pulmonary hyperplasia (underdeveloped lungs). CDH occurs in about one out of every 2,000 births.

• Urinary tract obstruction. The urethra (the tube that carries urine from the bladder to the outside of the body) may become obstructed *in utero* or fail to develop normally. When this happens, urine can back up into the kidneys and destroy tissue or cause the bladder to become enlarged. The amount of amniotic fluid also decreases because fetal urine is its major component. Pulmonary hypoplasia usually results because the lungs rely on amniotic fluid in their development.

• Twin/twin transfusion syndrome (TTTS). In some twin pregnancies, the two fetuses will share a placenta (called a monochorionic pregnancy). TTTS occurs in approximately 15% of these twins when blood volume between the fetuses is unequal, causing abnormally low blood volume in the donor twin and abnormally high blood volume in the recipient twin. There is often a large difference in size between the twins. Approximately 70–80% of fetuses suffering from TTTS will die without intervention.

• Acardiac twin. This condition also occurs in monochorionic pregnancies, but one twin develops normally while the other develops without a heart. The acardiac twin receives its blood supply from the normal twin, whose heart must now work harder to pump blood through both fetuses. Approximately 50–75% of acardiac twins will die as a result. An acardiac twin occurs in 1% of monochorionic pregnancies and one out of 35,000 overall pregnancies.

Demographics

External fetoscopy may be used to determine the fetal heart rate in any woman with a viable pregnancy, although certain circumstances may compromise its quality (a noisy environment, an obese mother, or hydramnios [excess amniotic fluid]).

No demographic data are available regarding patients undergoing operative fetoscopy, since it is a relatively new procedure being performed at only a handful of hospitals around the United States.

Description

The external fetoscope is used to listen to fetal heart tones for rate and rhythm. The earpieces and the headpiece allow auscultation (listening) via both air and bone conduction. External fetoscopy is inexpensive, noninvasive, and does not require electricity. It is difficult, however, to clearly hear the fetal heart tones prior to 18 to 20 weeks gestation. Doppler ultrasound can detect fetal heart tones around weeks 10 to 12.

Endoscopic fetoscopy uses a thin (1 mm) fiberoptic scope. Developed in the 1970s, the endoscope was originally inserted transabdominally to visualize the fetus for gross abnormalities suspected by ultrasound or to obtain tissue and blood samples. It was performed after about 18 weeks gestation. Even with practitioner expertise, associated fetal loss was 3–7%. During the 1980s, ultrasound-guided needle sampling of cord blood replaced fetoscopy when samples of fetal blood were required.

As laparoscopic and microsurgical techniques have become more common and the instrumentation has become more advanced technologically, fetoscopy has improved for fetal diagnostic and therapeutic purposes. Fetal surgery performed through an open maternal abdomen has a higher risk of such complications as infection, premature rupture of membranes, preterm labor, or fetal death. If surgery is performed via fetoscopy, which requires a very small transabdominal incision, the risks are much smaller. Techniques have advanced enough to allow some fetoscopy to be performed in the first trimester via the mother's cervix. The term "obstetrical endoscopy" may be used for surgery on the placenta, umbilical cord, or on the fetal membranes. The term "endoscopic fetal surgery" is used for such procedures as the repair of a fetal congenital diaphragmatic hernia or obstructed bladder.

Diagnosis/Preparation

The use of external fetoscopy requires access to the maternal abdomen, with the mother lying supine or in a semi-seated position. Afterwards, the mother is able to get up and resume a normal activity level.

Preparation for endoscopic fetoscopy will depend on the extent of the procedure, and whether it is performed transcervically or transabdominally. Obtaining a small fetal tissue sample is a smaller procedure by comparison to fetal surgery. Other factors include outpatient versus inpatient stay and anesthesia (both maternal and fetal). For some procedures medication may be administered to temporarily decrease fetal movement to lower the risk of fetal injury. Maternal anesthesia may be local, regional, or general.

Aftercare

External fetoscopy does not require aftercare. The care following fetal endoscopic use will depend on the extent of the procedure and the type of anesthesia used. If the procedure is done on an outpatient basis, the mother and fetus will be monitored for a period of time prior to discharge. More extensive surgery will require inpatient hospital **postoperative care**.

Risks

The only potential complication with external fetoscopy is the possibility of missing an abnormal heart

---

QUESTIONS TO ASK THE DOCTOR

- Why is fetoscopy recommended in my case?
- What alternatives to fetoscopy are available to me?
- For endoscopic fetoscopy, what will be the results if there is no medical intervention?
- For endoscopic fetoscopy, will the procedure be performed on an outpatient basis? What type of anesthesia will be used?

---

rate or rhythm. Its usefulness and accuracy depend on the skill of the practitioner.

Endoscopic fetoscopy has the potential for causing infection in the fetus and/or mother; premature rupture of the amniotic membranes; premature labor; and fetal death. When endoscopic fetal surgery is done instead of open-uterus fetal surgery, the risks to the mother and fetus are decreased. The risks are because the incision is significantly smaller, with less potential blood loss, decreased uterine irritability, and decreased risk of early miscarriage.

Normal results

The normal fetal heart rate is 120 to 160 beats per minute, regardless of the method used for auscultation (external fetoscopy or Doppler ultrasound). Some variability of fetal heart rate is expected, as the heart rate increases with fetal activity and slows with fetal rest.

Results expected using endoscopic fetoscopy will vary depending on the procedure undertaken. The goal is for the maximum benefit with the minimum of risk or complication to both the mother and fetus.

Morbidity and mortality rates

There is no morbidity or mortality associated with external fetoscopy. In the case of endoscopic fetoscopy, the risk of fetal loss is estimated to be between 3% and 5%. The procedure is therefore usually recommended only for the more severe cases of fetal disorders that may be treated during pregnancy.

Alternatives

A health care provider may listen to the fetal heart rate by means of a hand-held Doppler device, which uses ultrasound to amplify the heart beat. A continuous electronic fetal monitor may also be used to track the fetal

---

heart rate and maternal uterine contractions. It is held against the mother's abdomen by means of elastic straps.

Open fetal surgery is an alternative to internal fetoscopy. It is used for conditions that cannot be treated endoscopically. An incision is made through the abdomen and the uterus is partially removed from the body. Amniotic fluid is drained from the uterus and kept in a warmer for replacement after completion of the surgery. An incision is made in the uterus (called a hysterotomy). In order to minimize bleeding of the uterus, an instrument called a uterine stapler is used to make an incision while simultaneously placing staples around the perimeter of the incision to prevent bleeding. Surgery is then performed on the fetus through the opening in the uterus to locate the abnormality and remove or repair it. There is a greater risk of infection, premature labor, and leakage of amniotic fluid with open fetal surgery than there is with fetoscopy.

Resources

BOOKS

Creasy, Robert K., and Robert Resnik. *Maternal-Fetal Medicine,* 4th Edition. Philadelphia: W. B. Saunders Company, 1999.

Pillitteri, Adele. *Maternal & Child Health Nursing,* 3rd Edition. Philadelphia: Lippincott, 1999.

Scott, James R. et al., eds. *Danforth's Obstetrics and Gynecology.* Philadelphia: Lippincott Williams & Wilkens, 1999.

PERIODICALS

Gratacos, E. and J. A. Deprest. "Current Experience With Fetoscopy and the Eurofoetus Registry for Fetoscopic Procedures." *European Journal of Obstetrics, Gynecology, and Reproductive Biology* 92, no. 1 (September 2000): 151–159.

ORGANIZATIONS

American College of Obstetricians and Gynecologists. 409 12th St., SW, PO Box 96920. Washington, DC 20090-6920. <http://www.acog.com>.

Fetal Treatment Center. University of California San Francisco. 513 Parnassus Ave., HSW 1601, San Francisco, CA 94143-0570. (800) RX-FETUS. <http://www.fetus.ucsf.edu>.

OTHER

"The Fetal Treatment Center: Our Treatments." *University of California San Francisco.* 2001 [cited February 28, 2003]. <http://www.fetus.ucsf.edu/ourtreatments.htm>.

"Operative Fetoscopy." *Florida Institute for Fetal Diagnosis and Therapy* March 11, 2003 [cited March 12, 2003]. <http://www.fetalmd.com>.

Singh, Daljit. "Antenatal Testing." *eMedicine.* March 26, 2002 [cited March 12, 2003]. <http://www.emedicine.com/oph/topic485.htm>.

Esther Csapo Rastegari, R.N., B.S.N., Ed.M.
Stephanie Dionne Sherk

Fibrin sealants

Definition

Fibrin sealants are a type of surgical tissue adhesive derived from human and animal blood products. The ingredients in these sealants interact during application to form a stable clot composed of a blood protein called fibrin. Fibrin sealants are also called fibrin glues. They have been used in Japan and Western Europe since the 1980s, but were not approved for use in the United States until 1998 due to the Food and Drug Administration's (FDA) concerns about virus contamination. As of 2003, all fibrin sealants used in the United States are made from blood plasma taken from carefully screened donors and rigorously tested to eliminate hepatitis viruses, HIV-1, and parvovirus.

Purpose

Originally developed during World War II to stop bleeding from battle injuries, fibrin sealants are presently used during surgery for several different purposes:

- to control bleeding in the area where the surgeon is operating
- to speed wound healing
- to seal off hollow body organs or cover holes made by standard sutures
- to provide slow-release delivery of medications to tissues exposed during surgery

Fibrin sealants have several advantages over older methods of hemostasis (stopping bleeding). They speed up the formation of a stable clot; they can be applied to very small blood vessels and to areas that are difficult to reach with conventional sutures; they reduce the amount of blood lost during surgery; they lower the risk of postoperative inflammation or infection; and they are conveniently absorbed by the body during the healing process. They are particularly useful for minimally invasive procedures and for treating patients with blood clotting disorders. Fibrin sealants are, however, being replaced for some specialized purposes by newer wound adhesives known as cyanoacrylates.

Description

All fibrin sealants in use as of 2003 have two major ingredients, purified fibrinogen (a protein) and purified thrombin (an enzyme) derived from human or bovine (cattle) blood. Many sealants have two additional ingredients, human blood factor XIII and a substance called aprotinin, which is derived from cows' lungs. Factor XIII is a compound that strengthens blood clots by forming cross-links between strands of fibrin. Aprotinin is a protein that inhibits the enzymes that break down blood clots.

Preparation

The preparation and application of fibrin sealants are somewhat complicated. The thrombin and fibrinogen are freeze-dried and packaged in vials that must be warmed before use. The two ingredients are then dissolved in separate amounts of water. Next, the thrombin and fibrinogen solutions are loaded into a double-barreled syringe that allows them to mix and combine as they are sprayed on the incision. Pieces of surgical gauze or fleece may be moistened with the sealant solutions to cover large incisions or stop heavy bleeding.

As the thrombin and fibrinogen solutions combine, a clot develops in the same way that it would form during normal blood clotting through a series of chemical reactions known as the coagulation cascade. At the end of the cascade, the thrombin breaks up the fibrinogen molecules into smaller segments of a second blood protein called fibrin. The fibrin molecules arrange themselves into strands that are then cross-linked by a blood factor known as Factor XIII to form a lattice or net-like pattern that stabilizes the clot.

Fibrin sealants are undergoing rapid refinement as the result of recent advances in tissue adhesives in general. In 1997, the Tissue Adhesive Center was founded at the University of Virginia Health Sciences Center in order to develop and test new fibrin sealants and other surgical glues. Recent developments include a delivery system that forms a fibrin sealant from the patient's own blood within a 30-minute cycle, and uses a spraypen rather than a double-barreled syringe for applying the

sealant. The use of the patient's own blood lowers the risk of allergic reactions to blood products derived from animal or donated blood.

Normal results

Reports that have been published between 2001 and 2003 indicate that fibrin sealants are a safe and highly effective form of surgical adhesive. A survey done in 2000 at the University of Virginia hospital found that over 90% of the surgeons who had tried fibrin sealants were pleased with the results. Several American studies have reported that fibrin sealants have improved surgical outcomes significantly by shortening the time required for operations; lowering the rate of infections and other complications; minimizing blood loss during surgery; and reducing the amount of scar tissue formed over incisions. German researchers have found that fibrin sealants containing Factor XIII generally give better results than those that do not.

See also Stitches and staples; Transfusion.

Resources

BOOKS

"Hemostasis and Coagulation Disorders." Section 11, Chapter 131, *The Merck Manual of Diagnosis and Therapy.* Ed. Mark H. Beers, MD, and Robert Berkow, MD. Whitehouse Station, NJ: Merck Research Laboratories, 1999-2001.

PERIODICALS

Dickneite, G., H. J. Metzner, M. Kroez, et al. "The Importance of Factor XIII as a Component of Fibrin Sealants." *Journal of Surgical Research* 107 (October 2002): 186-195.

Dodd, R. A., R. Cornwell, N. E. Holm, et al. "The Vivostat Application System: A Comparison with Conventional Fibrin Sealant Application Systems." *Technology and Health Care* 10 (2002): 401-411.

Jackson, M. R. "Fibrin Sealants in Surgical Practice: An Overview." *American Journal of Surgery* 182 (August 2001) (2 Suppl): 1S-7S.

Mankad, P. S., and M. Codispoti. "The Role of Fibrin Sealants in Hemostasis." *American Journal of Surgery* 182 (August 2001) (2 Suppl): 21S-28S.

Morikawa, T. "Tissue Sealing." *American Journal of Surgery* 182 (August 2001) (2 Suppl): 29S-35S.

ORGANIZATIONS

Center for Biologics Evaluation and Research (CBER), U.S. Food and Drug Administration (FDA). 1401 Rockville Pike, Rockville, MD 20852-1448. (800) 835-4709 or (301) 827-1800. <www.fda.gov/cber>.

Tissue Adhesive Center. University of Virginia Health Sciences Center, MR4 Building, Room 3122, Charlottesville, VA 22908. (434) 243-0315. <www.hsc.virginia.edu/tac>.

OTHER

Food and Drug Administration (FDA) Talk Paper T98-22. *New Fibrin Sealant Approved to Help Control Bleeding in*

KEY TERMS

Aprotinin—A protein derived from cows' lungs included in some fibrin sealants to prevent the fibrin clot from dissolving.

Coagulation cascade—A term that refers to the process of blood clotting. The cascade itself is a series of chemical reactions involving blood proteins and enzymes that occurs wherever there is a break in a blood vessel. The end product of the cascade is a protein called fibrin.

Factor XIII—A substance found in blood that forms cross-links between strands of fibrin during the process of blood coagulation. Factor XIII is an ingredient in some types of fibrin sealants. It is also known as fibrin stabilizing factor.

Fibrin—A blood protein formed as the end result of the coagulation cascade. Fibrin is formed from fibrinogen when it interacts with thrombin.

Fibrinogen—A blood protein made in the liver that is broken up into shorter molecules by the action of thrombin to form fibrin.

Hemostasis—Stopping bleeding from a wound or incision. Fibrin sealants are used to speed up hemostasis.

Plasma—The liquid part of blood. Plasma is a clear pale yellow fluid composed primarily of water and dissolved minerals.

Thrombin—An enzyme found in blood plasma that helps to convert fibrinogen into fibrin.

Surgery. Rockville, MD: U. S. Department of Health and Human Services, May 1, 1998.

Smith, Andrew. "Use of Surgical Glue Takes Hold at Temple." *Temple Times*, May 18, 2000 [cited February 18, 2003]. <www.temple.edu/temple_times/5-18-00/glue.html>.

Rebecca Frey, Ph.D.

Fibroid surgery *see* **Myomectomy**

Finding a surgeon

Definitions

Finding a surgeon refers to the process of choosing a doctor with specialized training in one or more branches of surgery to perform a specific procedure. It is almost always done in the context of **elective surgery** rather than emergency operations.

Description

Recent changes in the healthcare professions

Choosing a surgeon is a relatively new development in health care. Until fairly recently, many people, particularly in rural areas in the United States and Canada, relied on one doctor who generally treated all members of the family for most illnesses and some surgical procedures, including **tooth extraction** and childbirth. These general practitioners often treated the same patients over a period of many years and consequently knew their medical histories quite well. Most hospitals were so-called general hospitals, and admitted patients for a wide variety of surgical procedures. Since World War II, however, advances in medical knowledge and technology have led to increasing specialization of both health care professionals and the facilities they work in. As of 2003, three members of a family, each scheduled for a different surgical procedure, might well be sent to three different hospitals or clinics in three different cities as well as having three different surgeons performing the operations. Under these circumstances, choosing a surgeon can seem both complicated and confusing.

Referral to a surgeon

In the United States, most people with health insurance belong to a health maintenance organization (HMO) or similar health care plan that either assigns them to a doctor or asks them to choose from a list of primary care physicians, or PCPs. PCPs are usually family practitioners, pediatricians, or internists, although some health care plans allow women to choose a gynecologist/obstetrician as their PCP. The PCP is sometimes referred to as a gatekeeper, because he or she makes decisions about referring patients to surgeons and other specialists. In some **managed care plans**, the PCP simply assigns patients to specific surgeons; in others, the patient may be given a list of surgeons to choose from. Many people use the PCP's list as a starting point for choosing their surgeon, and may ask the PCP for his or her opinion of the surgeons on the list. Such procedures as cosmetic surgery are not usually covered by HMOs, but many people will consult their primary care physician about this type of surgery anyway on the grounds that the PCP knows their medical history and may be able to give them a "short list" of local surgeons to consider.

In Canada, Australia, and other countries with publicly financed health care systems, patients usually have two options when surgery is considered. They may have the operation performed in a public hospital, in which case they are not likely to be able to choose their surgeon or even the date of the operation. Patients with private insurance, however, have the option of treatment in private clinics that give them some voice in selecting their surgeon. Private patients also do not have to wait as long for treatment; one Canadian study published in 2002 estimates that the average patient referred by a general practitioner for surgery in a public hospital waits an average of 16.5 weeks for admission, whereas the average waiting period for private patients is five weeks. Canadian medical journals have reported advertisements promoting surgery in the United States to Canadians who are frustrated by long waiting lists for certain operations.

Basic considerations in choosing a surgeon

TYPE OF PROCEDURE. Surgical procedures vary considerably in complexity and the length of specialized training needed to perform them. Some can be carried out by a general surgeon, who is a physician who has completed residency training and passed an examination given by the American Board of Surgery, or ABS. The ABS, which is one of 24 certifying boards that comprise the American Board of Medical Specialties (ABMS), provides a lengthy definition of the training and experience required of general surgeons. According to the ABS, a general surgeon should be competent to perform basic procedures in all of the following areas, though not necessarily the "full range and complexity of procedures" in each field.

The ABS defines the following fields as "essential in the comprehensive education of a broadly based surgeon":

• alimentary (digestive) tract

• abdomen and its contents

• breast, skin, and soft tissue

• the endocrine system

• head and neck surgery

• pediatric surgery

• critical care surgery

• surgical oncology (cancer treatment)

• organ transplantation

• trauma and burns

• vascular surgery

After certification by the ABS, a surgeon may undergo additional training in one of 10 surgical specialties as defined by the American Board of Medical Specialties (ABMS):

• colon and rectal surgery

• neurological (brain and nervous system) surgery

• obstetrics and gynecology

• ophthalmology (eye surgery)

• orthopedic (bone and joint) surgery

• otolaryngology (ear, nose, and throat surgery)

• pediatric surgery

• plastic surgery

• thoracic (chest) surgery

• urology

To complicate the picture even further, some surgical specialties are further divided into subspecialties. For example, plastic surgeons may specialize in plastic surgery of the hand, or plastic surgery of the face and neck. Similarly, some ear, nose and throat specialists specialize further in pediatric otolaryngology. For this reason, one of the first questions patients should ask their primary care provider in choosing a surgeon is the degree of specialization required to perform a specific procedure as well as the reasons for having the operation. Among other considerations, specialization will affect the range of choices available to the patient regarding the hospital or clinic where the operation is performed as well as choosing the operating surgeon. Some highly specialized procedures may require patients to travel long distances to a hospital or surgical center in another city.

ALTERNATIVES TO SURGERY. The Agency for Healthcare Quality and Research (formerly the Agency for Health Care Policy and Research) publishes a booklet called *Questions to Ask Your Doctor Before You Have Surgery*, which can be downloaded from the Agency's web site. The third question discussed in the booklet concerns such nonsurgical treatments as medications or changes in diet and lifestyle. Elective surgical procedures have potential risks as well as benefits, and patients should ask about both before committing themselves to having an operation. Some health care professionals advise exploring medical options first before agreeing to surgery when both types of treatments are available for a given condition and there is time to try nonsurgical approaches.

CREDENTIALS AND SKILL LEVEL. It is important for patients to check a surgeon's credentials and length of experience. After a doctor has received his or her MD or DO from an accredited school of medicine or osteopathy, he or she must pass a national licensure examination and a set of licensing procedures set by each state in order to practice general medicine or surgery in that state. Most surgeons have their medical school diploma and state licensing certificate framed and displayed on an office wall where patients can see them.

The American College of Surgeons recommends that patients look for the following credentials when they consult or are referred to a surgeon:

• Board certification. Board certification means that the surgeon has passed a rigorous examination administered by one of the specialty boards belonging to the ABMS. The ABMS publishes an annual directory of board certified medical specialists that can be found in many hospital libraries as well as university or medical school libraries. Patients can also call their local county medical society to verify a surgeon's specialty credentials.

• Fellowship in the American College of Surgeons. A surgeon with the letters FACS after his or her name is a Fellow of the ACS and is a board-certified surgeon.

• Approval for practice in accredited hospitals or other health care facilities. Patients can verify the accreditation status of the facility where the operation is to be performed by contacting the Joint Commission on Accreditation of Healthcare Organizations (JCAHO) for hospitals, or the Accreditation Association for Ambulatory Health Care (AAAHC) for **outpatient surgery** centers. These organizations are listed below under Resources.

An additional consideration is the number of procedures of a specific type that the surgeon performs on a regular basis. The more specialized the procedure, the more important it is for the surgeon to practice his or her skills. For example, the Johns Hopkins urology website states that a surgeon consulted for prostate surgery should have performed at least 150 prostate operations, and that it is preferable if he or she performs the same operation every day or several days a week. For some types of surgery, including joint replacement and cancer surgery, patients should look for a surgeon in high-volume medical centers where specialists have acquired a great deal of experience performing the specific procedure that the patient needs.

PERSONALITY ISSUES. In addition to a surgeon's level of skill and experience, his or her personality should be taken into consideration. Because many operations require dietary changes, certain types of **exercise**, or other detailed preparations, the patient should feel comfortable about talking to the surgeon—particularly when it comes to asking important questions about the operation itself or the surgeon's length of experience. Some patients are afraid to talk to surgeons because they have heard that surgeons have a reputation among other health professionals for being impatient, bossy, and generally lacking in "people skills." One popular article on doctors' personality styles describes the typical surgeon as fitting the "dictator" pattern, and several studies have reported that over 50% of doctors advised to seek anger management counseling are surgeons. As of 2003, however, a growing number of surgeons are recognizing that patients who take an active role in their treatment have better outcomes, and that a well-informed patient is their best ally. Patients should not hesitate to talk to several different surgeons in order to find one whose personality is a good fit with their own. One writer tells of an Australian patient who did some research at a nearby library on the operation he was going to have and then consulted two different surgeons. The first surgeon was pleased that the patient had taken the time to read about the operation, and was quite happy to answer a number of questions. The second surgeon brushed the patient aside. The patient told the writer, "[His attitude toward patients was to] keep them ignorant. Don't tell the patient a thing. I kept at him, and when I'd finished, I told him I didn't think much of his answers and that I wouldn't be back."

DISCIPLINARY HISTORY. Although only a small percentage of doctors in the United States have ever been disciplined by a professional peer review, sued for malpractice, or had their licenses suspended—about 0.5% per year—patients who are considering surgery should find out if any of the surgeons they have consulted have a history of disciplinary actions taken against them. The Federation of State Medical Boards has compiled a database called DocInfo that can be searched on the Federation's web site for information about a specific practitioner's record.

Preparation

Gathering information

Patients considering elective surgery should collect some information about the procedure in question and the qualifications required to perform it before they talk to a specific surgeon. People with Internet access can obtain information about surgical operations as well as credentialing processes on the web sites of the various surgical specialty associations. Links to these associations can be found on the ABMS web site. Many surgical specialty groups have patient education brochures and other informational material available for downloading free of charge. Most of these materials can also be obtained by writing, telephoning, or e-mailing the associations.

Other useful sources of information include hospital and outpatient surgery center web sites. These sites often have reader-friendly descriptions of specific procedures as well as information about the hospital or clinic's accreditation, location, and other important features.

Another good source of information about choosing a surgeon is first-person accounts of surgical procedures. There are a growing number of patient guides to plastic surgery, joint replacement surgery, oral and facial surgery, cancer surgery, and other procedures written by people who have had these operations. Most of these books include advice on finding one's way through the referral process as well as a list of specific questions to ask surgeons in particular specialties.

Getting recommendations

The next step in choosing a surgeon is asking other health professionals to recommend specific practitioners. As was mentioned earlier, most patients begin with their primary care doctor. Patients who have been treated recently by a medical specialist should also ask him or her for recommendations about surgeons. For example, someone who has been seeing a specialist in pulmonary (lung) medicine for asthma treatment will want to ask him or her for the names of good thoracic surgeons if an operation is recommended. One author of a popular patient guide suggests asking the PCP or medical specialist who they would ask to do the surgical operation if they themselves needed it.

Other sources of recommendations include home health care nurses or physical therapists, who are often familiar with the work of local surgeons. One expert in sports medicine has been quoted as saying, "If you want a good surgeon, ask a physical therapist. We see patients from all the surgeons. I see the same good surgeries come from the same good surgeons and the same lousy surgeries come from the same lousy surgeons. You see it all the time."

A third source of recommendations is other people who had the same procedure that the patient is considering and were pleased with the results.

Advertisements

As recently as the 1960s, it was considered unprofessional for doctors or dentists to advertise themselves except for brief listings of their specialties in professional association and local telephone directories. The spread of high-pressure advertising techniques that originated in the business world into medicine, however, has resulted in the production of web sites, radio announcements, and printed advertisements for doctors that can be confusing to patients who are looking for a surgeon. In particular, plastic surgeons who specialize in cosmetic procedures (face lifts, "tummy tucks," etc.) have been accused of exploiting people's vulnerabilities and fear of aging in their advertisements. The American Medical Association (AMA) has a set of guidelines issued in 1996 and updated in 2002 that warn doctors against using publicity containing deceptive or misleading claims. Patients looking for a surgeon should be wary of doctors who claim that they have unique skills, "secret" techniques, or an improbably large number of satisfied patients. In addition, an attractive web site or impressive advertisement should not be a substitute for a personal interview with the surgeon.

Second opinions

Patients who are considering surgery should not be shy about getting a **second opinion** if they feel unsure about having an operation after they talk to a surgeon. In fact, many health plans require patients to seek a second opinion for certain types of elective surgery before they will approve the procedure. Some insurance plans will reimburse patients for the cost of seeking a second opinion. The Centers for **Medicare** and **Medicaid** Services (CMS), formerly the Health Care Financing Administration (HCFA), publishes a brochure (Publication No. 02173) for Medicare patients on seeking second surgical opinions.

See also Elective surgery; Preparing for surgery.

Resources

BOOKS

Silber, Irwin. *A Patient's Guide to Knee and Hip Replacement: Everything You Need to Know.* New York: Simon & Schuster, 1999.

Trahair, Richard. *All About Hip Replacement: A Patient's Guide.* Melbourne, Oxford, and New York: Oxford University Press, 1998.

PERIODICALS

Johnston, C. "U.S. Ad Uses Lure of Prompt Treatment to Entice Canadians Needing Joint Replacement." *Canadian Medical Association Journal/Journal de l'Association medicale canadienne* 154 (April 1, 1996): 1071-1072.

Kaufmann, Michael. "Recognition and Management of the Behaviourally Disruptive Physician." *Ontario Medical Review* 78 (April 2001): 53-55.

Krauss, Clifford. "Long Lines Mar Canada's Low-Cost Health Care." *New York Times*, February 13, 2003 [March 1, 2003].

Ring, A. L. "Using 'Anti-Ageing' to Market Cosmetic Surgery: Just Good Business, or Another Wrinkle on the Face of Medical Practice?" *Medical Journal of Australia* 176 (June 17, 2002): 597-599.

Schwartz, R. W., J. R. Barclay, P. L. Harrell, et al. "Defining the Surgical Personality: A Preliminary Study." *Surgery* 115 (January 1994): 62-68.

Scurlock, William. "What Makes a General Surgeon." *Bulletin of the American College of Surgeons* 87 (May 2002): 24-25.

Spilson, S. V., K. C. Chung, M. L. Greenfield, and M. Walters. "Are Plastic Surgery Advertisements Conforming to the Ethical Codes of the American Society of Plastic Surgeons?" *Plastic and Reconstructive Surgery* 109 (March 2002): 1181-1186.

ORGANIZATIONS

Accreditation Association for Ambulatory Health Care (AAAHC). 3201 Old Glenview Road, Suite 300, Wilmette, IL 60091-2992. (847) 853-6060. <www.aahc.org>.

Agency for Healthcare Research and Quality (AHRQ). 2101 East Jefferson Street, Suite 501, Rockville, MD 20852. (301) 594-1364. <www.ahcpr.gov>.

American Board of Medical Specialties (ABMS). 1007 Church Street, Suite 404, Evanston, IL 60201. (866) ASK-ABMS. <www.abms.org>.

American Board of Surgery (ABS). 1617 John F. Kennedy Blvd., Suite 860, Philadelphia, PA 19103. (215) 568-4000. <www.absurgery.org>.

American College of Surgeons (ACS). 633 North Saint Clair Street, Chicago, IL 60611-3211. (312) 202-5001. <www.facs.org>.

Centers for Medicare and Medicaid Services (CMS). 7500 Security Boulevard, Baltimore, MD 21244-1850. (410) 786-3000. <cms.hhs.gov>.

Federation of State Medical Boards of the United States, Inc., P. O. Box 619850, Dallas, TX 75261-9850. (817) 868-4000. <www.fsmb.org>.

Health Canada/Santé Canada. A.L. 0900C2, Ottawa, Canada, K1A 0K9. (613) 957-2991. <www.hc-sc.gc.ca>.

Joint Commission on Accreditation of Healthcare Organizations (JCAHO). One Renaissance Boulevard, Oakbrook Terrace, IL 60181. (630) 792-5000. <www.jcaho.org>.

OTHER

Agency for Healthcare Research and Quality (AHRQ). *Questions to Ask Your Doctor Before You Have Surgery*. AHRQ Publication No. 95-0027. January 1995 [cited March 1, 2003]. <www.ahcpr.gov/consumer/surgery/htm>.

"In Search of the Right Surgeon." *Health Pages*. [cited February 28, 2003]. <www.thehealthpages.com/articles/ar-surgn.html>.

Shomon, Mary. "DoctorStyles: What Type of Doctor Do You Have? And What Style Do You Need?" *Thyroid-Info*. [cited February 28, 2003].<www.thyroid-info.com/articles/doctorstyles.htm>.

Rebecca Frey, Ph.D.

Finger reattachment

Definition

Finger reattachment (or replacement) is defined as reattachment of the part that has been completely amputated.

Purpose

Replantation refers to reattachment of a completely severed part, meaning there is no physical connection between the part that has been cut off and the person. Reattachment can be surgically performed for the finger and such other detached body parts, as the hand or arm.

Demographics

Good candidates for this procedure include persons with thumb or multiple digit **amputation**. Injury to multiple digits is an important patient selection criterion, since in some cases the least damaged digits may be shifted to the least injured or most useful stump. Patient exclusion is neither clear-cut nor absolute. Generally, severe crushing or avulsing (tearing away) injuries to the fingers may make replantation difficult, but venous grafts may help replace injured blood vessels. Additionally, older persons may have arteriosclerosis that frequently impairs function in blood vessels, especially in small vessels. Special efforts may be made to replant fingers if the person's livelihood (such as professional musical performance) depends on absolute finger control.

Description

To increase efficiency, the replantation team splits into two sub-teams. One sub-team in the **operating room** cleans the amputated finger with sterile solutions, places it on ice, and identifies and tags (with special surgical clips) nerves and blood vessels. Dead or damaged tissue is surgically removed with a procedure called **debridement**. The emergency room (ER) sub-team will assess the patient during a physical exam with x rays of the injured area, blood analysis, and cardiac (heart) monitoring. The patient is given fluids intravenously (IV), a tetanus injection, and **antibiotics**. Usually, most finger reattachments are performed with a local anesthetic such as bupivacaine and a nerve block to numb the affected arm. Maintaining a warm body temperature can enhance blood flow to the affected limb.

The surgical procedure consists of several stages. The bone in the amputated finger must be shortened and fixed, which means that the bone end is trimmed. After

The procedure is usually performed in a hospital operating room by a microsurgeon, who may be a plastic surgeon with five years of **general surgery** training, plus two years of plastic surgery training and another one or two years of training in microneurovascular surgery; or an orthopedic surgeon with one year of general surgery training, five years of **orthopedic surgery** training, and additional years in **microsurgery** training.

Hand with amputated fingers before finger reattachment surgery. *(Custom Medical Stock Photo. Reproduced by permission.)*

this process, the bone is stabilized with special sutures called K-wires, and fixed pins are placed in the bone after drilling a space to insert them. This process connects the two amputated bone fragments. After bone stabilization and fixation, the extensor and flexor tendons are repaired. This step is vital, since arteries, veins, and nerves should never be surgically connected under tension. Next, the surgeon must repair (suture) cut-off tendons, arteries, veins, and nerves. Healthy arteries and veins are sutured together without tension. A vein graft is used for blood vessels that cannot be reattached.

Nerve repair for finger reattachment is not difficult. Since the reattached bone parts are shorter than the original length, nerves can be reattached without tension. A microscope is used for magnified visualization of finger nerves during reattachment. When the severed ends of the nerve cannot be reattached, a primary nerve graft is performed. Finally, it is vital superficial veins on the affected finger (dorsal veins) to cover with a skin flap to prevent death of the venous vessels. The skin over the surgical field is loosely sutured with a few sutures. Any damaged tissue that may die (necrotic tissue) is removed. No tension should be placed on the skin fields during closure of the wound. Wounds are covered with small strips of gauze impregnated with petrolatum. The upper extremity is immobilized, and compression hand dressing and plaster splints are arranged to prevent slipping and movement of the affected arm.

Diagnosis/Preparation

The diagnosis is easily made by visual inspection since the finger(s) must be completely detached from the hand. The reattachment procedure is complex and involves the expertise and skill of a highly trained surgeon. There are several important factors necessary to successful replantation, including special instrumentation and transportation of the amputated finger. Surgical loupes (binocular-type eyepieces used by surgeons to magnify small structures during surgery) are necessary for this procedure. Instruments should be at least 3.9 in (10 cm) long to allow for proper positioning in the surgeon's hands. Special clips are used to help suture blood vessels together. The best method of saving and transporting the amputated finger is to wrap it with moistened cloth (Ringer's lactate solution or saline solution) and place it on ice. Generally, the tissues will survive for about six hours without cooling. If the part is cooled, tissue survival time is approximately 12 hours. Fingers have the best outcome for transportation survival, since digits (fingers) do not have a large percentage of muscle tissue.

Aftercare

Postoperative care is vital for successful finger reattachment. The hand is wrapped in a bulky compression dressing and usually elevated. If arterial flow is impaired, then the hand should be lowered, since this maneuver will promote blood flow from the heart to the reattached finger. If venous outflow is slow, the hand must be elevated. Medications to increase blood flow (peripheral vasodilators) and an anticoagulant (heparin) are used. A tranquilizer may be given to reduce unnecessary blood vessel movement (vasospasm) that can occur due to anxiety. Careful examination of the reattached digit(s) is necessary. The surgeon frequently monitors color, the capacity of blood vessels, capillary refill, and warmth to monitor replant progress. The YSI telethermometer monitors the digital (finger) temperature with small surface probes. Skin temperature falling below 86°F (30°C) indicates   poor blood perfusion

Finger reattachment

To save a detached finger for reattachment surgery, it should be wrapped in a moist paper towel and put on ice (A). First the surgeon will reattach the blood vessels and nerves of the finger (B). The bone may be repaired with wires (C), and tendons are repaired (D). Skin and muscle wounds are also closed during the procedure. *(Illustration by GGS Inc.)*

(poor blood and oxygen delivery to the affected area) of the replant. The cause of poor blood circulation must be investigated and corrected, if possible. The patient's room should be warm, and bed rest for two to three days is recommended. Patients must refrain from smoking and take antibiotics for one week after surgery. Follow-up consultations are necessary for continued wound care and rehabilitation.

Risks

The experienced surgeon can estimate the likelihood complications based on the nature of the injury. Replantations that are risky, such as those with circulatory perfusion problems, have lower success rates. Generally, the most difficult replantations are those that involve children under 10, injuries caused by a ring catching in machinery, and crush-and-tear injuries. Management of the difficult replant typically includes intravenous heparin to prevent clotting of the blood, and providing a continuous nerve block in either the median or ulnar nerve (depending on which fingers are reattached). A nerve block will cause vasodilatation, or expansion of the blood vessel. Vasodilatation will increase blood flow, bringing with it fresh oxygenated blood. Further evaluation should include checking the patient's dressing for constriction (i.e., if the dressing was placed too snugly and is constricting local blood vessels).

Normal results

Normal results may not seem encouraging. It must be considered that this is a major trauma and a highly complicated and intricate surgical repair. Generally, a normal result usually includes good nerve recovery; approximately 50% of normal for active range of joint motion; cold intolerance (usually reversed in about two years); and acceptable cosmetic results.

Morbidity and mortality rates

There are about 10,000 cases of job-related amputations in the United States each year; 94% of these involve fingers. Few statistics are available for the outcome of replantations.

Alternatives

The only alternative to this procedure is to lose the finger(s) entirely and manage the remaining hand injury.

Resources

BOOKS

American Society for Surgery of the Hand. *The Hand: Primary Care of Common Problems.* New York: Churchill Livingstone, 1990.

Green, David P. *Operative Hand Surgery,* Volume 1, 3rd Edition. New York: Churchill Livingstone, Inc., 1993.

Green, David P. *Operative Hand Surgery,* Volume 2, 3rd Edition. New York: Churchill Livingstone, Inc., 1993.

ORGANIZATIONS

American Association for Hand Surgery. 20 North Michigan Avenue, Suite 700, Chicago, Il 60602. (321) 236-3307; Fax: (312) 782-0553. E-mail: contact@handssurgery.org. <http://www.handsurgery.org>.

OTHER

"Superficial Fingertip Avulsion." National Center for Emergency Medicine Informatics. [cited June 2003] <http://www.ncemi.org/cse/cse1002.htm>.

"The V-Y Plasty in the Treatment of Fingertip Amputations." American Academy of Family Physicians. [cited June 2003] <http://www.aafp.org/afp/20010801/455.html>.

Laith Farid Gulli, MD, MS
Bilal Nasser, MD, MS
Robert Ramirez, BS

Fluoroquinolones

Definition

Fluoroquinolones are medications that kill bacteria or prevent their growth. Bacteria are one-celled disease-causing microorganisms that commonly multiply by cell division.

Purpose

Fluoroquinolones are a class of antimicrobials, which are medications used to treat infections caused by microorganisms. Physicians prescribe these drugs for bacterial infections in many parts of the body. For example, they are used to treat bone and joint infections, skin infections, urinary tract infections, inflammation of the prostate, serious ear infections, bronchitis, pneumonia, tuberculosis, some sexually transmitted diseases (STDs), and some infections that affect people with AIDS.

Although fluoroquinolones are normally used only to treat infections, and not for prophylaxis (prevention of infection), some of these compounds have been used before surgery, particularly if the patient is allergic to the antibiotic that is usually given. Fluoroquinolones have also been studied for their usefulness in eye surgery and surgery of the biliary tract.

Description

Fluoroquinolones are available only with a physician's prescription; they are sold in tablet and injectable forms. Examples of these medicines are moxifloxacin (Avelox), ciprofloxacin (Cipro), ofloxacin (Floxin), levofloxacin (Levaquin), lomefloxacin (Maxaquin), norfloxacin (Noroxin), enoxacin (Penetrex), gatifloxacin (Tequin), and sparfloxacin (Zagam).

Recommended dosage

The recommended dosage depends on the type and strength of fluoroquinolone, and the kind of infection for which it is being taken. Patients should consult the physician who prescribed the drug or the pharmacist who filled the prescription for the correct dosage.

To make sure an infection clears up completely, patients should take the full course of fluoroquinolone that their doctor prescribed. It is important to not stop taking the drug just because the symptoms begin to diminish.

Fluoroquinolones work best when they are at constant levels in the blood. To help keep blood levels constant, patients should take the medicine in doses spaced evenly through the day and night without missing any doses. For best results, these medications should be taken with a full glass of water, and the patient should drink several more glasses of water every day. Drinking plenty of water will help prevent some of the medicine's side effects. Some fluoroquinolones should be taken on an empty stomach; others may be taken with meals. Patients should read the directions on the package very carefully or ask the physician or pharmacist for instructions on the best way to take a specific medicine.

Precautions

The precautions described below are primarily applicable to the use of fluoroquinolones when they are prescribed to treat an infection for several days. Other than allergic reactions, few patients experience significant problems when they are given a single dose of a fluoroquinolone for surgical prophylaxis. The external use of these drugs—for example as eye drops—is also generally safe.

An important precaution to observe with any antimicrobial drug is that the unnecessary use or abuse of these medications can encourage drug-resistant strains of bacteria to develop and spread. These drug-resistant strains then become difficult or even impossible to treat. Bacteria found in hospitals appear to have become especially resilient, and are causing increasing difficulty for patients and the doctors treating them. One fear is that the overuse of fluoroquinolone medications could reduce their effectiveness against such infections as typhoid fever, hospital-acquired pneumonia, and others.

Research suggests that fluoroquinolones may cause bone development problems in children and teenagers. Infants, children, teenagers, pregnant women, and women who are breastfeeding should not take these drugs unless directed to do so by a physician.

Although such side effects are rare, some people have had severe and life-threatening reactions to fluoroquinolones. Patients should call their physician at once if they have any of the following signs:

- swelling of the face and throat
- problems swallowing
- shortness of breath
- rapid heartbeat
- tingling in the fingers or toes
- itching or hives
- loss of consciousness

Some fluoroquinolones may weaken the tendons in the shoulder, hand, or heel, making these fibrous bands of tissue more likely to tear. Anyone who notices pain or inflammation in these or other joints should stop taking the medicine immediately and call their physician. They should rest and avoid athletic activity or vigorous **exercise** until the physician determines whether the tendons have been damaged. Tendons that are torn may require surgical repair.

Fluoroquinolones make some people feel drowsy, dizzy, lightheaded, or less alert. Anyone who takes these drugs should not drive, use machines or do anything else that requires a high level of alertness until they have found out how the drugs affect them.

Fluoroquinolones may increase the skin's sensitivity to sunlight. Even brief exposure to sun can cause a severe sunburn or a rash. During treatment with these drugs, patients should avoid exposure to direct sunlight, especially high sun between 10 A.M. and 3 P.M.; wear a hat and tightly woven clothing that covers the arms and legs; use a sunscreen with a skin protection factor (SPF) of at least 15; protect the lips with a lip balm containing sun block; and avoid the use of tanning beds, tanning booths, or sunlamps.

Patients should not take antacids that contain aluminum, calcium, or magnesium at the same time as fluoroquinolones. The antacids may keep the fluoroquinolones from working as they should. If antacids are needed, they should be taken at least 2 hours before or 2 hours after taking norfloxacin or ofloxacin, and at least 4 hours before or 2 hours after taking ciprofloxacin. Patients who are taking sucralfate (Carafate), a medicine used to treat stomach ulcers and other irritations in the digestive tract and mouth, should follow the same instructions as for taking antacids.

Anyone who has had unusual reactions to fluoroquinolones or such related compounds as cinoxacin (Cinobac) or nalidixic acid (NegGram) in the past should let his or her physician know before taking the drugs again. The physician should also be told about any allergies to foods, dyes, preservatives, or other substances.

People with any of these medical problems should make sure their physicians are aware of their conditions before using fluoroquinolones:

- kidney disease
- liver disease together with kidney disease
- diseases that affect the brain or spinal cord, including hardening of the arteries in the brain; epilepsy; and other seizure disorders

Taking fluoroquinolones with certain other drugs may affect the way the drugs work or may increase the chance of side effects.

Side effects

The most common side effects are mild diarrhea, nausea, vomiting, stomach or abdominal pain, dizziness, drowsiness, lightheadedness, nervousness, sleep problems, and headache. These side effects occur in about 5% of patients taking fluoroquinolones. They usually go away as the body adjusts to the drug and do not require medical treatment unless they are bothersome.

More serious side effects are not common, but may occur. If any of the following side effects occur, the patient should consult a physician immediately:

- skin rash or such other skin problems as itching, peeling, hives, or redness
- fever
- agitation or confusion
- hallucinations
- shakiness or tremors
- seizures or convulsions
- tingling in the fingers or toes
- pain at the injection site that persists after the drug was injected
- pain in the calves that spreads to the heel area
- swelling of the calves or lower legs
- swelling of the face or neck
- difficulty swallowing
- rapid heartbeat
- shortness of breath
- loss of consciousness

Other rare side effects may occur. Anyone who has unusual symptoms after taking fluoroquinolones should consult his or her physician at once.

Interactions

Fluoroquinolones may interact with other medicines. When an interaction occurs, the effects of one or both of the drugs may change or the risk of side effects may be greater. Anyone who takes fluoroquinolones should give the doctor a list of all other medications that they take on a regular basis, *including over-the-counter drugs, herbal preparations, and traditional Chinese or other alternative medicines.* Drugs that may interact with fluoroquinolones include:

- antacids containing aluminum, calcium, or magnesium
- medicines that contain iron or zinc, including multivitamin and mineral supplements
- sucralfate (Carafate)
- caffeine
- such blood-thinning drugs as warfarin (Coumadin)
- drugs given to open the airway (bronchodilators), including aminophylline, theophylline (Theo-Dur and other brands), and oxtriphylline (Choledyl and other brands)
- didanosine (Videx), a drug used to treat HIV infection

The list above does not include every drug that may interact with fluoroquinolones. Patients should check

KEY TERMS

Bacterium (plural, bacteria)—A microscopic one-celled form of life that causes many diseases and infections.

Biliary tract—The part of the digestive system that conveys or stores bile, consisting of the bile ducts and the gallbladder.

Bronchitis—Inflammation of the air passages in the lungs.

Digestive tract—The stomach, intestines, and other parts of the body through which food passes.

Inflammation—A condition characterized by pain, redness, swelling, and warmth. Inflammation usually develops in response to an injury or infection.

Microorganism—An organism that is too small to be seen with the naked eye.

Pneumonia—A disease characterized by inflammation of the lungs. Pneumonia may be caused by bacteria, viruses, or other organisms, or by physical or chemical irritants.

Prophylaxis—A medical intervention intended to prevent disease.

Prostate—A donut-shaped gland in males below the bladder that contributes to the production of semen.

Sexually transmitted disease (STD)—A disease that is passed from one person to another through sexual intercourse or other intimate sexual contact.

Tendon—A tough band of tissue that connects muscle to bone.

Tuberculosis (TB)—An infectious disease that usually affects the lungs, but may also affect other parts of the body. Its symptoms include fever, weight loss, and coughing up blood.

Urinary tract—The passage through which urine flows from the kidneys to the outside of the body.

---

with a physician or pharmacist before combining fluoroquinolones with any other prescription or nonprescription (over-the-counter) medicine.

Resources

BOOKS

"Antibacterial Drugs: Fluoroquinolones." Section 13, Chapter 153 in *The Merck Manual of Diagnosis and Therapy*, edited by Mark H. Beers, MD, and Robert Berkow, MD. Whitehouse Station, NJ: Merck Research Laboratories, 1999.

Reynolds, J. E. F., ed. *Martindale: The Extra Pharmacopoeia*, 31st ed. London, UK: The Pharmaceutical Press, 1996.

Wilson, Billie Ann, RN, PhD, Carolyn L. Stang, PharmD, and Margaret T. Shannon, RN, PhD. *Nurses Drug Guide 2000*. Stamford, CT: Appleton and Lange, 1999.

ORGANIZATIONS

American Society of Health-System Pharmacists (ASHP). 7272 Wisconsin Avenue, Bethesda, MD 20814. (301) 657-3000. <www.ashp.org>.

United States Food and Drug Administration (FDA). 5600 Fishers Lane, Rockville, MD 20857-0001. (888) INFO-FDA. <www.fda.gov>.

OTHER

"Fluoroquinolones (Systemic)." National Library of medicine. <www.nlm.nih.gov/medlineplus/druginfo/fluoroquinolonessystemic202656.html>.

Rosalyn Carson-DeWitt, MD
Samuel Uretsky, PharmD

Forehead lift

Definition

A forehead lift is a cosmetic surgery procedure intended to improve a person's appearance by correcting the shape of the eyebrows and reducing horizontal wrinkles or furrows in the skin of the forehead. It is also known as a brow lift.

Purpose

The purpose of a forehead lift is improvement of the patient's external appearance, particularly with regard to the upper third of the face. Some people have clearly marked frown lines or drooping of the eyebrows or eyelid caused by loosening of the tissues and muscles around the eyes during the aging process. The drooping of the eyelid is sometimes referred to as ptosis, which comes from a Greek word meaning "fall." In some cases, these signs of aging make the person look angry, anxious, or sad. A forehead lift is not done to cure disease or repair a major wound or injury.

Demographics

Like other cosmetic surgery procedures, forehead lifts are performed much more frequently than they were even a decade ago. According to the American Society of Plastic Surgeons (ASPS), the number of forehead lifts performed in the United States has risen 172% since 1992. These changes are attributed in part to concerns about appearance in the so-called baby boomer generation. Adults born between 1945 and 1960 are now middle-aged or approaching retirement, and are generally more image-conscious than previous generations of Americans. In addition, newer surgical techniques have made forehead lifts less painful, easier to perform, and less likely to have complications.

Most plastic surgeons recommend that a forehead lift should be done when the patient is between 40 and 60 years old, although it is sometimes done on younger patients who have very deep frown lines due to stress or have inherited very low and heavy brows. In addition, people whose facial skin has aged prematurely due to sun exposure or heavy smoking may be candidates for a forehead lift in their mid-30s. In 2002, the average age of patients of either sex who had forehead lifts done in the United States was 47.

Statistics published by the American Academy of Cosmetic Surgery (AACS) in January 2003 indicate that although more men are choosing to have cosmetic surgery than in the past, the female:male ratio for forehead lifts is still 6:1. In 2002, surgeons who are AACS members performed 7,882 forehead lifts on women compared to 1,139 procedures on men. Forehead lifts account for a little less than 1% (0.96%) of all cosmetic surgery procedures performed each year in the United States and Canada.

Although most forehead lifts and other facial cosmetic procedures are still performed on Caucasian patients, this type of surgery is gaining rapidly in popularity among Hispanics, Asian Americans, and African Americans. Between 1999 and 2002, the proportion of cosmetic procedures performed on Hispanics has increased by 200%, on African Americans by 323%, and on Asian Americans by 340%. As of 2003, Caucasians account for only 77% of patients having elective facial surgery, compared to 83% in 1999.

Description

There are two main types of forehead lifts. The classic, or open, forehead lift involves a long incision along the top of the forehead and lifting of the skin of the forehead. The second type of forehead lift, known as an endoscopic lift, is performed with special instruments inserted through four or five small incisions behind the hairline.

In some cases, a forehead lift is combined with plastic surgery on the eyelids (**blepharoplasty**) or with a **face lift**.

Classic forehead lift

The classic forehead lift takes about one to two hours and may be performed with either general or local anesthesia. After the patient has been anesthetized, the surgeon makes a long incision across the top of the scalp from ear to ear. The exact location of the incision depends on the condition of the facial muscles to be removed or modified and the position of the patient's hairline. The most common type of incision in an open forehead lift is a coronal incision, which is made slightly behind the hairline. A second type of incision is called a pretrichial incision. It is similar to the coronal incision except that the central part of the incision lies directly on the hairline. A third type of incision, which is used mostly on male patients with very deep forehead creases, is placed directly inside the creases in the midforehead.

After the incision has been made, the surgeon lifts the skin of the forehead very carefully and cuts away excess underlying tissue. Some of the muscles that cause frowning may be loosened (released) or altered. If necessary, the brows will be lifted and excess skin along the line of the incision will be trimmed away. The incision is usually closed with stitches or staples, although some surgeons are now using tissue glues to hold the skin in place. The patient's face is then carefully washed to prevent infection and irritation. Some surgeons prefer to cover the incision with a gauze dressing held in place by an elastic bandage, but others do not apply any dressing.

One disadvantage of the classic forehead lift from the standpoint of male patients is that men's hairstyles will not usually cover the incision scar. It is easier for women, even those who prefer to wear their hair very short, to let the hair grow for several weeks before the procedure so that it will be long enough to cover the scar.

Endoscopic forehead lift

An endoscopic forehead lift is performed with the help of an endoscope, which is an instrument designed to allow the surgeon to see the tissues and other structures underneath the skin of the forehead. Instead of making one long incision, the surgeon makes four or five shorter incisions, each less than an inch (2.5 cm) long. The endoscope is inserted through one of these incisions; the others are used for the insertion of instruments for removing excess tissue and reshaping the facial muscles. If the eyebrows are being lifted, they may be kept in place in their new position by tiny stitches under the skin or fixation tacks placed behind the hairline. The incisions are closed and the patient's face washed and dressed in the same way as in the classic forehead lift.

Diagnosis/Preparation

Diagnosis

It is somewhat misleading to speak of diagnosis on the context of forehead lifts and similar procedures because cosmetic surgery is unique in one respect—it is the only type of surgery in which the patient initiates "treatment" rather than the doctor. This difference means that many plastic surgeons now screen patients for psychological stability as well as general physical fitness for surgery. Beginning in the 1970s and 1980s, psychiatrists began to see patients who were obsessed with a particular facial feature or other small part of their body, as distinct from overconcern about weight or general body shape. This condition, which is now called body dysmorphic disorder (BDD), became an official psychiatric diagnostic category in 1987. Patients with BDD frequently seek plastic surgery as a solution for their dissatisfaction with their looks. In many cases, however, the "flaw" that the patient sees in his or her face is either exaggerated or nonexistent. Ironically, although men are less likely than women to request facial surgery, a higher percentage of male cosmetic surgery patients are emotionally disturbed; one survey of plastic surgeons estimated that six out of every 100 female patients and seven out of every 100 male patients meet the diagnostic criteria for BDD.

When a person consults a plastic surgeon about a forehead lift or similar procedure, the doctor will spend some time talking with the patient about his or her motives for facial surgery as well as taking a general medical and surgical history. Good candidates for facial surgery are people who have a realistic understanding of the risks as well as the benefits of this type of surgery, and equally realistic expectations of the outcome. On the other hand, the following are considered psychological warning signs:

- The patient is considering surgery to please someone else, most often a spouse or partner.

- The patient expects facial surgery to guarantee career advancement.

- The patient has a history of multiple cosmetic procedures and/or complaints about previous surgeons.

- The patient thinks that the surgery will solve all his or her life problems.

- The patient has an unrealistic notion of what he or she will look like after surgery.

- The patient seems otherwise emotionally unstable.

If the surgeon thinks that the patient is a good candidate in terms of motivation, he or she will continue the diagnostic assessment by examining the patient's face at close range. To make an initial evaluation of the possible results of a forehead lift, the surgeon will gently lift the skin at the outer edges of the eyes above the brows in an upward direction. He or she may also ask the patient to look in a mirror and describe what they don't like about their face. Next, the surgeon will ask the patient to frown, smile, or make a variety of other facial expressions. This technique allows the surgeon to observe the activity of the patient's facial muscles. Depending on the amount of loose skin in the upper eyelid, the height of the patient's hairline, and the relative position of the eyebrows, the surgeon may recommend a blepharoplasty or other procedure instead of a forehead lift.

Preparation

Preparation for a forehead lift involves practical as well as medical concerns.

FINANCIAL CONSIDERATIONS. Most cosmetic facial procedures are not covered by health insurance because they are regarded as nonessential elective procedures. As a result, many cosmetic surgeons request that fees be paid in full before the operation. According to the AACS, 13.4% of cosmetic surgery patients take out loans to finance their procedure. In 2002, the average cost of a forehead lift was $3300.

MEDICAL AND HOME CARE ISSUES. A patient scheduled for a forehead lift will be asked to prepare for the operation by quitting smoking and discontinuing **aspirin** or any other medications that thin the blood. The surgeon will ask for a list of all medications that the patient is taking, including alternative herbal preparations as well as prescription drugs, to make sure that there will be no interactions with the anesthetic.

Patients are advised to have someone drive them home after the procedure and help them with routine chores for a day or two. If the forehead lift is combined with a face lift or blepharoplasty, the surgeon may have the patient remain in the hospital overnight. Although cosmetic surgery on the face does not interfere with walking or routine physical activity, most patients tire easily for the first few days after the procedure.

Aftercare

Classic forehead lift

Aftercare for a classic forehead lift is somewhat more complicated than for an endoscopic procedure. Pain or numbness around the incision is likely to last longer than for an endoscopic procedure. It is controlled with prescription medication. Patients are usually advised to keep the head elevated for two to three days after surgery to minimize swelling. Bandages are removed a day or two after the procedure; stitches or staples are taken out between 10 days and two weeks after surgery. The patient is asked to rest quietly for one or two days after surgery. Most patients can return to work after a week or 10 days.

Endoscopic forehead lift

Fixation devices around the eyebrows are usually removed within 10 days after endoscopic surgery. As of early 2003, however, new absorbable fixation tacks that do not require later removal are being used with good results.

Patients who have had either type of forehead lift should not wash their hair until the bandage or dressing is removed, usually within two days. Heavy lifting, vigorous athletic activity, sexual activity, or any type of exertion that raises the blood pressure should be avoided for five to six weeks after the surgery. The skin around the incision should be protected from direct exposure to the sun for at least six months, because the new tissue is much more vulnerable to sunburn than normal skin. Most surgeons advise patients to use a sunblock cream to protect the skin even after the first six months.

Patients can use a special camouflage makeup to cover the bruising or swelling that often occurs after surgery, although they should be careful to keep the makeup away from the incision. Most of the bruising and other signs of surgery will fade within about three weeks.

Risks

Major complications of a forehead lift are unusual. The most common risks from the procedure are as follows:

- Headaches for a day or two after surgery. This complication is much more common with a classic forehead lift than with endoscopic surgery.
- Mild pain around the incision for a few days after surgery.

QUESTIONS TO ASK THE DOCTOR

- How many forehead lifts have you performed?
- Should I consider combining the forehead lift with a face lift?
- Am I a candidate for an endoscopic forehead lift?
- Would I benefit from nonsurgical alternatives to a forehead lift?
- How long can I expect the effects of this surgery to last?

- Numbness or itching sensations on the top of the scalp. These may last for as long as six months after surgery.
- Mild bruising or swelling around the eyelids and cheeks.
- Hair loss or thinning in the area of the incision. The hair will usually regrow within a few weeks or months.
- A feeling of numbness or dryness in the eye.
- Loss of function of the eyelid. This complication is corrected by another operation.
- Bleeding or infection. These are rare complications with forehead lifts.

Normal results

Normal results of a forehead lift are an improvement in appearance that is satisfying to the patient. Specifically, the forehead should look less creased or wrinkled and frown lines should be lighter. The cosmetic effects of a forehead lift last between five and 10 years, depending on the person's age and the condition of their skin when the procedure was performed.

Morbidity and mortality rates

In general, mortality and morbidity rates for forehead lifts and similar facial cosmetic procedures are very low. Almost all cases of mortality following facial cosmetic surgery involve patients who were treated for facial disfigurement because they had been severely burned or attacked by animals. Moreover, many plastic surgeons do not consider morbidity and mortality rates to be as significant as other factors in evaluating the success of facial cosmetic procedures. One group of researchers at the University of Washington maintains that "[t]he most important measures of outcome in facial cosmetic surgery are quality of life and patient satisfaction,

KEY TERMS

Blepharoplasty—Plastic surgery performed on the eyelids.

Body dysmorphic disorder (BDD)—A psychiatric condition marked by excessive preoccupation with an imaginary or minor defect in a facial feature or localized part of the body. Many people with BDD seek cosmetic surgery as a treatment for their perceived flaw.

Botulinum toxin—A toxin produced by the spores and growing cells of *Clostridium botulinum*. Because it causes muscle paralysis, this toxin can be used to reduce frown lines in the face by temporarily paralyzing the muscles in the face that contract when a person frowns or squints.

Collagen—A type of protein found in connective tissue that gives it strength and flexibility. Collagen derived from cattle can be injected into wrinkles or lines in the face as an alternative to cosmetic surgery.

Cosmetic surgery—Surgery that is intended to improve a patient's appearance or correct disfigurement. It is also called aesthetic surgery.

Endoscope—An instrument that allows a surgeon to look underneath skin or inside a hollow organ while performing surgery.

Ptosis—The medical term for drooping of the upper eyelid.

---

in contrast to other, more objective measures such as complications or mortality rates."

Several American studies have reported that the rate of complications is no higher when a forehead lift is done in combination with other facial procedures than when it is done by itself.

Alternatives

Soft tissue fillers

Alternatives to surgical treatment for frown lines and wrinkles of the forehead include injections of filler materials under the skin to smooth wrinkles or injections of botulinum toxin to paralyze the facial muscles involved in frowning or brow wrinkling. The most commonly used filler materials are collagen and fat. Collagen is a protein found in human and animal connective tissue that makes the tissue strong and flexible. Most collagen that is used for cosmetic injections is derived from cattle, which produces allergic reactions in some people. Fat injections use fat taken from the patient's abdomen, thighs, or buttocks.

The fat is then reinjected under the skin of the forehead to smooth out lines and wrinkles.

One drawback of both collagen and fat injections is that the effects are not permanent. Some new injectable filler substances are said to be permanent wrinkle removers. They include Artecoll, which contains small plastic particles that supposedly stimulate the body to produce its own collagen; and Radiance, which is made of a chemical called calcium hydroxylapatite. Still other injectable tissue fillers are made from synthetic hyaluronic acid, which has been used for a number of years to treat joint pain. Since hyaluronic acid is produced naturally in the body, allergic reactions to this type of tissue filler are relatively rare.

Botulinum toxin

Botulinum toxin is a compound produced by the spores and growing cells of the organism that causes botulism, *Clostridium botulinum*. The toxin causes muscle paralysis. It was first used clinically in the 1960s to treat neurological disorders but also proved to be effective in paralyzing the facial muscles that cause "crow's feet" and frown wrinkles. Botulinum toxin, or Botox, was approved by the Food and Drug Administration (FDA) in April 2002 as a treatment for facial lines and wrinkles.

Both soft tissue fillers and Botox injections are regarded as effective though temporary alternatives to a forehead lift for reducing frown lines. Collagen injections must be repeated every three to six months, while Botox injections are effective for about four months.

Resources

PERIODICALS

Dayan, S. H., S. W. Perkins, A. J. Vartanian, and I. M. Wiesman. "The Forehead Lift: Endoscopic Versus Coronal Approaches." *Aesthetic Plastic Surgery* 25 (January-February 2001): 35–39.

De Cordier, B. C., J. I. de la Torre, M. S. Al-Hakeem, et al. "Endoscopic Forehead Lift: Review of Technique, Cases, and Complications." *Plastic and Reconstructive Surgery* 110 (November 2002): 1558–1568.

Landecker, A., J. B. Buck, and J. C. Grotting. "A New Resorbable Tack Fixation Technique for Endoscopic Brow Lifts." *Plastic and Reconstructive Surgery* 111 (February 2003): 880–886.

Most, S. P., R. Alsarraf, and W. F. Larrabee, Jr. "Outcomes of Facial Cosmetic Procedures." *Facial Plastic Surgery* 18 (May 2002): 119–124.

Namazie, A. R., and G. S. Keller. "Current Practices in Endoscopic Brow and Temporal Lifting." *Facial Plastic Surgery Clinics of North America* 9 (August 2001): 439–451.

Paul, M. D. "The Evolution of the Brow Lift in Aesthetic Plastic Surgery." *Plastic and Reconstructive Surgery* 108 (October 2001): 1409–1424.

Sclafani, Anthony J., MD, and Kyle S. Choe, MD. "Psychological Aspects of Plastic Surgery." *eMedicine*. June 24, 2002 [cited February 28, 2003]. <http://www.emedicine.com/ent/topic36.htm>.

Siwolop, Sana. "Beyond Botox: An Industry's Quest for Smooth Skin." *New York Times* March 9, 2003 [cited March 9, 2003. <http://www.nytimes.com/2003/03/09/business/09FACE.html>.

ORGANIZATIONS

American Academy of Cosmetic Surgeons (AACS). Cosmetic Surgery Information Service. 737 North Michigan Avenue, Suite 820, Chicago, IL 60611. (312) 981-6760. <http://www.cosmeticsurgery.org>.

American Academy of Facial Plastic and Reconstructive Surgery (AAFPRS). 310 South Henry Street, Alexandria, VA 22314. (703) 299-9291. <http://www.facemd.org>.

American Society of Plastic Surgeons (ASPS). 444 East Algonquin Road, Arlington Heights, IL 60005. (847) 228-9900. <http://www.plasticsurgery.org>.

OTHER

American Academy of Facial Plastic and Reconstructive Surgery. *2001 Membership Survey: Trends in Facial Plastic Surgery*. Alexandria, VA: AAFPRS, 2002.

"Browlift". American Society of Plastic Surgeons [cited March 11, 2003]. <http://www.plasticsurgery.org/public_education/procedures/Browlift.cfm>.

"Forehead Lift". American Society for Aesthetic Plastic Surgery [cited May 5, 2003]. <http://www.surgery.org/forehead_lift.html>.

Rebecca Frey, Ph.D.

Fracture repair

Definition

Fracture repair is the process of rejoining and realigning the ends of broken bones, usually performed by an orthopedist, general surgeon, or family doctor. In cases of an emergency, first aid measures should be used to provide temporary realignment and immobilization until proper medical help is available.

Purpose

Fracture repair is required when there is a need to restore the normal alignment and function of a broken bone. Throughout the stages of fracture healing, the bones must be held firmly in the correct position. In the event that a fracture is not properly repaired, misalignment of the bone may occur, resulting in possible physical dysfunction of the bone, adjacent joint, or region of the body.

WHO PERFORMS THE PROCEDURE AND WHERE IS IT PERFORMED?

Fracture repair is usually performed by an orthopedic surgeon, general surgeon, or family physician. In cases of an emergency, first aid measures should be used for temporary realignment and immobilization until proper medical help can be obtained. Relatively uncomplicated fractures may be immobilized in a physician's office. More commonly, fractures are treated in a hospital setting.

Demographics

The incidence of fractures that occur in the United States can only be estimated because fractures are not always reported. The average person sustains two to three fractured bones during the course of a lifetime. A reasonable estimate is approximately nine million fractures per year.

Fractures are slightly more common in children and adolescents than in young adults due to the levels and kinds of activities in which they engage. Fractures become more common in adults as they age, however, due to changes in bone structure and generally diminished levels of physical activity.

Description

Fracture repair is accomplished by means of applied **traction**, surgery, and immobilizing affected bones. The bone fragments are aligned as closely as possible to their normal position without injuring the skin. Metal wires or screws may be needed to align smaller bone fragments. Once the broken ends of the bone are set, the affected area is immobilized for several weeks and kept rigid with a sling, plaster cast, brace, or splint. With the use of traction, muscles pulling on the fracture site are neutralized by weights attached to a series of ropes running over pulleys. Strategically implanted electrical stimulation devices have proven beneficial in healing a fracture site, especially when the fracture is healing poorly and repair by other means is difficult.

Diagnosis/Preparation

Fractures are commonly diagnosed on the basis of history of trauma or the presence of pain. An x ray is usually taken to confirm the diagnosis.

Fracture repair

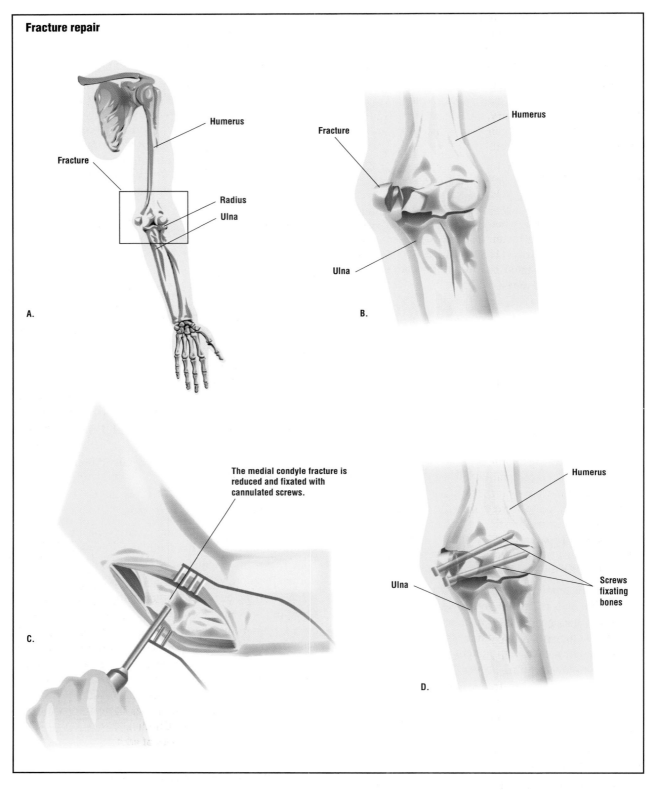

A.

Humerus

Fracture

Radius

Ulna

B.

Fracture

Humerus

Ulna

C.

The medial condyle fracture is
reduced and fixated with
cannulated screws.

D.

Humerus

Ulna

Screws
fixating
bones

In this patient, a fall has resulted in fractures in the bones of the elbow (B). To repair the fracture, an incision is made in the elbow area (C), and the bones are fixed with screws to aid proper healing (D). *(Illustration by GGS Inc.)*

Precautions for fracture repair include any relevant factors in an individual's medical condition and history. These include allergic reactions to anesthesia and the presence of bleeding disorders that may complicate surgery.

Preparation often begins with emergency splinting to immobilize the body part or parts involved. When fracture repair is necessary, the procedure is often performed in a hospital, but can also be successfully done in an outpatient surgical facility, doctor's office, or emergency room. Before any surgery for fracture repair, blood and urine studies may be performed. X rays may be obtained. It must be noted, however, that not all fractures are immediately apparent on an initial x-ray examination. In such a case, when a fracture is highly suspected, the extent of the fracture can be properly diagnosed by repeating the x rays 10–14 days later. Depending upon the situation, local or general anesthesia may be used during fracture repair.

Aftercare

Immediately following surgical repair of a fracture, x rays may be again taken through the cast or splint to evaluate whether the rejoined pieces are in good position for healing. The x ray can be performed either before the application of the splint or at least before an individual is awakened from the general anesthesia. Persons need to exercise caution and not place excess pressure on any part of the cast until it is completely dry. Excess pressure on the operative site should also be avoided until complete healing has taken place and the injury has been re-examined by the physician or surgeon. If the cast becomes exposed to moisture, it may soften and require repair. For this reason, plastic has largely replaced plaster as the casting material of choice. The injured region should be elevated or propped up whenever possible to reduce the possibility of swelling.

Risks

Surgical risks of fracture repair are greater in persons over 60 years of age because the bones often require more time to properly heal. Obesity may place extra stress on the fracture site, affecting healing and possibly increasing the risk of re-fracturing the same bone. The healing process after fracture repair may also be slowed by smoking, as well as by poor nutrition, alcoholism, and chronic illness. Some medications may affect the fracture site, causing poor union; such medications include antihypertensives and such steroids as cortisone.

Possible complications following fracture repair include excessive bleeding, improper fit of joined bone ends, pressure on nearby nerves, delayed healing, and a permanent incomplete healing (union) of the fracture. If

there is a poor blood supply to the fractured site and one of the portions of broken bone is not adequately supplied with blood, the bony portion may die and healing of the fracture will not take place. This complication is called aseptic necrosis. Poor immobilization of the fracture from improper casting that permits motion between the bone parts may prevent healing and repair of the bone, and result in possible deformity. Infection can interfere with bone repair. This risk is greater in the case of a compound fracture (a bone fracture involving a portion of bone that breaks through the surface of skin). Compound fracture sites provide ideal conditions for severe infections by *Streptococcus* and *Staphylococcus* bacteria. Occasionally, fractured bones in the elderly may possibly never heal properly. The risk is increased when nutrition is poor.

Normal results

Once the procedure for fracture repair is completed, the body begins to produce new tissue to bridge the fracture site and rejoin the broken pieces. At first, this tissue (called a callus) is soft and easily injured. Later, the body deposits bone minerals (primarily compounds containing calcium) until the callus becomes a solid piece of bone. The fracture site is thus further strengthened with extra bone. It usually takes about six weeks for the pieces of a broken bone to knit (heal) together. The exact time required for healing depends on the type of fracture and the extent of damage. Before the use of x rays, fracture repair was not always accurate and frequently resulted in crippling deformities. With modern x-ray technology, physicians can view the extent of the fracture, check the setting following the repair, and be certain after the procedure that the bones have not moved from their intended alignment. Children's bones usually heal more rapidly than do the bones of adults.

Morbidity and mortality rates

Morbidity associated with fracture repair includes damage to nerves or primary blood vessels that are adjacent to the fracture site. Improper alignment causing de-

KEY TERMS

Compound fracture—A fracture in which the broken end or ends of the bone have penetrated through the skin; also known as an open fracture.

Staphylococcal infection—An infection caused by any of several pathogenic species of *Staphylococcus,* commonly characterized by the formation of abscesses in the skin or other organs.

Streptococcal infection—An infection caused by a pathogenic bacterium of one of several species of the genus *Streptococcus* or their toxins. Almost any organ in the body may be involved.

formity is an abnormal outcome that is relatively rare due to presently available medical technology.

Mortality associated with fractures is also rare. It is usually associated with infections or contamination acquired during the fracture process.

Alternatives

There are no alternatives to proper fracture repair. Problems associated with allowing a fracture to heal without intervention include misalignment, deformity, loss of function, and pain.

Magnetic fields are occasionally used to stimulate healing when conventional techniques are not effective.

See also Bone grafting; Orthopedic surgery.

Resources

BOOKS

Browner, B., J. Jupiter, A. Levine, and P. Trafton. *Skeletal Trauma: Fractures, Dislocations, Ligamentous Injuries,* 3rd edition. Philadelphia: Saunders, 2002.

Canale, S. T. *Campbell's Operative Orthopedics.* St. Louis: Mosby, 2003.

Eiff, M. P., R. L. Hatch, W. L. Calmbach, and M. K. Higgins. *Fracture Management for Primary Care,* 2nd edition. Philadelphia: Saunders, 2002.

Staheli, L. T. *Fundamentals of Pediatric Orthopedics,* 3rd edition. Philadelphia: Lippincott, 2003.

PERIODICALS

Henry, B. J., et al. "The Effect of Local Hematoma Blocks on Early Fracture Healing." *Orthopedics* 25(11) 2002: 1259–1262.

Ong, C. T., D. S. Choon, N. P. Cabrera, and N. Maffulli. "The Treatment of Open Tibial Fractures and of Tibial Nonunion with a Novel External Fixator." *Injury* 33(9) 2002: 829–834.

Sammarco, V. J., and L. Chang. "Modern Issues in Bone Graft Substitutes and Advances in Bone Tissue Technology." *Foot and Ankle Clinics of North America* 7(1) 2002: 19–41.

Szczesny, G. "Molecular Aspects of Bone Healing and Remodeling." *Polish Journal of Pathology* 53(3) 2002: 145–153.

ORGANIZATIONS

American Academy of Orthopaedic Surgeons. 6300 North River Road, Rosemont, IL 60018-4262. (847) 823-7186 or (800) 346-2267. <http://www.aaos.org/wordhtml/home2.htm>.

American College of Surgeons. 633 North Saint Claire Street, Chicago, IL 60611. (312) 202-5000. <http://www.facs.org/>.

American Society for Bone and Mineral Research. 2025 M Street, NW, Suite 800, Washington, DC 20036-3309. (202) 367-1161. <http://www.asbmr.org/>.

Orthopedic Trauma Association. 6300 N. River Road, Suite 727, Rosemont, IL 60018-4226. (847) 698-1631. <http://www.ota.org/links.htm>.

OTHER

Evanston Northwestern Healthcare (Northwestern University), [cited February 28, 2003] <http://www.enh.org/surgery/100077.asp>.

International Society for Fracture Repair, [cited February 28, 2003] <http://www.fractures.com/isfr/>.

National Library of Medicine, [cited February 28, 2003] <http://www.nlm.nih.gov/medlineplus/ency/article/002966.htm>.

University of Maryland College of Medicine, [cited February 28, 2003] <http://www.umm.edu/news/releases/hip.html>.

L. Fleming Fallon, Jr, MD, DrPH

Functional endoscopic sinus surgery *see* **Endoscopic sinus surgery**

Fundoplication surgery *see* **Gastroesophageal reflux surgery**

Funnel chest repair *see* **Pectus excavatum repair**

Furosemide *see* **Diuretics**